CourseMate **Engaging. Trackable. Affordable.**

CourseMate brings course concepts to life with interactive learning, study, and exam preparation tools that support HLTH.

INCLUDES:
Integrated eBook, interactive teaching and learning tools, and **Engagement Tracker,** a first-of-its-kind tool that monitors student engagement in the course.

ON THE WEB

HLTH Are you in?

D1127332

ONLINE RESOURCES INCLUDED!

FOR INSTRUCTORS:
- First Day of Class Instructions
- Custom Options through 4LTR+ Program
- Instructor's Manual
- Test Bank
- PowerPoint® Slides
- Instructor Prep Cards
- Engagement Tracker

FOR STUDENTS:
- Interactive eBook
- Auto-Graded Quizzes
- Flashcards
- Crossword Puzzles
- BBC Videos
- Exercise Demonstration Videos
- Glossary
- Weblinks
- Health Checks
- Learning Objectives

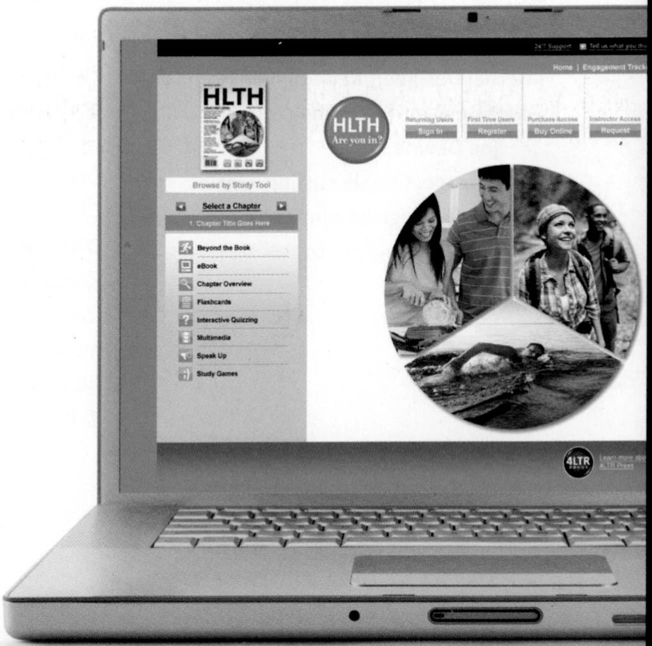

Students sign in at **login.cengagebrain.com**

WADSWORTH
CENGAGE Learning

HLTH

Jeffrey S. Nevid and Spencer A. Rathus

Executive Director, 4LTR Press: Neil Marquardt
Marketing Manager, 4LTR Press: Courtney Sheldon
Project Development Manager, 4LTR Press: Steven E. Joos
Associate Project Manager, 4LTR Press: Pierce Denny
Health Editor: Aileen Berg
Developmental Editor: Dana Freeman, B-books, Ltd.
Associate Development Editor: Samantha Arvin
Assistant Editor: Kristina Chiapella
Editorial Assistant: Shannon Elderon
Media Editor: Miriam Myers
Marketing Manager: Tom Ziolkowski
Marketing Assistant: Jing Hu
Marketing Communications Manager: Linda Yip
Production Director: Amy McGuire, B-books, Ltd.
Sr. Content Project Manager: Tanya Nigh
Design Director: Rob Hugel
Art Director: John Walker
Print Buyer: Karen Hunt
Production Service: B-Books, Ltd.
Rights Acquisitions Specialist: Don Schlotman
Photo Researcher: Charlotte Goldman
Text Permissions Researcher: Jennifer Wagner, PreMediaGlobal
Internal Designer: KeDesign, Mason, OH
Cover Designer: Red Hangar Design/Joe Devine
Cover Image: Couple cutting veggies: Getty Images; Swimmer: iStockphoto; Hikers: iStockphoto

Library of Congress Control Number: 2011941534

Student Edition ISBN-13: 978-1-111-98732-9
Student Edition ISBN-10: 1-111-98732-7

Wadsworth
20 Davis Drive
Belmont, CA 94002-3098
USA

Cengage Learning products are represented in Canada by Nelson Education, Ltd.

For your course and learning solutions, visit **www.cengage.com**
Purchase any of our products at your local college store or at our preferred online store **www.CengageBrain.com**

Design Photography Credits:
Chapter Opener and Learning Objectives: © iStockphoto.com/pixhook; Diversity icon: © iStockphoto.com/Mark Stay; Health Check icon: © iStockphoto.com/Victor Correia; Health Skills icon: © iStockphoto.com/ssstep; Prevention icon: © iStockphoto.com/Mark Stay; Question mark under magnifying glass: © iStockphoto.com/James E. Hernandez; Blue light bulb: © iStockphoto.com/kemie; Blue puzzle piece: © iStockphoto.com/kemie

Printed in the United States of America
1 2 3 4 5 6 7 15 14 13 12 11

HLTH Brief Contents

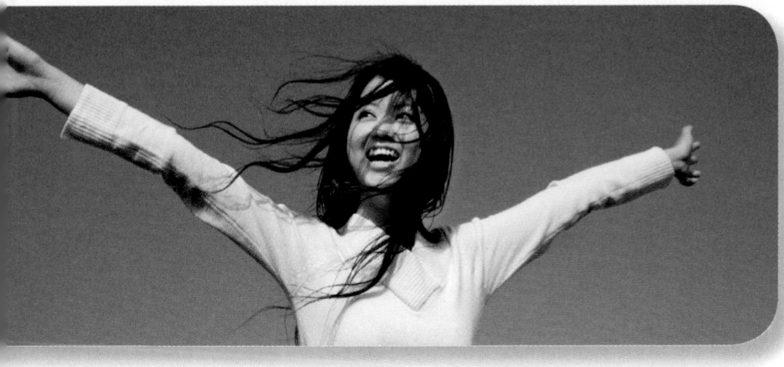

© iStockphoto.com/Nikada

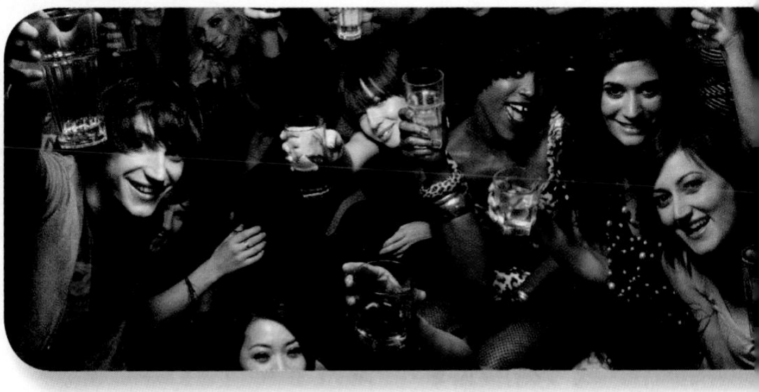

© Michael Blann/Lifesize/Jupiterimages

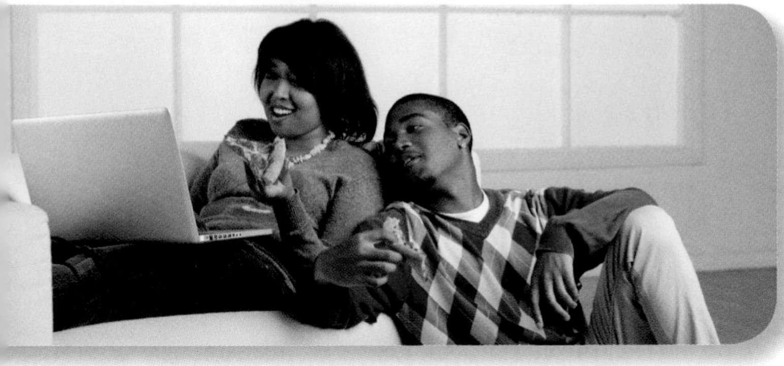

© iStockphoto.com/Blend_Images

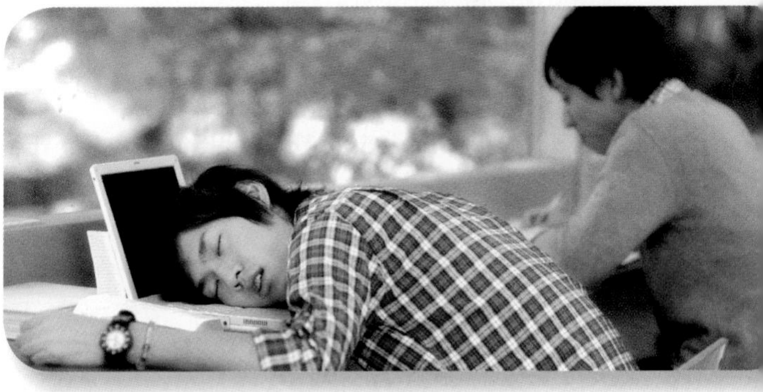

©iStockphoto.com/M. Eric Honeycutt

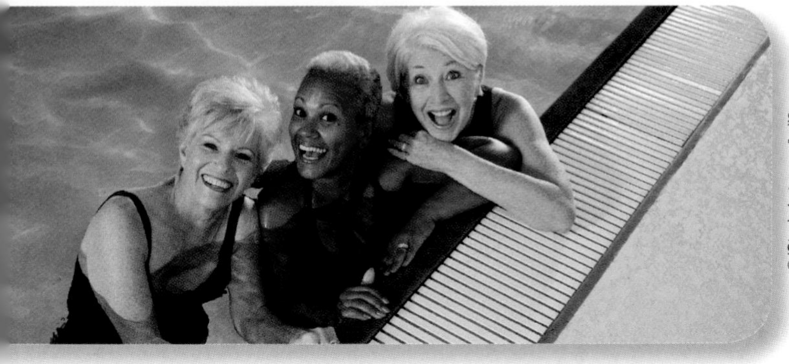

© iStockphoto.com/kali9

HLTH Contents

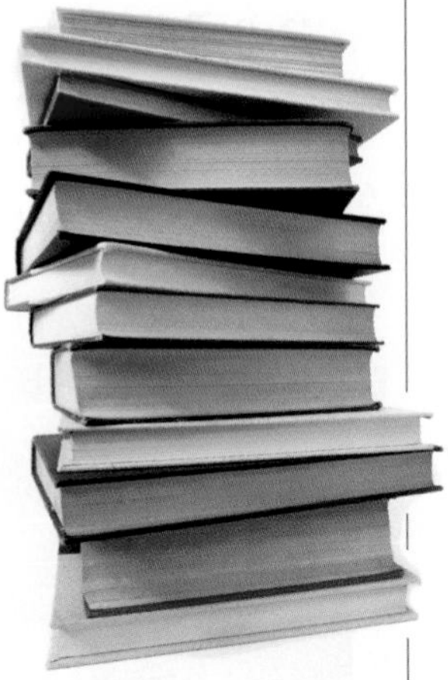

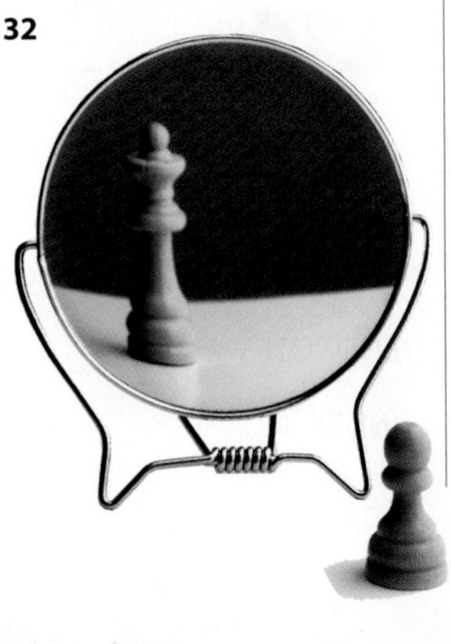

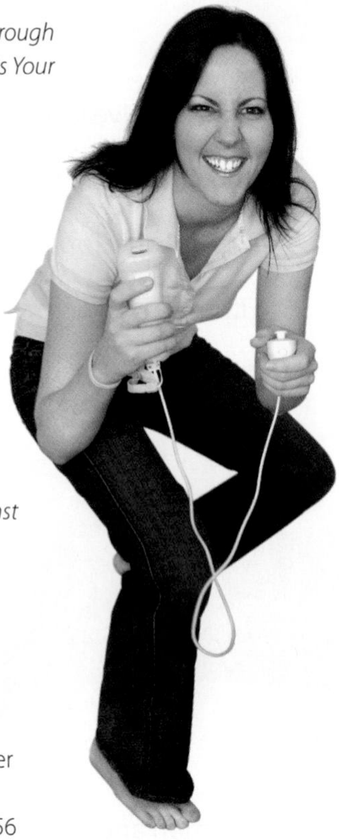

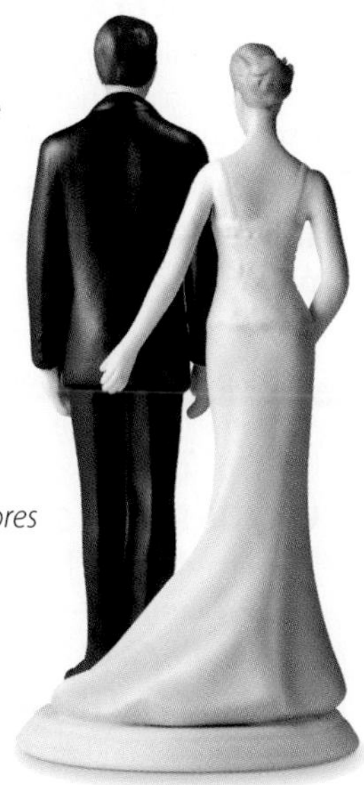

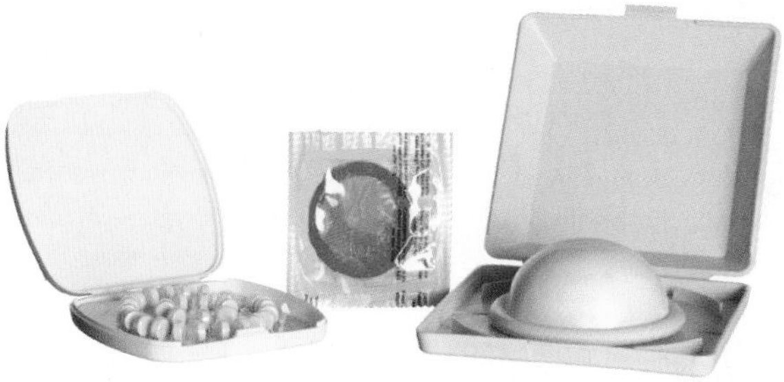

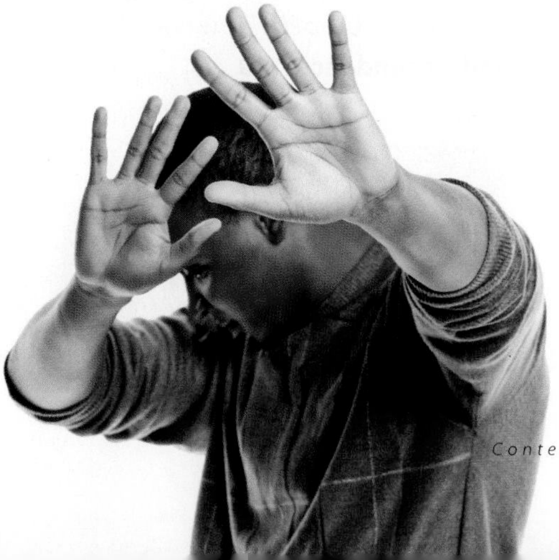

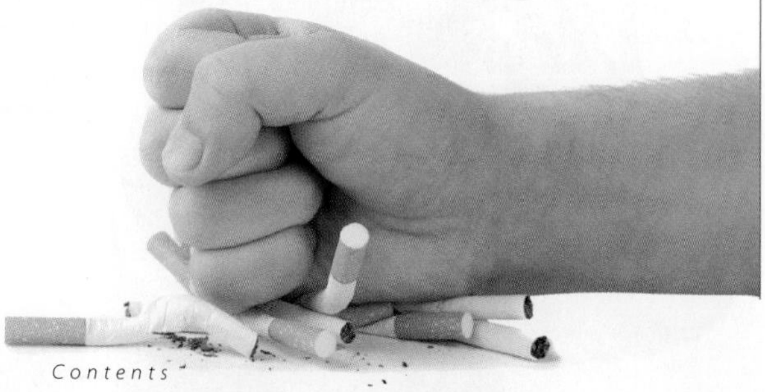

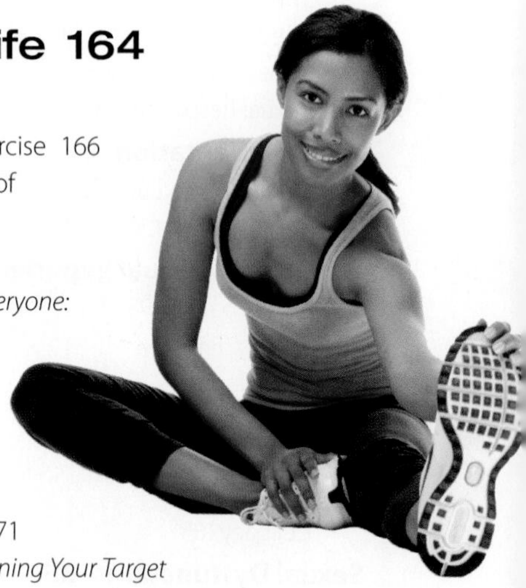

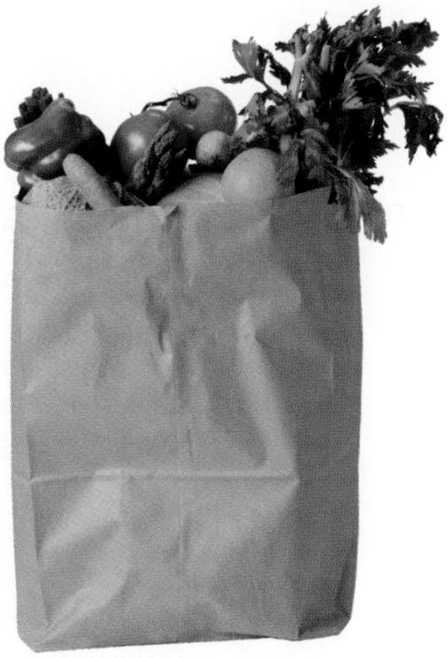

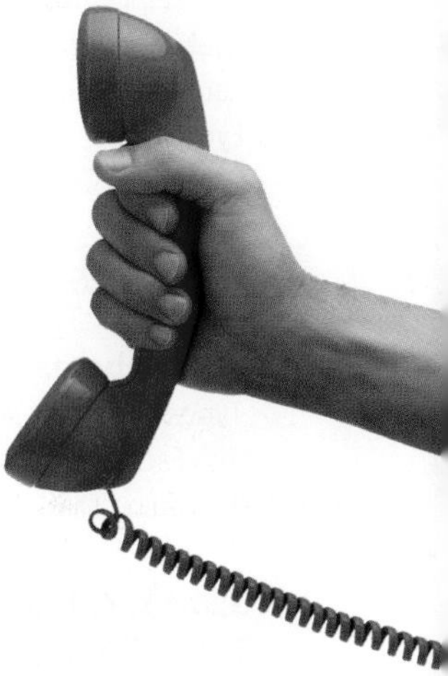

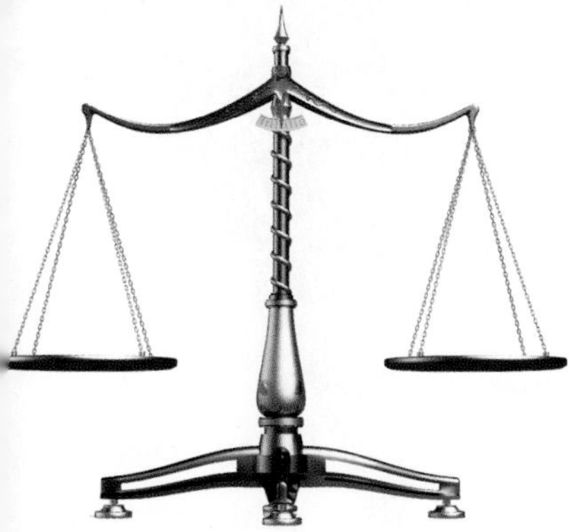

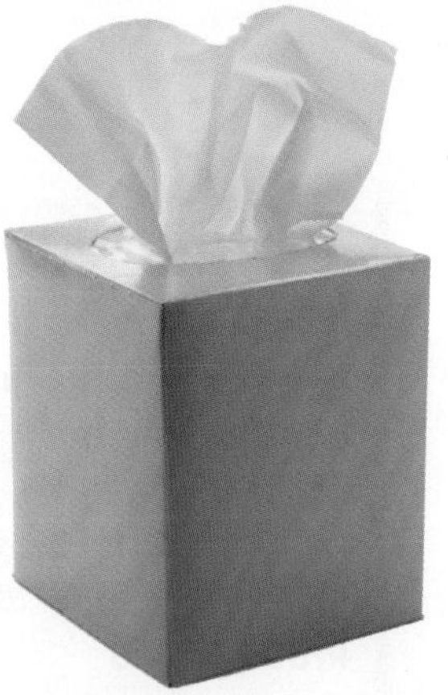

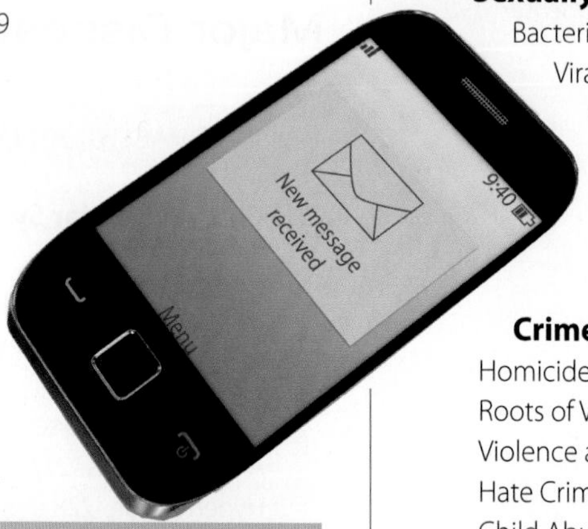

9:40
New message received
Menu

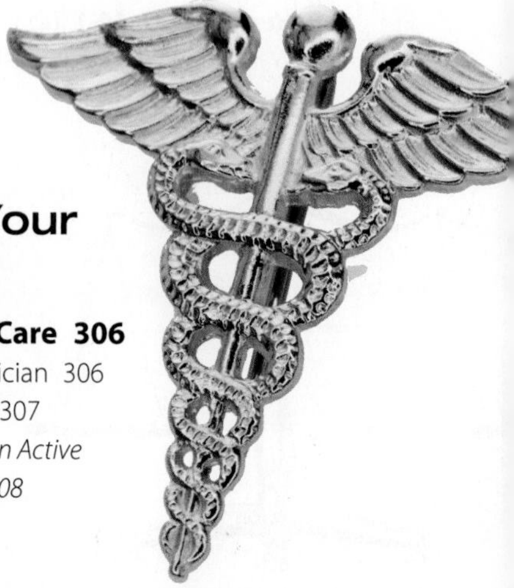

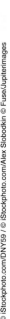

© iStockphoto.com/Bart Coenders / © iStockphoto.com/Jani Bryson

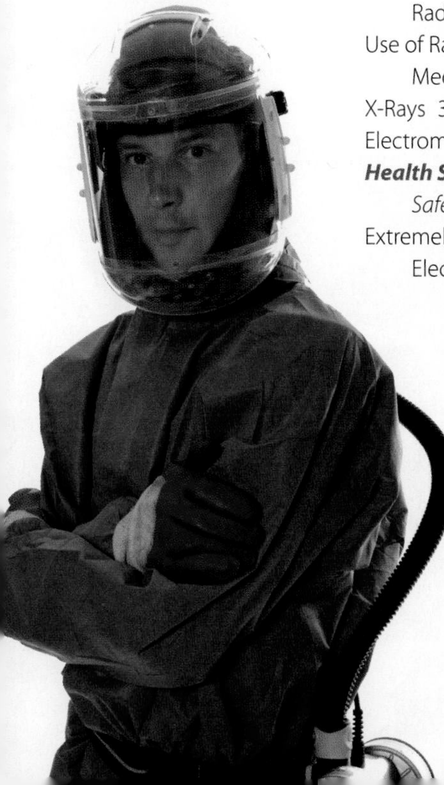

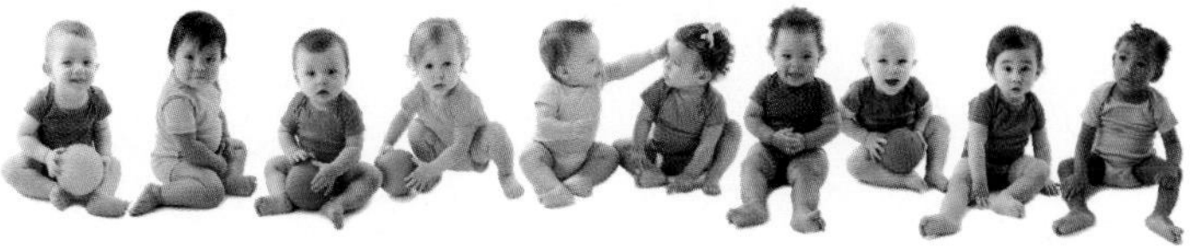

HLTH
Chapter 1

A Healthy You!

"This book is more about you than about medical science. It is about your role in protecting and enhancing your personal health."

We live in a time of great technological advances in medicine and other scientific fields. Doctors today can thread a tiny balloon into a clogged artery and then inflate it to clear away blockages that might otherwise lead to a heart attack or stroke. They can use viruses to ferry cancer-killing drugs directly to malignant tumors. They can transplant donated organs, literally giving recipients a new lease on life. New technologies offer promise of correcting genetic defects by substituting healthy genes for defective or missing genes. Other advances offer hope of slowing or even reversing some of the effects of aging. Altogether, technological advances raise hopes of curing or preventing many of the health problems that afflict us today and shorten our lives.

Throughout this text we introduce you to the latest medical advances. Yet, this book is more about you than about medical science. It is about your role in protecting and enhancing your personal health by taking charge of your health-related behavior.

The best way to safeguard your health and increase your chances of leading a healthier and longer life is to adopt a healthy lifestyle. Factors such as proper diet, weight control, exercise, and avoidance of harmful substances such as tobacco and drugs play critical roles in determining health and longevity. They are pivotal in influencing your risk of many diseases, including the nation's leading killers—heart disease, cancer, and stroke. Preventive health practices, such as keeping vaccinations up-to-date, also enhance your health. So too do early detection through medical checkups to detect serious diseases at their most curable stages. Avoiding unsafe sexual practices can protect you against sexually

LEARNING OUTCOMES

1 **Define health and wellness**

2 **Explain how to strive for wellness**

3 **Describe the health concerns of women and men from different racial and ethnic backgrounds**

4 **Describe the goals of the government project *Healthy People***

5 **Explain ways of thinking critically about health-related information**

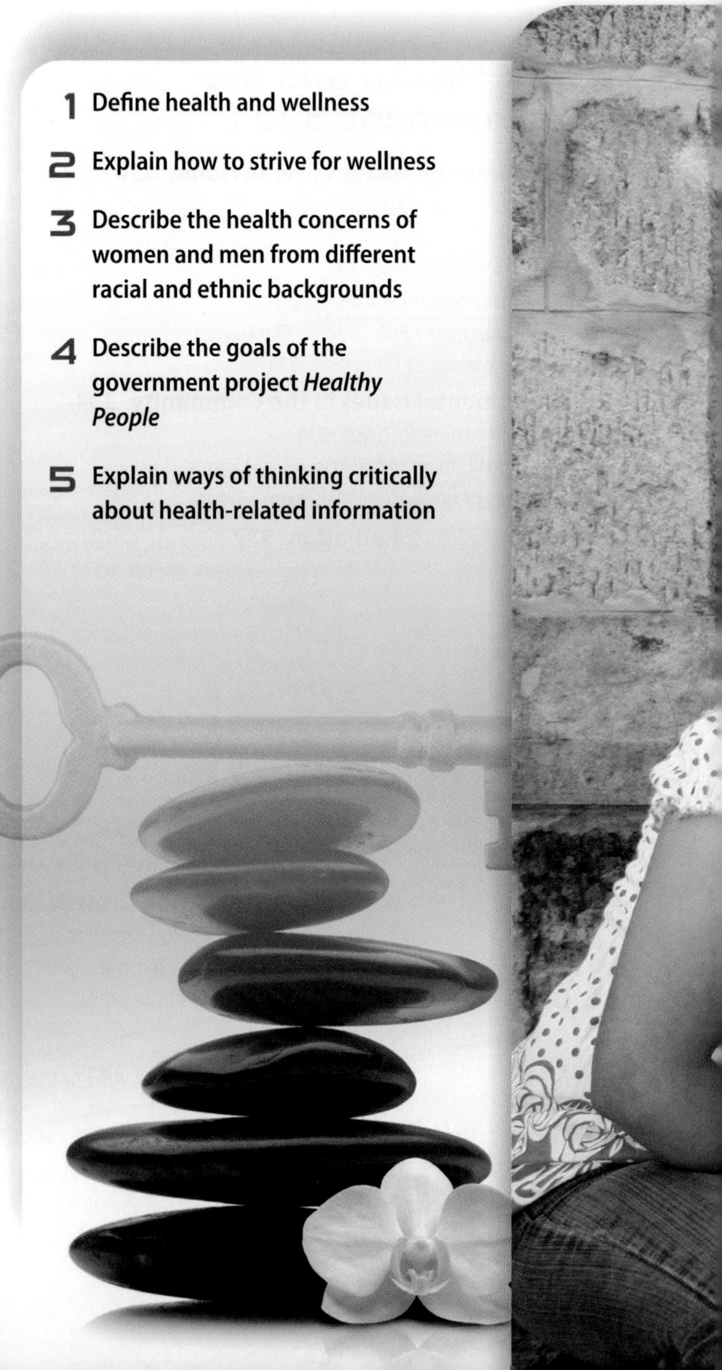

transmitted infections, including HIV/AIDS. Washing your hands regularly, especially after using the bathroom, can keep potentially dangerous microbes at bay. Taking precautions when hiking in the woods, or even when playing in the backyard, can help protect you and your family from Lyme disease.

This book focuses on ways to take charge of your health. The "Health Skills" features in each chapter and on the companion website describe specific ways you can put into practice the information in the chapter to help enhance your health. Taking charge of your health includes:

- *Becoming more aware of health risks.* A health risk is a factor that increases the chances of developing a health problem. You cannot control some factors, such as genetics—at least not yet. You can control others, such as diet and exercise. Knowing the risks associated with specific health problems can alert you to the steps you can take to reduce them. For example, the risks of certain birth defects are tied to a lack of folic acid, a B vitamin (see Chapter 5). Pregnant women can greatly reduce the risk of these birth defects by consuming 400 micrograms daily of the vitamin.

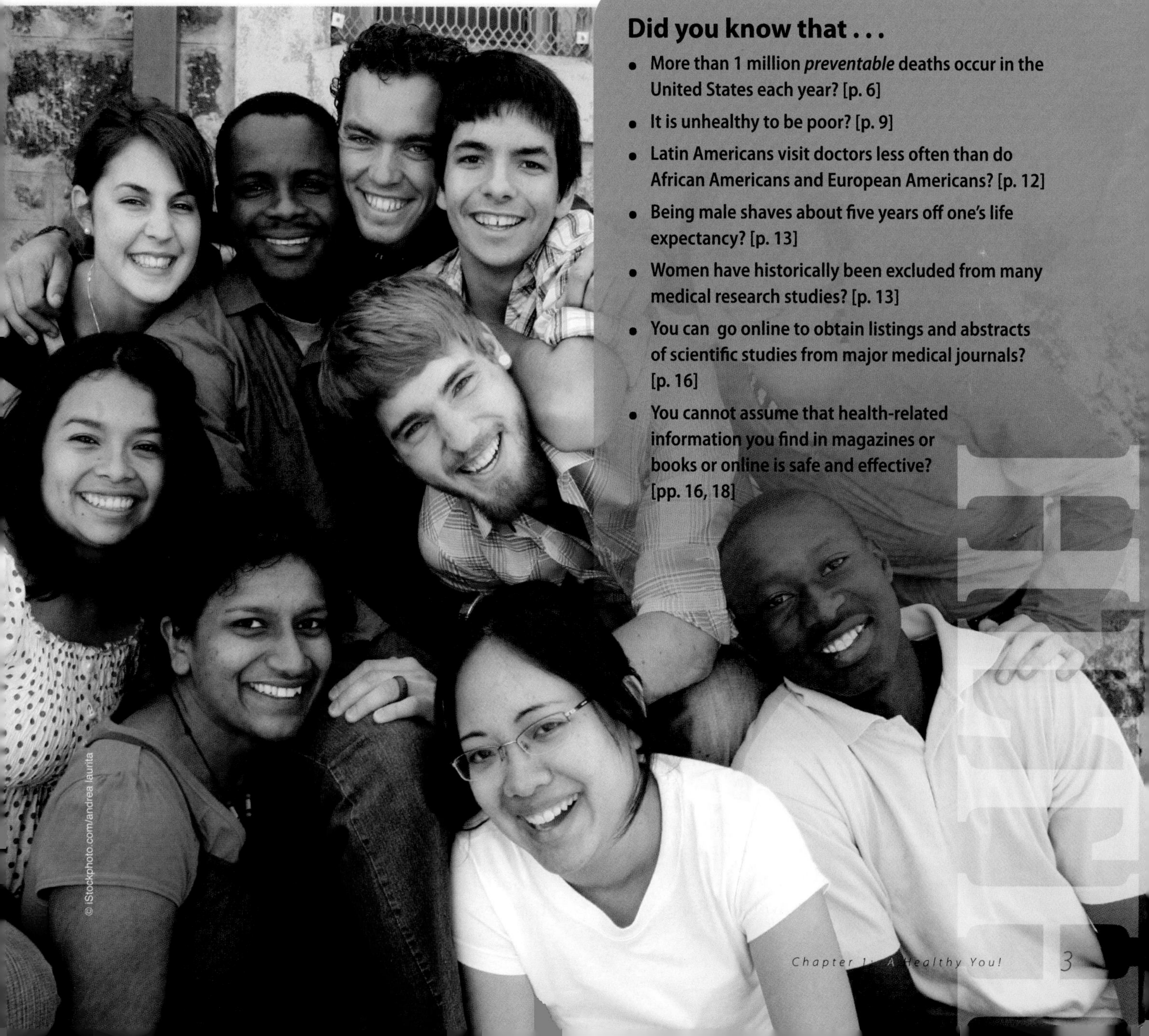

© iStockphoto.com/andrea laurita

Did you know that . . .

- More than 1 million *preventable* deaths occur in the United States each year? [p. 6]
- It is unhealthy to be poor? [p. 9]
- Latin Americans visit doctors less often than do African Americans and European Americans? [p. 12]
- Being male shaves about five years off one's life expectancy? [p. 13]
- Women have historically been excluded from many medical research studies? [p. 13]
- You can go online to obtain listings and abstracts of scientific studies from major medical journals? [p. 16]
- You cannot assume that health-related information you find in magazines or books or online is safe and effective? [pp. 16, 18]

- *Keeping informed.* Health developments are reported at a dizzying pace. Some information challenges long-held assumptions—for example, that vigorous, aerobic exercise is the only healthy form of exercise. (See Chapter 8 for a discussion of the benefits of regular moderate exercise.) Other developments reflect new directions in prevention and treatment, such as the finding that low daily doses of aspirin can reduce the risk of heart attacks (see Chapter 11). However, not all the information that reaches us through the popular media is trustworthy. We need to develop critical thinking skills—discussed later in this chapter—to separate the "wheat from the chaff."
- *Practicing prevention.* You may be familiar with the expression "An ounce of prevention is worth a pound of cure." Preventive health care incorporates regular screening examinations for health problems encountered by people of your age and sex, self-examinations (breast self-exams for women and testicular self-exams for men), keeping vaccinations current, exercising regularly, following a nutritionally sound diet, and avoiding unsafe behaviors such as reckless driving, smoking, excessive drinking, and risky sex. "Prevention" features in this text and on the companion website will inform you of specific steps to safeguard your health.
- *Becoming a knowledgeable consumer of health care services.* Do you have a primary care physician? Do you have health insurance, and, if so, do you know whether it provides adequate coverage? Do you know how to access health care services? Do you know how to obtain specialist services or emergency care? In the online feature "Health Skills 1-2" we offer suggestions for choosing a physician (see page 18). In Chapter 14, we discuss the health care system and the importance of becoming an active health care consumer.
- *Changing your health-related behavior.* Do you . . .
  — Avoid smoking?
  — Eat at least five helpings of fresh fruits and vegetables daily?
  — Drink alcohol responsibly?
  — Avoid unsafe sexual practices?
  — Avoid harmful drugs?
  — Use medicines as prescribed?
  — Have a carbon monoxide detector and a smoke detector in your home?
  — Maintain your weight at a healthy level?
  — Wear a seat belt in the car?

If you answered "no" to any of these questions, we invite you to take stock of your behavior and use this book to help change it.

health
Soundness of body and mind; a state of vigor and vitality that permits a person to function physically, psychologically, and socially.

physical health
Soundness of body, as represented by healthy physical functioning and the absence of disease.

emotional health
Emotional well-being and ability to share one's feelings with others.

social health
The ability to relate effectively to other people such as family members, intimate partners, friends, fellow students or workers, professors, and supervisors.

What Is Health?

Many people think of **health** as the absence of disease. True enough, but health involves more. It involves vitality, vigor, and general physical and mental well-being. Thus we need to speak not only of physical health but of other dimensions as well, including emotional, social, spiritual, intellectual, and environmental health. We can also speak about a dimension of health that relates to the relationship between the individual and his or her physical environment.

LEARNING OUTCOME 1

Define health and wellness

There are six dimensions of health (see Figure 1-1):

Physical health refers to "soundness of body." It involves such aspects of your physical being as the sharpness of your senses, the functioning of your body, and the presence—or absence—of disease or infirmity. Throughout this text we focus on aspects of our physical health such as nutrition, fitness, and weight management. We examine physical illnesses and what we can do to prevent them.

Emotional health involves many aspects of our emotional well-being, including the ability to maintain our emotions on an even keel, to share them with others, to feel good about ourselves and the future, to be generally happy, to manage stress, and to believe we can meet the demands of daily life.

Social health is the ability to relate effectively to other people such as family members, intimate part-

Figure1-1 Six Dimensions of Health

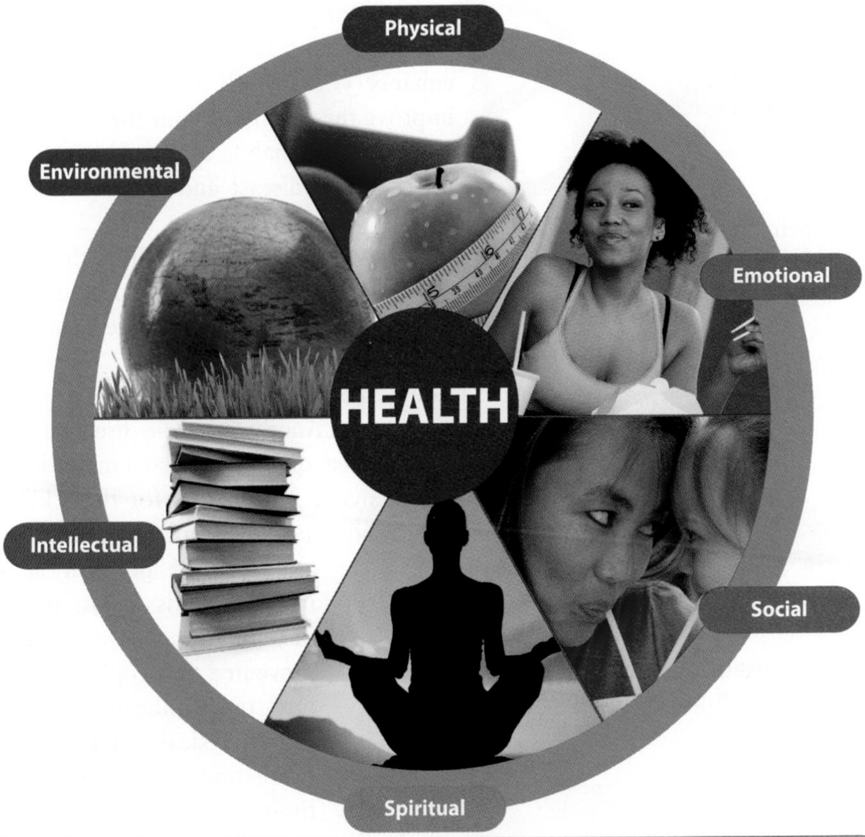

ners, friends, fellow students or workers, professors, and supervisors. To lead healthy and fulfilling lives, people need people. To paraphrase the sixteenth-century English poet John Donne, no man, and no woman, is an island, entire of itself. Social sources of stress, such as prolonged unemployment, marital separation or divorce, and loneliness, can impair the immune system, increasing our vulnerability to illness. Lack of social interaction can lead to depression. On the other hand, people may be better able to meet the challenges of coping with illness when they have social support.

Spiritual health refers to connectedness with a higher order or a purpose beyond oneself. For some, this involves a commitment to religion. For others, it involves a commitment to aesthetic values, such as the enjoyment or creation of music, poetry, or visual arts. For still others, spirituality involves a commitment to serving the needy or the community at large. Spiritual experience permits people to transcend the ordinary events of life. It imbues their lives with meaning and purpose.

Intellectual health involves the ability to use intellectual resources to meet challenges, to seek and gather information to make well-informed decisions, to pursue goals, to be open to new experiences and ways of thinking, to develop a set of personal values, to learn from experience, and to choose a healthy lifestyle. Intellectual health includes learning planning, creating, and thinking critically about the flood of health-related information to which you are exposed through the media and your life experience. Later in the chapter we see how critical thinking enables you to make healthier choices.

What do you envision when you think of the environment? Is it vast tracts of wilderness and deep, rolling oceans? Or do you think of endangered species and shorebirds enveloped in oil from oil spills? Do you conjure up visions of billowing summer storm clouds and refreshing rain, or do you imagine crowded sidewalks and acid rain? All these—the beauty and the horror—affect **environmental health**. Factors that threaten environmental health include extremes of temperature, pollution, exposure to lead and other toxic substances, and ultraviolet radiation.

Environmental health involves the relationship between the individual and the environment. The environment sustains us. Yet the environment can also threaten our health and our very survival. We have a reciprocal relationship with the environment: We affect the environment, for better or for worse, and the environment affects us. If we are to thrive, we need to preserve and protect the environment.

spiritual health
The attainment of connectedness to a higher order or purpose beyond oneself, such as commitment to a particular religion, aesthetic values, or community service.

intellectual health
The ability to use one's intellectual resources to solve problems, meet life challenges, develop personal values, and adopt healthy behaviors and lifestyles.

environmental health
The relationship between humans and other organisms and their physical environment that allows them to survive and flourish.

Completing the online feature "Health Check 1-1" will help you identify where you stand on these dimensions of health.

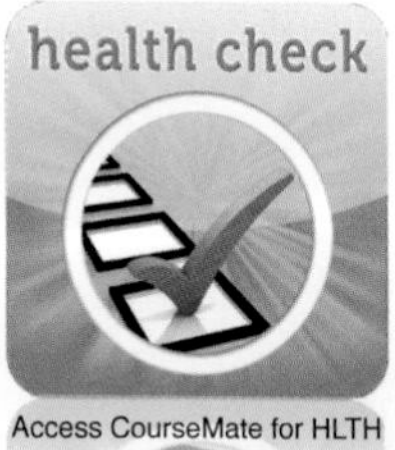

Access CourseMate for HLTH at www.cengagebrain.com.

Health and Wellness

Wellness refers to a state of optimum health. People who achieve wellness have developed a lifestyle that enhances their health, protects them from disease, and maximizes their physical, psychological, spiritual, social, intellectual, and environmental well-being.

wellness
A state of optimum health, as characterized by active efforts to maximize one's physical health and well-being

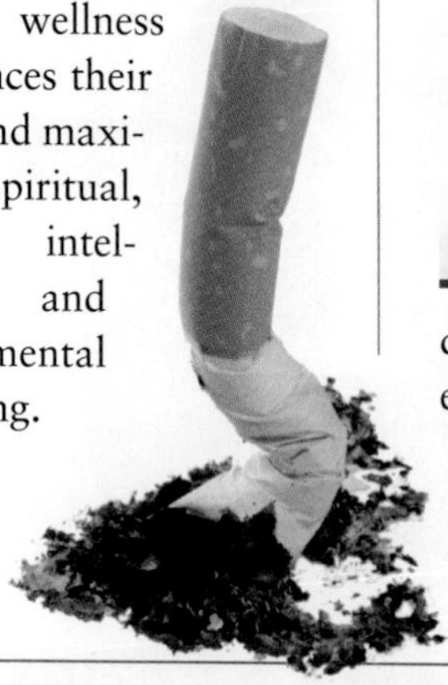

Striving for Wellness

Striving for wellness involves making changes in your lifestyle and behavior that enhance your health and well-being and improve the quality of your life.

Unhealthy habits are a major risk factor in serious disease and premature death. More than 2 million people die each year in the United States, and an estimated 1 million are in the process of dying. The leading causes of death overall are heart disease, cancer, and stroke. Another chronic disease a little further down on the list, diabetes, is also a major killer.

LEARNING OUTCOME 2

Explain how to strive for wellness

Many of the major risk factors for these killers are unhealthy habits such as smoking, overeating, and lack of physical activity. Hundreds of thousands of premature deaths could be prevented if people changed just two unhealthy behaviors—physical inactivity and overeating.[1] Hundreds of thousands more lives could be saved if people avoided smoking.[2] All in all, there are more than 1 million preventable deaths each year in the United States (see Figure 1-2). Developing healthier habits and practicing safer behaviors is a running theme throughout our study of health and wellness. Let's explore how you can make these changes.

Figure 1-2 Annual Preventable Deaths in the United States

Here we see a listing of the leading preventable causes of death in the United States—deaths that could be avoided if people adopted healthier lifestyles.

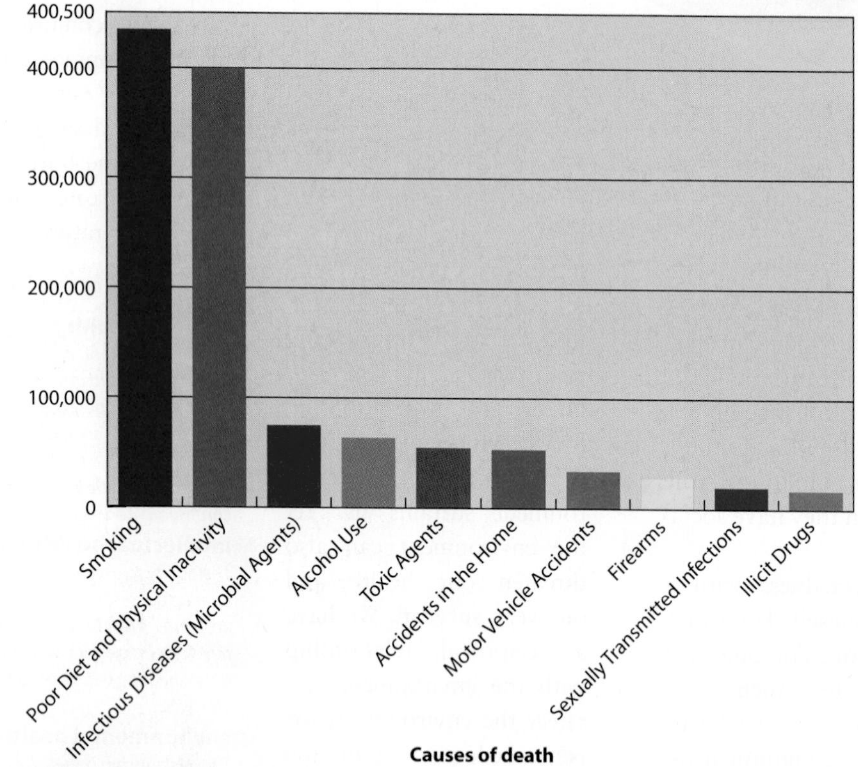

Note: Deaths due to alcohol-related motor vehicle accidents are included in the statistics given for motor vehicle crashes.

Sources: Danaei, G., et al. (2009). The preventable causes of death in the United States: Comparative risk assessment of dietary, lifestyle, and metabolic risk factors. *PLoS Medicine, 6*(4); Mokdad, A. H., et al. (2004). Actual causes of death in the United States, 2000. *Journal of the American Medical Association,* 291, 1238–1245; National Safety Council. *Summary from injury facts, 2010 edition,* Itasca, IL; White, J. B. (2010, December 15). New puzzle: Why fewer are killed in car crashes. *The Wall Street Journal,* p. D1.

Changing Unhealthy Habits

When asked about quitting smoking, the famed writer Mark Twain quipped that it was easy—he'd done it hundreds of times. Changing unhealthy behaviors may not be easy, but it is a challenge that can be met. Like Twain, people who succeed in making healthy changes often revert to their former unhealthy ways. Making changes in your health behavior, and maintaining these changes, depends on three sets of factors:

- Predisposing factors
- Enabling factors
- Reinforcing factors

Predisposing Factors

Predisposing factors either promote or hinder healthy changes in behavior. These factors include beliefs, attitudes, knowledge, expectancies, and values. For example, believing that smoking is dangerous only to people with a family history of lung cancer can hinder healthy changes in people without a family history of the disease. Similarly, young people who find smoking "cool" or glamorous are more likely to smoke than peers who view smoking as deviant.

Knowledge can lead to change. Millions of Americans quit smoking after the Surgeon General first reported the dangers of smoking. Knowledge about the risk factors in conditions such as heart disease and cancer can lead people to make changes that reduce their risks of these diseases. But knowledge is not always sufficient to change behavior. Most smokers today know of the dangers of smoking but continue to smoke. Most sexually active people know the dangers of unprotected sex (that is, sex without a condom), but many surrender to impulse.

Psychologists recognize that expectations play an important role in change. Young people who expect that drinking alcohol will make them popular, sexier, or more outgoing are more likely to drink than their peers who don't have these expectations.

Values are also a determinant of change. Young people who value their popularity over their future health are more likely to succumb to peer pressure to smoke than those who place a greater value on long-term health.

Enabling Factors

Factors that enable change include skills or abilities, physical and mental capabilities, and the availability and accessibility of resources. You are more likely to begin an exercise program, or stick with one, if there's a gym around the corner rather than a half-hour drive away, if you have developed the skills to accomplish the task (you can follow the steps in an aerobics dance class or serve a tennis ball), and if you possess the physical and mental capabilities required to perform the behavior (e.g., the strength, coordination, endurance, and concentration). Accessibility to health care services is another enabling factor. People who lack health insurance or access to health care facilities may not receive the care they need.

Reinforcing Factors

Reinforcing factors for healthy changes include praise and support—including self-praise. If you shrug off the changes you make (e.g., starting a beginner's exercise class) by saying to yourself, "It's no big deal," you'll be less likely to stick with it than if you credit yourself for getting started. You're more likely to continue making healthy changes if friends or loved ones make reinforcing comments than if your efforts go unnoticed. However, it's best if reinforcement becomes internalized. Whether it is losing weight, quitting smoking, or maintaining an exercise routine, you need to feel that what you are doing will ultimately lead you to feel better about yourself and to live a healthier life. Check out the feature "Health Skills 1-1" on the next page for some general guidelines for making healthful changes.

Human Diversity and Health

The population of the United States is growing increasingly diverse. Figure 1-3 on page 12 shows the current distribution of the population according to **ethnic group**—a group of people united by their cultural heritage, race, language, or common history. European Americans now constitute about 66% of the U.S. population. By contrast, European Americans constituted nearly 90% of the population in 1950, and African Americans were the largest minority group. Latin Americans (16% of the population) are currently the nation's largest minority group. By the year 2050, the number of European Americans will grow, but they will make up a much smaller percentage of the population than they do now. The percentage of Asian Americans is

☒ LEARNING OUTCOME 3

Describe the health concerns of women and men from different racial and ethnic backgrounds

ethnic group
A group of people who are united by their cultural heritage, race, language, and common history.

HEALTH SKILLS 1-1

Making Healthy Changes in Your Behavior

Following are some general guidelines for making healthy changes in behavior.

Set Reasonable Goals. Strive toward achieving attainable goals. For most of us mere mortals, that may mean taking a brisk walk or swimming 30 minutes several times a week, not training to qualify for the next Olympics. If you are overweight, set a goal for achieving a healthy weight, not an unrealistic or dangerously thin weight.

Approach Goals Gradually. Nibble, don't bite. Begin an exercise program easily, working up gradually to meet your training goals. Don't overtax your muscles or your endurance. Develop a timetable for approaching your goals. You can jot down specific weekly goals and post them on the refrigerator as a reminder.

Identify Specific Behaviors You Want to Change. Rather than thinking "I need to follow a healthier diet," lay out a specific menu plan that meets the nutritional guidelines described in Chapters 9 and 10. Rather than saying, "I need to do more exercise," set specific goals: "I plan to work out on the treadmill for 30 minutes three times a week," or "I plan to go to an aerobics class twice a week."

Track Your Problem Behavior. Want to change unhealthy habits, like excessive snacking? Use a diary (see Chapter 10) to track the problem behavior for a week or two, noting where it took place, when it occurred, who you were with, and how you felt beforehand and afterwards. Notice patterns that emerge, such as tendencies to overeat when you have time on your hands. Develop a plan of action based on what you've learned. You might fill in those empty hours with productive activities.

Acquire the Information You Need. Use this textbook and other resources (such as your college library, your instructor, and the Internet) to obtain the information you need to change your behavior. Chapter 8 will help you start designing an exercise program you can live with. Chapter 9 will provide guidelines for a nutritional diet. Other chapters provide information about stress management (Chapter 3), healthy relationships (Chapter 4), safer sex (Chapter 5), anger management (Chapter 13), and protecting yourself from chronic diseases such as heart disease and cancer (Chapter 11).

continued

expected to more than double by 2050, making them the most rapidly growing ethnic group in the United States.

Nations within Nations

Each country is really a collection of nations within a nation. The United States, for example, is composed of many ethnic groups drawn from many parts of the world. Americans differ according to religion as well as race. Yet classifying people according to racial categories is blurred by the growing numbers of people who identify themselves as biracial, multiracial, or multiethnic. President Barack Obama, golfer Tiger Woods, baseball player Derek Jeter, and singer Mariah Carey are not easily classified by traditional racial distinctions. More than 5 million Americans describe themselves as multiracial.[3] Multiracial Americans have become the nation's fastest growing demographic group. [4]

When it comes to our health, we are also nations within a nation. Wide differences exist in the health status and life expectancy of the majority European American population and ethnic minority groups. Differences also exist in the health status and longevity of men and women. There are key ethnic and gender differences in health status and utilization of health care services.

Health, Gender, and Ethnicity

The life expectancy of the average African American is shorter than that of the average European American.[5] European American males born today can expect to live about 75.7 years, as compared to about 69.7 years for African American males (see Table 1-1). Euro-

Adopt an Internal Locus of Control. Who's in charge of your life? The answer can be *you,* if you decide it will be you. People with an **internal locus of control** believe they are in control of what happens to them, for better or for worse. They believe they can take steps to promote their health and prevent disease. Some health outcomes may be beyond our control; we may be exposed to harmful germs or inherit a health problem. But if you believe your health is at least in part affected by your behavior, you are more likely to take steps to prevent disease and enhance your well-being. By contrast, people with an **external locus of control** believe their fates are largely out of their hands. They take a "whatever happens, happens" attitude toward their health, believing that health and illness are largely determined by the shifting sands of luck and fortune.

The feature "Health Check 1-2" on page 10 will provide insight as to whether or not you feel you are in charge of what happens to you. If you tend more toward the "external," consider an attitude shift in the other direction. Ask yourself, "What can I do to enhance my health?" There may be no guarantees of good health and long life, but you can help shift the odds in your favor by determining what you will eat and drink, whether you smoke, whether you exercise, and whether you get regular medical check-ups.

Challenge Negative Thinking. Negative thoughts and beliefs such as "can't succeed" and "Nothing ever changes" can undermine your confidence and motivation. Replace negative thoughts with rational alternatives such as "Take it a step at a time" and "If I work at this, I can do it." Negative beliefs about yourself ("I'm stupid"), your world ("This school is awful"), and the future ("Nothing will ever work out for me") can become a recipe for depression and hopelessness. Identify and correct these self-defeating beliefs (see Chapter 2) to boost your psychological health and help stay motivated to achieve your health goals.

Don't Give Up When You Give In. Don't give up if you occasionally slip up. Anyone can miss an exercise class or lose a battle with a chocolate chip cookie. Despairing when you experience a setback can lead you to give up on achieving your goals. An occasional slip-up is inevitable for most of us. Nobody's perfect. The best response is to pick yourself up and get back on track.

Make Healthy Habits a Part of Your Lifestyle. Make your exercise routine a regular part of your weekly schedule. Climb stairs rather than using the elevator to get to class or work. Park at the farther end of the lot, and walk briskly to class or to the mall. Make unhealthy behavior difficult or impossible. You can't reach for the donuts in your refrigerator if you have left them at the supermarket (that is, not bought them).

Table 1-1 Life Expectancies of European American and African American Men and Women

	MALE	FEMALE
European American	75.7 years	80.6 years
African American	69.7 years	76.2 years

Source: Arias, E. (2010, June 8). *National Vital Statistics Reports, Vol. 58, No. 21. United States life tables,* Centers for Disease Control and Prevention, National Center for Health Statistics, National Vital Statistics System.

pean American females born today have an average life expectancy of about 80.6 years as compared to 76.2 years for African American females. How might we account for these differences? A primary factor is not race per se, but differences in **socioeconomic status**, which encompasses income and educational level.[6]

African Americans, Latin Americans, and Native Americans are more likely than European Americans to live below the poverty line, and people on the lower rungs of the socioeconomic ladder have average life spans about seven years less than those of more affluent people. Better-educated and wealthier people tend to take better care of themselves (they exercise more, are less often overweight, are less likely to smoke, and consume less fat in their diets) than do poorer or less-educated people. African Americans also tend to have less access to health

internal locus of control
The belief that one can control the outcomes that one experiences in life.

external locus of control
The perception that a person's future is determined by forces beyond his or her control.

socioeconomic status
Relative position in terms of education and income level.

Locus of Control Scale

Do you believe that your health and well-being lies within your control? Or do you believe that what happens to you in life depends on the whims and fancies of others or just blind luck? To find out, select "Yes" or "No" in the corresponding column for each question. Then total your score and interpret your results using the key provided at the end of the scale.

		YES	NO
1.	Do you believe that most problems will solve themselves if you just don't fool with them?	_____	_____
2.	Do you believe that you can stop yourself from catching a cold?	_____	_____
3.	Are some people just born lucky?	_____	_____
4.	Most of the time, does getting good grades means a great deal to you?	_____	_____
5.	Are you often blamed for things that just aren't your fault?	_____	_____
6.	Do you believe that if somebody studies hard he or she can pass any subject?	_____	_____
7.	Do you feel that most of the time it doesn't pay to try hard because things never turn out right anyway?	_____	_____
8.	Do you feel that if things start out well in the morning, it's going to be a good day, no matter what you do?	_____	_____
9.	Do you feel that most of the time parents listen to what children have to say?	_____	_____
10.	Do you believe that wishing can make good things happen?	_____	_____
11.	When you get punished, does it usually seem to be for no good reason at all?	_____	_____
12.	Most of the time, do you find it hard to change a friend's opinion?	_____	_____
13.	Do you think cheering more than luck helps a team win?	_____	_____
14.	Do you feel that it is nearly impossible to change your parents' minds about anything?	_____	_____
15.	Do you believe that parents should allow children to make most of their own decisions?	_____	_____
16.	Do you feel that when you do something wrong there's very little you can do to make it right?	_____	_____
17.	Do you believe that most people are just born good at sports?	_____	_____
18.	Are most other people your age stronger than you are?	_____	_____
19.	Do you feel that one of the best ways to handle most problems is just not to think about them?	_____	_____
20.	Do you feel that you have a lot of choice in deciding who your friends are?	_____	_____
21.	If you find a four-leaf clover, do you believe that it might bring you good luck?	_____	_____
22.	Do you often feel that whether or not you do your homework has much to do with what kind of grades you get?	_____	_____
23.	Do you feel that when a person your age is angry with you, there's little you can do to stop him or her?	_____	_____
24.	Have you ever had a good-luck charm?	_____	_____
25.	Do you believe that whether or not people like you depends on how you act?	_____	_____
26.	Do your parents usually help you if you ask them to?	_____	_____
27.	Do you ever feel that when people are angry with you, it is usually for no reason at all?	_____	_____

continued

		YES	NO
28.	Most of the time, do you feel that you can change what might happen tomorrow by what you do today?	____	____
29.	Do you believe that when bad things are going to happen they are just going to happen no matter what you try to do to stop them?	____	____
30.	Do you think that people can get their own way if they just keep trying?	____	____
31.	Most of the time, do you find it useless to try to get your own way at home?	____	____
32.	Do you feel that when good things happen, they happen because of hard work?	____	____
33.	Do you feel that when somebody your age wants to be your enemy there's little you can do to change matters?	____	____
34.	Do you feel that it's easy to get friends to do what you want them to do?	____	____
35.	Do you usually feel that you have little to say about what you get to eat at home?	____	____
36.	Do you feel that when someone doesn't like you, there's little you can do about it?	____	____
37.	Did you usually feel it was almost useless to try in school, because most other children were just plain smarter than you were?	____	____
38.	Are you the kind of person who believes that planning ahead makes things turn out better?	____	____
39.	Most of the time, do you feel that you have little to say about what your family decides to do?	____	____
40.	Do you think it's better to be smart than to be lucky?	____	____

Scoring Key

Place a check mark in the blank space in the scoring key each time your answer agrees with the answer in the key. The number of check marks is your total score.

1. Yes____	9. No ____	17. Yes____	25. No ____	33. Yes____
2. No ____	10. Yes____	18. Yes____	26. No ____	34. No ____
3. Yes____	11. Yes____	19. Yes____	27. Yes____	35. Yes____
4. No ____	12. Yes____	20. No ____	28. No ____	36. Yes____
5. Yes____	13. No ____	21. Yes____	29. Yes____	37. Yes____
6. No ____	14. Yes____	22. No ____	30. No ____	38. No ____
7. Yes____	15. No ____	23. Yes____	31. Yes____	39. Yes____
8. Yes____	16. Yes____	24. Yes____	32. No ____	40. No ____

Total Score ______

Interpreting Your Score

Low scorers (0–8): About one person in three earns a score of 0 to 8. These people typically have an internal locus of control. They see themselves as responsible for their fate and for the success or failure they experience in life.

Average scorers (9–16): Most respondents earn from 9 to 16 points. Average scorers may see themselves as partially in control of their lives. Perhaps they see themselves as in control at work, but not in their social lives—or vice versa.

High scorers (17–40): About 15% of respondents attain scores of 17 or above. High scorers largely tend to see life as a game of chance, and success as a matter of luck or the generosity of others.

Figure 1-3 Ethnic/Racial Breakdown of the U.S. Population

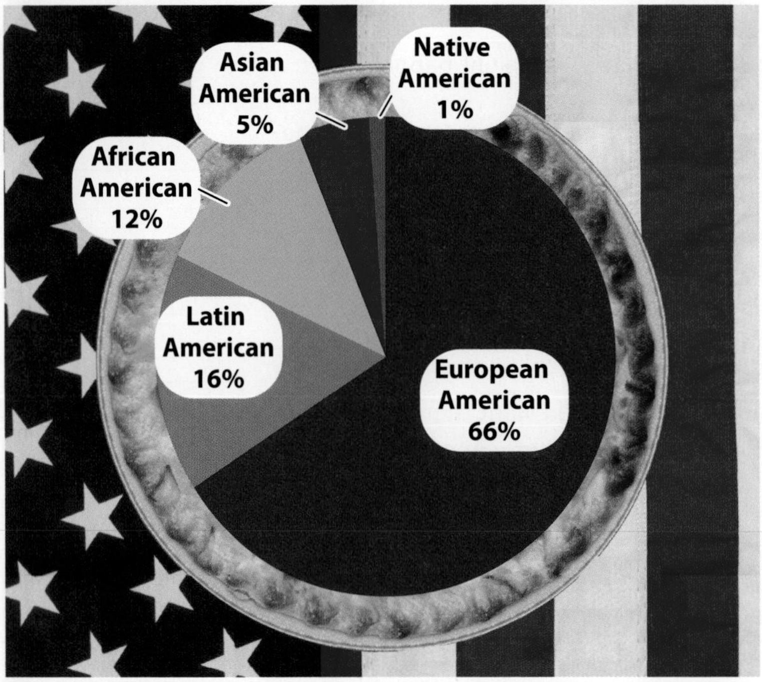

Note: Percentages are based on population estimates of single-racial identification for European Americans, African Americans, Native Americans, Asian Americans, and Latin Americans.
Source: U.S. Census Bureau, Population Division, Population Projections Branch. (2010, June). *Annual estimates of the resident population by sex, race, and Latin American origin for the United States: April 1, 2000 to July 1, 2009* (NC-EST2009-03).

care than European Americans.[7] Furthermore, African Americans are more likely to be exposed to life stressors that can have a negative impact on health, such as overcrowded housing, poverty, crime, and racism.[8] Chronic stress can contribute to health problems, including heart disease.

Genetic factors also play a role in ethnic group differences in health. The incidence of **sickle-cell anemia** is highest among African Americans and Latin Americans. The incidence of **Tay-Sachs disease** is greatest among Jews of Eastern European origin.

African Americans are also much more likely to be overweight and to have **hypertension** (high blood pressure), two of the major risk factors for heart disease and stroke.[9] Interestingly, African Americans are more likely to have hypertension than are Black Africans, suggesting that environmental factors affecting many African Americans—such as stress, diet, and smoking—contribute to their increased risk of hypertension.[10]

sickle-cell anemia
An inherited blood disorder that mostly affects African Americans and is characterized by the presence of crescent- or sickle-shaped red blood cells.

Tay-Sachs disease
A fatal neurological disorder that primarily affects Jews of eastern European origin.

hypertension
High blood pressure.

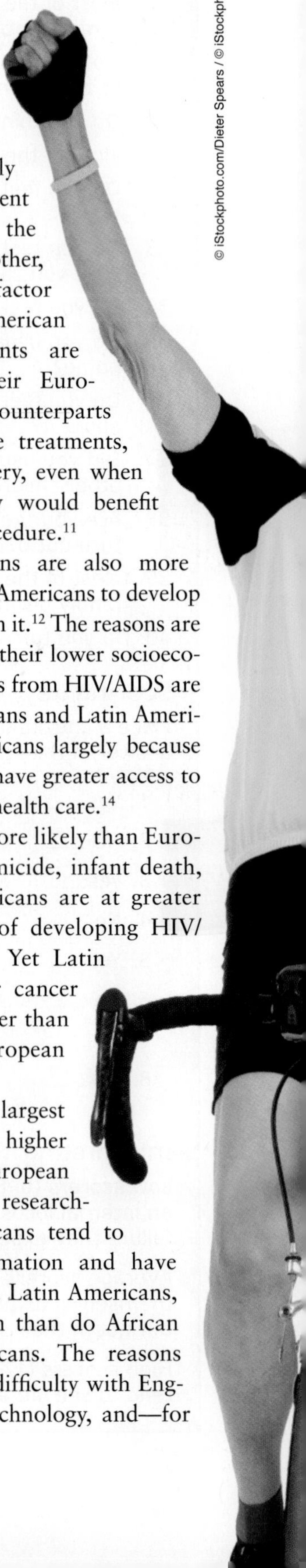

African Americans are more likely than European Americans to suffer heart attacks and strokes and to die from them. Early diagnosis and treatment might help reduce the racial gap. But another, often unrecognized factor is that African American heart disease patients are less likely than their European American counterparts to receive aggressive treatments, such as bypass surgery, even when it appears that they would benefit equally from the procedure.[11]

African Americans are also more likely than European Americans to develop cancer and to die from it.[12] The reasons are apparently related to their lower socioeconomic status.[13] Deaths from HIV/AIDS are also higher among African Americans and Latin Americans than among European Americans largely because European Americans, on average, have greater access to health insurance and high-quality health care.[14]

African Americans are also more likely than European Americans to die from homicide, infant death, diabetes, and AIDS. Latin Americans are at greater risk than European Americans of developing HIV/AIDS and adult-onset diabetes. Yet Latin Americans generally have lower cancer rates and death rates due to cancer than either African Americans or European Americans.

Mexican Americans, the largest group of Latin Americans, have higher rates of heart disease than European Americans. The major reasons, researchers say, is that Mexican Americans tend to receive less health-related information and have less access to health care services. Latin Americans, overall, visit physicians less often than do African Americans and European Americans. The reasons include lack of health insurance, difficulty with English, misgivings about medical technology, and—for

Did You Know That... Being male shaves about five years off a person's life expectancy.

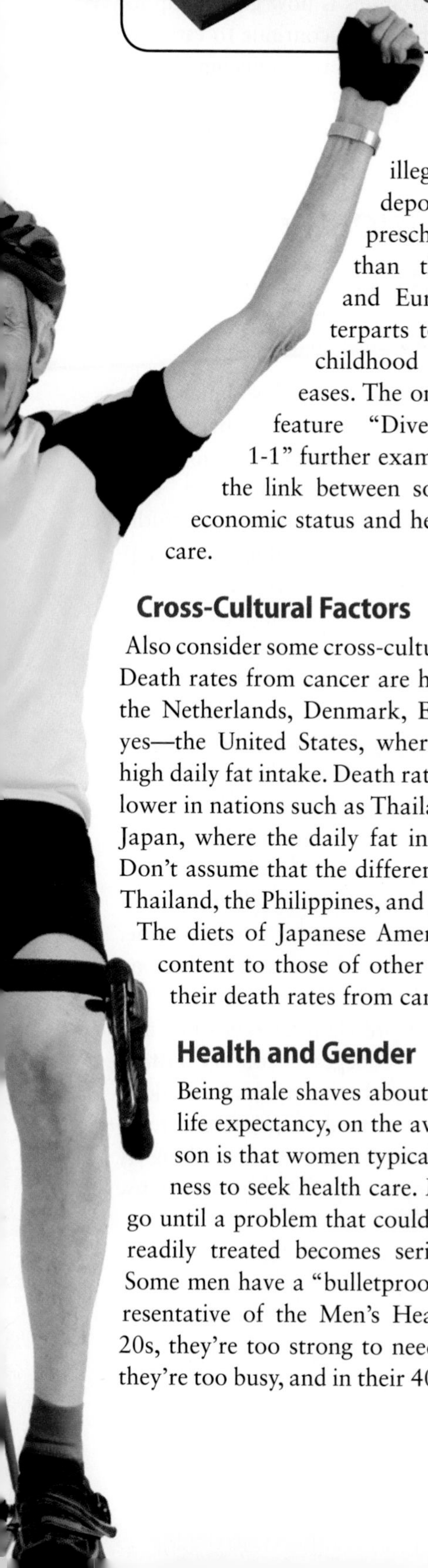

illegal immigrants—fear of deportation. Latin American preschoolers are also less likely than their African American and European American counterparts to be immunized against childhood diseases. The online feature "Diversity 1-1" further examines the link between socioeconomic status and health care.

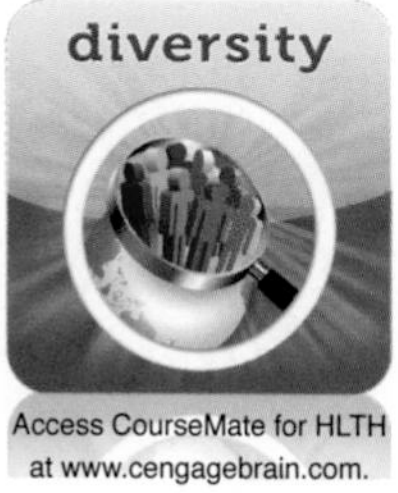
diversity
Access CourseMate for HLTH at www.cengagebrain.com.

Cross-Cultural Factors

Also consider some cross-cultural differences in health. Death rates from cancer are higher in nations such as the Netherlands, Denmark, England, Canada, and—yes—the United States, where the population has a high daily fat intake. Death rates from cancer are much lower in nations such as Thailand, the Philippines, and Japan, where the daily fat intake is markedly lower. Don't assume that the difference is racial just because Thailand, the Philippines, and Japan are Asian nations. The diets of Japanese Americans are similar in fat content to those of other Americans—and so are their death rates from cancer!

Health and Gender

Being male shaves about five years off a person's life expectancy, on the average.[15] Why? One reason is that women typically show greater willingness to seek health care. Men often let symptoms go until a problem that could have been prevented or readily treated becomes serious or life-threatening. Some men have a "bulletproof" mentality. Says a representative of the Men's Health Network: "In their 20s, they're too strong to need a doctor; in their 30s, they're too busy, and in their 40s, too scared."[16] Women are similarly much more likely to examine themselves for signs of breast cancer than men are to examine their testicles for signs of cancer.

Men and women are also at different risks for various kinds of health problems. Men are at higher risk than women for certain diseases, including coronary heart disease. Women are apparently protected from heart disease by high levels of estrogen, at least until menopause. After menopause, women's risk of heart disease increases dramatically so that gender differences disappear by about age 65.

Women are at higher risk for many serious chronic conditions, such as **arthritis** and **osteoporosis**. Severe or moderately reduced bone density affects 7 out of 10 women over age 50. Arthritis affects one-third of women age 45 to 64 years and half of women age 65 years and older. Women, particularly poor women, are much more likely than men to be victims of sexual violence and of violent crime committed by an intimate (a current or former partner) or relative.

Women have also been underrepresented as subjects of health research, and have sometimes even been excluded from participating. The online feature "Diversity 1-2" explains why this is so and what has been done about it.

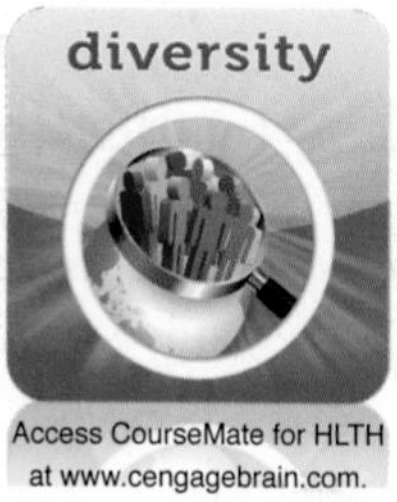
diversity
Access CourseMate for HLTH at www.cengagebrain.com.

Healthy People 2000 and Beyond

The U.S. government embarked upon an ambitious effort in the 1990s to promote health and prevent disease among all Americans. This project, called *Healthy People*, was based on the vision of a society in which all people live long, healthy lives.[17] Three goals to promote health were identified:

arthritis
Inflammation of a joint, typically accompanied by pain, stiffness, and swelling; results from a number of conditions affecting the structures inside and surrounding the joint.

osteoporosis
Condition of generalized bone loss, making bones more brittle and subject to breakage.

LEARNING OUTCOME 4

Describe the goals of the government project *Healthy People*

- *To increase the span of* healthy *life for all Americans.* Expanding the number of years lived by the typical American is not enough. The goal is to increase the number of healthy, fulfilling years. On average, the U.S. population lives only 64 healthy years, which is lower than the life expectancy of 76. For African Americans, the figure is even lower—56 years. Thus, many people survive for a number of years in a state of declining health and poor quality of life.
- *To reduce the health discrepancies among Americans.* Some ethnic groups are more vulnerable to certain diseases than others because of differences in lifestyle, access to health care, and possible genetic factors. The goal is to reduce those discrepancies that can be reduced, such as differences in access to health care.
- *To achieve access to preventive services for all Americans.* Some groups, especially ethnic minorities, have less access to preventive health care than others do.[18] Partly because of limited access, they tend to suffer more health problems and stand a greater risk of early death. Again, a major goal is to remove barriers to prevention and treatment.

Midcourse Update and *Healthy People 2010*

The first leg of the project, *Healthy People 2000*, set 300 specific health objectives. A review in the mid-1990s showed progress toward meeting more than two-thirds of the objectives on which data have been collected, including declines in deaths due to heart disease, cancer, and stroke—the three leading causes of death. Fewer Americans are dying prematurely, in part because of improvements in medical care, but also because of changes in lifestyle, such as quitting smoking and reducing fat intake. Americans are also exercising more and watching their weight more closely. With gains in health and improvements in health care, life expectancy continues to increase, although differences remain across races and genders.

critical thinking
The adoption of a questioning attitude characterized by careful weighing of evidence and thoughtful analysis and probing of the claims and arguments of others.

Healthy People 2010 built upon the framework of *Healthy People 2000* in setting health objectives for Americans. It specified two familiar overall goals: to increase quality and years of healthy life, and to eliminate health disparities.

Progress has been made on achieving most objectives identified in *Healthy People 2010*, but more needs to be done to achieve the vision of improved health of all Americans. The United States is now gearing up for *Healthy People 2020*, which will continue to establish objectives for promoting health and reducing disease through the end of the decade.[19]

Thinking Critically about Health-Related Information

LEARNING OUTCOME 5

Explain ways of thinking critically about health-related information

We are flooded with so much information about health that it is difficult to sort facts from fiction. Some reports contradict each other. Others contain half-truths, or draw misleading or unsupported conclusions. In some cases, we are bewildered because health professionals do not agree among themselves. Sadly, most of us take certain "truths" for granted. We tend to assume that authority figures like doctors and government officials provide us with accurate information and are qualified to make decisions that affect our lives. However, when two doctors disagree on the need for a hysterectomy or whether people should take megadoses of antioxidant vitamins, we wonder how they can both be correct.

To help students evaluate claims, arguments, and widely held beliefs, most colleges encourage **critical thinking.** Becoming a critical thinker means being skeptical of things that are presented in print or uttered by authority figures or celebrities, or passed along by friends. Critical thinkers never say, "This is true because so-and-so says that it is true."

Another aspect of critical thinking is thoughtful analysis of claims and arguments. It means looking carefully at both sides of the argument. Critical thinking requires willingness to challenge the conventional wisdom and common knowledge that many of us take for granted. It means scrutinizing definitions of terms and finding *reasons* to support beliefs, rather than relying on feelings or "gut impressions." Critical thinkers maintain open minds. They suspend their beliefs until they have obtained and evaluated evidence that either supports or refutes them.

Throughout this book we raise issues that demand critical thinking. These issues may stimulate you to analyze and evaluate your beliefs and attitudes about the health choices available to you in the light of scientific evidence. For example, there are controversies over use of hormone replacement therapy by postmenopausal women. Other issues invoke moral values. There is controversy over whether or not governments should issue needles to drug addicts to prevent them from sharing needles and possibly infecting one another with bloodborne health problems such as HIV/AIDS. What of the issue of abortion? Should health professionals be permitted to help terminally ill people end their lives painlessly by administering lethal drugs? Critical thinkers know that while scientific knowledge can help inform their decisions, many decisions require consideration of their moral and ethical issues.

Features of Critical Thinking

Critical thinkers maintain a healthy skepticism. When they hear arguments and claims, they examine definitions of terms, carefully consider evidence, and decide whether arguments are valid and logical. Here are some suggestions for thinking critically about health information:

Be skeptical. Politicians, religious leaders, and other authority figures attempt to convince you of their points of view. Even researchers and authors may hold certain biases. Adopt the attitude of accepting nothing as true—including the comments of the authors of this text—until you have weighed the evidence.

Examine definitions of terms. Some statements are true when a term is defined in one way but not true when it is defined in another. Consider the statement, "Stress is bad for you." If we define stress in terms of hassles and work or family pressures that stretch our ability to cope to the max, this statement may have substance. However, if we define stress more broadly to include any factors that impose a demand on us to adjust, including events such as a new marriage or the birth of a child, certain stressors can be good.

Recognize that correlation is not causation. Suppose we find that people whose diets contain higher levels of vitamin X have lower rates of death from heart disease than people whose diets contain lower levels of vitamin X. In other words, a correlation (a mathematical relationship) exists between death rates from heart disease on the one hand and dietary intake of vitamin X on the other. Does this mean vitamin X plays a *causal role* in lowering death rates from heart disease? Critical thinkers recognize the limits of their knowledge claims. They realize they cannot determine from a correlational relationship alone whether two variables (intake of vitamin X and death rates from heart disease) are causally connected. It is possible that other ingredients in foods containing high levels of vitamin X deserve the credit. Or perhaps people who consume high levels of vitamin X engage in other behaviors that explain their good fortune. To determine cause and effect, scientists need to conduct experiments in which they manipulate the variable of interest (the vitamin, in this case) and study its effects while controlling other factors, such as diet and lifestyle.

Consider the quality of the evidence upon which conclusions are based. Some conclusions, even seemingly "scientific" ones, are based on anecdotes and personal endorsements. They are not founded on sound research.

Do not oversimplify. Consider the statement, "Alcoholism is inherited." Genetic factors may create a predisposition to alcoholism, but the origins of alcoholism and many other health problems involve a complex interplay of biological and environmental factors. People may inherit a predisposition to heart disease but never develop it if they watch their diet, exercise regularly, and learn to manage stress. On the other hand, people may develop heart problems if they overeat, smoke, and fail to exercise, even if there is no family history of the disease.

Do not overgeneralize. Certain chemicals in our environment pose health risks. Some of these chemicals can be dangerous or deadly at high levels of exposure. But they may not pose a significant risk to a typical person who is exposed to very small levels of them. Therefore, the evidence might not support the views that the environment must be completely cleansed of the chemicals.

For tips on how to apply critical thinking when evaluating health-related articles in magazines and self-help books, check out the online feature "Prevention 1-1."

prevention

Access CourseMate for HLTH at www.cengagebrain.com.

Thinking Critically about Online Health-Related Information

The Internet offers a world of health information literally at your fingertips. If you have access to the Internet, you can obtain information relating to:

- Listings and abstracts (brief descriptions) of scientific studies published in leading health and medical journals. Much of this information is provided free of charge.
- Information about medications, medical treatments, and medical conditions.
- Consumer-oriented material, such as the latest health-related reports from *Consumer Reports*.
- Electronic encyclopedias that contain entries for thousands of health-related terms.
- Listings of thousands of medical service providers, including leading hospitals, clinics, and health organizations.
- Forums and message boards that bring together people who share medical concerns or interests.
- Vendors who supply a range of medical products and services.
- Information provided by federal health agencies, including the National Cancer Institute and the National Institute on Aging.
- Information from leading national health organizations, such as the American Heart Association, the American Diabetes Association, and the American Lung Association.

Are you interested in learning more about the relationship between hypertension and stress? You could enter the term "hypertension" in an online search engine, such as Google.com. This would retrieve every site indexed to hypertension, perhaps thousands. To narrow your search, input key terms, such as "hypertension" and "stress." In this case, only sites containing references to both terms, hypertension and stress, would be retrieved. Once you've landed on a website, you may find links to related information of interest to you.

You can also go to particular websites. Table 1-2 on the next page provides examples of reliable health-related Internet sites.

Should I Believe It?

Although there is a great deal of reliable health-related information on the Internet, you can't believe everything that is posted. Anyone can post information on the Internet, so the casual user may not know how to distinguish accurate, scientifically-based information from misinformation.[20] Here are some tips for thinking critically about online health-related information:

1. *Check out the credentials of the source.* Who is posting the material? Is it a well-respected medical or scientific institution, or an individual or group that has no scientific credentials, or even a person with an ax to grind with the scientific or medical establishment?

   The most reliable sources are scientific journals that are subject to peer review, a process by which other scientists carefully scrutinize each potential contributor's work before publication. In addition to scientific journals, the more reliable sources of health and medical information are those that are frequently updated. Examples include websites maintained by government agencies, such as the National Institutes of Health and its many divisions, as well as those sponsored by leading medical organizations, such as the American Medical Association, the American Heart Association, the American Lung Association, and the American Dental Association (see Table 1-2).
2. *Look for citations.* Scientists back up what they say with citations to the original scientific sources. For example, the references at the end of this book represent the sources your authors used in preparing it. If the authors cite findings from the scientific literature, you should expect them to supply some of the references they use, such as the journals or other periodicals in which the studies were published, including the year, volume, and page numbers. This information allows the reader to check accuracy by referring to the original sources. In some cases, however, scientific organizations such as the National Institutes of Health and leading medical schools and medical centers prepare information for the general public that is accurate but not annotated with source notes or references.
3. *Beware of product claims.* Many commercial organizations use the Internet to tout or sell

Table 1-2 Reliable Health-Related Internet Sites

HEALTH RESOURCE	WHO THEY ARE/ WHAT THEY DO	INTERNET ADDRESS
National Institutes of Health (NIH)	Gateway to information on the latest biomedical research from its many institutes	www.nih.gov
U.S. Department of Agriculture (USDA), Food and Nutrition Information	Food and nutrition information people can use to make healthier food choices	www.usda.gov
American Heart Association (AHA)	Information on fighting heart disease and stroke	www.amhrt.org
American Cancer Society (ACS)	Information about cancer and its treatment	www.cancer.org
Food & Drug Administration (FDA)	Information about food and drug safety	www.fda.gov
Environmental Protection Agency (EPA)	Citizen information about threats to the environment; EPA publications, programs, and initiatives	www.epa.gov
Centers for Disease Control and Prevention (CDC), a federal agency	Information about diseases and health risks	www.cdc.gov
Mayo Clinic	Information about diseases and health conditions	www.mayoclinic.com
National Center for Health Statistics (NCHS), a division of the CDC	Statistical information about diseases and health care	www.cdc.gov/nchs
National Center for Infectious Disease (NCID)	Information on infectious diseases ranging from STIs to Lyme disease	www.cdc.gov/ncidod/about.htm
National Women's Health Resource Center	Health information specifically focusing on women's health issues	www.healthywomen.org
American Psychological Association	Information on psychology for the general public	www.apa.org
American Psychiatric Association	Information on mental health, including online pamphlets on topics such as depression, phobias, and Alzheimer's disease	www.psych.org
HealthFinder.gov	Tips on healthy living from government health experts	www.healthfinder.gov

health-related products. Don't assume such product claims are scientifically valid. Think of them as electronic advertising—an Internet version of a TV commercial. Take them with a grain of salt, and keep a tight grip on your wallet. Don't be misled by a money-back guarantee. These do not guarantee that the product will work. Rather, they claim that you'll get your money back if they don't succeed. Sometimes you will.

Recognize too that information from the Internet is no substitute for consulting your personal physician about any health-related concerns. Surf the net for health-related information, but check with your primary health care provider before changing your lifestyle or health-related habits.

The "Health Skills" features throughout this book and on the companion website help you apply the material to your own life so that you can optimize your health. The online feature "Health Skills 1-2" focuses on an important element of achieving wellness—practicing self-care. It covers the following topics:

health skills

Access CourseMate for HLTH at www.cengagebrain.com.

- Choosing a primary care physician
- Putting prevention first
- Replacing patterns of abuse with healthier habits
- Practicing dental self-care
- Keeping a home health record
- Keeping abreast of developments in health

HEALTH APPS: YOUR LINK TO ONLINE HEALTH APPLICATIONS

health check

The Dimensions of Health: Where Do You Stand? All of us want to be healthy and achieve wellness, but many of us have not taken stock of our health habits. "Health Check 1-1" will help you examine your behavior with respect to each of the dimensions of health.

diversity

Socioeconomic Status: The Rich Get Richer and the Poor Get . . . Sicker Socioeconomic status (SES) and health have been intimately connected throughout history. Generally speaking, people higher in SES levels enjoy better health and live longer. "Diversity 1-1" explains why.

diversity

Women's Health Research: A History of Exclusion Women have long been underrepresented as subjects of health research, and have sometimes even been excluded from participating. "Diversity 1-2" explores reasons and solutions for this problem.

prevention

Debunking Miracle Cures and Quick Fixes from the Self-Help Aisle Self-help books have flooded the marketplace in recent years, promising everything from easy and quick weight loss to power fitness in as little as five minutes a day. How can consumers know what to buy? How can they separate helpful information from useless or harmful chatter? Go online to read "Prevention 1-1" to learn how to use critical thinking to evaluate health-related articles in magazines and the self-help books.

health skills

Practicing Self-Care "Health Skills 1-2" focuses on some very important elements of achieving wellness, such as choosing a physician and putting prevention first.

Go to the CourseMate for HLTH at www.cengagebrain.com for additional resources including flashcards, games, self-quizzing, review exercises, web exercises, learning checks, and more.

Psychological Health

"A sound mind in a sound body is a short but full description of a happy state in this World."
—John Locke

The people of the classical period of ancient Greece and Rome understood the close relationship between a healthy mind and a healthy body. As the Roman poet Juvenal put it, "You should pray for a sound mind in a sound body." The seventeenth-century philosopher John Locke offered this prescription for a good life: "A sound mind in a sound body, is a short, but full description of a happy state in this World: he that has these two, has little more to wish for; and he that wants either of them, will be little the better for anything else." This prescription for a good life still rings true today.

Psychological health, or soundness of mind, is as important to our well-being as soundness of body (physical health). Our physical health is also closely intertwined with our psychological health. Physical illness can impact us psychologically, leading to psychological problems such as depression and anxiety, or making it difficult to maintain an active social life. Psychological factors can also impair our physical health. Persistent negative emotions, especially anger, can increase the risks of developing heart disease or suffering a heart attack. Negative feelings can also make us more vulnerable to physical health problems by impairing the body's immune system.

psychological health
Soundness of mind, characterized by the absence of significant psychological problems and by the ability to function effectively in meeting life demands and to derive satisfaction from work, social relationships, and leisure pursuits.

LEARNING OUTCOMES

1 Describe the elements of psychological health

2 Explain what is meant by the mind–body connection

3 Discuss the contribution of spiritual health to psychological health

4 Discuss psychological disorders, focusing on anxiety and depression

5 Describe ways of treating psychological disorders

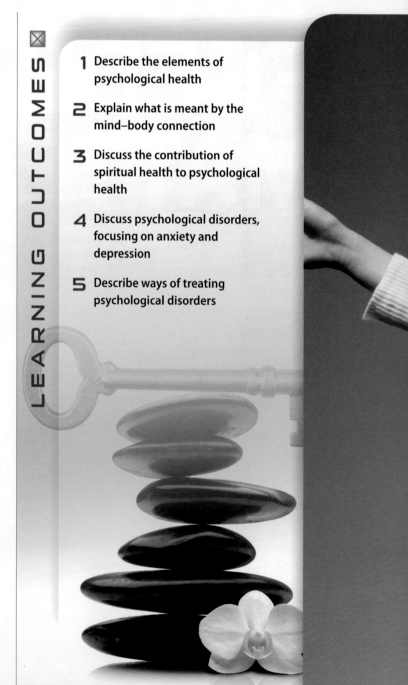

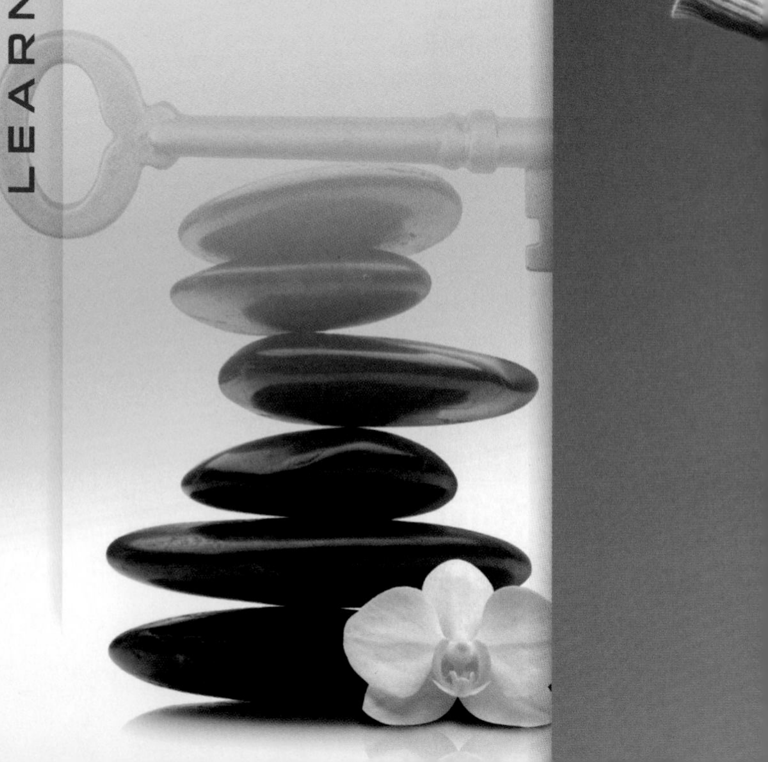

The Elements of Psychological Health

Just what is psychological health? Health is more than the absence of illness. Psychological health is more than the absence of psychological disorders. Psychological health also involves the ability to meet the challenges we face in life, to think clearly, and to derive satisfaction from our work, social relationships, and leisure activities.

LEARNING OUTCOME 1

Describe the elements of psychological health

Psychological health is also characterized by self-esteem, self-confidence, and ego identity—a firm sense of who you are and where you are headed in life. Psychological health involves being in touch with your needs and goals. Psychological health also has a spiritual dimension: finding—or creating—meaning in life.

No two of us are quite alike. You are unique, let us consider the elements of psychological health so that you can assess whether or not you are psychologically healthy.

Did you know that . . .

- An average student might have higher self-esteem than a respected scientist? [p. 24]
- Optimists tend to return more quickly to their normal lives following coronary artery bypass surgery than pessimists do? [p. 28]
- The wealthiest Americans are only a tiny bit happier than other Americans? [p. 28]
- Within a year of striking it rich, lottery winners are generally no happier than they were before hitting the jackpot? [p. 28]
- Despite the myth to the contrary, people who threaten suicide are quite likely to be serious about taking their lives? [p. 37]

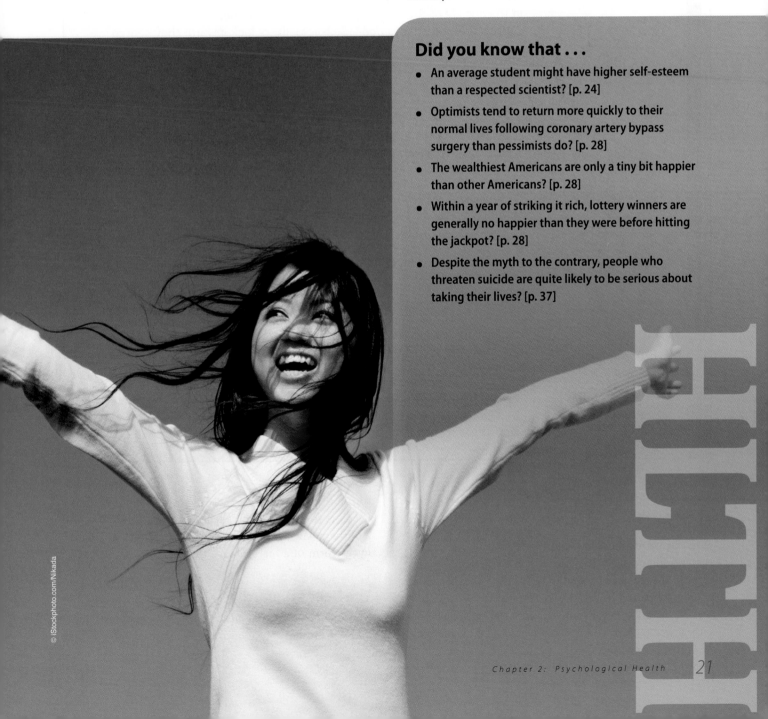

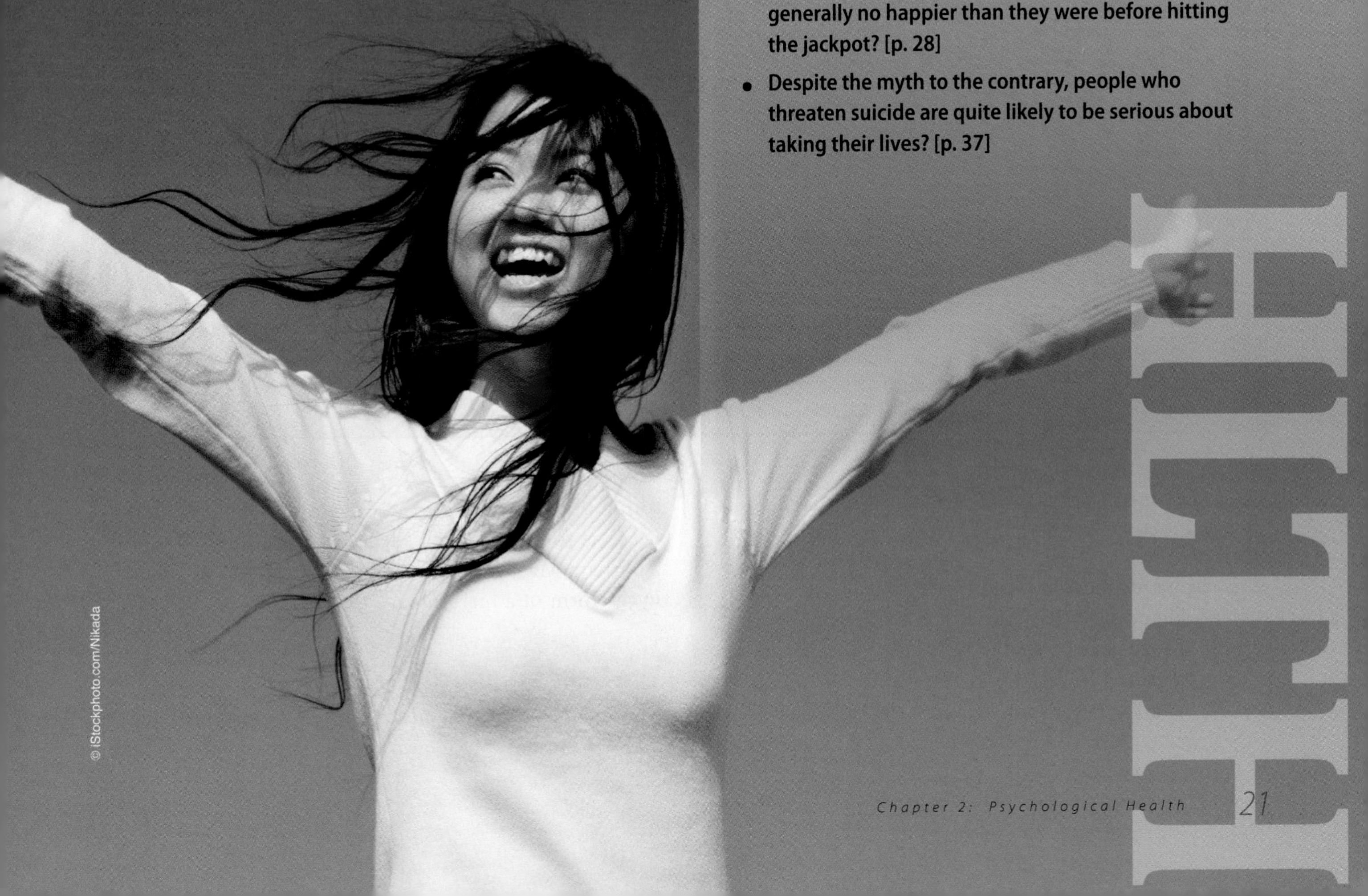

© iStockphoto.com/Nikada

HEALTH CHECK 2-1

Do You Strive to Be All That You Can Be?

Are you a self-actualizer? Do you strive to be all that you can be? Maslow attributed the following characteristics to the self-actualizing person. How many of them describe you? Why not undertake some self-evaluation?

YES **NO**

_____ _____ 1. *Do you fully experience life in the present—the here and now?* (Self-actualizers do not focus excessively on the lost past or wish their lives away as they strive toward distant goals.)

_____ _____ 2. *Do you make growth choices rather than fear choices?* (Self-actualizers take reasonable risks to develop their unique potentials. They do not bask in the dull life of the status quo. They do not "settle.")

_____ _____ 3. *Do you seek self-knowledge?* (Self-actualizers look inward; they search for values, talents, and meaningfulness. The questionnaires in this book offer a jumping-off point for getting to know yourself. It might also be enlightening to take an "interest inventory"—a test frequently used to help make career decisions—at your college testing and counseling center.)

_____ _____ 4. *Do you strive toward honesty in interpersonal relationships?* (Self-actualizers strip away the social facades and games that stand in the way of self-disclosure and the formation of intimate relationships.)

_____ _____ 5. *Do you behave assertively and express your own ideas and feelings, even at the risk of occasional social disapproval?* (Self-actualizers do not bottle up their feelings for the sake of avoiding disapproval.)

_____ _____ 6. *Do you strive toward new goals? Do you strive to be the best that you can be in a chosen life role?* (Self-actualizers do not live by the memory of past accomplishments. Nor do they present second-rate efforts.)

_____ _____ 7. *Do you seek meaningful and rewarding life activities?* Do you experience moments of actualization that Maslow referred to as *peak experiences?* (Peak experiences are brief moments of rapture filled with personal meaning. Examples might include completing a work of art, falling in love, redesigning a machine tool, suddenly solving a complex problem in math or physics, or having a baby. Again, we differ as individuals, and one person's peak experience might be boring to another.)

_____ _____ 8. *Are you open to new experiences?* (Self-actualizers do not hold themselves back for fear that novel experiences might shake their views of the world, or their views of right and wrong. Self-actualizers are willing to revise their expectations, values, and opinions.)

"Scoring" the Health Check: The more "yeses" you checked, the farther along you are on the road to self-actualization. Self-actualization is a continuing process of psychological growth and realization, more a path than a destination.

Needs: What Do You Need to Feel Fulfilled?

What are your most important needs? To achieve status and financial security? To make a difference in the world? To achieve something that no one has ever achieved before? To eat, drink, and be merry?

Needs are the wellsprings of motivation. When you experience a need, you feel motivated to do something to fulfill it or satisfy it. A useful way of thinking about needs is to use a model suggested by the psychologist Abraham Maslow, who believed that needs are ordered in the form of a hierarchy.

The Needs Hierarchy

Maslow believed that needs run up a ladder, or hierarchy, from basic biological needs, such as hunger and

Figure 2-1 Maslow's Hierarchy of Needs

What do you do when you're no longer hungry? Do you nap until it's time to eat again, or do you seek to satisfy higher-level needs? According to Maslow, once we satisfy lower-level needs, we seek to meet higher needs. Where would you place yourself in the hierarchy?

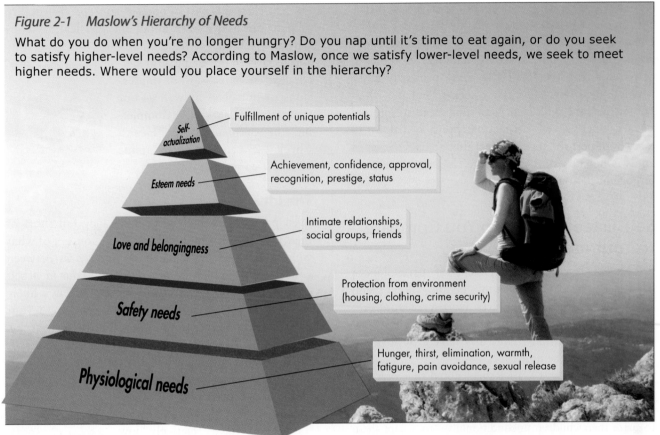

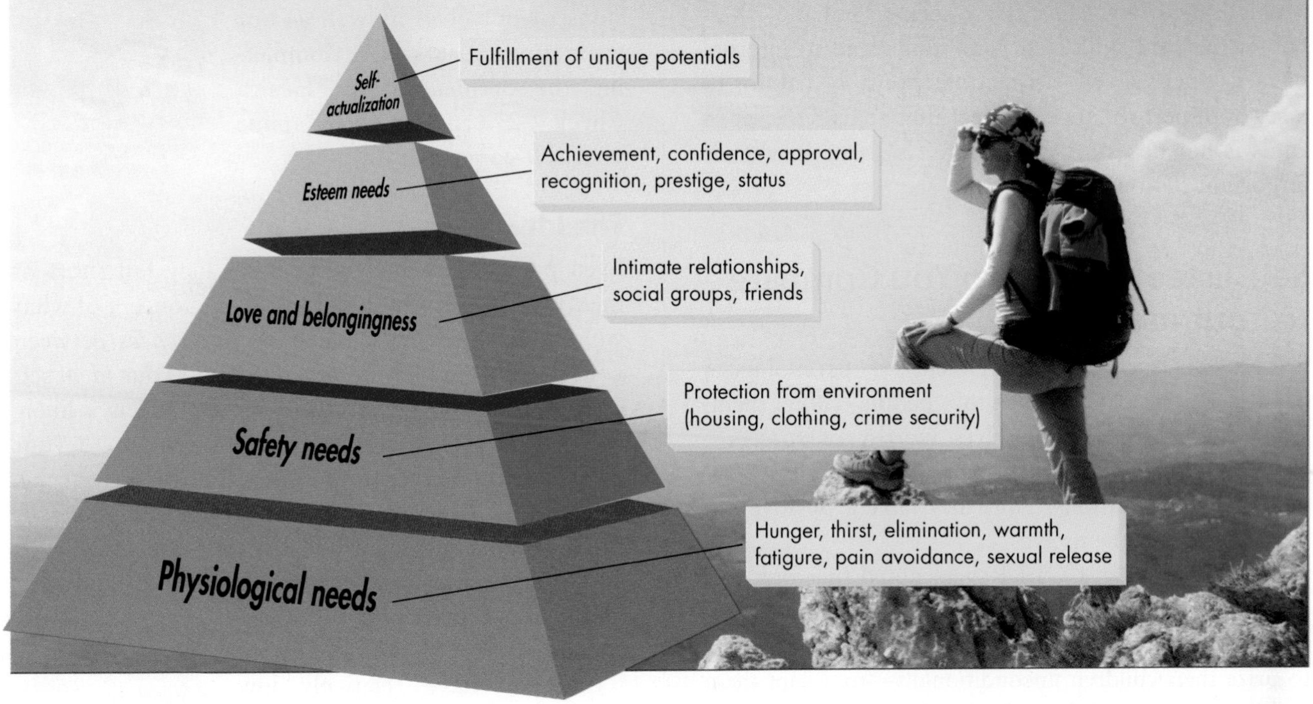

thirst, to psychological needs, such as self-esteem and self-actualization (see Figure 2-1). The hierarchy of needs teaches that people usually try to fulfill needs in an ordered way. Once lower-level needs are satisfied, people strive to meet higher-level needs. Once our bellies are full, we don't just snooze until we're hungry again. Rather, we experience higher needs.

The highest need in the hierarchy is **self-actualization**, the need to become all that you are capable of being. Self-actualizing people are continually growing and developing, achieving some goals and striving to achieve others. Life is motion and the self-actualizing person does not stand still. Since no two people are alike, self-actualization takes many forms, from creating works of art to becoming an accomplished athlete, theologian, or military officer. Maslow believed that people are basically good and that, if given the opportunity, people will strive to achieve higher goals relating to love, esteem, and self-actualization.

In a relatively affluent society like ours, most people satisfy basic physiological and safety needs. They have food on the table and a roof over their heads. Struggles for love and belongingness often take center stage. Maslow noted that many people feel psychologically fulfilled even if they don't reach the pinnacle of the hierarchy. Psychological health means recognizing and seeking to satisfy the needs that are important to the individual.

Are you a self-actualizing person? Self-actualization does not depend on how much money you make or how many friends you have. It is more closely related to your approach to life, to whether you are open to experiences and opportunities that help you fulfill your potential. Maslow identified eight qualities of the self-actualizing individual, which we have represented in form of personal reflection questions posed in Health Check 2-1.

Need for Achievement

Psychologically healthy people set challenging but attainable goals. They feel motivated to achieve success in their chosen walk of life, but don't set the bar so high that they will inevitably fall short.

People with a strong *need for achievement* tend to earn higher grades than people who have comparable ability but a lower need for achievement. They are more likely to earn high salaries and be promoted. People who have strong needs for achievement take risks and make decisions. They may enter business or establish businesses of their own.

self-actualization
Self-initiated tendency to strive to realize one's potential.

The need for achievement can be driven by different forces. Some students are mainly driven by *performance goals*. They seek tangible, external rewards—a good job, entry into graduate school, the approval of parents or professors. Others are primarily motivated by *learning goals*. They seek to enhance their knowledge and skills. Learning goals lead to internal rewards such as self-satisfaction. Many of us aim to meet both performance and learning goals. One set of goals is not necessarily superior. The issue is what is important to you.

Self-Esteem: How Do You Compare to Your Ideal Self?

Self-esteem is a core component of psychological health. Psychologically healthy people value themselves and consider themselves worthy of success—however they define success. They also recognize their deficits and limitations. Thus they have a positive but realistic view of themselves.

The psychologist Carl Rogers noted that our self-esteem first mirrors the value placed on us by others. For this reason, Rogers believed it is crucial for parents to prize their children unconditionally—to accept them children as worthwhile and valuable regardless of their behavior at any moment in time. Unfortunately, many parents show approval only when their children behave "properly." Children may thus come to regard themselves as worthwhile only when they behave in approved ways. Consequently, they may develop a distorted self-concept, disowning the parts of themselves that differ from what others—especially their parents—value.

Rogers did not suggest that parents accept all of their children's behavior. Parents can correct children's misbehavior without damaging their self-concepts. However, parents need to make it clear that it is the behavior that is being rejected, not the child.

ideal self
The mental image corresponding to what we believe we ought to be like.

Self-esteem is part of our *self-concept*, the totality of perceptions we have about the physical, psychological, spiritual, intellectual, and social parts of our being. Our self-concept encompasses our impressions of ourselves as well as our evaluation of ourselves. Completing the online feature "Health Check 2-2" can help you examine your self-concept.

health check
Access CourseMate for HLTH at www.cengagebrain.com.

The Ideal Self

Even people with high self-esteem may fall short of their ideal selves. Our **ideal self** is our concept of what we ought to be. The greater the *differences* between your perception of your *actual* self and your *ideal* self on important traits, the *lower* your self-esteem is likely to be. The *closer* your self-perceptions are to your ideal self, the *higher* your self-esteem is likely to be. Therefore, an average student might have higher self-esteem than a respected scientist. Self-esteem depends on the difference between your self-concept and your ideal self in terms of highly valued traits.

If you have relatively low self-esteem, don't give up the ship. This chapter's online feature "Health Skills 2-1" and the following section focus on ways to enhance self-esteem.

health skills
Access CourseMate for HLTH at www.cengagebrain.com.

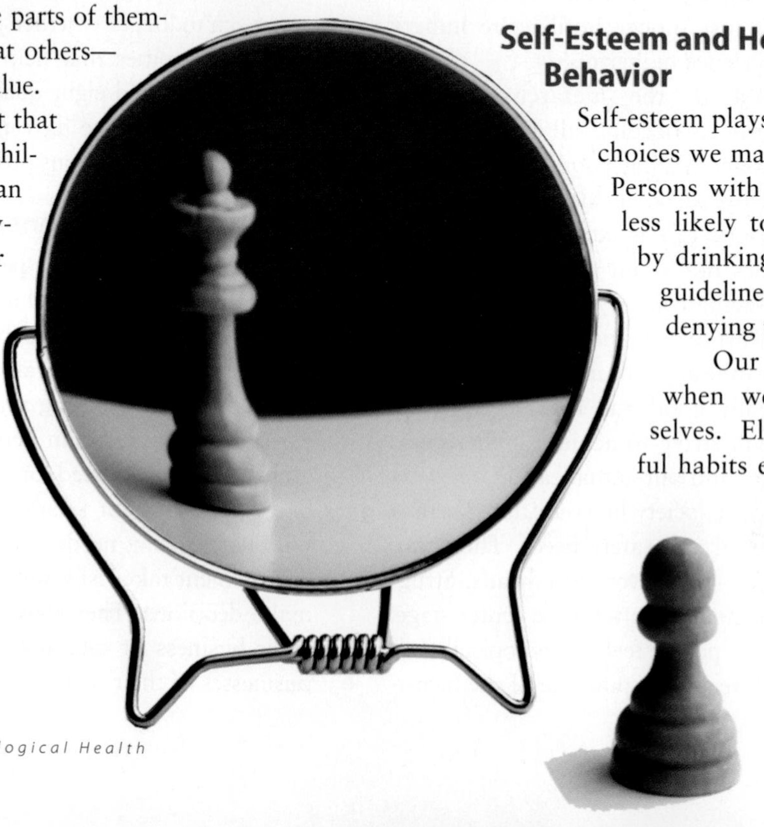

Self-Esteem and Healthful Behavior

Self-esteem plays a critical role in the choices we make about our health. Persons with high self-esteem are less likely to abuse their health by drinking to excess, ignoring guidelines for safer sex, or denying the signs of illness.

Our self-esteem also rises when we are good to ourselves. Eliminating unhealthful habits enhances self-esteem. Virtually all former smokers feel better about themselves than they did when they were smoking.

So do people who eat a balanced diet and exercise regularly.

Self-Confidence: The Little Engine that Could?

Psychologically healthy people not only have high self-esteem, but they also have self-confidence. They believe in their ability to accomplish what their goals, such as completing a college course or doing a flip off a diving board. Self-confident people are more likely to face the challenges of life than to retreat from them. They are more likely to grasp opportunities, such as gaining a foothold in a new career, taking up a new sport or hobby, or making healthful changes such as quitting smoking. They are more likely to stick to their efforts.

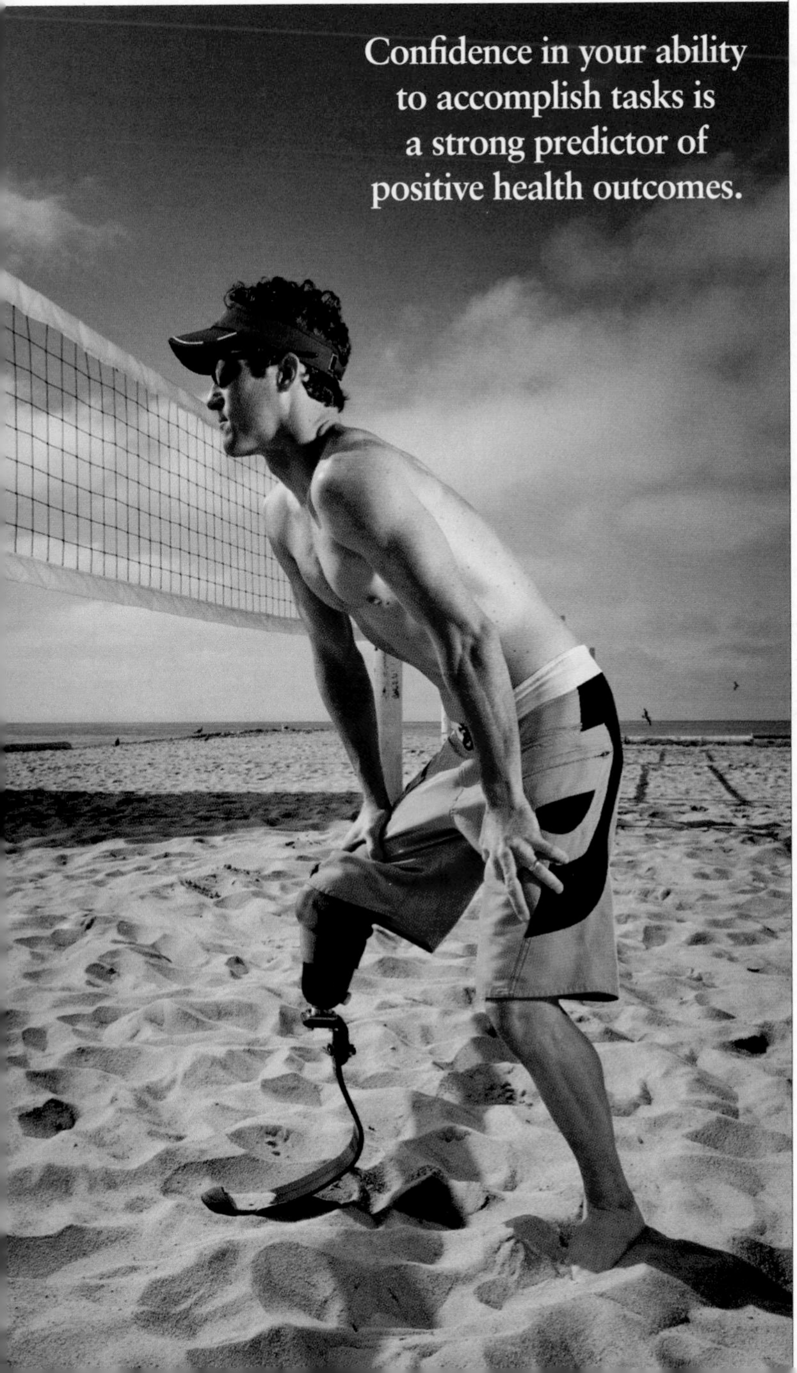
Confidence in your ability to accomplish tasks is a strong predictor of positive health outcomes.

© iStockphoto.com/MichaelSvoboda

Confidence in your ability to accomplish tasks is a strong predictor of positive health outcomes. Among diabetic patients, this quality predicts adherence to medical directives given by their doctors.[1] It also predicts the likelihood of sticking with an exercise program, and for ex-smokers, preventing a relapse.[2] Self-confidence also predicts recovery from the trauma of calamities such as natural disasters and terrorist attacks.[3]

Self-confidence is generally higher among people who are free of psychological disorders, such as anxiety or mood disorders. Life is not necessarily a bowl of cherries for people with self-confidence. But if they should need psychological help for emotional problems, they are more likely than people lacking self-confidence to benefit from psychotherapy.

Self-confidence and success go hand in hand. People with self-confidence are more likely to succeed, and success boosts self-confidence. "Success experiences" are so important to children and adults alike.

Self-Assertiveness: Expressing Yourself

Self-assertiveness is the expression of a person's genuine feelings and beliefs. An assertive individual communicates who she or he is as a person. Assertiveness means taking an active rather than a passive approach to life. It is learned behavior that is largely shaped by early experiences.

Assertiveness is not aggressiveness. Assertive people are not bossy or belligerent. They don't have a chip on their shoulder. They don't put other people down. Assertive people express positive feelings as well as personal grievances. They respect the rights and feelings of others, even when they disagree with them.

You can learn how assertive you are compared to other students by completing the feature "Health Check 2-3" on the next page. You can then go online to read "Health Skills 2-2" for tips on being more assertive.

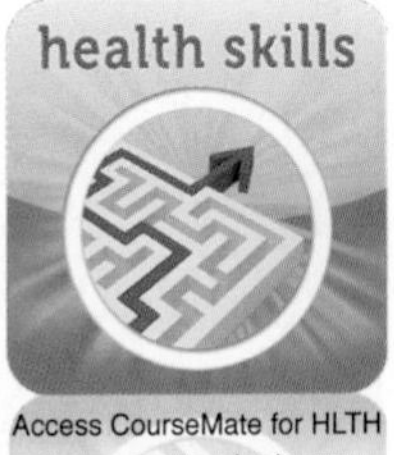
health skills

Access CourseMate for HLTH at www.cengagebrain.com.

Shyness is a roadblock to self-assertion. Shy people are bashful or retiring. Their anxiety or fear in social interactions may lead them to avoid such situations. Their fears may be so intense that they fail to develop intimate relationships. Fortunately, many people can overcome shyness by practicing assertive behavior.

Do You Speak Your Mind or Do You Wimp Out? The Rathus Assertiveness Schedule

What about you? Do you enrich the pockets of every telemarketer, or do you say no? Do you stick up for your rights, or do you allow others to walk all over you? Do you say what you feel or what you think other people want you to say? Do you initiate relationships with attractive people, or do you shy away from them?

One way to gain insight into how assertive you are is to take the following assertiveness schedule. Once you have finished, use the Scoring Key that follows to find out how to calculate your score; then you can compare your assertiveness to that of a sample of 1,400 students drawn from 35 college campuses across the United States.

If you believe that you are not assertive enough, why not take the quick course in self-assertion in the online feature, Health Skills 2-2, Assert Yourself!

Directions: Indicate how well each item describes you by using this code:

3 = very much like me
2 = rather like me
1 = slightly like me
–1 = slightly unlike me
–2 = rather unlike me
–3 = very much unlike me

______ 1. Most people seem to be more aggressive and assertive than I am.*
______ 2. I have hesitated to make or accept dates because of "shyness."*
______ 3. When the food served at a restaurant is not done to my satisfaction, I complain about it to the waiter or waitress.
______ 4. I am careful to avoid hurting other people's feelings, even when I feel that I have been injured.*
______ 5. If a salesperson has gone to considerable trouble to show me merchandise that is not quite suitable, I have a difficult time saying "No."*
______ 6. When I am asked to do something, I insist upon knowing why.
______ 7. There are times when I look for a good, vigorous argument.
______ 8. I strive to get ahead as well as most people in my position.
______ 9. To be honest, people often take advantage of me.*
______ 10. I enjoy starting conversations with new acquaintances and strangers.
______ 11. I often don't know what to say to people who are sexually attractive to me.*
______ 12. I will hesitate to make phone calls to business establishments and institutions*
______ 13. I would rather apply for a job or for admission to a college by writing letters than by going through with personal interviews.*
______ 14. I find it embarrassing to return merchandise.*
______ 15. If a close and respected relative were annoying me, I would smother my feelings rather than express my annoyance.*
______ 16. I have avoided asking questions for fear of sounding stupid.*
______ 17. During an argument I am sometimes afraid that I will get so upset that I will shake all over.*
______ 18. If a famed and respected lecturer makes a comment which I think is incorrect, I will have the audience hear my point of view as well.
______ 19. I avoid arguing over prices with clerks and salespeople.*
______ 20. When I have done something important or worthwhile, I manage to let others know about it.
______ 21. I am open and frank about my feelings.
______ 22. If someone has been spreading false and bad stories about me, I see him or her as soon as possible and "have a talk" about it.

continued

______ 23. I often have a hard time saying "No."*
______ 24. I tend to bottle up my emotions rather than make a scene.*
______ 25. I complain about poor service in a restaurant and elsewhere.
______ 26. When I am given a compliment, I sometimes just don't know what to say.*
______ 27. If a couple near me in a theater or at a lecture were conversing rather loudly, I would ask them to be quiet or to take their conversation elsewhere.
______ 28. Anyone attempting to push ahead of me in a line is in for a good battle.
______ 29. I am quick to express an opinion.
______ 30. There are times when I just can't say anything.*

Source: Reprinted from *Behavior Therapy*, Volume 4 (3), Spencer A. Rathus, A 30-item schedule for assessing assertive behavior, pp. 398-406. © 1973, with permission from Elsevier.
*These asterisks are explained in the answer key.

Scoring Key

For those items followed by an asterisk (*), change the signs (plus to minus; minus to plus). For example, if the response to an asterisked item was 2, place a minus sign (–) before the two. If the response to an asterisked item was –3, change the minus sign to a plus sign (+) by adding a vertical stroke. Then add up the scores of the 30 items.

Scores on the assertiveness schedule can vary from +90 to –90. The following table will show you how your score compares to those of 764 college women and 637 men from 35 campuses across the United States. For example, if you are a woman and your score was 26, it exceeded that of 80% of the women in the sample.

Percentiles for Scores on the RAS

Women's Scores	Percentile	Men's Scores
55	99	65
48	97	54
45	95	48
37	90	40
31	85	33
26	80	30
23	75	26
19	70	24
17	65	19
14	60	17
11	55	15
8	50	11
6	45	8
2	40	6
–1	35	3
–4	30	1
–8	25	–3
–13	20	–7
–17	15	–11
–24	10	–15
–34	5	–24
–39	3	–30
–48	1	–41

Source: Reprinted from *Behavior Therapy*, Volume 9 (4), Nevid, J. S. & Rathus, S. A., Multivariate and normative data pertaining to the RAS with the college population, p. 675. © 1978, with permission from Elsevier.

Ego Identity: Who Are You? What Do You Stand For?

Psychologically healthy people have **ego identity**, a firm sense of who they are, what they stand for, and where they are headed in life. Ego identity is based on understanding or creating personal needs and life goals. It involves developing values that reflect the importance we place on objects, principles, ideals, and goals. Achievement of ego identity is a key developmental task of adolescence and young adulthood.

Many college students undergo a period of serious self-examination in which they actively seek to construct ego identity. This period of soul-searching has been called an **identity crisis**. Though an identity crisis may be stressful—which is why it's dubbed a crisis—it is a normal part of developing psychological health.

People who fail to develop ego identity lack clear values and goals. They may drift without a rudder. They may be especially vulnerable to negative peer influences that can affect their health, such as illicit drug use. Although achieving direction in life is a key goal of adolescence or early adulthood, many middle-aged and older adults also undergo periods of self-reflection about the future or grapple with their beliefs and values.

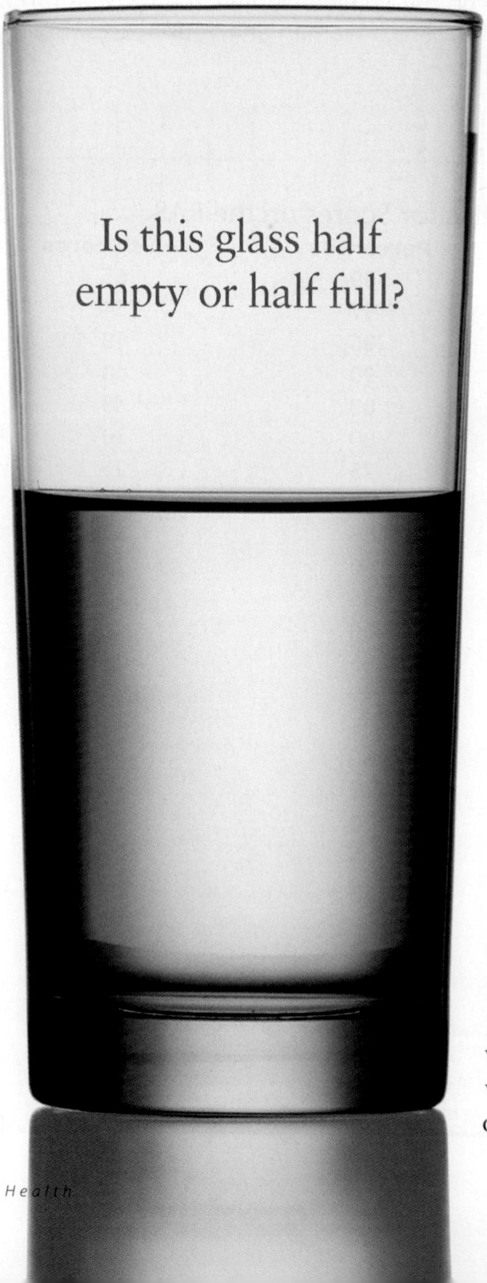

Is this glass half
empty or half full?

© Mike Kemp/Rubberball/Jupiterimages

Optimism: Do You See the Cup as Half Empty or Half Full?

Psychologically healthy people are optimists. They believe their prospects are bright and the future holds promise, even in difficult times. Because they are hopeful, optimists are more likely than pessimists to make the most of opportunities and bounce back from disappointments.

Researchers find that *optimism* is connected with positive health outcomes. For example, more optimistic women tend to have lower rates of heart disease and to live longer than pessimistic women.[4] In one study, college students took an optimism scale, the Life Orientation Test (LOT) (see "Health Check 2-4"). They were asked to track their physical symptoms for one month. Students scoring higher on the optimism scale reported fewer physical symptoms such as dizziness, fatigue, muscle soreness, and blurred vision.[5]

health check

Access CourseMate for HLTH at www.cengagebrain.com.

Optimists tend to be more resilient in the face of illness. They experience less distress when they incur heart disease. Optimism is linked to less distress and pain in cancer patients.[6] Among pregnant women, optimism is linked to better birth outcomes, such as high infant birth weight, and to a lower risk of postpartum depression, a type of depression that affects many women after giving birth.[7]

Optimism is even linked to faster recovery from surgery. In a study of people recovering from coronary artery bypass surgery, optimists were up and about their rooms more quickly than pessimists, and returned more quickly to family and work.[8]

Happiness: What Makes You Happy?

Personal happiness is another aspect of psychological health. What makes people happy? Happiness does not necessarily depend on the size of your bank account. Although extreme poverty dampens happiness, there is little evidence that happiness increases as wealth rises above a subsistence level. Members of the affluent *Forbes* 400—the nation's wealthiest individuals—are only a bit happier than the public at large.[9] Even lottery winners who get an emotional boost after their windfall generally return to their previous level of happiness within a year of cashing in.[10]

ego identity
The sense of who one is and what one stands for.

identity crisis
A period of serious soul-searching and self-examination in an effort to achieve ego identity.

Marriage also makes only a small contribution to happiness.[11] Although married people report being happier than single people[12], it is not clear that marriage is the cause of happiness. Happier people might also be more likely to get married or stay married, and the bounce in happiness reported by many newlyweds is actually short-lived.[13]

All in all, it seems that people have a "set point" for happiness, a general disposition that remains fairly stable throughout their lives, despite their ups and downs. Some people are generally happy despite misfortune, and others seem to be unhappy even when fortune shines on them. Even people who suffer catastrophes such as developing cancer or losing a loved one tend to bounce back eventually.

Interestingly, there is evidence for a genetic contribution to happiness. But even if genes are involved, there is still much we can do to increase our level of happiness. For example: [14]

- Expressing gratitude increases feelings of happiness. Pay a visit to someone who has had a large impact on your life but whom you never really thanked. Gratitude visits can be infectious, leading the person you visited to think of people they'd like to thank.
- Before going to bed, reflect on three things that went right during the day. They can be small things, like the (small) dog sitting on your lap.
- Think of the times in your life when a door closed because of death or loss, but another door opened later on. You may come to better appreciate the ebb and flows of life.
- Plan a perfect day and share it with someone.

Happiness is not so much a function of what you have as what you make of it. Happiness is less likely to be found in the pursuit of material things as in finding meaningful work, investing in family and community life, and developing strong spiritual or personal values.

DID YOU KNOW THAT . . .

Within a year of striking it rich, lottery winners are generally no happier than they were before hitting the jackpot?

The Mind–Body Connection: The Healthy Body for the Healthy Mind

Your self—your psychological sense of being you and of journeying through life—is based in the functioning of your brain. Every thought and feeling you have is made possible by the activity of cells in your brain. Your thoughts and feelings also affect the health of your body. In Chapter 3 we'll see that stress can dampen the functioning of your immune system, leaving you vulnerable to illnesses that might otherwise not affect you. The health of your body, especially of your nervous system, also affects your psychological health.

LEARNING OUTCOME 2

Explain what is meant by the mind–body connection

The nervous system is the body's information superhighway, a network of nerve cells that gives rise to our thoughts, feelings, and behavior. The nervous system includes the brain, the spinal cord, and nerve pathways that carry messages back and forth between the brain and the rest of the body. Nerve pathways from the brain and spinal cord cause muscles to contract and command glands to secrete hormones. Health professionals are interested in the links between the nervous system and our health. They use techniques such as CT scans and PET scans to locate brain tumors and to see which parts of the brain are affected in psychological disorders.

Neurons (nerve cells) are the basic building blocks of the nervous system. Some neurons regulate the heart rate. Others release sugar from the liver during times of threat. Still others regulate sexual responses and other body functions. Neurons in the brain allow us to think, to dream, and to experience the world around us through the processing of messages from our sensory organs.

Neurons use chemical messengers called **neurotransmitters** to transmit messages that are released by the transmitting neuron and when taken up by other neurons. Imbalances of neurotransmitters have been linked to a wide variety of psychological

neuron
A nerve cell.

neurotransmitter
Chemical substance that transfers neural impulses from one neuron to another.

disorders, including depression, eating disorders, Alzheimer's disease, and schizophrenia. Neurons are microscopic in width, and neurons in the brain may be only a few thousandths of an inch long. Other neurons, such as those that run from your spinal cord to your toes, are several feet long. In the disease *multiple sclerosis*, the coating of neurons degenerates and is replaced by tough fibrous tissue that throws off the timing of messages and impairs muscular control. If neurons that regulate breathing are affected, a person may suffocate.

Health professionals are also concerned with the influences of hormones and genes on our physical and psychological functioning. **Hormones** are chemical substances secreted by glands into the bloodstream. The hormone *prolactin*, for example, stimulates the production of milk. *Oxytocin* is a hormone that stimulates labor in pregnant women. Sex hormones stimulate development of the sex organs and regulate the menstrual cycle. Stress hormones enhance our resistance to stress. Excesses and deficiencies in hormone levels are connected with many physical and psychological disorders. For example, excess thyroid hormones are linked to anxiety and restlessness, while thyroid deficiencies are linked to sluggishness and weight gain, and—in children—intellectual deficiency.

Genes, the basic units of heredity, are located within the cell's **chromosomes**. Chromosomes are rod-shaped structures housed in the cell nucleus that consist of large molecules of **deoxyribonucleic acid (DNA)**. The normal human cell contains 46 chromosomes organized into 23 pairs, each of which carries more than 1,000 genes (see Figure 2-2). A child normally inherits one member of each pair of chromosomes from each parent. Genetic factors contribute not only to physical traits, but also to many psychological traits, including sociability, emotional stability, sensation-seeking, aggressiveness, leadership, even feelings of happiness.[15] Genetic factors also play a role in psychological disorders, such as anxiety disorders, addictive disorders, mood disorders, and schizophrenia.[16] Moreover, genetic factors can increase the risks for many physical health problems, including coronary heart disease and cancer.

hormones
Chemicals that are secreted by endocrine glands and are involved in the regulation of a wide range of body processes, including reproduction and growth.

gene
The basic unit or building block of heredity that contains the genetic code.

chromosomes
Rod-shaped structures in the cell's nucleus that house the organism's genes.

deoxyribonucleic acid (DNA)
The chemical substance in chromosomes that carries the organism's genetic code.

Figure 2-2 Chromosomes

People normally have 46 chromosomes arranged in 23 pairs. Each parent contributes one member of each pair. The unnumbered pair shown here are the sex chromosomes—in this case, a male set composed of one X and one Y chromosome. Females have two X chromosomes.

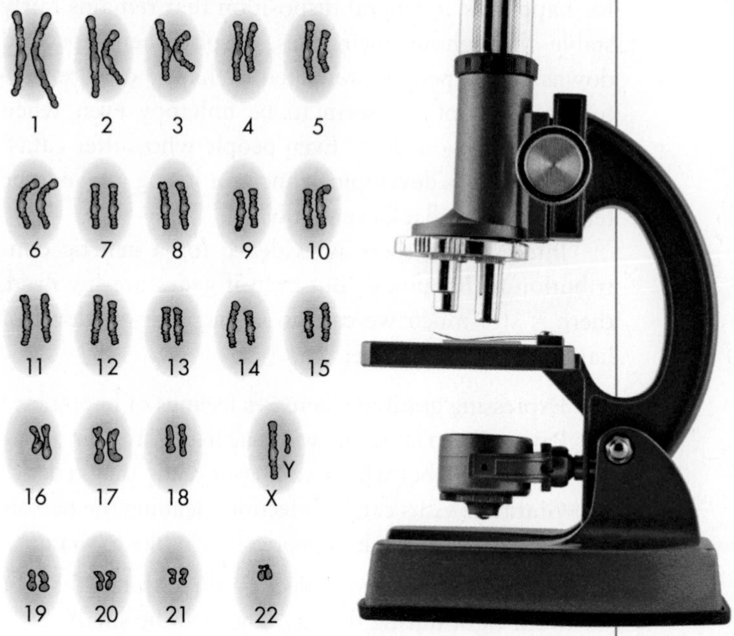

Changing the Unchangeable: Is Biology Destiny?

What can people do who possess unfortunate personality traits, such as shyness and nervousness, which are at least partly inherited? Is it healthful to accept biology as destiny and say, "That's me," or to try to change self-defeating behavior patterns, such as social withdrawal and the tendency to avoid challenging situations?

And what of people who inherit tendencies toward obesity or heart disease? Should they throw up their hands and say, "What will be, will be"? Or should they eat properly and exercise to maximize their chances of averting these health problems? (We think you know the answer.)

By focusing on changing their health-related *behavior*—for example, by following the suggestions for enhancing self-esteem discussed in the online feature "Health Skills 2-1" (see page 24)—people can take greater control over their lives and not simply accept their traits as "part of their nature." Simply put, biology need not be destiny.

The Spiritual Dimension

A sense of meaning and purpose is another aspect of psychological health. Psychologically healthy people do not see life as a matter of muddling through each day. Rather, each day allows for the expression of inner purpose.

LEARNING OUTCOME 3

Discuss the contribution of spiritual health to psychological health

People find many different kinds of meaning in life—many different purposes. For some, meaning takes on a spiritual quality. They find meaning in connecting themselves spiritually to something larger—whether it be God, a specific religion, or the cosmos.

Other people find meaning in their community, which may consist of people who share a common ethnic identity and cultural heritage. In this case, the development of ethnic pride can help boost self-esteem. Or, a person's community may be a religious congregation. Some people take civic pride, finding meaning in their neighborhoods and good works. Many people find meaning in love and family. Their partners and children provide them with fulfillment.

Still other people find meaning in their work. Work not only brings home the bacon (or the kosher chicken)—it also satisfies many internal motives. It provides an opportunity to engage in stimulating and satisfying activities. People's identities and social roles become wrapped up in their work. They do not think, "I teach." They think, "I *am* a teacher," "I *am* a nurse," or "I *am* an architect." Work not only provides a living—it helps give life meaning and direction.

Religion

If increased wealth isn't the ticket to happiness, what is? Psychologists have identified two factors that consistently link to personal happiness: having friends (a big plus) and having a religious commitment. [17]

Religion involves beliefs and practices centered on claims about the nature of reality and moral behavior, usually codified as rituals, religious laws, and prayers. Religions also usually encompass cultural traditions, faith, spiritual experience, and communal as well as private worship. Religion often involves participating in the social, educational, and charitable activities of a congregation, as well as worshiping. Therefore, religion and religious activities provide a vast arena for social networking.

Researchers find that religious involvement in late adulthood is usually associated with less depression and more life satisfaction.[18] Frequent churchgoing has also been shown to be associated with fewer problems in the activities of daily living among older people.[19] Here, of course, we can assume that there are benefits for social networking as well as for church attendance per se.

One study focused on religion and longevity in African Americans. African Americans who attend religious services more than once a week outlive African Americans who never attend by an average of 13 to 14 years![20] This difference in longevity sounds rather "miraculous," and the authors of the study allow that "the power of prayer" itself could have a role. But the authors also found other reasons that church attendance was connected with longevity: churchgoers were also more likely than non-churchgoers to avoid becoming involved in violence, to avoid dealing with stress by drinking, and to reap the benefits of social support—including getting to the doctor when needed—found in active involvement with a congregation.

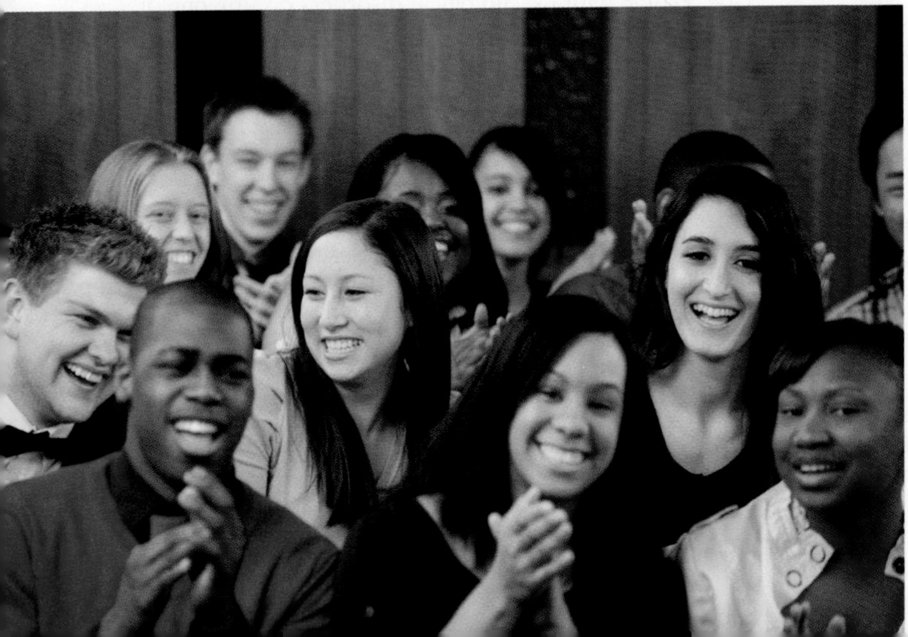

© iStockphoto.com/Christopher Futcher

Prayer

Most Americans believe in a higher being, so it is not surprising that many turn to prayer when they encounter health problems. There has been a good deal of research on the roles of prayer and religion in health. One study, for example, surveyed some 5,100 Americans age 40 and above and found that 47.2% of them reported that they pray for health.[21] Of this number, some 90% believed that prayer had a positive effect on their health. The researchers found that those who reported praying for health also gave God a helping hand; that is, they were less likely to abuse alcohol and smoke than those who did not pray, were more likely to have a primary care physician, make preventive care visits, obtain vaccinations, and eat fruits and vegetables.

We can't say whether links between religion, life satisfaction, and longevity have to do with religious belief per se. Religious traditions also help provide people with a sense of purpose and meaning. For those who belong to congregations, social connectedness to other religious followers and involvement in religious activities are likely providers of health benefits. In any event, the spiritual dimension appears to be a key contributor to psychological and physical health.

Psychological Disorders

Not everyone achieves psychological health. Some people, in fact, are psychologically unhealthy. Some of them are in such trouble that they are labeled as having psychological disorders.

☒ LEARNING OUTCOME 4

Discuss psychological disorders, focusing on anxiety and depression

Just what is a **psychological disorder**? One category of psychological disorders—also called *mental disorders,* or *mental illnesses*—is anxiety disorders, but aren't most of us anxious now and then? Isn't it normal to be anxious before a job interview or a final exam? Depression is another psychological disorder, but isn't it appropriate to feel down if you have suffered a disappointment, such as flunking a test?

Where, then, do we draw the line between *normal* and *abnormal* behavior? Anxiety and depression are recognized as abnormal, or as signs of psychological disorders, when they are not appropriate to the situations we face. Although it is normal to feel down or depressed for a time because of a poor performance on a test, it is *not* normal to be depressed when things are going well. Yes, it is normal to be anxious before meeting a new date, but it is *not* normal to be anxious when you are looking out of a sixth-story window or about to receive a harmless vaccination. The magnitude and persistence of the problem also indicate whether it represents a psychological disorder. Although anxiety about a job interview is normal, feeling that your heart is pounding so fiercely that it might leap out of your chest—and then avoiding the interview—are not. Nor is it normal to be depressed for a prolonged period of time or to become so depressed that you can't meet your usual responsibilities.

psychological disorder
An abnormal behavior pattern associated with significant personal distress, impaired functioning, or disturbed thinking, perceptions, or emotions. Also called mental disorder *or* mental illness.

How Many People Are Affected?

Psychological disorders might seem to affect only a few of us. After all, relatively few people are diagnosed with a severe psychological disorder such as schizophrenia or bipolar disorder. Fewer still need to be hospitalized in a psychiatric facility. Most people never consult a psychiatrist or psychologist.

Yet psychological disorders affect virtually all of us in one way or another. In the United States, about half of all adults develop a diagnosable psychological or mental disorder at some point in their lives.[22] About three of ten adults are affected in any given year.[23] Even if we do not develop a psychological disorder, we are affected by the psychological health problems of family members, friends, and co-workers. If we also consider the economic costs to society of treating psychological disorders, *virtually all of us are affected.* Nearly all of us cover the costs of treatment for psychological disorders through payments for taxes and health insurance.

Psychological disorders also affect our physical health and wellness. Suicide is typically associated with depression and is among the leading causes of death in the United States. It is the third leading cause of death among people age 15 to 24, after accidents and homicide. People with psychological disorders occupy one of every four hospital beds in the United States. The costs for caring for people with psychological disorders represent one of every ten dollars spent on health care. In terms of lost productivity and treatment, the costs for depression alone equal if not exceed the costs of heart disease, the leading cause of death in the United States.[24]

Let's take a closer look at three of the major types of psychological disorders: anxiety disorders, mood disorders, and schizophrenia.

Anxiety Disorders

There is much to be anxious about—our health, our jobs, our families, the state of the nation and the world. Anxiety can be adaptive in that it can motivate us to study before an exam or to seek medical checkups. But when anxiety is out of proportion to the situation or impairs our ability to function, it may reflect a psychological disorder.

Anxiety is a feeling of uneasiness or apprehension that something bad is about to happen. It is accompanied by physical symptoms such as sweaty palms, jitteriness, a pounding heart, and feelings of tightness in the pit of the stomach or chest. **Anxiety disorders** include phobic disorders (phobias), panic disorder, generalized anxiety disorder, obsessive-compulsive disorder, and post-traumatic stress disorder (see Chapter 3). Are you troubled by anxiety? The online feature "Health Check 2-5" will help you determine how often you experience symptoms of anxiety.

health check

Access CourseMate for HLTH at www.cengagebrain.com.

Heredity plays a role in the development of many psychological disorders, including anxiety disorders, mood disorders, and schizophrenia.[25] Genetic factors create a vulnerability or predisposition that makes it more likely that a disorder will develop, especially in the face of stressful life experience.

In anxiety disorders, the brain may not be sensitive enough to the neurotransmitter **gamma-aminobutyric acid (GABA)**. GABA plays a role in calming anxiety reactions by curbing excess firings of neurons in the nervous system. Drugs such as *Valium* and *Xanax* reduce anxiety by increasing the brain's sensitivity to GABA.

Phobias

Phobias are irrational or excessive fears of particular objects or situations. In social phobia, a person shows an extreme fear of social interactions—perhaps when speaking in front of a group, meeting new people, going on a date, or even interacting with peers. **Specific phobias** involve fears of specific situations, such as heights (*acrophobia*) or enclosed spaces (*claustrophobia*), or objects such as insects or particular animals. Even though people with phobias usually recognize that their fears are irrational or excessive, they are still not able to face them.

Some phobias are learned. A person who was bitten by a dog at a young age may learn to fear dogs or other small animals. Someone trapped in an elevator for hours may acquire a fear of elevators or of confinement in other enclosed spaces. Cognitive (thinking) factors also play a role.

Panic Disorder

People with **panic disorder** have sudden attacks with powerful physical symptoms: profuse sweating, choking sensations, nausea, numbness or tingling, flushes or chills, trembling, chest pain, shortness of breath, and pounding of the heart. People experiencing a panic attack may think they are about to die from a heart attack, go crazy, or lose control. The attack may last a few minutes or more than an hour.

People who have panic attacks tend to misinterpret relatively minor changes in their body as signs of imminent catastrophe, such as a heart attack. Their thoughts may race out of control, which heightens bodily sensations of anxiety, leading to more catastrophic thinking, and so on, in a vicious cycle.

Panic attacks seem to come "out of the blue." Yet

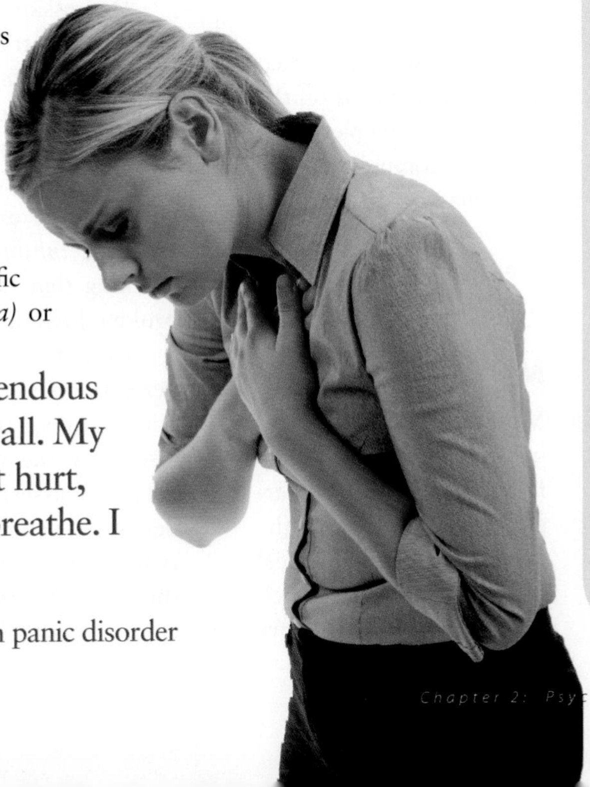

"All of a sudden, I felt a tremendous wave of fear for no reason at all. My heart was pounding, my chest hurt, and it was getting harder to breathe. I thought I was going to die."

—A person with panic disorder

anxiety
Emotional state characterized by body arousal, feelings of nervousness or tension, or a sense of apprehension about the future.

anxiety disorders
Category of psychological disorders involving excessive or inappropriate anxiety reactions.

gamma-aminobutyric acid (GABA)
A neurotransmitter that helps calm anxiety reactions by inhibiting excess firing of neurons.

phobia
An excessive or irrational fear.

specific phobia
Phobia involving specific objects or situations, such as fear of enclosed spaces (claustrophobia) or fear of small animals or insects.

panic disorder
Type of anxiety disorder characterized by episodes of sheer terror, called panic attacks, and by the resultant fear of such attacks occurring again.

they can become connected with situations in which they occur, such as shopping in a crowded department store or riding on a train. *Agoraphobia*, or fear of open or public places, may develop if the person fears having another attack and being away from a secure place.

Generalized Anxiety Disorder

People with **generalized anxiety disorder** experience persistent "free-floating" anxiety, which is anxiety that is not specific to any object or situation. People with the disorder worry excessively, even about trifles that other people shrug off. Symptoms include shakiness, inability to relax, fidgeting, sweating, and feelings of dread and foreboding.

Obsessive-Compulsive Disorder

People with **obsessive-compulsive disorder (OCD)** have recurrent obsessions and/or compulsions. Obsessions are intrusive, nagging thoughts that the person feels unable to control. Compulsions are repetitive behaviors or rituals that the person feels compelled to perform. A person may be obsessed with the thought that his or her skin is contaminated by germs, and spend hours each day compulsively washing his or her hands or showering. One compulsive hand washer, who spent 3 to 4 hours daily washing her hands, complained, "My hands look like lobster claws." Another person with OCD may spend hours each night checking and rechecking whether or not he or she has locked the doors or turned off the appliances. People with obsessive-compulsive disorder may become trapped in a vicious cycle of obsessive thinking and compulsive behavior.

Mood Disorders

Most of us have occasional ups and downs. We may feel unmotivated, lethargic, or just down in the dumps for a time. We feel sad if we have a setback at work or school or are rejected by Mr. or Ms. Right. We feel elated when we get a good grade or land a job, or when the person we are attracted to returns our interest. It is normal to feel sad when unfortunate events occur and to feel uplifted when fortune shines on us. In the case of **mood disorders**, we may feel down when things are going right. Or we may remain down following a misfortune long after others would have snapped back. Some people with mood disorders have wild mood swings. For no apparent reason, their moods alternate between dizzying heights and abysmal depths.

Depression

Depressed people often experience feelings of hopelessness and worthlessness along with periods of sadness. They may withdraw from friends and family, and find little interest in things they used to enjoy. People with depression may not be able to get out of bed to face the day. They may be unable to make decisions, even about small things, like what to have for dinner. They may be unable to concentrate. They may feel helpless to change their life situation, or they may say they no longer care. They may have recurrent thoughts of suicide or attempt suicide. Depression may also be associated with physical symptoms, such as changes in appetite and sleep patterns and feelings of lethargy. Women are more likely than men to be depressed, as you will read in the online feature "Diversity 2-1."

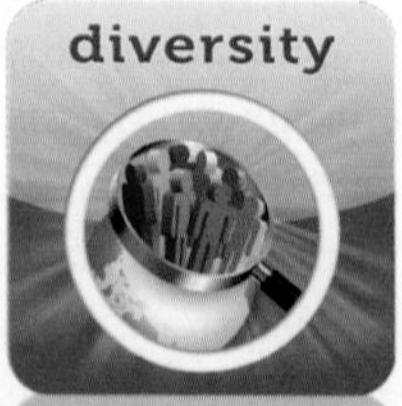

Access CourseMate for HLTH at www.cengagebrain.com.

Depression is linked to lower-than-normal levels of certain neurotransmitters, especially **serotonin**, a chemical that plays an important role in regulating appetite and mood states, among other functions. Drugs that help relieve depression, called **antidepressants**, increase the activity of neurotransmitters in the brain. The most widely used antidepressants are *selective serotonin reuptake inhibitor*s (SSRIs; e.g., *Prozac* and *Zoloft*), meaning that they help prevent serotonin from being broken down in the brain.

Cognitive factors can contribute to depression. Perfectionists can set themselves up for depression with unrealistic self-demands. Depressed people also view the world and themselves through "blue-colored glasses." Psychiatrist Aaron Beck believes that depressed people filter their experiences through three types of cognitive distortions: (1) a negative view of the self ("I'm worthless"); (2) a negative view of the environment ("This job is awful"); and (3) a negative

generalized anxiety disorder
Type of anxiety disorder characterized by high levels of anxiety that is not limited to particular situations and by general feelings of worry, dread, and foreboding.

obsessive-compulsive disorder (OCD)
Type of anxiety disorder characterized by obsessions (nagging, intrusive thoughts or images) and/or compulsions (repetitive behaviors that the person feels compelled to perform).

mood disorder
Disturbances of mood that affect the individual's ability to function effectively, are unduly prolonged or severe, or are out of keeping with the events the person has encountered.

serotonin
A type of neurotransmitter that is involved in regulating appetite and mood states and is linked to depression.

antidepressant
Drug that combats depression by altering the action of neurotransmitters in the brain.

view of the future ("Nothing will ever work out for me"). When you check out the online feature "Health Skills 2-3" on alleviating depression, you will see examples of cognitive distortions that might help you assess your own style of thinking. "Health Check 2-6" can help increase your awareness of the warning signs of depression and of concerns you may wish to share with a helping professional.

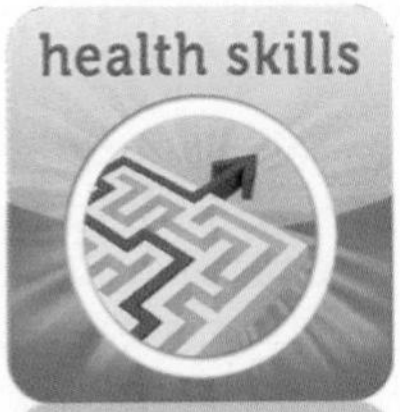

Access CourseMate for HLTH at www.cengagebrain.com.

Depression and Suicide

Did you know that most people entertain thoughts of suicide, now and then, when they are under great stress? A national survey reported that about one in seven adults (13%) in the United States had experienced suicidal thoughts; nearly one in twenty (4.6%) reported making a suicide attempt.[26] Most people do not act on suicidal thoughts. Still, about one million Americans attempt suicide each year and about 33,000 commit suicide.[27] An estimated 24,000 college students attempt to take their own lives each year, and more than 1,000 "succeed."[28] Suicide is the second leading cause of death among college students, after motor vehicle accidents.

Why Do People Take Their Lives? Suicide is motivated by the attempt to end unendurable psychological pain. It is usually brought on by feelings of

HEALTH CHECK 2-6

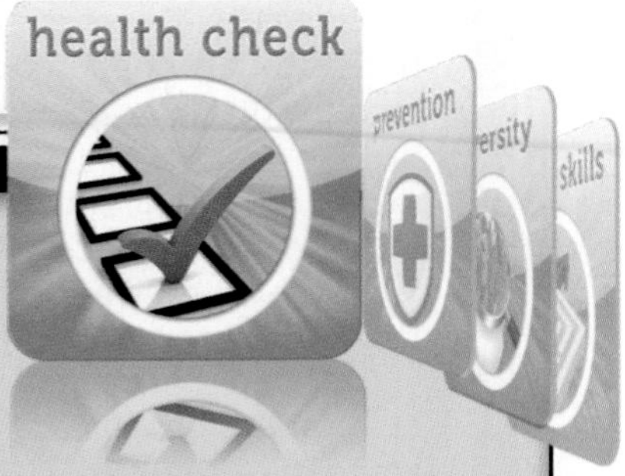

Are You Depressed?

Many people suffer depression in silence out of ignorance or shame. They believe that depression is not a real problem because it doesn't show up on an X-ray or CT scan. But depression is all too real. The loss of appetite, the disruption of sleep patterns, and the lethargy are real. Fortunately, depression can be treated successfully, but only if the individual obtains help.

The following test was developed to help make people more aware of the warning signs of depression. It should not be used for self-diagnosis, but rather to raise awareness of concerns that you might choose to discuss with a health professional.

YES	NO	
______	______	1. I feel downhearted, blue, and sad.
______	______	2. I don't enjoy the things that I used to.
______	______	3. I feel that others would be better off if I were dead.
______	______	4. I feel that I am not useful or needed.
______	______	5. I notice that I am losing weight.
______	______	6. I have trouble sleeping through the night.
______	______	7. I am restless and can't keep still.
______	______	8. My mind isn't as clear as it used to be.
______	______	9. I get tired for no reason.
______	______	10. I feel hopeless about the future.

If you answered "yes" to at least five of the statements, including either item 1 or 2, and if these complaints have persisted for at least 2 weeks, then professional help is strongly recommended. If you answered "yes" to the third statement, we suggest that you immediately consult a health professional. Irrespective of your particular score, we suggest you contact a helping professional if you've experienced any significant change in your mood that has lasted beyond 2 weeks. Contact your college or university counseling or health center.

DIVERSITY 2-2

Who Is at Risk of Committing Suicide?

Suicide prediction is far from perfect. Even trained professionals find it difficult to predict who is likely to commit suicide. Most suicides are linked to depression, but the great majority of depressed people do not attempt to end their lives. Yet many people who commit suicide signal their intentions, such as telling others about their suicidal thoughts or intentions. Changes in behavior may also be suggestive of possible suicidal intent, such as suddenly disposing of one's possessions or drafting a will or buying a cemetery plot. But see Table 2-1 for some myths about suicide.

Suicide cuts across every stratum of society, but certain groups in our society are at increased risk:

Age. Adolescent suicides may seem hard to understand, since young people have "everything to live for." Tragically, many of them come to the opposite conclusion. Yet, suicide rates are higher among older adults, especially older white males.

Gender. More women attempt suicide, but more men complete the act.[29] Men commit four times as many suicides as women. How do we explain these differences? Men tend to use more lethal means, especially firearms. Women are more apt to use pills, poison, or other means that may be less lethal.

Ethnicity. European Americans and Native Americans are more likely to take their lives than African Americans or Hispanic Americans. Two of the groups most at risk of suicide are young Native Americans and older White men.[30] Overall, about one in six Native American teenagers attempts suicide. This rate is four times the national average.[31] Among some tribes, the rate is even higher.

How do we account for the high rate of suicide among Native Americans? One answer is the widespread sense of hopelessness that arises from lack of opportunity and being segregated from the dominant culture. Such factors also set the stage for alcohol and drug abuse, which often become preludes to depression and suicide.

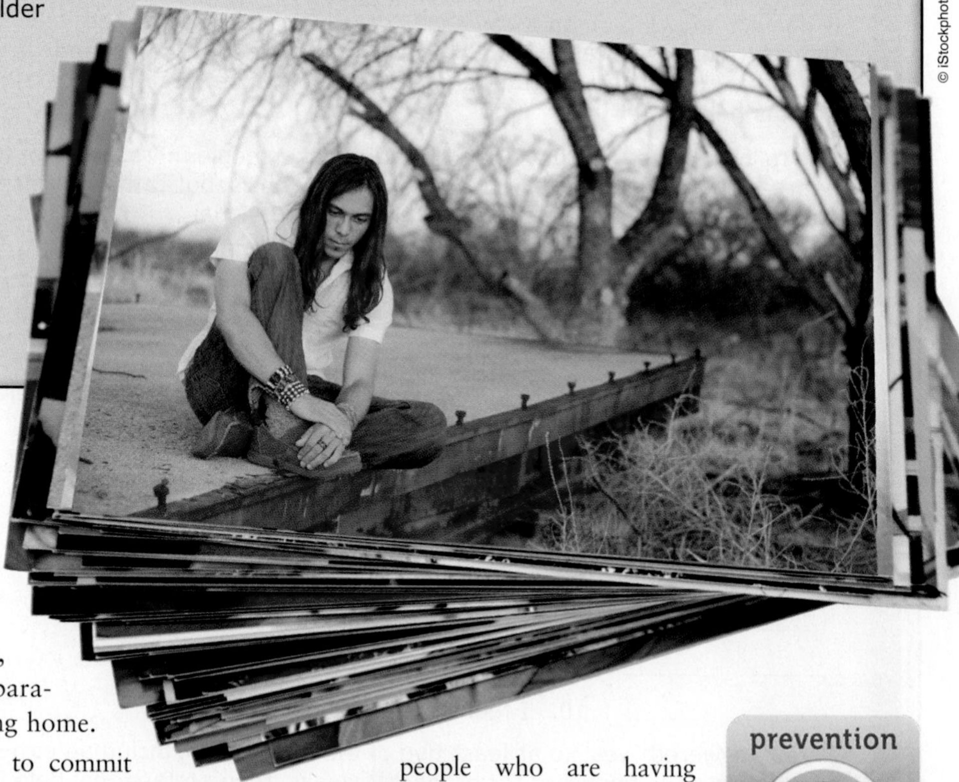

© iStockphoto.com/Scott Griessel / © iStockphoto.com/Michael Bodmann

helplessness and hopelessness, which are features of depression (see Diversity 2-2). Suicide attempts often follow stressful life events, especially *exit events*, which involve loss of social support, as through death, divorce or separation, or a family member's leaving home.

Teenagers have been known to commit copycat suicides in the wake of widely publicized suicides in their communities. This tendency has been called the "cluster effect." The sensationalism that attends a teenage suicide may make it seem a romantic or courageous statement to impressionable young people who are having problems.

What would you do if someone you knew threatened suicide? The online feature "Prevention 2-1" offers some suggestions.

prevention

Access CourseMate for HLTH at www.cengagebrain.com.

Table 2-1 Myths about Suicide

MYTH	FACT
People who threaten suicide are only seeking attention.	Not so. Researchers report that most people who have committed suicide gave prior indications of their intentions or consulted a health provider beforehand.
A person must be insane to attempt suicide.	Most people who attempt suicide may feel hopeless, but they are not insane (i.e., out of touch with reality).
Talking about suicide with a depressed person may prompt the person to attempt it.	An open discussion of suicide with a depressed person does not prompt the person to attempt it. In fact, extracting a promise that the person will not attempt suicide before calling or visiting a mental health worker may well *prevent* a suicide.
People who attempt suicide and fail aren't serious about killing themselves.	Most people who commit suicide have made previous unsuccessful attempts.
If someone threatens suicide, it is best to ignore it so as not to encourage repeated threats.	Although some people do manipulate others by making idle threats, it is prudent to treat every suicidal threat as genuine and to take appropriate action.

Bipolar Disorder

Depression is *unipolar.* That is, a person's mood changes in a single direction: *down*. People with **bipolar disorder** (formerly called *manic-depression*) have mood swings between depression and mania. **Manic episodes** are periods of extreme excitability and elation that occur for no apparent reason. People in a manic episode may become very excited and argumentative, and show poor judgment. They may spend lavishly, drive recklessly, destroy property, or become involved in sexual escapades that appear out of character from their usual personalities. Even people who love them may find them abrasive. Other symptoms are *pressured speech* (talking too rapidly), *rapid flight of ideas* (flitting from topic to topic), and an inflated sense of self-worth (grandiosity). Manic people may even become delusional, as in believing that they have a special relationship with God. They may have boundless energy and show little need for sleep. Then, when their moods sink into depression, they may feel hopeless and despairing. Some people with bipolar disorder commit suicide on the way down, to avert the depths of depression they have learned to expect.

Schizophrenia

Schizophrenia is the disorder that most closely corresponds to the popular concepts of "madness" or "lunacy." The word *schizophrenia* comes from Greek roots meaning "split brain." In schizophrenia, psychological functioning is "split." Emotional reactions are split off from external events. The individual may giggle in the face of disaster, or fail to react to tragic events.

Schizophrenia is a **psychotic disorder**, meaning that it involves a break with reality. Confusion reigns. The individual may not know the time of day, or what day or year it is. Or where she or he is. Or *who* she or he is. The break with reality may involve **hallucinations**, such as hearing voices or seeing things that are not there. Or it may involve **delusions**. Some of the more common types of delusions include *delusions of persecution* (believing that one is being persecuted by demons or by the Mafia) and *delusions of grandeur* (believing that one is Jesus or has superhuman powers).

People with schizophrenia show confused thinking that is characterized by a *loosening of associations.* Normally, our thoughts are tightly connected—that is, one thought follows another in a logical sequence. But

bipolar disorder
Type of mood disorder characterized by mood swings between severe depression and mania.

manic episode
Episode of extremely inflated mood and excitability.

schizophrenia
An enduring type of psychotic disorder involving disturbances in thought processes, perception, emotion, and behavior.

psychotic disorder
A psychological disorder involving a break with reality.

hallucinations
Perceptual distortions that occur in the absence of external stimuli and are confused with reality, such as "hearing voices" or seeing things that are not there.

delusions
False, unshakable beliefs.

people with schizophrenia often think in a confused, disconnected manner with no logical connections between their thoughts. They may form meaningless words or mindless rhymes. Their speech may become incoherent. They may jump from topic to topic but communicate no useful information.

Schizophrenia typically affects young adults just at the point in their lives when they are beginning to make their way in the world. Although the condition typically lasts the rest of their lives, antipsychotic medications, combined with rehabilitation services and psychological counseling, can help people with schizophrenia live more productive lives in the community.

Schizophrenia is currently thought of as a disease of the brain. Brain imaging especially connects the problems we find in schizophrenia with dysfunction in the frontal part of the brain, where we engage in logical thinking and make plans and decisions. There is a loss of gray matter, which is needed for higher mental functions such as thinking (see Figure 2-3). Brain imaging has also shown that people with schizophrenia tend to have larger ventricles—open areas in the brain—than other people, suggestive of loss of brain tissue. Schizophrenia has also been linked to overutilization of a neurotransmitter called *dopamine*.[32] So-called *anti-psychotic* drugs work by blocking the action of dopamine.

Research evidence suggests that there are a number of biological risk factors for schizophrenia, such as genetics and complications during prenatal development and childbirth.

Mental health problems such as anxiety disorders, mood disorders, and schizophrenia are not rooted in any one cause. Many factors play roles in their development, including biological and psychological factors that interact in complex ways we are only beginning to understand.

Treating Psychological Disorders

People seeking help for psychological problems face a bewildering array of choices. Not only are there many different types of available treatments, but also different types of therapists and helping professionals. Nor is professional treatment necessary for everyone. Many people with psychological disorders turn to clergy or trusted friends. Self-help groups or support groups also help many people who are experiencing psychological problems. These groups include Alcoholics Anonymous, Overeaters Anonymous, and Gamblers Anonymous. When problems become overwhelming or persistent, or when people seem to be at risk of harming themselves or others, professional help is indicated.

LEARNING OUTCOME 5

Describe ways of treating psychological disorders

Figure 2-3 Average Rates of Loss of Gray Matter among Normal Adolescents and Adolescents Diagnosed with Schizophrenia

High-resolution brain scans show rates of gray matter loss in normal 13- to 18-year-olds and among adolescents of the same age diagnosed with schizophrenia. Maps of brain changes reveal profound, progressive loss in schizophrenia (right). Loss also occurs in normal adolescents (left) but at a slower rate.

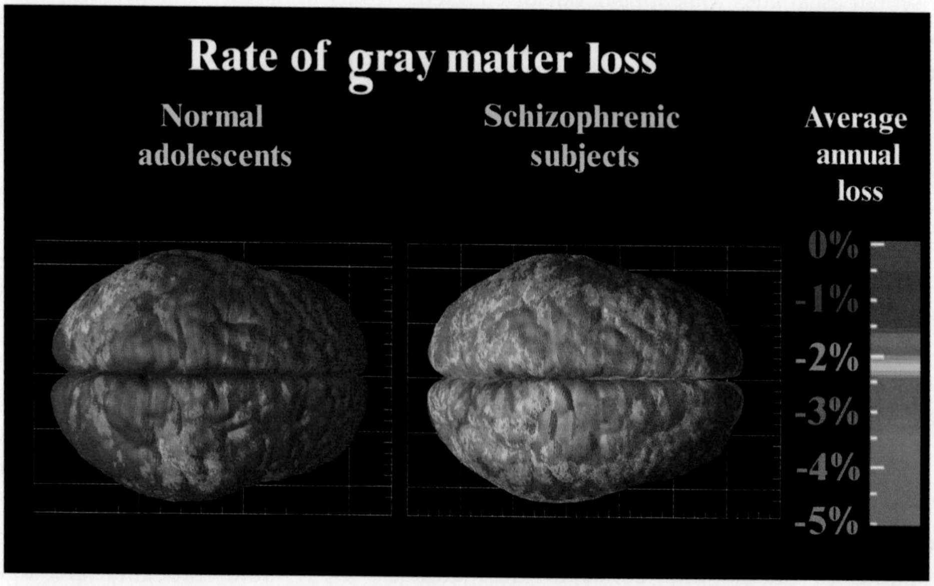

Source: P. M. Thompson, et al. Mapping Adolescent Brain Change Reveals Dynamic Wave of Accelerated Gray Matter Loss in Very Early-Onset Schizophrenia. *Proceedings of the National Academy of Sciences of the USA, 98* (2001), 11650–11655. Copyright 2001 National Academy of Sciences, U.S.A.

Table 2-2 A Who's Who of Psychological Health Professionals

Different kinds of professionals treat psychological disorders. Many people who do not have psychological disorders also seek out health professionals to help them gain better insight into themselves or reach their full potential.

PROFESSION	ACADEMIC DEGREE	COMMENTS
Psychiatrists	M.D.s or D.O.s	Psychiatrists and other health professionals use psychotherapy to help people cope with psychological disorders. As licensed physicians, psychiatrists can prescribe drugs and use other medical techniques, such as electroconvulsive therapy or ECT (discussed later in the chapter). Many psychiatrists also complete more extensive training in psychoanalysis or other psychotherapeutic approaches.
Psychologists	Ph.D., Psy.D., Ed.D.	Psychologists diagnose psychological disorders—using psychological tests when desirable—and treat them with psychotherapy.
Counselors	Master's degree	Counselors work in many settings, including public schools, college testing and counseling centers, and hospitals and health clinics. Many specialize in academic, vocational, marital, or family counseling. Other counselors specialize in career development or treatment of milder psychological disorders, such as adjustment disorders.
Social workers	Master's degree (M.S.W.)	Clinical social workers provide counseling or psychotherapy and utilize their knowledge of community agencies and organizations to help people obtain the services they need. For example, they may help people with schizophrenia adjust more successfully to the community once they leave the hospital. Like counselors, many social workers also specialize in marital or family therapy.

Table 2.2 offers a "Who's Who" of psychological health professionals.

Psychological Therapies

Psychological therapies involve different forms of **psychotherapy.** These forms of therapy differ in techniques and theoretical frameworks, yet they all apply psychological principles to help people overcome psychological and interpersonal problems. Here we focus on the major types of psychotherapy in use today: psychoanalysis, behavior therapy, cognitive therapy, eclectic therapy, and group, family, and couple therapy.

Psychoanalysis

Psychoanalysis is the form of therapy originated by Sigmund Freud. It probes possible childhood roots of psychological problems. Freud's followers believe that psychological problems are rooted in *unconscious* psychological conflicts that can be traced to childhood. They assume that insight into the nature of these conflicts helps resolve them and restores psychological health.

Freud believed that these unconscious conflicts are basically sexual or aggressive in nature. Their true nature is kept hidden from consciousness by psychological defenses, such as **repression** (motivated forgetting). For example, people may develop a fear of knives because of a hidden (repressed) desire to harm themselves or others. Psychoanalysis is a sort of mental detective work intended to help people ferret out unconscious conflicts and work them through in the context of their adult personality.

Freud used the method of **free association.** He instructed clients to say anything that crossed his or her mind with the assumption that these associations would find their way into emotionally laden issues that touched upon unconscious material. Freud also used **dream analysis**, or the interpretation of the hidden meaning of dreams to shed light on unconscious conflicts.

psychotherapy
A verbal form of therapy, or "talk therapy," based on the application of psychological principles and techniques.

psychoanalysis
Type of therapy developed by Sigmund Freud that helps people achieve insight into unconscious processes and conflicts believed to give rise to psychological problems.

repression
In Freudian theory, the process of motivated forgetting by which the unconscious mind banishes from awareness troubling ideas or impulses.

free association
Technique used in psychoanalysis in which the patient is encouraged to verbalize any thoughts that come to mind, free of conscious efforts to censure or edit them.

Behavior Therapy

Behavior therapists assume that psychological disorders are largely learned and can therefore be unlearned. Psychoanalysis focuses on helping people gain insight into the root causes of their behavior and thereby overcome psychological problems. Behavior therapists focus on directly changing problem behavior.

Learning principles are applied to problem behavior. One technique, **systematic desensitization**, helps people overcome phobias by guiding them through a series of imaginal encounters with increasingly fearful stimuli while they remain deeply relaxed.

Behavior therapists also use a technique of real-life exposure to fearful situations, usually arranged according to a stepwise or graduated program of exposure to increasingly fearful stimuli in people's environment. By confronting fearful situations or objects gradually but directly, people learn to tolerate them.

Cognitive Therapy

Cognitive therapies focus on helping people change the thoughts and attitudes that can lead to disorders such as anxiety disorders and depression. Two of the major forms of cognitive therapy were developed by psychologist Albert Ellis and psychiatrist Aaron Beck. Ellis's **rational-emotive behavior therapy (REBT)** shows people how irrational beliefs, such as the demand for perfection and excessive need for approval, can lead to psychological problems like anxiety and depression in the face of disappointing life experiences. Beck's **cognitive therapy** focuses on identifying and correcting cognitive distortions, such as tendencies to magnify the importance of disappointing events ("making mountains out of molehills"). People are taught more adaptive, flexible, and realistic ways of thinking.

dream analysis
Technique used in psychoanalysis in which the symbolic meaning of dreams is believed to reflect upon unconscious material.

behavior therapy
Type of therapy involving the systematic application of learning-based techniques to help people change problem behaviors.

systematic desensitization
Behavior therapy technique that attempts to help a person overcome a phobia by staging a series of imagined encounters with feared objects or stimuli while the person remains deeply relaxed.

rational-emotive behavior therapy (REBT)
Type of cognitive therapy developed by Albert Ellis that focuses on helping people dispute and correct irrational thinking.

cognitive therapy
Type of psychotherapy developed by Aaron Beck that helps clients identify and correct dysfunctional thinking patterns.

psychotropic drugs
Drugs used to treat psychological or mental disorders.

Eclectic Therapy

Some therapists adopt an eclectic orientation, meaning that they use techniques from several different therapeutic approaches. Depending on a patient's needs, an eclectic therapist might use behavior therapy to help change problem behavior and psychodynamic techniques to help the person acquire insight into underlying conflicts.

Group, Family, and Couple Therapy

Some forms of therapy expand the focus of treatment beyond the individual client.

Group therapy brings people together in small groups to explore and cope with their problems. Group therapy is less costly than individual therapy. It is particularly helpful for interpersonal problems such as loneliness, shyness, and low self-esteem. Individuals learn how other group members cope with similar problems, and offer each other social support. The give-and-take of the group also improves social skills.

Family therapy helps troubled families communicate and resolve their differences. Most family therapists view the family unit as a complex social system in which individuals play certain roles. For instance, there is often an "identified patient" whom the family brands as the source of the family's problems. The family operates according to the "bad apple" myth, believing that if they can change the bad apple, the barrel will become functional. Family therapists show how the problems of the identified patient are symptomatic of a breakdown in the whole family system, not just one individual.

Couple therapy helps couples build healthier relationships by enhancing their communication skills and helping them cope with conflicts. The couple therapist encourages partners to share their feelings and needs in ways that do not put one another down.

Biomedical Therapies

Remarkable gains have been made in treating a wide range of psychological disorders with psychotherapeutic drugs, called **psychotropic drugs**. Psychotropic drugs include antidepressants (e.g., *Prozac* and *Zoloft*), antianxiety agents (e.g., *Valium* and *Xanax*), stimulants (e.g., *Ritalin*), and antipsychotic drugs (e.g., *Thorazine* and *Zyprexa*).

Psychotropic drugs can help relieve emotional distress and enable people to cope more effectively, but they are not cure-alls. For one thing, when drugs are withdrawn, symptoms often return. Drugs can also produce adverse side effects, ranging from drowsiness (antianxiety drugs) to muscular tremors and even movement disorders (antipsychotic drugs). Furthermore, drugs do not teach patients any new skills they can use to overcome their problems. Some drugs, such as the antianxiety drug *Valium*, can lead to psychological and physical dependence (addiction). *Valium* can also be dangerous if taken in overdoses or mixed with alcohol or other drugs.

Another biomedical form of treatment is **electroconvulsive therapy (ECT)**, which is commonly called *shock therapy*. The very idea of sending an electrical current or shock through the brain may send shudders down your spine. But although the procedure may sound barbaric, it often produces dramatic relief from severe depression and can be life-saving when depressed people are suicidal. ECT produces significant levels of improvement in many cases of depression, including those that have failed to respond to antidepressant medication or other forms of treatment.[33] It is not clear how ECT works, but it may help normalize the levels of neurotransmitters in the brain.

ECT is effective, but it can produce loss of memory, especially for events that occurred shortly before or after the ECT.[34] Because of its extreme nature, many health professionals view ECT as a treatment of last resort.

electroconvulsive therapy (ECT)
Form of therapy for severe depression involving the administration of brief pulses of electricity to the patient's brain.

HEALTH APPS: YOUR LINK TO ONLINE HEALTH APPLICATIONS

health check

Getting in Touch with Your Self-Concept What do you really think of yourself? Are you pleased with the person you see in the mirror? Or do you put yourself down at every opportunity? Complete "Health Check 2-2" to gain insight into the answers.

health skills

Enhancing Self-Esteem Self-esteem is at the heart of psychological health. "Health Skills 2-1" proposes some ways that self-esteem can be improved.

health skills

Assert Yourself! Assertive behavior involves the expression of one's genuine feelings, standing up for one's legitimate rights, and refusing unreasonable requests. It means resisting undue social influences, disobeying *arbitrary* authority figures, and resisting conformity to *arbitrary* group standards. Check out "Health Skills 2-2" for hints on becoming more assertive.

health check

Are You an Optimist or a Pessimist? Do you see a silver lining behind every cloud, or do you see more clouds darkening the horizon? Do you believe that things will work out well, or do you expect the worst? "Health Check 2-4" will provide insight into whether you see the cup half full or half empty.

health check

Are You Anxious? Completing "Health Check 2-5" will help you determine how often you experience symptoms of anxiety.

diversity

The Case of Women and Depression Women are about twice as likely as men to be diagnosed with depression. "Diversity 2-1" discusses the reasons.

health skills

Do You Need to Get out of the Dumps? "Health Skills 2-3" has some advice for alleviating depression.

prevention

Suicide Prevention: Helping A Friend in Crisis If a friend tells you he or she is thinking of committing suicide, would you know what to do? Read "Prevention 2-1" for some ideas.

Go to the CourseMate for HLTH at www.cengagebrain.com for additional resources including flashcards, games, self-quizzing, review exercises, web exercises, learning checks, and more.

Stress and Your Health

"The stress of a life change reflects its meaning to the individual. The stress of pregnancy is connected with desire for a baby and readiness to care for it."

Which straw will break the camel's back? The final straw, of course. *Stressors* (sources of stress) are like straws. They can accumulate gradually until there is one too many. A heavy load of stress may not literally break our backs. However, it can tax our coping ability and impair the functioning of our immune system.

In the science of physics, stress is the pressure or force placed upon a body. When boulders crash in a landslide, they exert pressure or stress on the valley floor. With people, **stress** is the pressure we experience when a demand is placed upon us that requires us to adjust or adapt. Sources of stress include occupational or academic demands, time pressures, parental responsibilities . . . even the neighbor's stereo.

People actually need some stress to help them stay active, alert, and energized. Without it, we might become stagnant and bored. Although the word "stress" sounds bad, positive events can also be sources of stress, such as graduating from school, getting married, or having a baby. Positive events place demands that require us to adjust or adapt and can strain our ability to cope (ask any new parent!). Some stressors, such as calamitous or traumatic events, threaten our well-being, even our survival. Intense or prolonged stress can overtax our ability to adjust and lead to health problems. Even people who are generally resilient to stress may buckle under the strain of chronic or prolonged stress. Learning to manage stress is one of the keys to achieving and maintaining wellness.

stress
A pressure or force placed upon a body or an object. In human terms, it refers to a demand placed upon a person to adjust.

Learning Outcomes

1. Describe various sources of stress
2. Describe the effects of stress on the body
3. Explain the effects of stress on the immune system
4. Explain how stress affects your health
5. Discuss the problem of insomnia and ways of getting your *Z*s.
6. Describe ways of managing stress

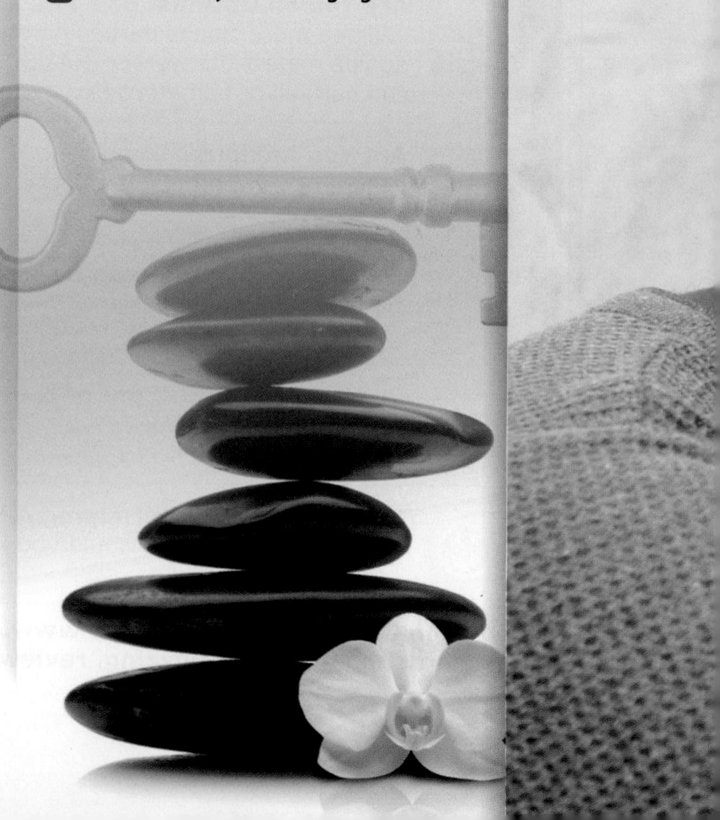

Stress in America

What stresses you out? A bad grade? Worrying about whether you will get a job, or keep it? Arguments with a partner or a friend? Health problems?

Each year, the American Psychological Association commissions a survey of stress in America among a nationally representative sample of Americans. In 2010, as you see in Figure 3.1 on the next page, the respondents overwhelmingly reported that money and work were their major sources of stress.

LEARNING OUTCOME 1

Describe various sources of stress

We will see later that job strain is a key contributor to heart disease. When we add in the costs of housing, which are mentioned by nearly half the sample, we find another area in which finances contribute to stress. Health is another major area of concern, mentioned in various ways by more than half of the sample. Finally, Figure 3-1 shows that close personal relationships are also a source of stress for more than half of the sample. One might think that intimate relationships would serve as a buffer against

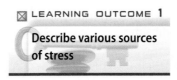

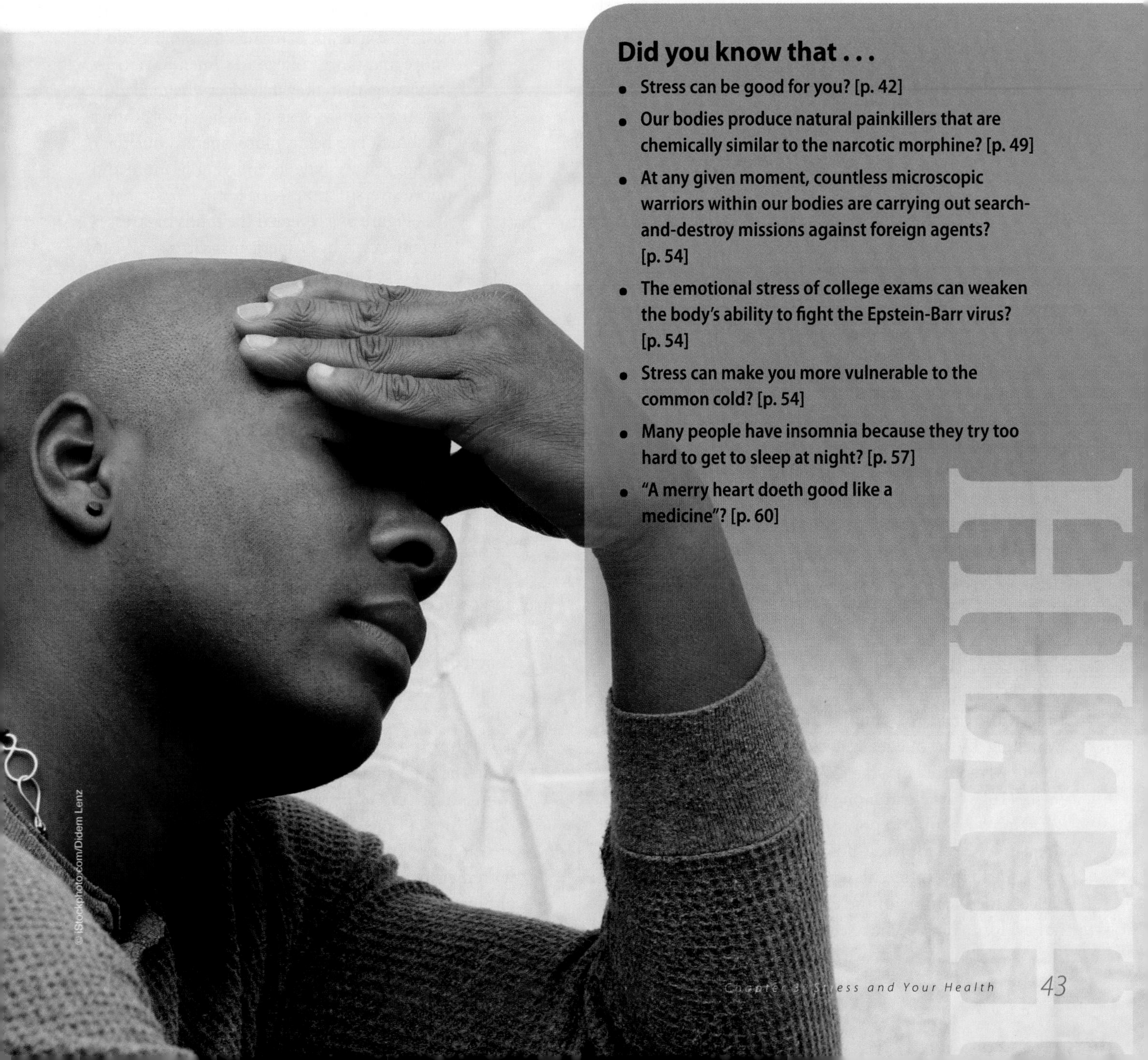

Did you know that . . .

- Stress can be good for you? [p. 42]
- Our bodies produce natural painkillers that are chemically similar to the narcotic morphine? [p. 49]
- At any given moment, countless microscopic warriors within our bodies are carrying out search-and-destroy missions against foreign agents? [p. 54]
- The emotional stress of college exams can weaken the body's ability to fight the Epstein-Barr virus? [p. 54]
- Stress can make you more vulnerable to the common cold? [p. 54]
- Many people have insomnia because they try too hard to get to sleep at night? [p. 57]
- "A merry heart doeth good like a medicine"? [p. 60]

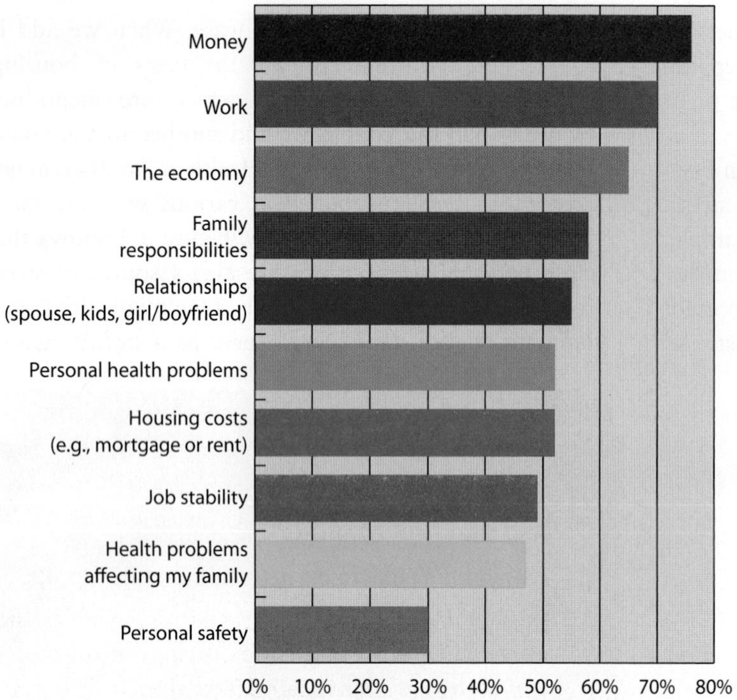

Figure 3-1 Sources of Stress

Percent of respondents who say that the source of stress is somewhat or very significant.

Source: American Psychological Association. (2010). *Stress in America 2011: Executive Summary.* Retrieved from http://www.apa.org/news/press/releases/stress-exec-summary.pdf. Page 8. Reprinted by permission.

external sources of stress for people, *and perhaps they do*. (Life is complex.) However, these relationships can also contribute to stress.

Respondents reported many symptoms of stress, both physical and psychological. Nearly half the respondents (45%) reported that stress made them irritable or angry. Stress made more than two in five respondents (41%) tired, and more than one-third (36%) reported having headaches. More than one in four (26%) had indigestion, and almost one in four (23%) felt tense. About one-third felt depressed (34%) or as though they could cry (30%).

Figure 3-2 shows that the most commonly reported methods of coping with stress were listening to music (49%), exercising or going for walks (48%), spending time with friends or family (46%), and reading (45%). Watching TV or movies was close behind (38%). About one-third reported praying (37%) or napping (34%). One in six (16%) drank, and one in seven (13%) smoked.

Not all people report that the same events cause them stress, of course. And as we see, they respond to stress in many different ways. The stress of an event reflects the meaning of the event to an individual. Pregnancy, for example, may seem like a blessing to a well-established couple who has been trying to have a child for many years, but it may seem disastrous to a single teenager without resources. We appraise events, and our responses depend on their perceived danger, our values and goals, our beliefs in our coping ability, and our social situations.

College freshmen have been experiencing many of the stresses surveyed by the American Psychological Association. A study by the UCLA Higher Education Research Institute found that college freshmen are now encountering a record level of stress. Figure 3-3 shows that over the past 25 years, fewer and fewer college freshmen have been reporting that their emotional health is above average. During the same period, more and more college freshmen have been reporting that they felt overwhelmed during their senior year at high school. Either freshmen are being more open about their feelings or we have been living in more and more stressful times—or both.

Figure 3-1 revealed the kinds of stresses experienced by Americans. Stressors can also be categorized as daily hassles, life changes, frustration and conflict, burnout, Type A personality, and pain.

Daily Hassles

Hassles are the common annoyances of everyday life. No doubt you will recognize most, if not all, of the following daily hassles:

1. *Household hassles*, such as making meals, shopping, and housecleaning, are significant sources of stress. They especially affect women, who typically shoulder a disproportionate burden of household and child care responsibilities.
2. *Health hassles*, such as minor illnesses, difficulty contacting a health professional, and side effects of medications, are common examples of sources of stress.
3. *Time-pressure hassles*, such as having too little time to do the things you need to do, can be a major source of stress. At the other extreme is having too much "down time" on your hands. College students are often pressured to balance their need to study with their personal needs, such as socializing and family responsibilities. Procrastination—putting off tasks and decisions until the last minute—can

Figure 3-2 How Americans Handle Stress

Percent of respondents who say they use one of these techniques to manage stress.

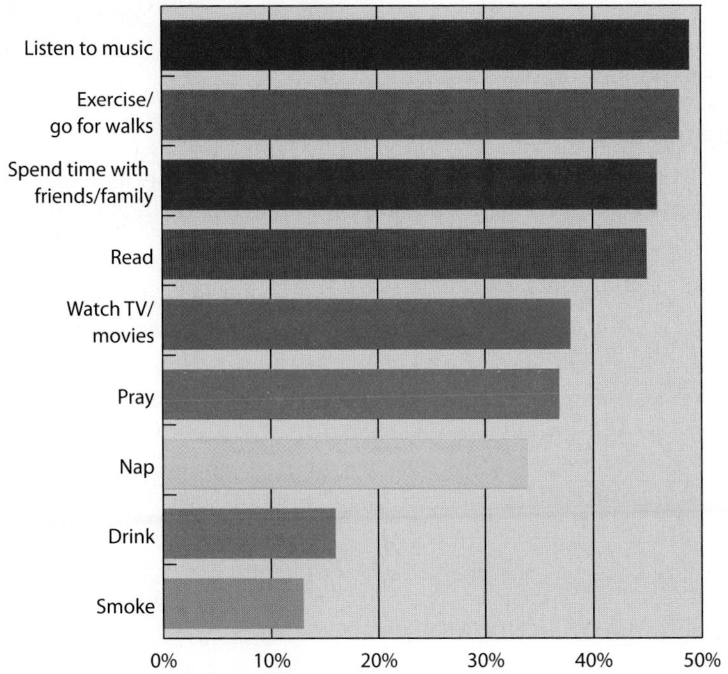

also become a source of stress. You can reduce time-pressure hassles by stating what you want to accomplish, creating a schedule, and sticking to it.

4. *Inner-concern hassles* such as feelings of loneliness, fears of social confrontations, and doubts about the value of what we are doing with our lives. Loneliness is common for college students who have left friends and family behind and not yet established a new support network.
5. *Environmental hassles* such as air and noise pollution, traffic congestion, neighborhood deterioration, and fear of crime are environmental hassles.
6. *Financial-responsibility hassles* such as concerns about debts and other financial matters can create chronic stress.
7. *Work hassles* such as dissatisfaction on the job, job strain, and problems with supervisors and co-workers. Other daily hassles can converge at work. Time hassles, such as pressures to get reports in on schedule, are additional sources of job stress.

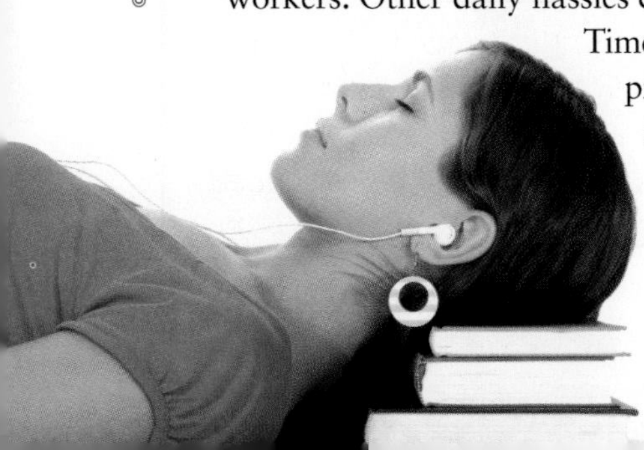

8. *Future security hassles* such as concerns about job security, property investments, taxes, vacillations in the stock market, and getting by in retirement.

Life Changes

Changes in life circumstances, even positive life changes, can create stress. Daily hassles are all negative events, but many life changes are beneficial and attractive, such as getting married or receiving a promotion. "Health Check 3-1" on the next page helps you examine the level of change-related stress in your life.

We all face situations involving change. Leaving school, getting a job, moving to another town or state, becoming spouses and parents, illness, and losses are life changes. Each transition challenges us to cope. Feelings of optimism and of being in control help us meet the challenges posed by life changes.

The stress of a life change reflects its meaning to the individual. The stress of pregnancy is connected with a couple's desire for a baby and their readiness to care for it. The same event or source of stress is less taxing for people who find it meaningful and believe they can cope with it. Similarly, whether you perceive your job to be stressful may depend on whether you feel rushed or overwhelmed by the demands placed on you

Figure 3-3 College Freshmen's Emotional Health

Freshmen's self-assessment of their emotional health hit a 25-year low in 2010. A much larger share of students said they had felt frequently overwhelmed with all they had to do as high school seniors. Women were twice as stressed as men.

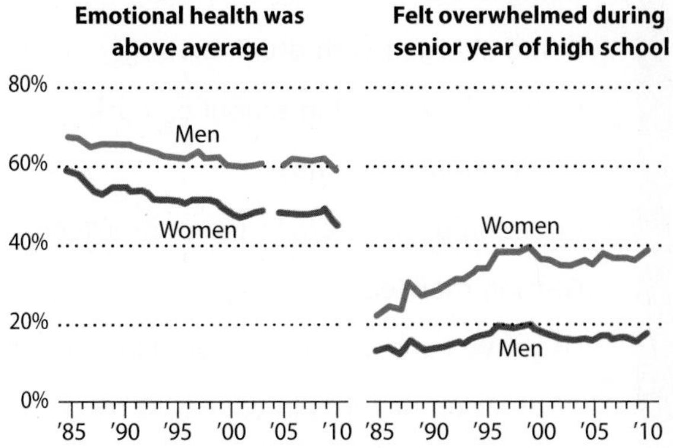

Source: Lewin, T. (2011, January 26). Record level of stress found in college freshmen. *The New York Times*, p. A1.

health check

Going through Changes: How Stressful Is Your Life?

The College Life Stress Inventory measures the level of life stress experienced by college students. The inventory consists of various life events or life changes that are scaled according to their perceived degrees of stress.

To evaluate your own level of stress, select the items in the inventory that you have experienced during the past year. Then calculate your overall stress level by adding up the stress ratings of the selected items.

Event	(√) Experienced during Past Year	Stress Rating
Being raped	______	100
Finding out that you are HIV-positive	______	100
Being accused of rape	______	98
Death of a close friend	______	97
Death of a close family member	______	96
Contracting a sexually transmitted infection (other than HIV/AIDS)	______	94
Concerns about being pregnant	______	91
Finals week	______	90
Concerns about your partner being pregnant	______	90
Oversleeping for an exam	______	89
Flunking a class	______	89
Having a boyfriend or girlfriend cheat on you	______	85
Ending a steady dating relationship	______	85
Serious illness in a close friend or family member	______	85
Financial difficulties	______	84
Writing a major term paper	______	83
Being caught cheating on a test	______	83
Being charged with drunk driving	______	82
Sense of overload in school or work	______	82
Two exams in one day	______	80
Cheating on your boyfriend or girlfriend	______	77
Getting married	______	76
Negative consequences of drinking or drug use	______	75
Depression or crisis in your best friend	______	73

continued

Event	(√) Experienced during Past Year	Stress Rating
Difficulties with parents	______	73
Talking in front of a class	______	72
Lacking sleep	______	69
Changing your housing situation (hassles, moves)	______	69
Competing or performing in public	______	69
Getting into a physical fight	______	66
Difficulties with a roommate	______	66
Job changes (applying, new job, work hassles)	______	65
Declaring a major or having concerns about future plans	______	65
A class you hate	______	62
Drinking or using drugs	______	61
Confrontations with professors	______	60
Starting a new semester	______	58
Going on a first date	______	57
Registration	______	55
Maintaining a steady dating relationship	______	55
Commuting to campus or work, or both	______	54
Peer pressures	______	53
Being away from home for the first time	______	53
Getting sick	______	52
Concerns about your appearance	______	52
Getting straight A's	______	51
A difficult class that you love	______	48
Making new friends; getting along with friends	______	47
Fraternity or sorority rush	______	47
Falling asleep in class	______	40
Attending an athletic event (e.g., football game)	______	20

Source: Renner, M. J. and Mackin, R. S. 1998. A life stress instrument for classroom use. *Teaching of Psychology*, 25: 46–48. Reprinted by permission of the publisher (Taylor & Francis Group, http://www.informaworld.com).

Scoring Key

Compare your total stress rating (total score) with those of a sample of 257 introductory psychology students. The average (mean) score in the sample was 1,247. About two out of three of the students obtained stress rating scores ranging from 806 to 1,688. Your total stress score can help you gauge how stressful your life has been during the preceding year, but it cannot reveal how stress may be affecting you.

or hold a position that combines heavy demands with little control over how and when you do your work.

Frustration and Conflict

We feel *frustration* when our efforts to achieve our goals are thwarted. The seeds of frustration are obvious enough. Adolescents are frustrated when they are told they are too young to drive, date, wear makeup, drink, spend money, or hold a job. A person who wants to go away to college may be frustrated by lack of money or concern about leaving home. We can frustrate ourselves by setting goals too high or demanding perfection.

Conflict is a state of tension brought about by competing motives. People in conflict feel "damned if they do and damned if they don't." People may know that eating fattening food is harmful yet be tempted by the flavor. Students may feel torn ("in conflict") about whether to pursue further training in graduate school or enter the job market. The longer they remain in conflict, the more stressed and frustrated they feel.

The way out of conflict is to make decisions. Making decisions means we need to:

- Sort out our competing values and needs, and identify meaningful, attainable goals.
- Make plans to attain those goals.
- Try out the plans.
- Evaluate the results.

Burnout

Burnout is a state of exhaustion caused by the stress of excessive commitment to one's work or other causes. People can experience burnout when they overextend themselves. Workaholics may become so consumed by their work that they neglect social relationships and leisure activities. Burnout typically arises from imbalances between work and other activities; it is not caused by hard work per se.

Burnout is common in people who face competing demands for their time. They feel pulled in several directions at once. Other people burn out because they do not say no. They accumulate ever-increasing responsibilities. Still others burn out because they are uncertain of what other people expect of them. Thus, they work hard at trying to be all things to all people.

Type A personality
A personality type characterized by impatience, time urgency, competitiveness, and hostility.

The signs of burnout may not appear for years, but they tend to include:

- Loss of energy and feelings of exhaustion, both physical and mental
- Increased irritability and shortness of temper
- Stress-related problems, such as depression, headaches, backaches, or general malaise
- Difficulty concentrating at work or feeling disengaged from your work
- Loss of motivation in someone who was previously enthusiastic
- Lack of satisfaction or a sense of accomplishment in your work
- Loss of concern about work in someone who previously was enthusiastic and committed to the work
- Feeling that you have nothing left to give

Whether or not you notice any early signs of burnout, the suggestions offered in the online feature "Prevention 3-1" might help you prevent burnout.

prevention

Access CourseMate for HLTH at www.cengagebrain.com.

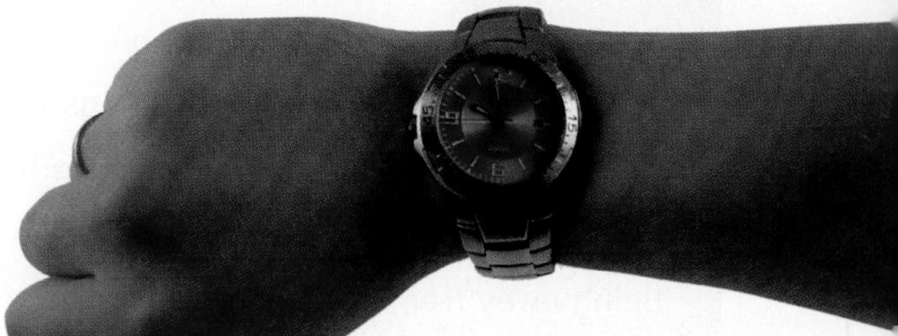

©iStockphoto.com/Joni Rantasalo

Type A Personality

Your personality style may also be a source of stress. Are you hard-driving, competitive, and impatient? Does waiting in line or getting stuck in traffic lead you to pull your hair out or pound your fists? If so, you probably fit the profile of a **Type A personality.**

Type A people have a strong sense of time urgency. They keep one eye glued to the clock. They tend to arrive promptly for appointments, and are often early. They talk, walk, and eat fast. They quickly become impatient and even hostile toward others who work slowly or fail to meet their expectations. They are intense, even at play. On the tennis court, they are not content to bat around the ball for enjoyment. Instead, they scrutinize every stroke, constantly polishing their form and demanding self-improvement. By contrast, Type B people are relaxed and easy-going and consistently take life at a slower pace.

Type A personality is modestly associated with increased risk of heart disease.[1] Hostility, a component of Type A personality, and proneness to anger are more strongly linked to heart disease.[2] Angry people secrete higher levels of the stress-related hormones *epinephrine* and *norepinephrine.* Elevated secretions of these hormones over time may eventually damage the cardiovascular system. Gain insight into whether you have a Type A personality by filling out the online feature "Health Check 3-2."

health check

Access CourseMate for HLTH at www.cengagebrain.com.

Pain

Pain can be unpleasant and even excruciating. Nagging pain can be a significant source of stress. But pain is also necessary for survival. Pain alerts us to danger. It signals that something is wrong in the body and prompts us to seek the source of the problem. When you stub your toe, nerves in your toe send pain messages through the spinal cord to the brain, where that discomfort is registered.

Analgesic drugs, such as aspirin and ibuprofen, are pain-relieving drugs that reduce inflammation and fever as well as pain. But did you know that your brain produces natural painkillers of its own? **Endorphins** are neurotransmitters that are released in response to pain. The word *endorphin* is a contraction of the words *endogenous* (meaning "coming from within") and *morphine* (a narcotic drug that deadens pain). Endorphins are similar in chemical structure to narcotic drugs like morphine and heroin. Like these drugs, endorphins deaden pain by fitting into receptor sites for neurotransmitters that carry pain messages, in effect locking out signals that lead to sensations of pain.

The brain is a marvel of engineering. By allowing us to experience the first pangs of pain, we are alerted to danger. Otherwise, we might not pull our hand away from a hot object in time to prevent burns. Then, by releasing endorphins, the brain gradually shuts the gate on pain. But in some injuries and chronic diseases, endorphins are not enough to shut the gate.

Most pain quickly diminishes or disappears. However, for some 11 million Americans, pain is a constant, unwelcome companion. Chronic pain can last for months or years. It severely drains the pleasure from life and saps our vitality. Sources of chronic pain include back problems, migraines, pain in the jaw, and pain from diseases such as cancer. See the online feature "Health Skills 3-1" to learn more about pain relief.

Stress and the Body: The War Within

health skills

Access CourseMate for HLTH at www.cengagebrain.com.

What happens in the body in response to stress? Although the body reacts differently depending on the type of stressor (cold versus heat, for instance), layered over these distinct reactions is a more general response to stress dubbed the **general adaptation syndrome (GAS).**

LEARNING OUTCOME 2

Describe the effects of stress on the body

The General Adaptation Syndrome (GAS)

The GAS, also called the *stress response,* is characterized by three stages. During the first stage, called the *alarm reaction*, the body mobilizes its resources in the face of stress. If the source of stress persists, the body attempts to conserve its reserves during the resistance stage. But under persistent stress, our bodies are like clocks with alarm systems that do not shut off until their energy is depleted—sometimes dangerously so, as happens during the third stage, which is called the *exhaustion stage.* Let's look more closely at what happens in the body during each of these stages.

The Alarm Reaction—Fight or Flight?

When people encounter a stressor, the nervous system sets off an **alarm reaction** that mobilizes the body's resources. Imagine that a car in front of you on the road swerves out of control. You immediately take defensive action to avoid a collision. Afterward, you notice that beads of sweat are dripping down your forehead and your heart is pounding. These are features of the alarm reaction.

Endorphins
Neurotransmitters that have opiate-like effects of deadening pain and producing states of pleasure by directly stimulating pleasure pathways in the brain.

general adaptation syndrome (GAS)
The body's three-phase general response to persistent or intense stress.

alarm reaction
The first stage of the general adaptation syndrome; it describes the body's initial response to stress, consisting of activation of the sympathetic nervous system and release of stress hormones.

During the alarm reaction stage, we experience strong physiological and psychological arousal. Our muscles tense, and we are flooded with strong emotions such as terror, anxiety, and anger. The alarm reaction mobilizes the body's defenses to prepare for action—to fight or to flee. For this reason, the response to stress has also been labeled the *fight-or-flight reaction.* The strength of the reaction depends on the degree to which the event is perceived as threatening. For example, the alarm reaction in a person with a strong fear of rejection may be set off whenever she or he is introduced to a new person. Another person's alarm may be triggered by taking a test. In such cases, a psychological threat (rejection or failure), rather than a physical stressor, invokes the stress reaction, but the body's response is the same. Learn more about the fight-or-flight reaction by reading the online feature "Diversity 3-1."

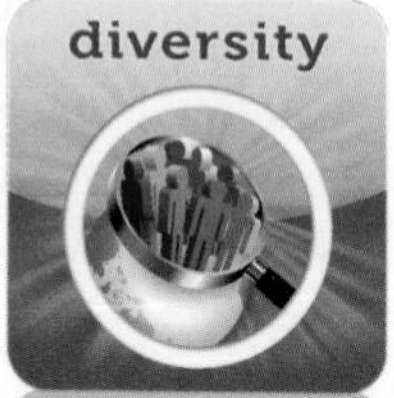

Access CourseMate for HLTH at www.cengagebrain.com.

The alarm reaction is wired into the nervous system. The wiring is a legacy we inherited from our earliest ancestors, who faced life-threatening stressors. For them, the alarm may have been triggered by the sight or sound of a predator lurking in a thicket. The alarm reaction did not last long. Our ancestors either fought off the predator or fled. If they survived and were free of the immediate threat, the "alarm" was turned off, and their body returned to normal. If they failed to fend off the threat, or get away, they perished.

A sensitive alarm system may have kept our ancestors alive. Today, however, it can be a handicap. The stresses of modern life can be recurring or enduring, exciting our alarm systems day after day, year after year. Our ancestors did not have to juggle school and jobs to make ends meet, or struggle to make their sales quota each month, or write term papers.

resistance stage
The second stage of the general adaptation syndrome, during which the body attempts to renew and conserve its resources in order to cope with prolonged stress. Also called the adaptation stage.

exhaustion stage
The third and final stage of the general adaptation syndrome; characterized by depletion of body resources and lowering of resistance to stress-related illness.

homeostasis
The maintenance of a steady state in the body.

Resistance Stage

When a stressor is intense and persistent, the body progresses to the next stage of the GAS, the **resistance stage** (also called the *adaptation stage*). In this stage, the body tries to renew spent energy and repair damage. It seeks to restore the normal biological state. In the resistance stage, body arousal remains high, but not as high as during the alarm reaction. Prolonged body arousal may become expressed in the form of emotions such as anger, fatigue, irritability, and impatience.

Exhaustion Stage

If stressors continue to persist, the body's resources become seriously depleted. The body enters the final stage of the GAS—the **exhaustion stage**. Now the heart rate and respiration rate decrease to conserve body resources.

Some of us are hardier than others, but relentless, intense stress can eventually exhaust any of us. If stress still endures, we may develop stress-related disorders, ranging from an allergic reaction to a potentially fatal condition such as coronary heart disease. Health experts estimate that 60%–90% of all doctor visits involve stress-related problems.[3]

Intense or persistent stress affects **homeostasis**, the body's tendency to maintain processes such as body temperature and blood sugar at a steady state. A state of equilibrium or balance is necessary for health. Under great stress, however, the body can no longer maintain a homeostatic balance, which makes us more vulnerable to stress-related disorders.

During the resistance stage, the body attempts to restore homeostasis—its steady state. Whether the body succeeds in restoring homeostasis depends on whether the stressor is removed or otherwise managed effectively. "Diversity 3-2" explains how strong social networks of friends and family help some ethnic minorities cope with the stress of racism.

The Role of the Nervous System

The body's response to stress is regulated by the nervous system, the communication and control system that comprises the brain, the spinal cord, and the network of nerves that convey messages between the brain and spinal cord

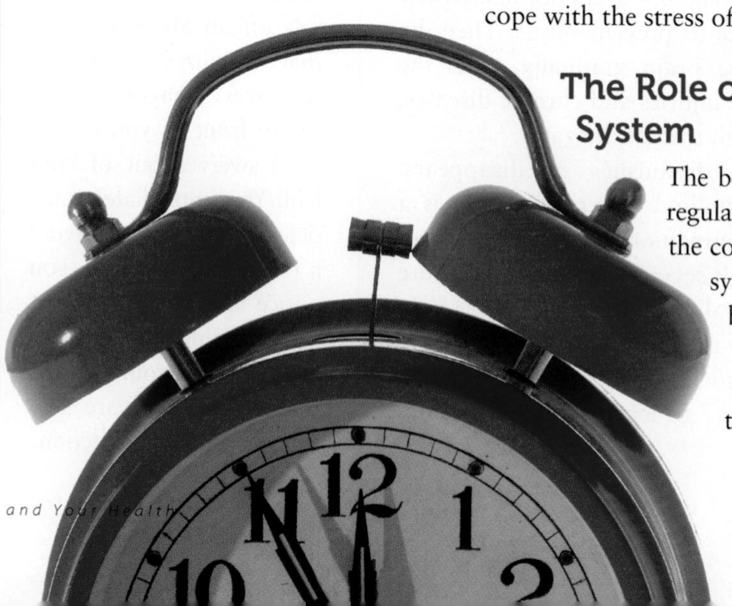

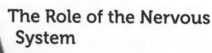

© iStockphoto.com/Udo Kroener

DIVERSITY 3-2

diversity

Ethnic Identity—A Buffer Against Stress

African Americans have higher rates of a number of health problems than European Americans, including hypertension, heart disease, diabetes, and certain types of cancer. The experience of prejudice and racism is a significant source of stress for many African Americans and other ethnic minority groups, heightening the risks of health problems. Many African Americans also face the stresses of poverty, violence, and overcrowded living conditions. Yet, despite these many sources of stress, African Americans as a group show a high degree of resilience in coping with stress.[3] Strong social networks of family and friends, beliefs in their ability to handle stress, and effective coping skills buffer the effects of stress for many.

A strong sense of ethnic identity also bolsters ability to cope with stress.[4] Ethnic pride is a stronger predictor of psychological well-being among African Americans than European Americans.[5] On the other hand, young people of color who become alienated from their cultural heritage tend to develop a more negative self-image and stand greater risks of developing both physical and psychological disorders.[6]

to other parts of the body. The nervous system has two parts, the *central nervous system* and the *peripheral nervous system*. The **central nervous system** consists of the brain and spinal cord. The **peripheral nervous system** connects the central nervous system to other parts of the body and to the world outside. It receives and transmits sensory messages—such as nerve impulses from the eyes and ears—to the central nervous system, and carries nerve impulses from the brain and spinal cord to the muscles, causing them to contract, and to glands, causing them to secrete hormones. The peripheral nervous system is further divided into two major divisions, the *somatic nervous system* and the *autonomic nervous system (ANS)*.

The Somatic Nervous System

The **somatic nervous system** is responsible for transmitting messages between your brain and your sense organs (eyes, ears, tongue, nose, and skin). The somatic nervous system enables us to perceive the world, to contract our muscles to move our limbs, and to maintain our posture and balance. Nerve impulses travel from the brain to the spinal cord and through the somatic nervous system to the muscles that control body movement.

The Autonomic Nervous System

The **autonomic nervous system (ANS)** controls involuntary body activities, such as heartbeat, respiration, digestion, and dilation of the pupils of the eyes. Because it works automatically, the ANS regulates these vital processes without your having to think about them. Your ANS is at work even while you sleep.

The ANS has two branches, the *sympathetic nervous system* and the *parasympathetic nervous system* (see Figure 3-4 on the next page). These two branches have largely opposite effects. The **sympathetic nervous system** accelerates body processes such as heart rate and respiration. The **parasympathetic nervous system** slows them, which helps conserve and replenish vital body resources. The sympathetic system is most active when we are engaged in vigorous physical activities or experiencing strong emotions (which is why our hearts beat faster when we are anxious). The parasympathetic system controls processes that restore spent supplies of energy, such as digestion.

During the alarm reaction of the GAS, the sympathetic nervous system takes command. It accelerates the heart and respiration rates, helping the body contend with the stressor—to flee from it, or if

central nervous system
The central part of the nervous system, consisting of the brain and spinal cord.

peripheral nervous system
The part of the nervous system comprising a system of nerves that connect the brain and spinal cord to the other body parts, including sensory organs, muscles, and glands.

somatic nervous system
The part of the peripheral nervous system that involves the voluntary control of skeletal muscles and feeds information from the sense organs to the brain.

autonomic nervous system (ANS)
The part of the peripheral nervous system that functions "automatically" (without awareness or voluntary control) to control internal body processes such as heart rate, respiration, and endocrine functioning.

sympathetic nervous system
The branch of the autonomic nervous system that accelerates body processes and releases stores of energy needed for physical exertion. The sympathetic branch is activated as part of the alarm reaction in response to stress.

parasympathetic nervous system
Branch of the autonomic nervous system involved in body processes, such as digestion, that preserve and replenish the body's stores of energy.

need be, to fight it off. During the exhaustion stage, the parasympathetic nervous system dominates. Body processes slow down to conserve energy and replenish spent resources.

The Role of the Endocrine System

The autonomic nervous system also regulates the **endocrine system**. The endocrine system consists of glands located throughout the body that secrete hormones directly into the bloodstream (see Figure 3-5). The word *hormone* is derived from Greek roots meaning "to set in motion." As you learned in chapter 2, hormones are chemical substances that regulate and coordinate the functions of organs and body cells.

A pea-sized structure in the brain, the **hypothalamus**, helps coordinate the body's response to stress. The hypothalamus secretes releasing hormones that cause other glands to release their own hormones. The process is akin to a series of falling dominoes.

Under stress, **corticotropin-releasing hormone (CRH)** is released by the hypothalamus. CRH in turn stimulates the **pituitary gland**, which lies just below the hypothalamus. The pituitary is sometimes referred to as the "master gland" because it plays a role in many body processes. Pituitary hormones spur the growth of muscles and bones. They also stimulate the production of sperm in the male and ova (egg cells) in the female.

Figure 3-4 The Sympathetic and Parasympathetic Branches of the Autonomic Nervous System (ANS)

The autonomic nervous system is divided into the sympathetic and parasympathetic nervous systems, which have generally opposing effects. The sympathetic nervous system accelerates the heart and respiration rates, helping the body cope with stress, whereas the parasympathetic nervous system slows these responses and helps restore bodily resources.

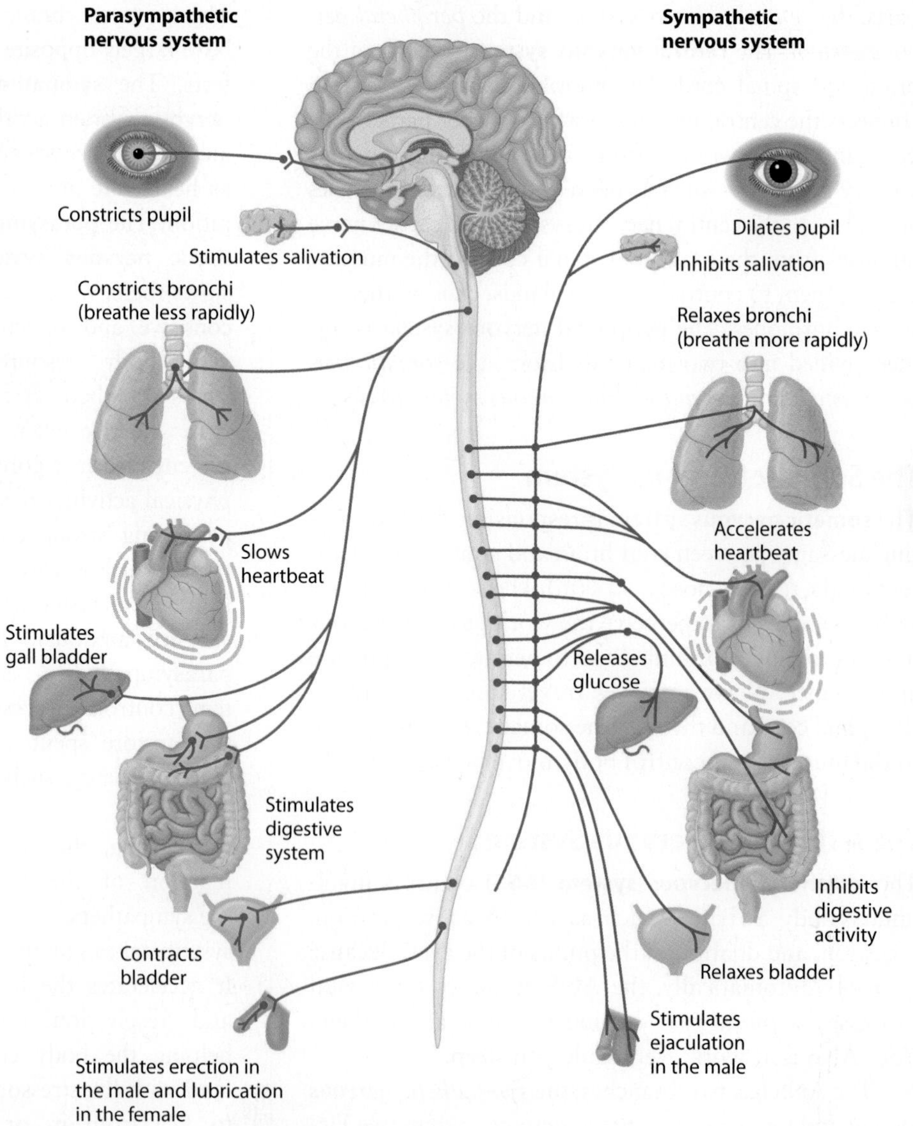

endocrine system
A system of glands that secrete hormones directly into the bloodstream, rather than by means of ducts.

hypothalamus
The small brain structure in the lower middle part of the brain that is involved in regulating a range of body processes, including motivation, emotion, and body temperature.

corticotropin-releasing hormone (CRH)
Substance produced by the hypothalamus that causes the pituitary gland to release adrenocorticotropic hormone (ACTH).

pituitary gland
A structure in the brain dubbed the "master gland" because of its key role in many body processes, including growth and the formation of sperm and egg cells.

Figure 3-5 Major Glands of the Endocrine System

The endocrine system consists of ductless glands that release hormones directly into the bloodstream.

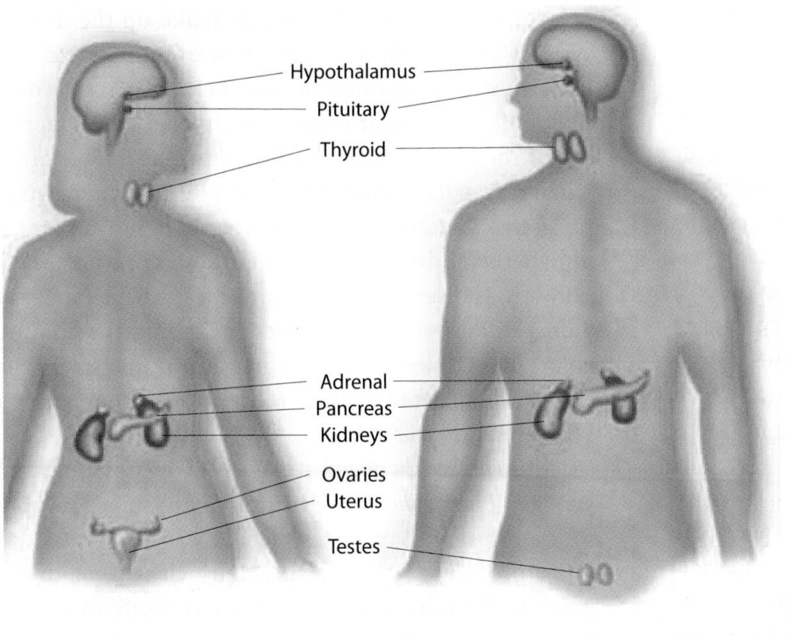
Hypothalamus
Pituitary
Thyroid
Adrenal
Pancreas
Kidneys
Ovaries
Uterus
Testes
© Cengage Learning 2013

Figure 3-6 The Body's Response to Stress

The body responds to stress by releasing stress hormones epinephrine and norepinephrine from the adrenal medulla and corticosteroids from the adrenal cortex. These hormones mobilize the body to cope. Stress hormones increase the heart and respiration rates, elevate the blood pressure, suppress digestion, and dilate (expand) the pupils of the eyes. Corticosteroids spark the release of stored reserves of energy.

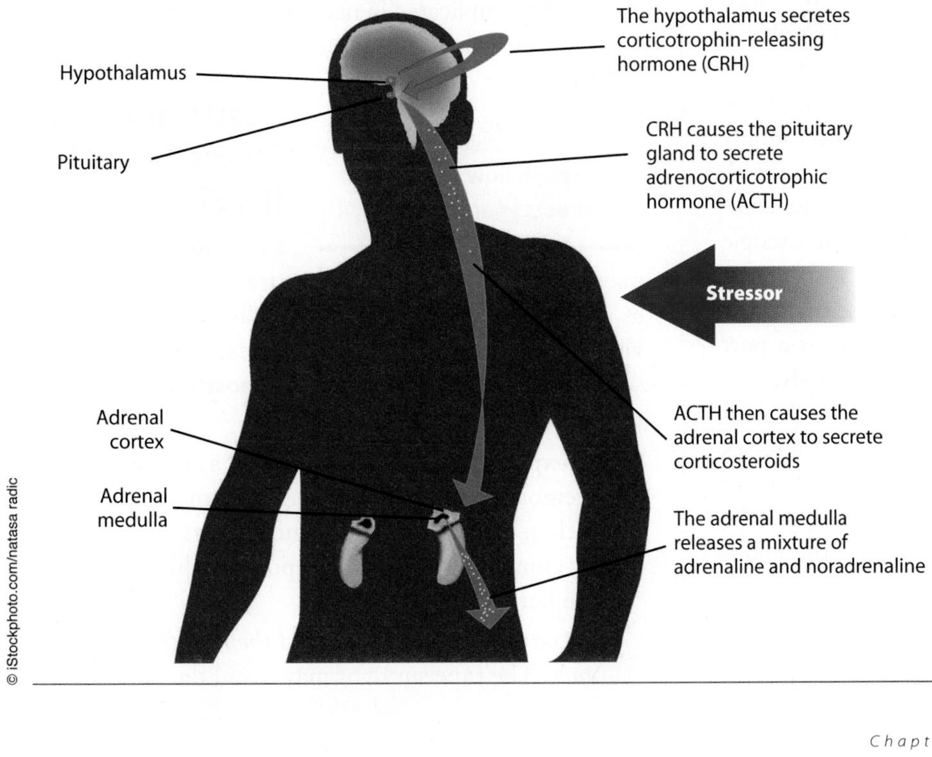
The hypothalamus secretes corticotrophin-releasing hormone (CRH)
Hypothalamus
Pituitary
CRH causes the pituitary gland to secrete adrenocorticotrophic hormone (ACTH)
Stressor
Adrenal cortex
Adrenal medulla
ACTH then causes the adrenal cortex to secrete corticosteroids
The adrenal medulla releases a mixture of adrenaline and noradrenaline
© iStockphoto.com/natasa radic

In response to CRH, the pituitary gland secretes **adrenocorticotropic hormone (ACTH)**. ACTH stimulates the **adrenal glands**, a pair of small endocrine glands located just above the kidneys, to secrete stress hormones that help the body deal with stress. The outer layer of the adrenal glands, the *adrenal cortex*, releases stress hormones called **corticosteroids** (or *cortical steroids*) that help the body resist stress by stimulating the liver to release stores of sugar. More energy thus becomes available to face threats. Steroids also promote muscle development and combat allergic reactions and inflammation.

The sympathetic nervous system also kicks into gear in response to a stressor by activating the inner layer of the adrenal glands, the *adrenal medulla*, to secrete its own cocktail of stress hormones—*epinephrine* (also called *adrenaline*) and *norepinephrine* (also called *noradrenaline*). These hormones accelerate processes such as heart and respiration rates, which cause more oxygen-rich blood to flow to the extremities where muscles are preparing to flee from a threatening stressor or fight it off. The "racing heart" we feel under stress is caused by this surge of epinephrine and norepinephrine. Figure 3-6 illustrates the body's response to stress.

adrenocorticotropic hormone (ACTH)
Hormone produced by the pituitary gland that activates the adrenal cortex (outer layer) to secrete corticosteroids (cortical steroids).

adrenal glands
A pair of endocrine glands that lie just above the kidneys and produce various stress hormones.

corticosteroids
Steroidal hormones released by the adrenal cortex that increase resistance to stress by fending off allergic reactions and reducing inflammation. Also called cortical steroids.

Stress and the Immune System

Researchers study the **immune system** because it has several functions that combat disease. One of these is the production of white blood cells, technically called *leukocytes*, which engulf and kill pathogens such as bacteria, fungi, viruses, worn-out body cells, and cancerous cells. Leukocytes conduct microscopic warfare. They engage in search-and-destroy missions in which they "recognize" and eradicate foreign agents and unhealthy cells.

LEARNING OUTCOME 3

Explain the effects of stress on the immune system

Leukocytes recognize foreign substances by their shapes. The foreign substances are termed *antigens* because the body reacts to them by generating specialized proteins, or **antibodies.** Antibodies attach themselves to the foreign substances, deactivating them and marking them for destruction. The immune system "remembers" how to battle antigens by maintaining their antibodies in the bloodstream, often for years.*

Inflammation is another function of the immune system. When injury occurs, blood vessels in the area first contract (to stem bleeding) and then dilate. Dilation increases the flow of blood, bringing chemical substances to the damaged area that cause the redness, swelling, and warmth that characterize inflammation. The increased blood supply also floods the region with white blood cells to combat invading microscopic life forms such as bacteria, which otherwise might use the local damage as a port of entry into the body.

The field of *psychoneuroimmunology* addresses the relationships among psychological factors, the nervous system, the endocrine system, the immune system, and disease. One of its major concerns is the effect of stress on the immune system. Research shows that stress suppresses the immune system, as measured by the presence of various substances in the blood that make up the immune system. One of the reasons stress eventually exhausts us is that it stimulates the production of corticosteroids. These steroidal hormones suppress the functioning of the immune system. They have negligible effects when secreted occasionally, but under continuing stress, persistent secretion of these steroidal hormones can impair the ability of the immune system to protect the body from disease. As a consequence, we become more vulnerable to various illnesses, including the common cold.[8] By weakening the immune system, stress may also be connected with a more rapid progression of HIV infection to AIDS.[9]

Studies with college students have shown that the stress of exams weakens the immune system's response to the Epstein-Barr virus, which causes fatigue and other problems.[10] The Epstein-Barr virus remains dormant in 90% of people who recover from an episode. Persistent stress keeps blood levels of stress hormones elevated, which heightens the probability that the virus will be reactivated.[11]

immune system
The body's system for identifying and eliminating disease-causing agents, such as bacteria and viruses, and for ridding the body of diseased, mutated, or worn-out cells.

antibody
Specialized protein produced by white blood cells that attaches itself to invading microbes and other foreign bodies, inactivates them, and marks them for destruction.

posttraumatic stress disorder (PTSD)
Type of psychological disorder involving a maladaptive reaction to a traumatic experience. The disorder may not begin until months or years following the traumatic event and may last for years after its onset.

* A vaccination introduces a weakened form of an antigen (usually a bacteria or a virus) into the body to stimulate the production of antibodies. Antibodies can confer immunity for many years, in some cases for a lifetime.

Stress and Health

Stress is a fact of life. But when it overtaxes our ability to adjust, it can affect our psychological and physical health. Stress is implicated in many health-related problems, such as those listed in Table 3-1.

LEARNING OUTCOME 4

Explain how stress affects your health

Posttraumatic Stress Disorder (PTSD)

Psychological disorders may arise following exposure to traumatic events, such as combat and warfare, natural catastrophes, crimes of violence, or witnessing the violent death of another person. People may be diagnosed with **posttraumatic stress disorder (PTSD)** when they:

- *Reexperience the traumatic event* as intrusive memories or images, dreams, nightmares, or the feeling that the event is recurring—as experienced by combat veterans who report "flashbacks" to the battlefield.
- *Avoid situations that remind them of the experience.* The rape survivor may avoid the part of

Table 3-1 Stress-Related Health Problems

BIOLOGICAL PROBLEMS	PSYCHOLOGICAL PROBLEMS
• Tension or migraine headaches	• Overeating
• Painful menstruation	• Fatigue
• Allergic reactions	• Depression
• Back pain, especially low back pain	• Anger
• High blood pressure	• Resentment
• Skin inflammations (such as hives and acne)	• Feeling short-tempered
• Rheumatoid arthritis (painful inflammation of the joints)	• Irritability
• Nausea and vomiting	• Anxiety
• Sleep problems	• Difficulty concentrating
• Upset stomach or indigestion	• Feeling overwhelmed
• Shortness of breath	• Alcohol or substance abuse
• Ulcers	
• Regional enteritis (inflammation of the intestine, especially the small intestine)	
• Ulcerative colitis (inflammation and open sores of the colon, or large intestine)	
• Asthma	
• Cardiac problems, such as tachycardia (rapid heartbeat), arrhythmia (irregularity in the rhythm of the heart), angina pectoris (recurrent pain in the chest and the left arm, caused by sudden decrease in the blood supply to the heart), and cardiospasm (sudden contractions of the heart muscle)	
• Frequent urination or diarrhea	
• Skin rashes	

town where the rape took place. The combat veteran may avoid his service buddies so that he need not talk about his experiences.

- *Maintain high levels of body arousal* as in feeling keyed up or on edge and having difficulty relaxing or getting to sleep. The person may seem always on guard and jumpy in response to sudden noises.
- *Experience emotional numbing* as in having difficulty feeling love or other strong emotions.
- *Exhibit impaired functioning and significant emotional distress* as in having difficulty meeting responsibilities as a worker, student, spouse, or parent. She or he may be bothered by feelings of depression or anxiety.

Not everyone who experiences a traumatic event develops PTSD, but many do. Firefighters regularly come across fires, accidents, stabbings, shootings, suicides, medical emergencies, bombs, and hazardous material explosions. One firefighter in six can be diagnosed with PTSD. Vulnerability to PTSD depends on such factors as the severity of the trauma, individual differences in biological reactivity and coping ability, and the availability of social support.

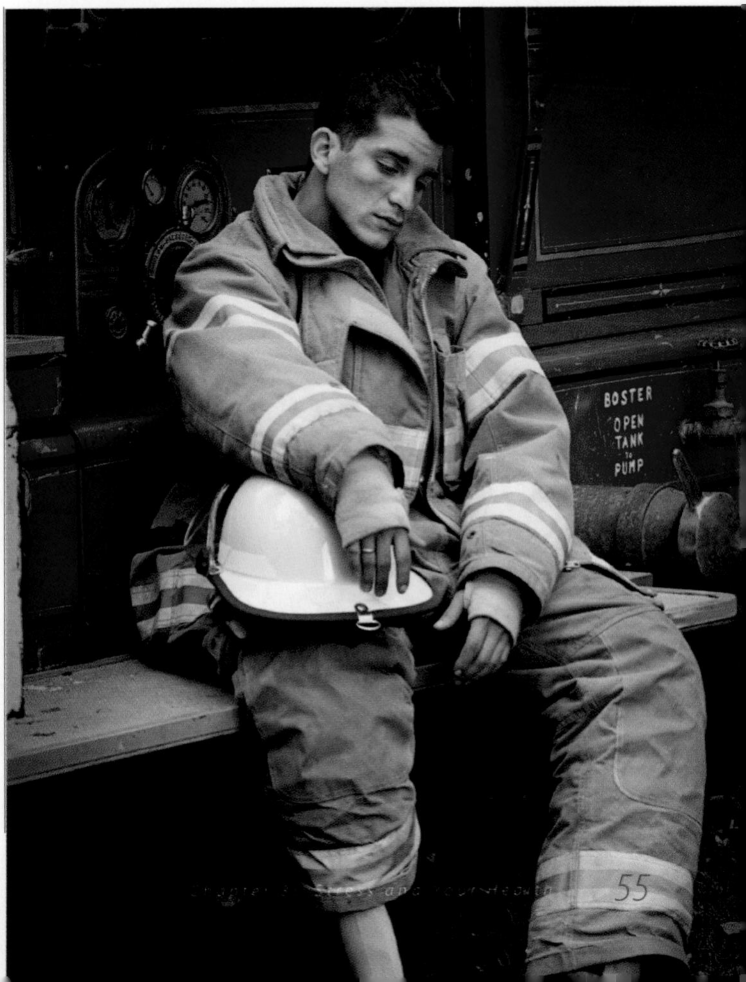

Stress and Physical Health

Links between stress and physical health have been documented for many disorders, including hypertension, heart disease, and asthma. Though the release of the stress hormones epinephrine and norepinephrine helps prepare the body to cope with a stressor, continued secretion in response to persistent stress may compromise the cardiovascular system. These hormones accelerate the heart rate, raise blood pressure, and increase the strength of heart contractions, all of which can burden the cardiovascular system. Stress hormones, especially epinephrine, make clotting factors in the blood stickier, raising the risk that blood clots will form in arteries and lead to heart attacks or strokes.

Stress on the job also may increase the risk of cardiovascular problems, especially for people in high-strain jobs—highly repetitive, time-pressured jobs that allow little decision-making latitude but require high standards of performance. People in high-strain jobs include waiters and waitresses, telephone operators, and cooks. Workers in these jobs stand about one and one-half times greater risk of developing coronary heart disease than those in low-strain jobs.

The scientific jury is still out on the question of whether stress makes us more vulnerable to developing cancer. Conceivably, persistent stress may weaken the immune system, making it less capable of ridding the body of cancerous cells. Yet, research evidence linking exposure to stressful life events and risk of cancer remains inconclusive.[12] The possible relationship between stress and cancer deserves further study.

insomnia
Difficulty falling asleep, remaining asleep, or achieving restorative sleep.

One of the best ways to cope with the stresses of daily life is to ensure that you get enough sleep. Unfortunately, stressors such as financial hassles can keep you awake at night.

Stress and Sleep: Getting Your *Zs*

Most people need between six and eight hours of sleep nightly to feel refreshed and to handle the stresses of everyday life. Yet many of us get too little sleep. We may go to bed later than we should or get up earlier than we'd like. For parents of young children, a full night's rest is a wistful memory. Many people are also troubled by **insomnia**, a sleep disorder characterized by persistent or recurring problems falling asleep, remaining asleep, or achieving restorative sleep—the type

LEARNING OUTCOME 5

Discuss the problem of insomnia and ways of getting your *Zs*.

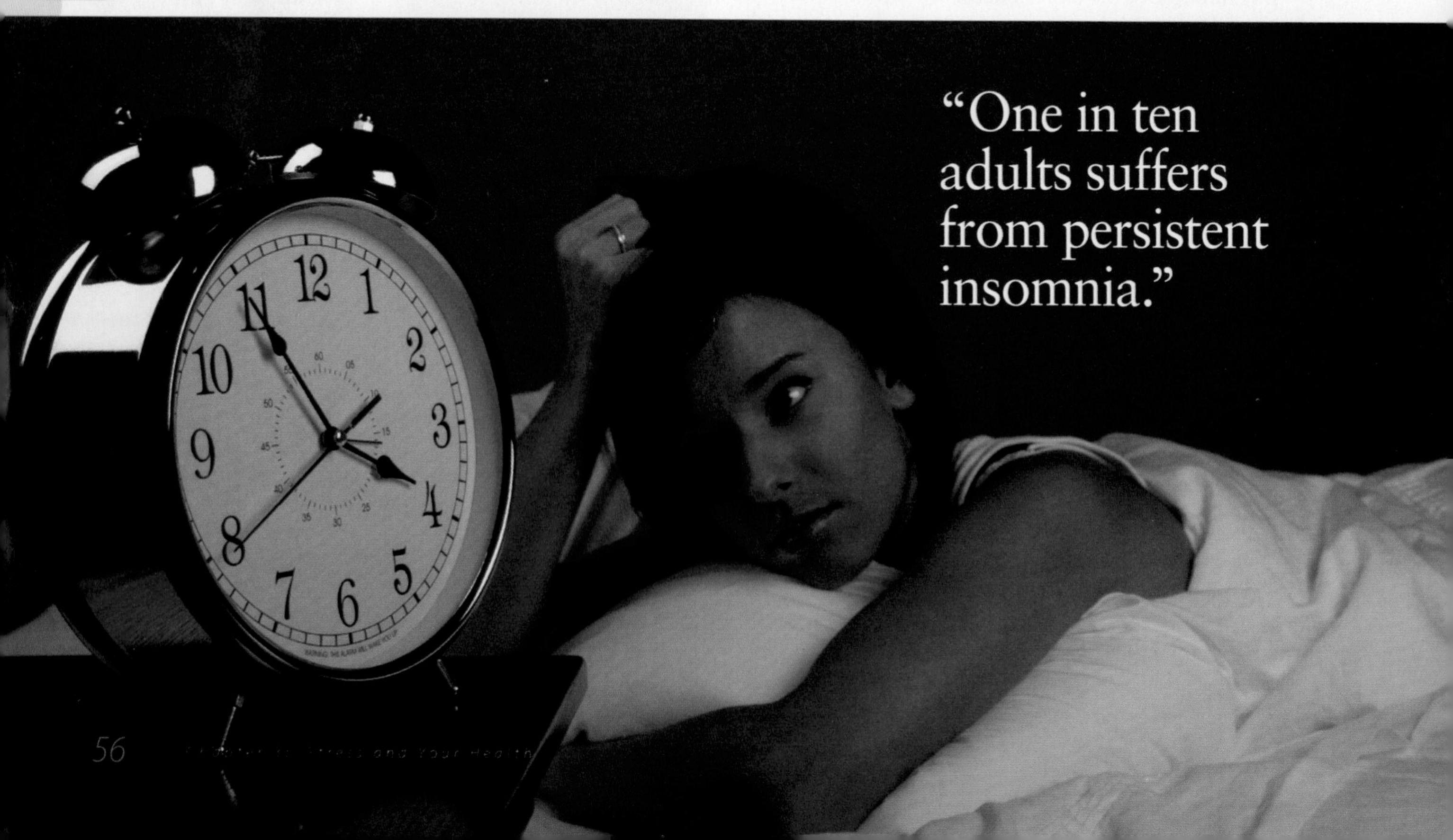

"One in ten adults suffers from persistent insomnia."

© iStockphoto.com/Justin Horrocks

of sleep that leaves you feeling refreshed and alert in the morning.

Occasional difficulty falling or remaining asleep, especially during times of stress, is normal. However, about one in ten adults suffers from persistent insomnia.[13] In many cases, the sleep problem is actually a sign of an underlying physical cause, such as drug or alcohol abuse, or a psychological disorder, such as depression. If the underlying problem is successfully resolved, chances are good that normal sleep patterns can be restored. In other cases, the sleep problem itself is considered the primary problem.

The risk of insomnia increases with age and is greater among women than men. For younger people, insomnia usually takes the form of difficulty falling asleep, while older people are typically bothered by awakening during the night or too early in the morning.

Insomnia may have biological causes (such as changes in the brain mechanisms controlling sleep and waking cycles as we age), but psychological problems also play a prominent role. People with chronic insomnia tend to bring their worries to bed with them, which raises their anxiety and the accompanying body arousal to a level that prevents natural sleep. They may then worry about not getting enough sleep, which bumps up their arousal level even more. They may try to concentrate really hard on falling asleep, which usually backfires by creating even more pressure and tension, making sleep even less likely to occur.

According to the National Sleep Foundation, more than half of American adults experience occasional insomnia in any given year. Are you getting enough sleep at night? Take the quiz in "Health Check 3-3" below if you're not sure. If you decide you want more sleep and are having trouble getting it, you can then explore the online feature "Health Skills 3-2" for suggestions on getting those Zs back.

health skills

Access CourseMate for HLTH at www.cengagebrain.com.

HEALTH CHECK 3-3

health check

Sleep Quiz: Are You Getting Your *Zs*?

This questionnaire can help you learn whether you are getting enough sleep. Circle the *T* if an item is true or mostly true or the *F* if an item is false or mostly false for you. Then check the meaning of your answers below.

T	F	1.	I'm tired, cranky, and stressed out all week long.
T	F	2.	I know I look tired . . . I've even got dark circles under my eyes.
T	F	3.	My memory is shot and it's hard to concentrate.
T	F	4.	Without a nap, I just can't get through the day.
T	F	5.	I feel really slow when I'm trying to solve a problem or be creative.
T	F	6.	Driving makes me feel drowsy.
T	F	7.	I'm so relaxed after dinner, I can curl up and go right to sleep!
T	F	8.	Falling asleep in front of the TV is normal for me.
T	F	9.	I can't keep my eyes open after a heavy meal or a couple of drinks.
T	F	10.	Once I crawl into bed it only takes me a few minutes to fall asleep.
T	F	11.	It's a real struggle every morning to get out of bed.
T	F	12.	Without my alarm clock, I'd never wake up in time for class.
T	F	13.	I hit the snooze button over and over to try to get more sleep.
T	F	14.	I sleep in on the weekends and on my days off—sometimes for hours!

Scoring Key

An answer of "true" to two or more of these statements may be a sign of a sleep problem.

Stress Management: Taking the Distress Out of Stress

Stress is a part of life. Whereas some stress is good for you, keeping you active and alert, excesses of stress are discomforting in themselves and connected with health problems. There are two major ways of coping with stress: *problem-focused coping* and *emotion-focused coping*.

LEARNING OUTCOME 6

Describe ways of managing stress

Problem-focused coping seeks to manage stress directly either by changing the stressor itself or the ways we respond to the stressor. If you are having difficulty with a college subject, you can study harder or more efficiently, talk to your professor to find ways to perform better, or consult a tutor. If you're involved in arguments with a roommate or a partner, you can hold discussions aimed at getting at the roots of the problems and finding ways to solve them.

Developing time-management skills is a fine example of problem-focused coping. Organize your time more efficiently. Use a monthly calendar. Fill in appointments and important events (e.g., upcoming exams, doctor's visits, family get-togethers, etc.). Make sure there's a time for everything, and everything is in its time. You can also use prioritized to-do lists. Start each day with a list of things you feel you need to do. Then prioritize them, using a three-point code. Assign a 1 to things you absolutely must get done today. Assign a 2 to things you'd like to get done today, but don't absolutely need to get done. Then give a 3 to things you'd like to get done today if time allows. Also, break down larger tasks into smaller, manageable jobs. Take that term paper that's been staring you in the face. Don't try to finish it off in just one or two marathon sittings. Break it down into smaller pieces, and then tackle them one by one.

Emotion-focused coping attempts to reduce the effects of a stressor by avoiding it, ignoring it, or managing the emotional needs connected with your reaction to the stressor. Some people, sadly, choose to drink alcohol to lower the reactivity of the nervous system when faced with a stressor. The emotional benefits of drinking are short-lived and do nothing to remove the stressor or respond to it in a more productive way. Some students drop out of college when they encounter academic or social stress. Other students, more usefully, seek out their friends and families to help them manage their emotional needs.

Because stress depresses the functioning of the immune system, it may be that alleviating stress has beneficial effects on the immune system, thus making us less vulnerable to some health problems. Health professionals have devised a number of methods collectively referred to as *stress management*. Stress management is not always the cure-all, but it at least reduces feelings of stress! Moreover, the strategies for preventing and coping with stress, headaches, heart disease, and cancer involve significant improvements in your lifestyle. By following them, there is an excellent chance that you will live longer. It is almost a certainty that you will live *better*.

Next we will discuss stress management techniques that are examples of problem-focused coping—ways of changing your responses to stressors.

Control Irrational Thoughts—Changing Your Mind for the Better

People often feel stressed because of their own thoughts. Consider the following experiences:

1. You have difficulty with the first item on a test and become convinced that you will flunk.
2. You want to express your genuine feelings but think that if you do so you might make another person angry or upset.
3. You haven't been able to get to sleep for 15 minutes and assume that you will lie awake all night and feel "wrecked" in the morning.
4. You're not sure what decision to make, so you try to put the problem out of your mind by going out, playing cards, or watching TV.
5. You decide not to play tennis because your form isn't perfect and you're in less-than-perfect condition.

If you have had these or similar experiences, it may be because you are overly concerned about the approval of others (item 2 in the preceding list) or perfectionistic (item 5). How do we change the irrational thoughts that create and compound stress? The answer is deceptively simple: We just change them. However, this may require work. Moreover, before we can change our thoughts, we must become aware of them. Table 3-2 will help you become aware of irrational beliefs and how to change them.

Here are ways for controlling the irrational or catastrophizing thoughts that often accompany feelings of anxiety, conflict, or tension:

1. Develop awareness of the thoughts that seem to be making you miserable by careful self-examination. Study the examples at the beginning of this section or in the table below to see if they apply to you. In addition, when you encounter anxiety or frustration, pay close attention to your thoughts.
2. Evaluate the accuracy of your thoughts. Are they guiding you toward a solution, or are they compounding your problems? Do they reflect reality, or do they blow things out of proportion? Do they misplace the blame for failure or shortcomings?
3. Prepare thoughts that are incompatible with the irrational or catastrophizing thoughts and practice saying them firmly to yourself.
4. Reward yourself with a mental pat on the back for making effective changes in your beliefs and thought patterns.

Lower Arousal: Turning Down the Inner Alarm

Stress can trigger intense activity in the sympathetic branch of the autonomic nervous system—that is, overarousal. Overarousal is a sign that something may be wrong. It is a message telling us to solve a problem—to

Table 3-2 Thoughts that Blow Stressors Out of Proportion and Rational Alternatives

THOUGHTS THAT BLOW STRESSORS OUT OF PROPORTION	RATIONAL ALTERNATIVES THAT HELP KEEP THINGS IN PERSPECTIVE
"Oh my God, it's going to be a mess! I'm losing all control!"	"This is annoying and upsetting, but I haven't lost all control and I'm not going to."
"This is awful. It'll never end."	"It's bad, but it doesn't have to get the best of me. And upsetting things do come to an end, even if that's sort of hard to believe right now."
"I just can't stand it when Mom (Dad/my roommate/my date) gives me that look."	"Life is more pleasant when everyone is pleased with me, but I have to be myself. That means that other people are going to disagree with me from time to time."
"There's no way I can get up there and perform/give that speech! I'll look like an idiot."	"So I'm not perfect; that doesn't mean I'm going to look like an idiot. And so what if someone thinks I look bad? It doesn't mean I *am* bad. And if I am bad, so what? I can live with that, too. I don't have to be perfect every time. So stop being such a worrywart and get up and have some fun."
"My heart's beating a mile a minute! It's going to leap out of my chest! How much of this can I take?"	"Take it easy! Hearts don't jump out of chests. Just slow down a minute—stop and think. I'll find a way out. And if I don't for the time being, I'll survive. Some day I'll look back on this and laugh at how upset I got myself."
"What can I do? I'm helpless! It's just going to get worse and worse."	"Take it easy. Just stop and think for a minute. Just because there's no obvious solution doesn't mean I won't be able to do anything about it. Just take it minute by minute for the time being until I figure it out."

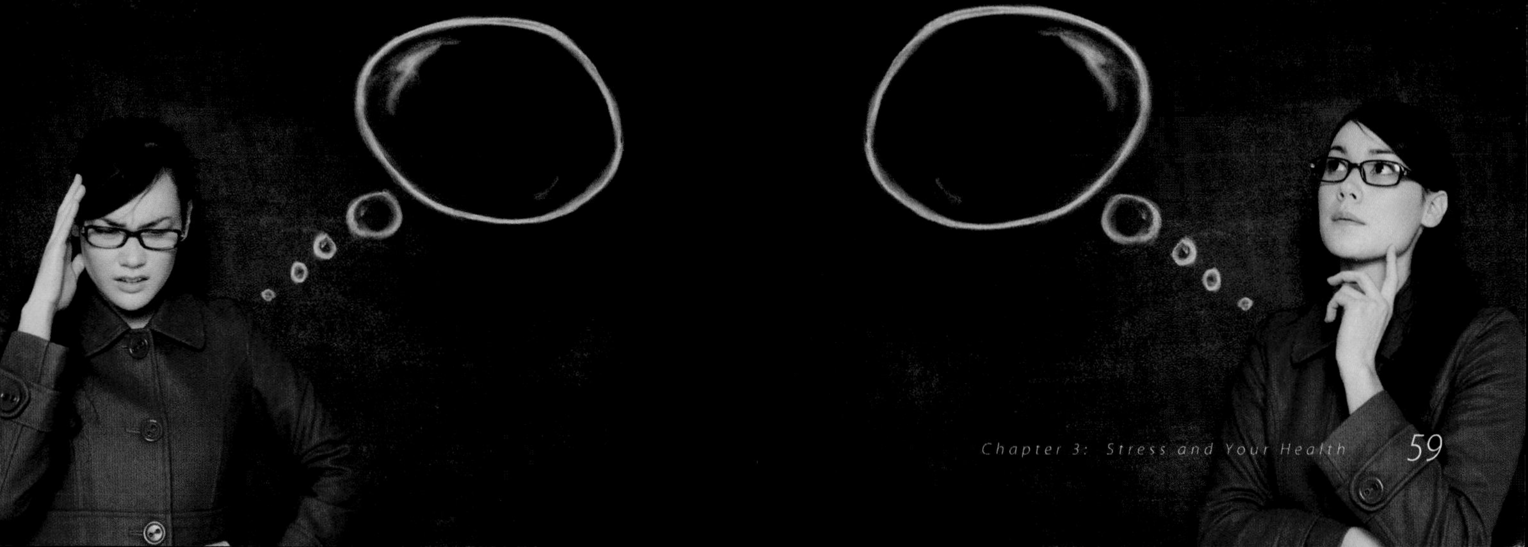

survey the situation and take appropriate action. But once we are aware that a stressor is acting on us and have developed a plan to cope with it, it is no longer helpful to have blood pounding fiercely through our arteries.

There are many methods for reducing arousal. These include progressive relaxation and meditation. In progressive relaxation, people purposefully tense a particular muscle group before relaxing it. This sequence allows them to develop awareness of their muscle tensions and also to differentiate between feelings of tension and relaxation.

The following instructions will help you try meditation as a means for lowering the arousal connected with stress:

1. Begin by meditating once or twice a day for 10 to 20 minutes.
2. In meditation, what you *don't* do is more important than what you *do* do. Adopt a passive, "what happens happens" attitude.
3. Create a quiet, nondisruptive environment. For example, don't face a light directly.
4. Do not eat for one hour beforehand; avoid caffeine for at least two hours.
5. Assume a comfortable position. Change it as needed. It's okay to scratch or yawn.
6. As a device to aid concentrating, you may focus on your breathing or seat yourself before a calming object such as a plant or burning candle. Think or silently repeat the word *one* on each outbreath. Or think or silently repeat the word *in* as you inhale and *out* as you exhale. Elongate the sounds in your mind.
7. If you are using a mantra (like the syllable "om," pronounced *oammm*), you can prepare for meditation and say the mantra out loud several times. Enjoy it. Then say it more and more softly. Close your eyes and only think the mantra. Allow yourself to perceive, rather than actively think, the mantra. Again, adopt a passive attitude. Continue to perceive the mantra. It may grow louder or softer, disappear for a while, and then return.
8. If disruptive thoughts enter your mind as you are meditating, you can allow them to pass through. Don't get wrapped up in trying to squelch them, or you may raise your level of arousal.
9. Allow yourself to drift. What happens happens.
10. Above all, take what you get. You cannot force the relaxing effects of meditation. You can only set the stage for them and allow them to happen.

Reach Out and Be Touched by Someone

People are social beings, and social support seems to act as a buffer against the effects of stress. How can you broaden your own social support network? The Social Support Inventory in Table 3-3 offers ideas for getting the kinds of social support that people rely upon, especially in times of stress. There are also likely to be numerous clubs and organizations on your campus or in your community that can provide opportunities to make new friends. Check with your office of student life or college counseling services.

Try a Little Humor: It's Good Medicine

Humor can help buffer the effects of stress. The notion that humor eases life's burdens is an ancient one. We find references to humor's tonic effect in the biblical adage, "A merry heart doeth good like a medicine" (Proverbs 17:22). By making us laugh, humor can get our minds off our troubles, at least for a time. A regular dose of humor makes stress more bearable. In one study, stress had less impact on college students who had a good sense of humor, especially among those who were able to bring themselves to laugh in the face of adversity. You might try a dose of something amusing tonight, a comedy perhaps.

Reduce Type A Behavior

People with the Type A personality pattern continually place pressure on themselves to accomplish as much as possible in as little time as possible. Can Type A personalities learn to reduce or relieve their sense of time urgency and take things more slowly? Yes, if they follow some suggestions for changing their behavior. The following stress-busting suggestions may be helpful to you even if you are not a bona fide Type A personality:

- Spend more time socializing with friends and family.
- Take a few minutes each day to think about your earlier life experiences. Pore through old photos.
- Read books for pleasure's sake—fiction, biography, literature. (Avoid books on succeeding in business or climbing the corporate ladder.)

Table 3-3 Social Support Inventory: What It Is, How to Get It

TYPE OF SUPPORT	WHAT IT IS	HOW TO GET IT
Emotional concern	Having others available who will listen to your problems and express understanding, sympathy, caring, and reassurance	Develop friendships and maintain relationships with current friends and family members. Make contact with trusted advisors in your community, such as your local priest, minister, or rabbi. Get involved in social organizations or community activities that provide opportunities to expand your social network.
Instrumental aid	Having the material assistance and services needed to support adaptive behavior in times of stress.	Learn about the resources in your community that assist people in times of need. Become acquainted with government support programs and the work of voluntary support agencies.
Feedback	Having feedback from others that tells us how we're doing when we're under stress	Develop a give-and-take relationship with several people whose opinions you trust.
Socializing	Having opportunities to socialize with others in our free time	Invite friends and family members to get together with you on a regular basis, perhaps organized around enjoyable activities like playing cards, going to dinner or shows, or bowling.

- Spend time visiting museums and art galleries. Examine works of art for their beauty, not their prices.
- Take enjoyable extension courses—not career-related courses.
- Take up a hobby or learn to play the piano or violin.
- Attend the theater, ballet, or concerts. Or take in a movie.
- Write to old friends and family members.
- Lighten up on yourself. Don't impose impossible demands to complete all your projects by a certain date.
- Take time around the dinner table to ask your roommates or family members how they spent their day. Actually listen to the answers without interrupting or finishing their sentences for them.
- Don't overschedule yourself. Don't cram all your courses into one school day.
- Don't wolf down your food. Relax while you eat. Make meals an occasion.
- Take things more slowly. The posted speed limit tells you the maximum allowable driving speed, not the minimum. Walk around the campus for the sake of enjoying the day, not just to rush from one class to another. Read a newspaper or magazine for enjoyment.

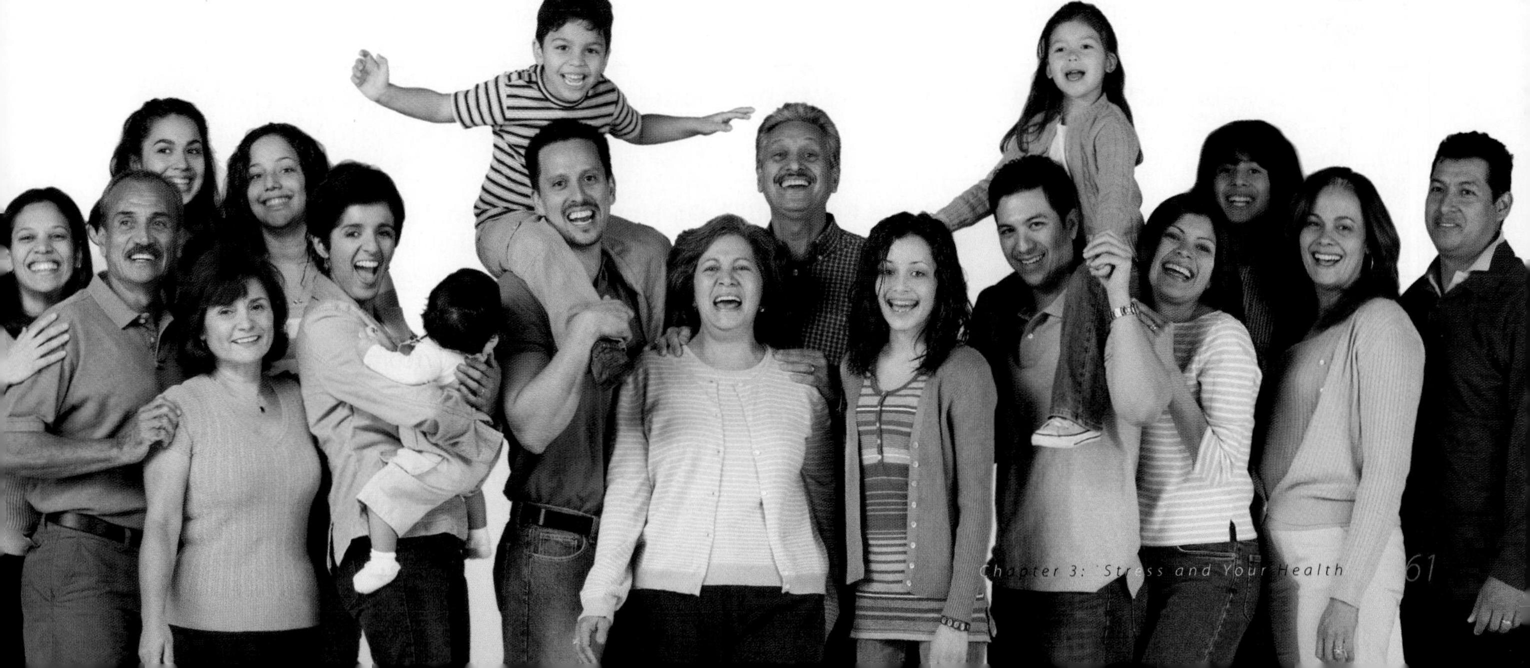

"I like long walks, especially when they are taken by people who annoy me."

Fred Allen

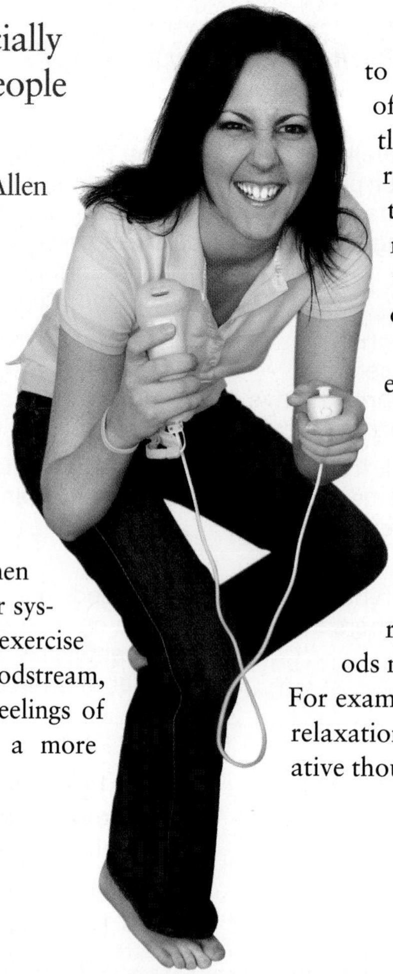

© iStockphoto.com/Beano5

Work It Out by Working Out

Exercise not only builds up your physical resources—it can also combat stress. Many people work off the tensions of the day with a game of racquetball, a run around the park, or laps in the pool.

Regular exercise can help strengthen body systems, such as the cardiovascular system, that are affected by stress. Vigorous exercise raises the levels of endorphins in the bloodstream, which can counter stress by inducing feelings of well-being. Exercise can help restore a more relaxed state of mind and body.

You need not push your body to extremes to benefit from the stress-reducing effects of exercise. Even mild exercise—a gentle swim, a brisk walk in the park—can relieve stress. Regardless of the reasons that exercise relieves stress, exercise has a remarkable effect on our moods. It calms us down and improves our psychological outlook.

Choose a physical activity that you enjoy. (Pushing yourself to do something you detest will only increase your stress.)

Coping with Headaches

Because many headaches are related to stress, one way to fight headaches is to reduce the stress in your life. All the methods mentioned in this chapter may be of help. For example, headache sufferers may benefit from relaxation training, meditation, and changing negative thoughts into coping thoughts.

HEALTH APPS: YOUR LINK TO ONLINE HEALTH APPLICATIONS

prevention

Ten Ways to Prevent Burnout People may become burned out when they are overextended. Yet, burnout is not inevitable. "Prevention 3-1" has some suggestions for preventing burnout.

health check

Are You Type A? Are you always pushing? Does waiting in line make you pull your hair out? You can gain insight into whether you have a Type A personality by completing "Health Check 3-2."

health skills

Pain, Pain, Go Away—Don't Come Again Another Day Is life a pain? For relief, check out "Health Skills 3-1."

diversity

"Fight or Flight" or "Tend and Befriend"? Do Men and Women Respond Differently to Stress? Is the fight-or-flight reaction for men only? You can find answers to these questions and more in "Diversity 3-1."

health skills

Overcoming Insomnia According to the National Sleep Foundation, more than half of American adults and about two-thirds of older adults are affected by insomnia in any given year. If you decide you want more sleep, and are having trouble getting it, "Health Skills 3-2" has suggestions on how to reclaim those *Zs*.

Go to the CourseMate for HLTH at www.cengagebrain.com for additional resources including flashcards, games, self-quizzes, review exercises, web exercises, learning checks, and more.

HLTH
Chapter 4

Intimate Relationships and Sexuality

"Social relationships are important to our physical and psychological health."

Will you, won't you, will you, won't you, will you join the dance?

—Lewis Carroll, *Alice in Wonderland*

No man is an island, entire of itself.

—John Donne

Yes, no man—and no woman—is an island. We're all social creatures. Social relationships are important to our physical and psychological health. Many people suffer health problems when they undergo the stress of divorce or separation. Moreover, married people—men, especially—tend to be healthier and live longer than single people.

Forming Relationships

There are many types of relationships—relationships with parents, children, friends, neighbors, and even the shopkeepers in your neighborhood. In this chapter we focus on the development of an intimate, romantic relationship, the type of relationship we have, or hope to have, with a special person in our lives—a partner or lover. Relationships typically begin with feelings of attraction, so that is where we begin as well.

LEARNING OUTCOME 1

Describe the formation of intimate relationships

LEARNING OUTCOMES

1. **Describe the formation of intimate relationships**
2. **Discuss contemporary lifestyles, from being single to cohabitation to marriage and parenting**
3. **Discuss factors in unhealthy relationships**
4. **Describe female and male sexual anatomy and related health issues**
5. **Discuss sexual orientation**
6. **Discuss different types of sexual behaviors**
7. **Discuss sexual dysfunctions and sex therapy**

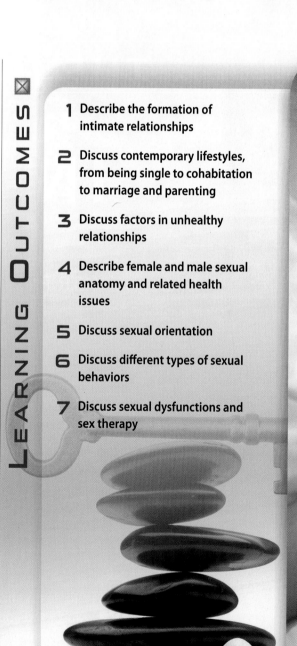

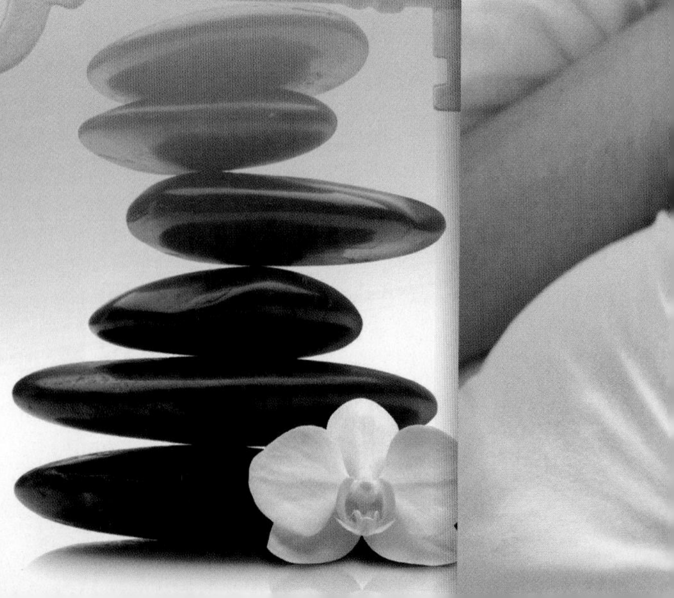

Attraction

Attraction occurs when two people become aware of each other and find one another appealing or enticing. We may find ourselves attracted to an enchanting person "across a crowded room," in a nearby office, or in a new class. We may meet others through blind dates, speed dates, introductions by friends, or simply by accident. Many people also meet via online dating and social networking sites, such as Facebook, but networking sites are used mainly to share information in established relationships.

Married people are most likely to have met their spouses through mutual friends (35%) or by self-introductions (32%)[1] (see Figure 4-1 on the next page). Other common sources of introductions are family members (15%) and co-workers, classmates, or neighbors (13%).

Physical Attractiveness: How Important Is Looking Good?

We might like to think that we are attracted to people because of what's on the inside, not how they look on the outside. However, evidence shows that physical appearance is the key factor in determining initial attraction—whom we date and with whom we form

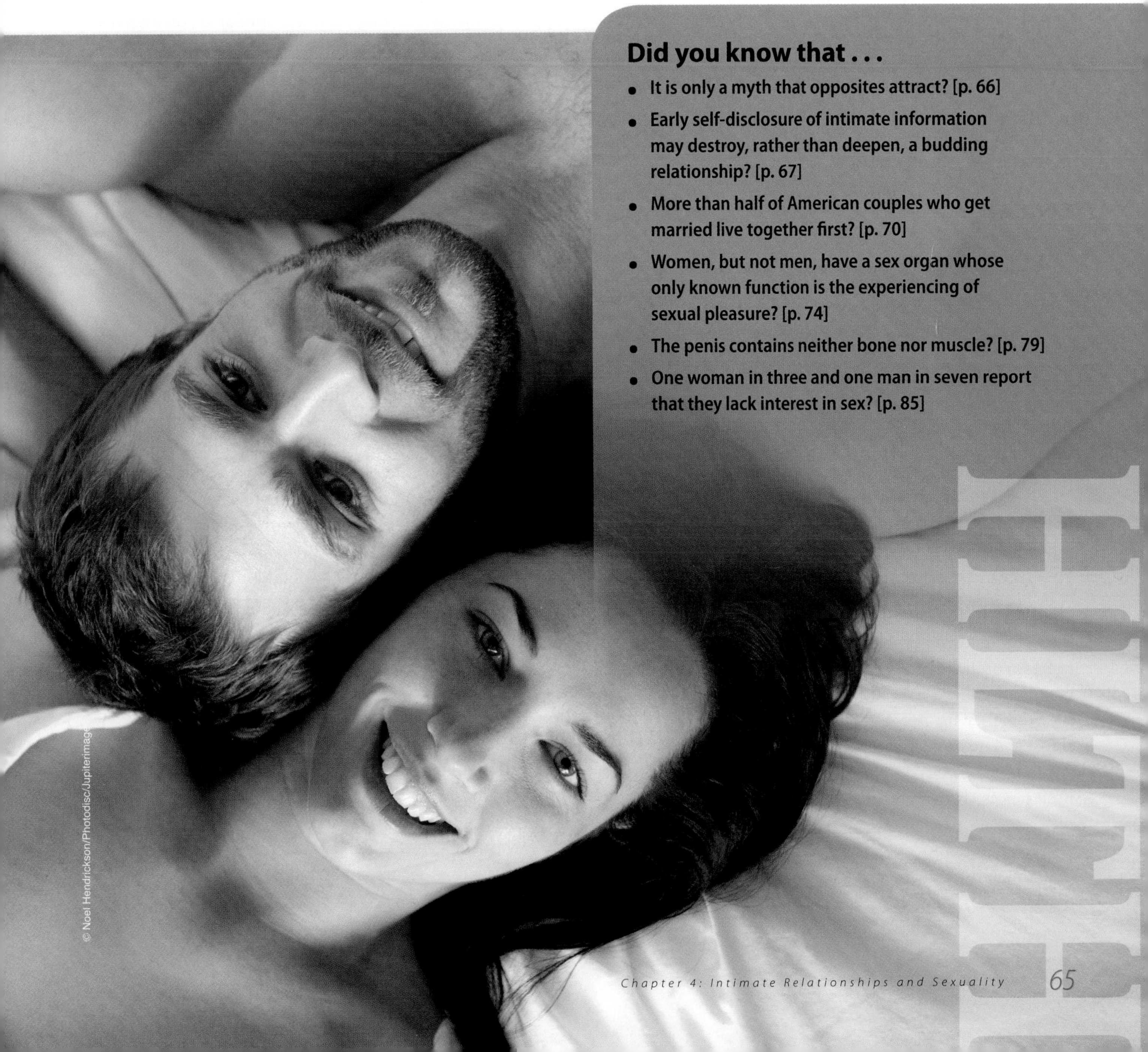

© Noel Hendrickson/Photodisc/Jupiterimage

Did you know that . . .

- It is only a myth that opposites attract? [p. 66]
- Early self-disclosure of intimate information may destroy, rather than deepen, a budding relationship? [p. 67]
- More than half of American couples who get married live together first? [p. 70]
- Women, but not men, have a sex organ whose only known function is the experiencing of sexual pleasure? [p. 74]
- The penis contains neither bone nor muscle? [p. 79]
- One woman in three and one man in seven report that they lack interest in sex? [p. 85]

Figure 4-1 How We Meet

Spouses are most likely to have met through mutual friends or self-introductions.

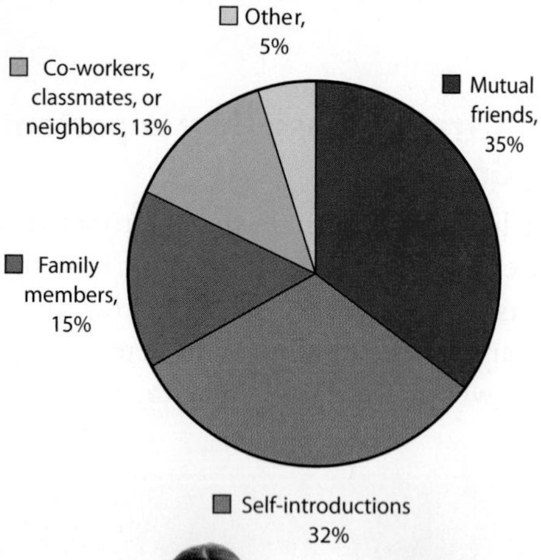

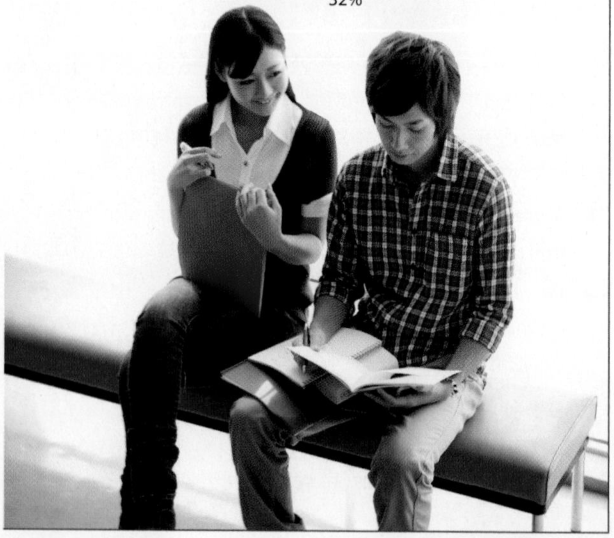

© iStockphoto.com/subman

relationships.[2] Other qualities are also important, but we may never learn about them if we are not initially attracted on the basis of physical appearance.

What do we find physically attractive? Both males and females in our culture find slenderness attractive, especially in females. The female hourglass figure and the V-tapered male physique tend to be favored.[3] Women prefer taller men, and college men tend to prefer women who are a few inches shorter.[4] The online feature "Diversity 4-1" explores the differences in preferences for mates across 37 different cultures.

diversity

Access CourseMate for HLTH at www.cengagebrain.com.

Women tend to place greater emphasis in prospective partners than men do on vocational status, earning potential, kindness, dependability, and fondness for children. Men give relatively more emphasis than do women on youth and physical attractiveness.

What do you do when you see someone who appeals to you? The online feature "Health Skills 4-1" offers suggestions for jump-starting a relationship.

health skills

Access CourseMate for HLTH at www.cengagebrain.com.

Attraction and Similarity: Do "Opposites Attract" or Do "Birds of a Feather Flock Together"?

Do not despair if, along with most of us mere mortals, you are less than exquisite in appearance. You may be saved by the *attraction–similarity hypothesis*, which expresses the tendency for people to develop romantic relationships with those who are similar to themselves in physical attractiveness rather than with James Franco or Zoe Saldana look-alikes. One motive for seeking people similar to ourselves is fear of rejection by more attractive people.

We also tend to favor people who think like we do and hold similar attitudes. We and our partners are more likely to be birds of a feather than opposites.

Intimacy

Intimacy is a trademark of healthy relationships and more than skin-deep. It involves a sense of trust, caring, acceptance, and willingness to share innermost thoughts and feelings with a partner. It is not necessary for people to be *sexually* intimate to have an emotionally intimate relationship. Nor does sexual intimacy automatically produce emotional intimacy. People who are sexually involved may still fail to touch one another's lives in emotionally intimate ways. Sometimes people share greater intimacy with their friends than with their lovers.

Consider some factors that build intimacy:

- *Knowing and liking yourself.* An initial step toward intimacy with others involves getting to know and liking yourself. Self-knowledge enables you to identify your needs and develop the security to share them.
- *Self-disclosure: You tell me and I'll tell you . . . carefully.* Opening up, or *self-disclosure,* is central to building intimate relationships. Yet, we should refrain from disclosing certain types of information, such as our sexual histories, too rapidly. People who divulge too much too soon are perceived as less mature, secure, and genuine than other people.
- *Trust and caring.* When partners trust one another, they feel secure that disclosing intimate feelings will

not lead to ridicule or rejection. Trust usually builds gradually, as partners learn whether or not it is safe to share confidences.

- *Honesty.* Honesty is a core feature of intimacy. Without honesty, partners see only one another's facades.
- *Commitment.* An intimate relationship is a commitment to work to overcome problems rather than running for the exit at the first sign of trouble.

Love, Sweet Love

As relationships deepen, feelings of attraction can turn into love. Most Americans believe that love is a prerequisite for marriage. So what is love? A leading psychologist, Robert Sternberg,[5] believes that love has three components:

1. *Intimacy.* Feelings of closeness; sharing innermost feelings.
2. *Passion.* Intense romantic or sexual desire.
3. *Commitment.* The commitment to maintain the relationship through good times and bad.

Sternberg conceptualizes love as a triangle, with each vertex representing a basic element of love (see Figure 4-2). Various combinations of the elements of love characterize different love relationships. Infatuation (passionate love) is typified by strong sexual desire, but not by intimacy and commitment. Infatuation may be a passing fancy, but now and then it leads to deeper feelings of intimacy and commitment.

Liking is akin to friendship. It consists of feelings of closeness and emotional warmth without passion or commitment. People often feel close enough to friends to share innermost feelings and thoughts.

Romantic love has passion and intimacy but lacks commitment. Romantic love may burn brightly, then flicker out. Or it may develop into a more complete love—consummate love—in which all three components blossom. Consummate love is the ideal sought by many people.

In companionate love, intimacy and commitment are strong, but passion is lacking. This form of love typifies long-term (platonic) friendships and partnerships in which passion has ebbed but a deep and abiding friendship remains.

Are you in love? How do you know? You can gather insight into your own feelings toward other people or potential partners by completing "Health Check 4-1."

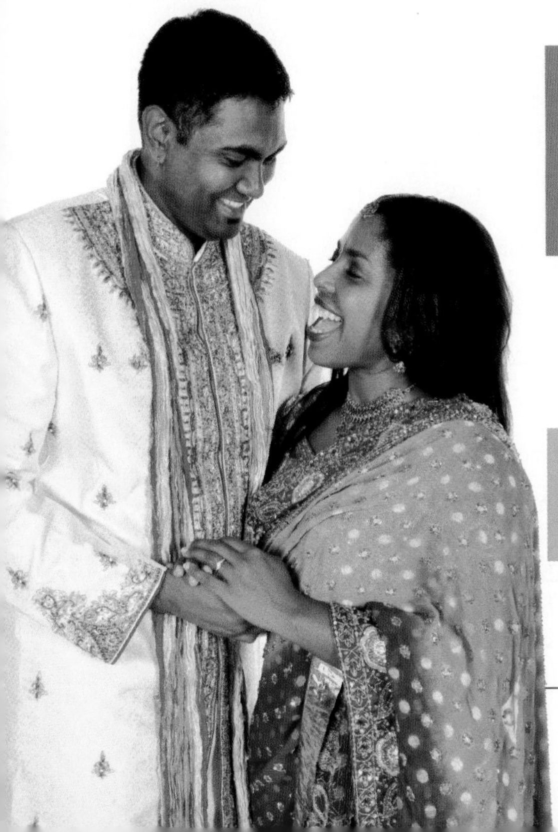

Figure 4-2 The Love Triangle

Researcher Robert Sternberg conceptualizes love as a triangle. Each vertex represents one of these basic elements of love: intimacy, passion, and commitment.

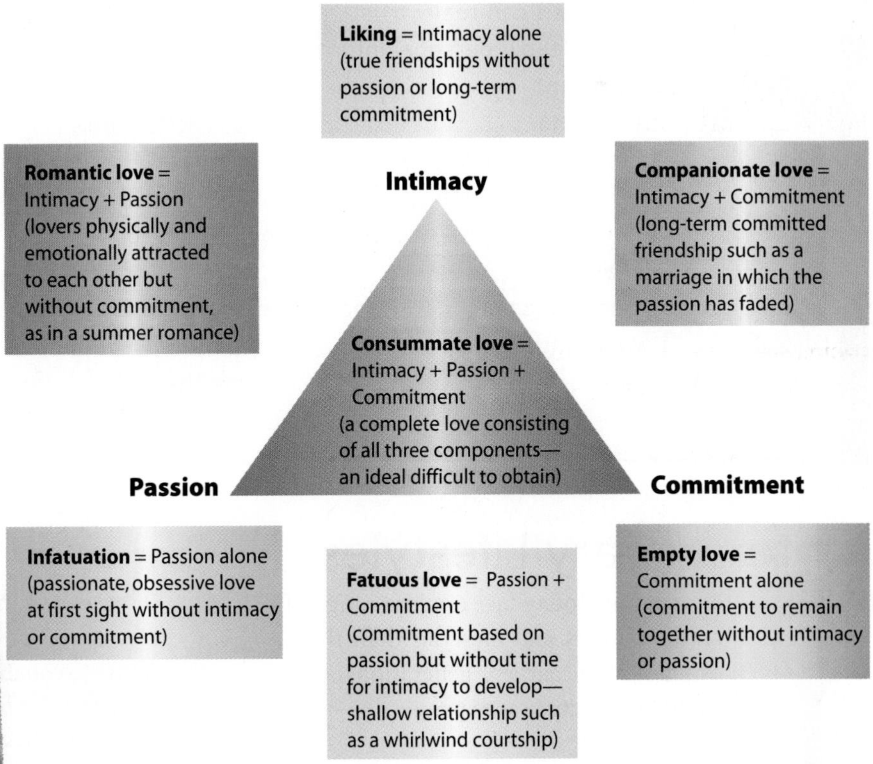
Liking = Intimacy alone (true friendships without passion or long-term commitment)
Romantic love = Intimacy + Passion (lovers physically and emotionally attracted to each other but without commitment, as in a summer romance)
Intimacy
Companionate love = Intimacy + Commitment (long-term committed friendship such as a marriage in which the passion has faded)
Consummate love = Intimacy + Passion + Commitment (a complete love consisting of all three components—an ideal difficult to obtain)
Passion
Commitment
Infatuation = Passion alone (passionate, obsessive love at first sight without intimacy or commitment)
Fatuous love = Passion + Commitment (commitment based on passion but without time for intimacy to develop—shallow relationship such as a whirlwind courtship)
Empty love = Commitment alone (commitment to remain together without intimacy or passion)

HEALTH CHECK 4-1

Has Cupid Shot His Arrow into Your Heart? The Love Scale

Which are the strongest components of your love relationship(s)? Intimacy? Passion? Commitment? Two of these? All three?

Complete the following scale by filling in the blank spaces with the other person's name. Then rate your agreement with each item by using a 9-point scale in which 1 = "not at all," 5 = "moderately," and 9 = "extremely." Use points in between to indicate intermediate levels of agreement between these values. Then check the scoring key below.

Intimacy Component

____ 1. I am actively supportive of ____________________'s well-being.
____ 2. I have a warm relationship with ____________________.
____ 3. I am able to count on ____________________ in times of need.
____ 4. ____________________ is able to count on me in times of need.
____ 5. I am willing to share myself and my possessions with ____________________.
____ 6. I receive considerable emotional support from ____________________.
____ 7. I give considerable emotional support to ____________________.
____ 8. I communicate well with ____________________.
____ 9. I value ____________________ greatly in my life.
____ 10. I feel close to ____________________.
____ 11. I have a comfortable relationship with ____________________.
____ 12. I feel that I really understand ____________________.
____ 13. I feel that ____________________ really understands me.
____ 14. I feel that I can really trust ____________________.
____ 15. I share deeply personal information about myself with ____________________.

Passion Component

____ 16. Just seeing ____________________ excites me.
____ 17. I find myself thinking about ____________________ frequently during the day.
____ 18. My relationship with ____________________. is very romantic.
____ 19. I find ____________________ to be very personally attractive.
____ 20. I idealize ____________________.
____ 21. I cannot imagine another person making me as happy as __________ does.
____ 22. I would rather be with ____________________ than anyone else.
____ 23. There is nothing more important to me than my relationship with __________.

continued

Contemporary Lifestyles

Young adults today face a wider range of sexual choices and lifestyles than those available to earlier generations. We begin our discussion as people do—with being single.

LEARNING OUTCOME 2

Discuss contemporary lifestyles, from being single to cohabitation to marriage and parenting

Being Single

An increasing number of young people choose to remain single as a way of life, not merely as a way station preceding the arrival of Mr. or Ms. Right. Being single,

___ 24. I especially like physical contact with ___________________.
___ 25. There is something almost "magical" about my relationship with ___________.
___ 26. I adore ___________________.
___ 27. I cannot imagine life without ___________________.
___ 28. My relationship with ___________________ is passionate.
___ 29. When I see romantic movies and read romantic books, I think of ___________.
___ 30. I fantasize about ___________________.

Commitment Component

___ 31. I know that I care about ___________________.
___ 32. I am committed to maintaining my relationship with ___________________.
___ 33. Because of my commitment to ___________, I would not let other people come between us.
___ 34. I have confidence in the stability of my relationship with ___________________.
___ 35. I could not let anything get in the way of my commitment to ___________________.
___ 36. I expect my love for ___________________ to last for the rest of my life.
___ 37. I will always feel a strong responsibility for ___________________.
___ 38. I view my commitment to ___________________ as a solid one.
___ 39. I cannot imagine ending my relationship with ___________________.
___ 40. I am certain of my love for ___________________.
___ 41. I view my relationship with ___________________ as permanent.
___ 42. I view my relationship with ___________________ as a good decision.
___ 43. I feel a sense of responsibility toward ___________________.
___ 44. I plan to continue my relationship with ___________________.
___ 45. Even when ___________ is hard to deal with, I remain committed to our relationship.

Source: From *The Triangle of Love: Intimacy, Passion, Commitment* by Sternberg, Robert J. Copyright 1998. Reproduced with permission of ROBERT J. STERNBERG in the format Textbook via Copyright Clearance Center.

Scoring Key

First add your scores for the items on each of the three components—Intimacy, Passion, and Commitment—and divide each total by 15. This procedure will yield an average rating for each subscale. An average rating of 5 on a particular subscale indicates a moderate level of the component represented by the subscale. A higher rating indicates a greater level. A lower rating indicates a lower level. Examining your ratings on these components will give you an idea of the degree to which you perceive your love relationship to be characterized by these three components of love. For example, you might find that passion is stronger than commitment, a pattern that is common in the early stages of an intense romantic relationship. You might find it interesting to complete the questionnaire a few months or perhaps a year or so from now to see how your feelings about your relationship change over time. You might also ask your partner to complete the scale so that the two of you can compare your respective scores. Comparing your ratings for each component with those of your partner will give you an idea of the degree to which you and your partner see your relationship in a similar way.

not married, is now the most common lifestyle among people in their 20s. Marriages may be made in heaven, but many Americans are saying heaven can wait.

Several factors contribute to the increased numbers of singles today. More young people are postponing marriage to pursue educational and career goals. Many are deciding to live together (cohabit), at least for a while, rather than get married. As career options for women have expanded, women are not as financially dependent on men as their mothers and grandmothers were. Single people face less social stigma today, and some haven't yet found the partner they want. Also, people are getting married later. The typical American man gets married at about age 28 today compared with age 23 some 50 to 60 years earlier. The typical woman gets married today at about age 26 compared with age

20 in 1960. The increased prevalence of divorce also swells the ranks of single adults.

There is no single "singles scene." Single people differ in their sexual interests and lifestyles. Most, but not all, are sexually active. Many sexually active singles practice **serial monogamy**—that is, they become involved in one exclusive relationship after another rather than having multiple sexual relationships at the same time. Some have casual relationships with "friends with benefits" (FWBs)—people with whom they have sexual relationships, not necessarily with expectations of future cohabitation or marriage—that might coexist with other relationships. Also known as *friends with privileges* or *cut friends*, these are friends who are also partners in casual sexual relationships. Friends with benefits are usually intended to meet singles' sexual needs rather than their romantic needs. Relationships with FWBs are usually intended to be temporary and to end when either partner wishes it to do so.

Cohabitation: "Darling, Would You Be My POSSLQ?"

POSSLQ? POSSLQ is the abbreviation introduced by the U.S. Bureau of the Census to refer to **cohabitation**. It stands for "People of Opposite Sex Sharing Living Quarters" and applies to unmarried heterosexual couples who live together. The majority of American young adults cohabit at some time.[6] The numbers of households consisting of cohabitors in the United States has increased more than ten-fold since 1960, from fewer than half a million couples to nearly 5 million couples today. Another half million households consist of same-sex partners. More than half of marriages are preceded by a period of cohabitation.

People cohabit for many reasons. Cohabitation is an alternative to living alone (read about loneliness and health in the online feature "Health Skills 4-2.") Partners may have deep feelings for each other but not be ready to get married. Some couples prefer cohabitation because it provides an abiding relationship without the legal entanglements of marriage. Willingness to cohabit is related to more liberal attitudes toward sexual behavior, less traditional views of marriage, and less traditional views of gender roles.

health skills

Access CourseMate for HLTH at www.cengagebrain.com.

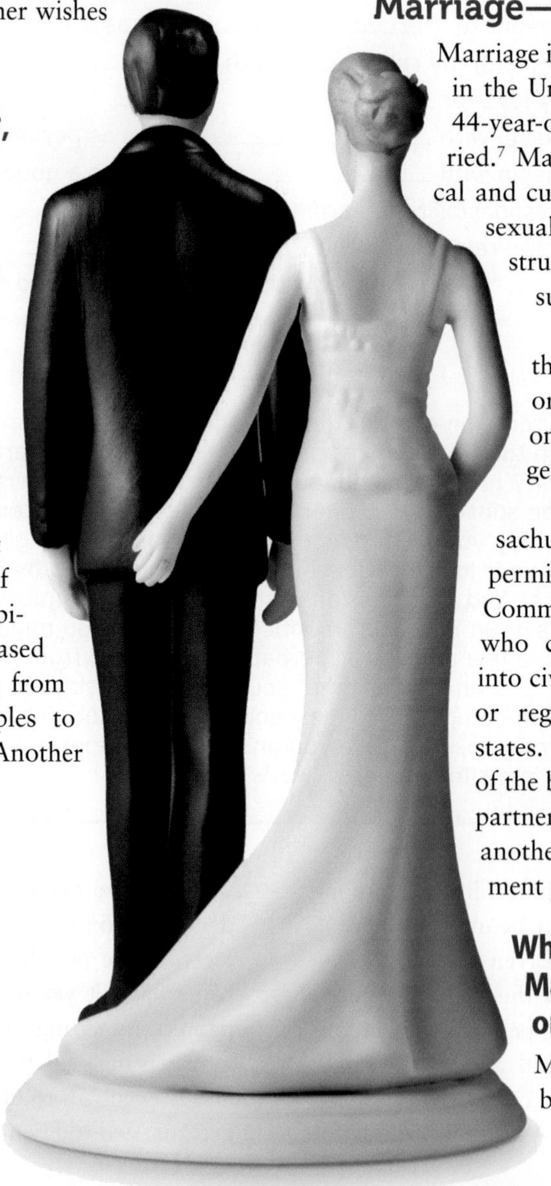
© iStockphoto.com/malerapaso

Marriage—Tying the Knot

Marriage is the most common adult lifestyle in the United States. Two of three 35- to 44-year-olds in the United States are married.[7] Marriage meets various psychological and cultural needs, such as legitimizing sexual relations and providing a social structure in which children can be supported and reared. Unless one signs a prenuptial agreement to the contrary, marriage permits the orderly transmission of wealth from one family to another and from one generation to another.

Several states, including Massachusetts, Connecticut, and Iowa, permit same-sex couples to marry. Committed gay and lesbian couples who cannot legally marry can enter into civil unions, domestic partnerships, or registered partnerships in various states. These arrangements offer many of the benefits of marriage. For example, partners can typically benefit from one another's health insurance and retirement plans.

Whom Do We Marry? Are Marriages Made in Heaven or in the Neighborhood?

Marriages are made in the neighborhood, not in heaven. We tend to marry people who are similar

serial monogamy
A pattern of involvement in one exclusive relationship after another, as opposed to engaging in multiple sexual relationships at the same time.

cohabitation
Living together as though married but without legal sanction.

to ourselves in race, ethnic background, age, level of education, religion, attitudes, and outlooks on life. The concept of "like marrying like" is termed **homogamy**. One reason for like marrying like is that people tend to select mates from the same schools and neighborhoods, and people from similar backgrounds tend to hold similar attitudes and tastes as well.[8] Storybook marriages like Cinderella's are the exception to the rule. Moreover, young adults are more often than not similar to their chosen mates in age, height, weight, personality traits, intelligence, and even in use of alcohol and tobacco.[9] Yet more than one-third of Asian Americans and Latin Americans marry outside their racial/ethnic groups, along with about 13% of African Americans and 7% of European Americans.

Parenthood

Just as people today are first getting married in their later 20s or 30s, so too are they delaying parenthood.[10] Many women do not bear children until they are in their 30s, some in their 40s. Becoming a parent is a major life event that requires changes in nearly every sphere of life: personal, social, and financial. In fact, many people no longer think of parenthood as a necessary part of marriage or a relationship.[11] Most couples today report that they choose to have children for reasons of personal happiness or fulfillment, not out of a sense of obligation.

Single Parenthood

The public image of the single parent is probably quite distorted. In many ways, single parents have a great deal in common with cohabiting or married parents. There are nearly 17 million single parents in the United States today, and they are rearing about 25 million children—more than one child in four.[12] Five of six single parents are mothers, and one of six is a father. Nearly half are separated or divorced, and about one-third have never married. Four single mothers out of five are in the workforce, and half of them work full time. Ninety percent of single fathers also work. Only one single mother in four or five receives public assistance.

Single parents must usually survive on one income. When it comes down to getting to work and getting the children to school, they learn quickly that if something needs to get done, they have to do it for themselves. Children in single-parent families tend to learn to assume responsibilities earlier than children in two-parent families. The upside is that they develop maturity more quickly.

Satisfaction and Dissatisfaction in Relationships

LEARNING OUTCOME 3

Discuss factors in unhealthy relationships

The quality of our intimate relationships is linked to our physical and psychological health; not surprisingly, people in more satisfying personal relationships tend to report better health than those in troubled relationships.[13] Intimacy, which is fueled by trust, honesty, and the sharing of innermost feelings, is strongly connected with satisfaction in relationships.[14] So is the psychological support of one's spouse (read Diversity 4-2 on the next page). Satisfaction with one's career is positively correlated with satisfaction in relationships, and both forms of satisfaction are related to general satisfaction with life.[15]

Jealousy: "The Green-Eyed Monster"?

> O! beware, my lord, of jealousy;
> It is the green-ey'd monster . . .
>
> —William Shakespeare, *Othello*

Thus was Othello, the Moor of Venice, warned of jealousy in the Shakespearean play that bears his name. Yet, Othello could not control his feelings and ended up killing his beloved wife, Desdemona.

Lovers can become jealous when others show interest in their partners or when their partners show interest in someone else. Jealousy damages relationships by causing loss of affection, insecurity and rejection, and mistrust of a person's partner and potential rivals. Jealousy is one of the commonly mentioned reasons relationships fail. On a personal level, jealousy is associated with loss of self-esteem, anxiety, and depression. In extreme cases, jealousy can give rise to partner abuse, suicide, or even, as with Othello, murder.

Ironically, milder forms of jealousy may serve a positive function by revealing how much one cares

homogamy
The practice of marrying people who are similar in social background and standing. (From Greek roots meaning "same" [homos] *and "marriage"* [gamos].*)*

DIVERSITY 4-2

Gay and Lesbian Relationships: On Household Chores and Power

When it comes to factors determining relationship satisfaction in heterosexual and homosexual couples, the interesting finding is that we are hard pressed to find differences. Both heterosexual and homosexual couples are more satisfied when they receive social support from their partners, when there is sharing of power in the relationship, when they fight fair, and when they perceive their partners to be committed to the relationship.[16] One difference that stands out favors the stability of homosexual couples: They tend to distribute household chores evenly, rather than based on gender-role expectations and stereotypes.[17] But there are differences that favor stability in the relationships of heterosexual couples: They are more likely to have the support of their families and less likely to be stigmatized by society at large.

for one's partner. For this reason, some investigators distinguish between "normal jealousy," which reflects occasional self-doubts and the belief that one's partner is attractive, and "obsessional jealousy," in which the individual, like Othello, is consumed by his or her fears of interference in the relationship.[18]

Many lovers play jealousy games. They let their partners know that they are attracted to other people. They flirt openly or manufacture tales to make their partners pay more attention to them, to test the relationship, to inflict pain, or to take revenge for a partner's disloyalty. But such "games" can be hurtful and contribute to dissatisfaction in a relationship.

Drawing to the Close of a Relationship

Failure to share power, failure to provide emotional support, reluctance to discuss innermost feelings, unjustified jealousy—these and other negative factors cause dissatisfaction and can lead to the end of a relationship. Relationships tend to draw to a close when the partners glean little satisfaction from them and when the barriers to breaking up are low—that is, when the social, religious, and financial constraints are manageable. Troubled relationships tumble down especially when alternate partners are available.

Some couples prevent a deteriorating relationship from ending by reinvesting in it. Troubled relationships can be salvaged and made more satisfying when the couple works on their differences, sometimes with the help of a professional counselor. But at other times the swan song of a relationship is the most healthful outcome. When people are incompatible—and when efforts to preserve the relationship have failed—ending can offer each partner a chance to find satisfaction with someone else.

Divorce: Breaking Bonds

Between 40% and 50% of American marriages end in divorce. The high number of divorces has been attributed to such factors as the relaxation of legal restrictions on divorce, the increased economic independence of women, and the widespread view of marriage as an alterable condition—even though most people who get married intend to remain married at the time. Moreover, Americans today hold high expectations for marriage; that is, they expect marriage to be personally fulfilling, not just serve as a basis for raising children. The most common reasons given for a divorce are problems in communication and lack of understanding. In times past, the reason was more likely to be lack of financial support.

Divorce is often associated with financial difficulties and health problems such as anxiety, depression, physical ailments, and even suicide. When a household splits, the resources available often cannot maintain the earlier standard of living for both partners. Divorced mothers often face the sole responsibility for rearing the children and the need to increase their incomes to make ends meet. Single mothers—including divorced and never-married mothers—are more likely to feel depressed and dissatisfied with life than are single fathers or married parents.

Most divorced people eventually remarry. But remarriages are even more likely than first marriages to end in divorce. People who get divorced in the first place may be less inclined than other people to persist in a troubled marriage.

Children of Divorce

Children suffer in divorce as well as in troubled marriages.[19] Marital problems can spill over into parent–child relations and affect the children's emotional health. Boys tend to have more trouble adjusting to marital conflict or divorce, as shown by conduct problems at school and increased anxiety and dependence.

Should bickering parents remain together for the sake of the children? The answer seems to depend on how they behave in front of the children. Parental fighting in front of the children is linked to the same kinds of problems children experience when their parents are separated or divorced.[20] Moreover, exposure to marital conflict is a source of continuing stress, which over time may weaken children's immune systems, leaving them more vulnerable to health-related problems. Read more about resolving conflicts in relationships in the online feature "Health Skills 4-3."

health skills

Access CourseMate for HLTH at www.cengagebrain.com.

Sexual Anatomy and Physiology

Our sexual anatomy includes external and internal organs and structures that bring us pleasure and provide the biological means of reproduction. (If reproduction were a painful or unpleasant process, none of us might be here to tell the story.) Here we take a quick tour of our sexual anatomy and functioning.

LEARNING OUTCOME 4

Describe female and male sexual anatomy and related health issues

Female Sexual Anatomy

The external reproductive structures of the female are termed the pudendum, or **vulva**. The vulva consists of the *mons veneris*, the *labia majora* and *minora* (major and minor lips), the *clitoris*, and the vaginal opening (see Figure 4-3, part A).

The adjustment of children in divorced families can be enhanced when parents

- set aside their differences long enough to agree upon child-rearing practices.
- encourage each other to continue to play important roles in their children's lives.
- avoid saying negative things about each other in front of the children.

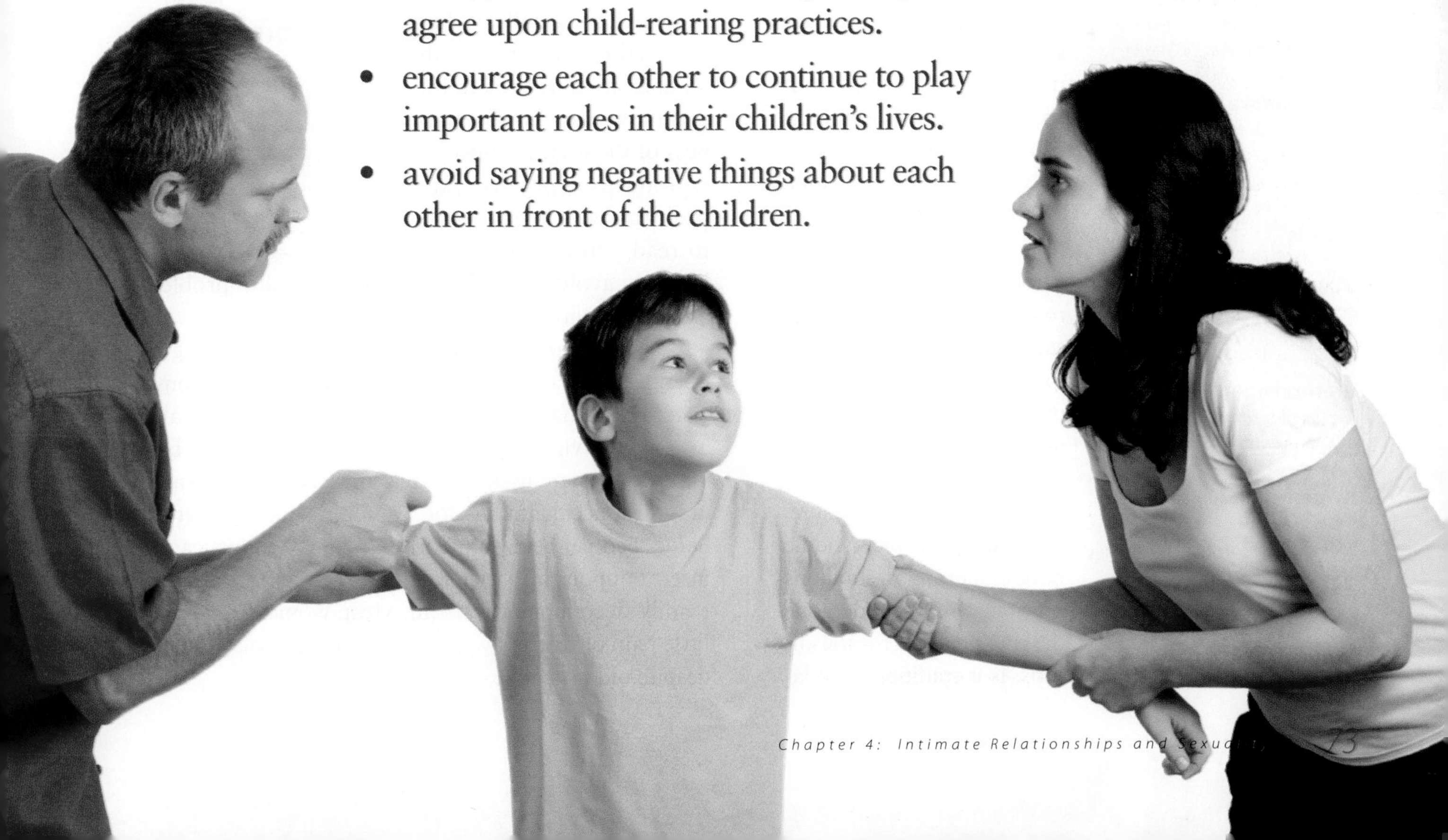

Figure 4-3 Female Sexual Organs

A. External organs **B. Internal organs**

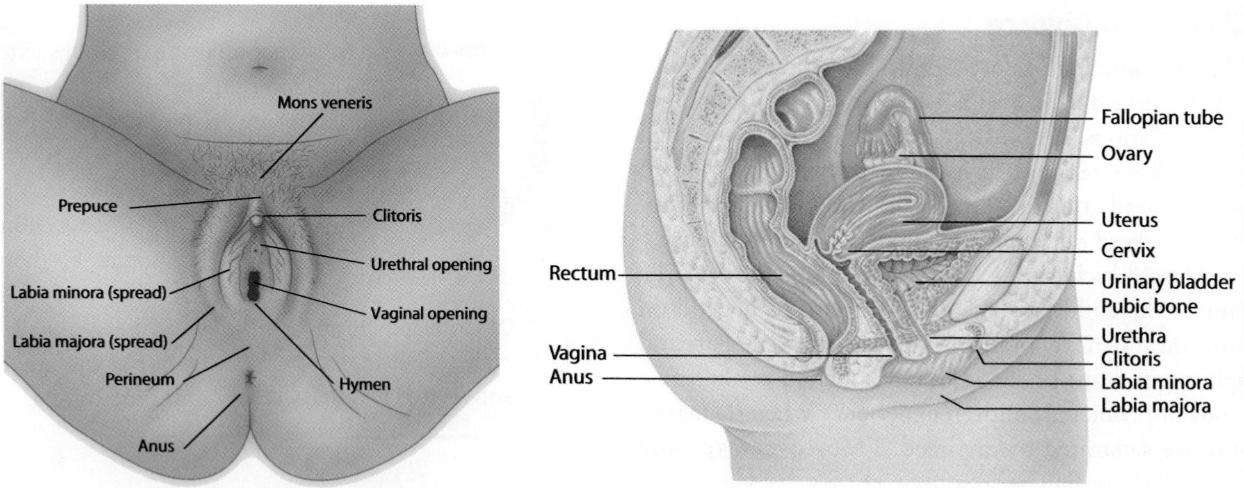

Part A: The external female reproductive organs, with the labia opened to reveal the urethral and vaginal openings.

Part B: The internal sexual organs that make up the female reproductive system include the vagina, uterus, and ovaries.

The *mons veneris* consists of fatty tissue that covers the joint of the pubic bones in front of the body, below the abdomen and above the clitoris. The mons cushions a woman's body during sexual intercourse. The **labia majora** and **labia minora** surround the urethral and vaginal openings and are sensitive to sexual stimulation. The body of the **clitoris**, termed the *clitoral shaft*, contains spongy masses that fill with blood and become enlarged or erect in response to sexual stimulation. The clitoral *glans* is a smooth, round knob or lump of tissue that is highly sensitive to touch. The clitoris is a unique sex organ. It serves no known purpose other than enabling women to experience sexual pleasure. In Africa and the Middle East, hundreds of millions of women have undergone the ritual removal of the clitoris. Is it tradition, mutilation, or both? Decide for yourself after reading the online feature "Diversity 4-3."

vulva
The external sexual structures of the female.

labia majora
Large folds of skin that run downward from the mons along the sides of the vulva. (Latin for "large lips" or "major lips.")

labia minora
Hairless, light-colored membranes, located between the labia majora. (Latin for "small lips" or "minor lips.")

clitoris
A female sex organ consisting of a shaft and glans located above the urethral opening. It is extremely sensitive to sexual sensations.

urethral opening
The opening through which urine passes from the female's body.

hymen
A fold of tissue across the vaginal opening that is usually present at birth and remains at least partly intact until a woman engages in coitus. (Greek for "membrane.")

diversity
Access CourseMate for HLTH at www.cengagebrain.com.

Urine passes from the female body through the **urethral opening**, which is connected by a short tube called the *urethra* to the urinary bladder (see Figure 4-3, part B), where urine collects. In women, the urethral opening, urethra, and bladder are unrelated to the reproductive system; however, the closeness of the urethral opening to the reproductive organs can create problems with infection. Go online to read "Prevention 4-1" to learn how to avoid infection and other health problems associated with the female anatomy.

prevention
Access CourseMate for HLTH at www.cengagebrain.com.

The **hymen** is a fold of tissue across the vaginal opening. It may remain partly intact until a woman becomes sexually active. Its presence has been taken as proof of virginity. However, some women are born with incomplete hymens, while other women's hymens are torn accidentally—for example, during exercise. Some people believe incorrectly that virgins cannot insert tampons into their vaginas, but most hymens will readily accommodate them. Most women experience little pain or distress when they become sexually active, despite old horror stories.

The internal reproductive organs of the female include the innermost parts of the **vagina**, the *cervix*, the *uterus*, the *ovaries*, and the *fallopian tubes* (see Figure 4-3, part B). These structures make up the woman's internal reproductive system. Women are advised to have an internal pelvic examination at least once a year by the time they reach their late teens, or earlier if they have become sexually active (read more in the online feature "Prevention 4-2").

prevention

Access CourseMate for HLTH at www.cengagebrain.com.

Menstrual flow passes out of the body from the uterus through the vagina. The penis is contained within the vagina during sexual activity. When at rest, the walls of the vagina touch like a deflated balloon, but the vagina expands during sexual arousal and to accommodate a baby's head and shoulders during childbirth.

The vaginal walls secrete substances that help maintain the vagina's normal acidity (pH 4.0 to 5.0). Douching or spraying may alter the natural chemical balance of the vagina, which can increase the risk of vaginal infections. Feminine deodorant sprays can irritate the vagina and evoke allergic reactions. The normal, healthy vagina cleanses itself through regular chemical secretions, evidenced by a mild white or yellowish discharge.

The **cervix** is the lower end of the uterus. Following intercourse, sperm pass from the vagina to the uterus through the cervical canal. During childbirth, babies pass from the uterus to the vagina through the same opening.

The **uterus**, or womb, is the pear-shaped organ in which a fertilized egg cell implants and develops until birth. The inner layer of the uterus is called the **endometrium**. Endometrial tissue is discharged through the cervix and vagina during menstruation. In some women, endometrial tissue may also grow in the abdominal cavity or elsewhere in the reproductive system. This condition, called *endometriosis*, is most commonly characterized by menstrual pain. If left untreated, endometriosis may lead to infertility.

One woman in three in the United States has a **hysterectomy** by the age of 60, making it the second most commonly performed operation in the country. (Cesarean sections are the most common.) A hysterectomy may be performed when a woman develops a disease that causes pain or excessive uterine bleeding or cancer of the uterus, ovaries, or cervix. A complete hysterectomy is the surgical removal of the ovaries, fallopian tubes, cervix, and uterus. It is usually performed to reduce the risk of cancer spreading throughout the reproductive system. A partial hysterectomy removes the uterus but spares the ovaries and fallopian tubes, allowing the woman to continue to ovulate and produce female sex hormones.

The hysterectomy has become steeped in controversy. In many cases, less radical medical interventions might successfully treat the problem. Women whose physicians recommend a hysterectomy are advised to seek a second opinion before proceeding.

The two fallopian tubes extend from the upper end of the uterus toward the almond-shaped **ovaries** (see Figure 4-3, part B). Egg cells (ova) pass through the fallopian tubes to the uterus. Two ovaries lie on either side of the uterus. The ovaries produce egg cells and the female sex hormones estrogen and progesterone. During a woman's reproductive years, about one egg cell per month is released by its follicle for possible fertilization. Estrogen promotes the changes of puberty and regulates the menstrual cycle.

The Breasts

In some cultures, the breasts are just a means for feeding infants. In Western culture, however, breasts have also achieved erotic significance. In fact, a woman's self-esteem may become linked to her feelings about her bustline.

The breasts contain milk-producing **mammary glands**. Each gland opens at the nipple through its own duct. The mammary glands are separated by soft, fatty tissue. The amount of fatty tissue, not the amount of glandular tissue, determines the size of the breasts. Women vary little in their amount of glandular tissue. Thus, breast size does not determine the quantity of milk that can be produced.

The nipple contains smooth muscle fibers that make it become erect when they contract. Nipples are also richly endowed with

vagina
The tubular female sex organ that contains the penis during sexual intercourse and through which a baby is born. (Latin for "sheath.")

cervix
The lower end of the uterus. (Latin for "neck.")

uterus
The organ in which a fertilized ovum implants and develops until birth. Also called the womb.

endometrium
The innermost layer of the uterus. (From Latin and Greek roots meaning "within the uterus.")

hysterectomy
Surgical removal of the uterus.

ovaries
Almond-shaped organs that produce ova and the hormones estrogen and progesterone.

mammary glands
Milk-secreting glands. (From the Latin mamma, which means both "breast" and "mother.")

nerve endings, so that stimulation of the nipples heightens sexual arousal for many women.

The Menstrual Cycle

Menstruation is the cyclical bleeding that stems from shedding of the uterine lining (endometrium). Menstruation takes place when an egg cell (ovum) goes unfertilized. The word *menstruation* derives from the Latin *mensis*, meaning "month." The menstrual cycle averages 28 days in length.

The menstrual cycle is divided into four phases (see Figure 4-4). The first phase, or **proliferative phase**, begins with the end of menstruation and lasts 9 or 10 days in a 28-day cycle. Low levels of estrogen and progesterone are circulating in the blood as menstruation draws to an end. When the hypothalamus senses a low level of estrogen in the blood, it triggers the pituitary gland to release follicle-stimulating hormone (FSH). When FSH reaches the ovaries, it stimulates some follicles to mature. As the follicles ripen, they produce estrogen, which further ripens ova within their follicles. During this phase, the endometrium develops, or "proliferates."

The second phase is the **ovulatory phase. Ovulation** is triggered by peak estrogen levels. The hypothalamus detects these estrogen levels and triggers the pituitary to release ample amounts of FSH and *luteinizing hormone (LH)*. The surge of LH triggers ovulation, which usually begins 12 to 24 hours after the peaking of LH. A mature ovum is released *near* a fallopian tube, not *into* a fallopian tube. If two ova are released during ovulation and both are fertilized, fraternal (nonidentical) twins develop. Identical twins develop when one fertilized ovum divides into two separate embryos.

A woman's *basal body temperature (BBT)*, taken by oral or rectal thermometer, dips slightly at ovulation (see Figure 4-5) and rises by about 1° F on the day after. Many women use BBT to help them conceive or avoid conceiving. Some women have discomfort or cramping during ovulation, termed *mittelschmerz.* Mittelschmerz is sometimes confused with appendicitis. However, Mittelschmerz may occur on either side of the abdomen, depending on which ovary is releasing an egg cell, whereas a ruptured appendix always hurts on the right side.

The third phase of the cycle, called the **secretory phase** or *luteal phase*, begins right after ovulation and continues through the beginning of the next cycle. The term *luteal phase* is derived from the follicle that

proliferative phase
The first phase of the menstrual cycle, which begins with the end of menstruation and lasts about 9 or 10 days. During this phase, the endometrium proliferates.

ovulatory phase
The second stage of the menstrual cycle, during which a follicle ruptures and releases a mature ovum.

ovulation
The release of an ovum from an ovary.

secretory phase
The third phase of the menstrual cycle, which follows ovulation. Also referred to as the luteal phase, after the corpus luteum, which begins to secrete large amounts of progesterone and estrogen following ovulation.

Figure 4-4 The Four Phases of the Menstrual Cycle

The menstrual cycle consists of proliferative, ovulatory, secretory (luteal), and menstrual phases.

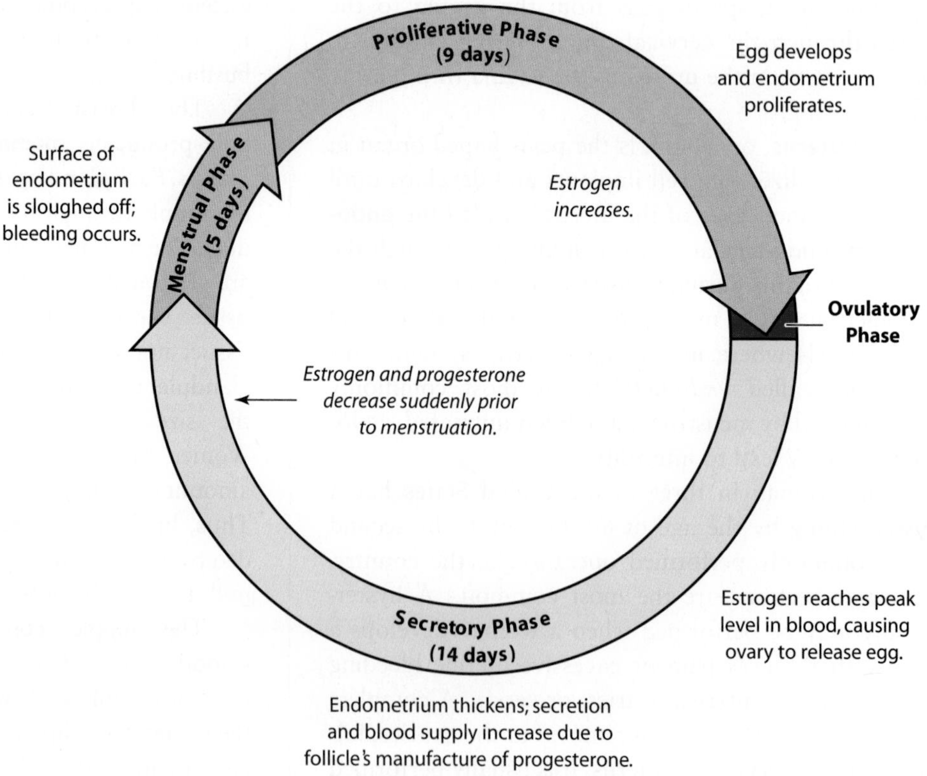
Proliferative Phase
(9 days)
Egg develops and endometrium proliferates.
Surface of endometrium is sloughed off; bleeding occurs.
Menstrual Phase
(5 days)
Estrogen increases.
Ovulatory Phase
Estrogen and progesterone decrease suddenly prior to menstruation.
Secretory Phase
(14 days)
Estrogen reaches peak level in blood, causing ovary to release egg.
Endometrium thickens; secretion and blood supply increase due to follicle's manufacture of progesterone.

Figure 4-5 Physiological Changes over the Course of the Menstrual Cycle

This illustration shows five categories of biological changes: (a) changes in the development of the lining of the uterus (endometrium), (b) changes in the follicle, (c) changes in the levels of ovarian hormones in the blood, (d) changes in the levels of pituitary hormones in the blood, and (e) changes in basal body temperature. Note the dip in temperature associated with ovulation.

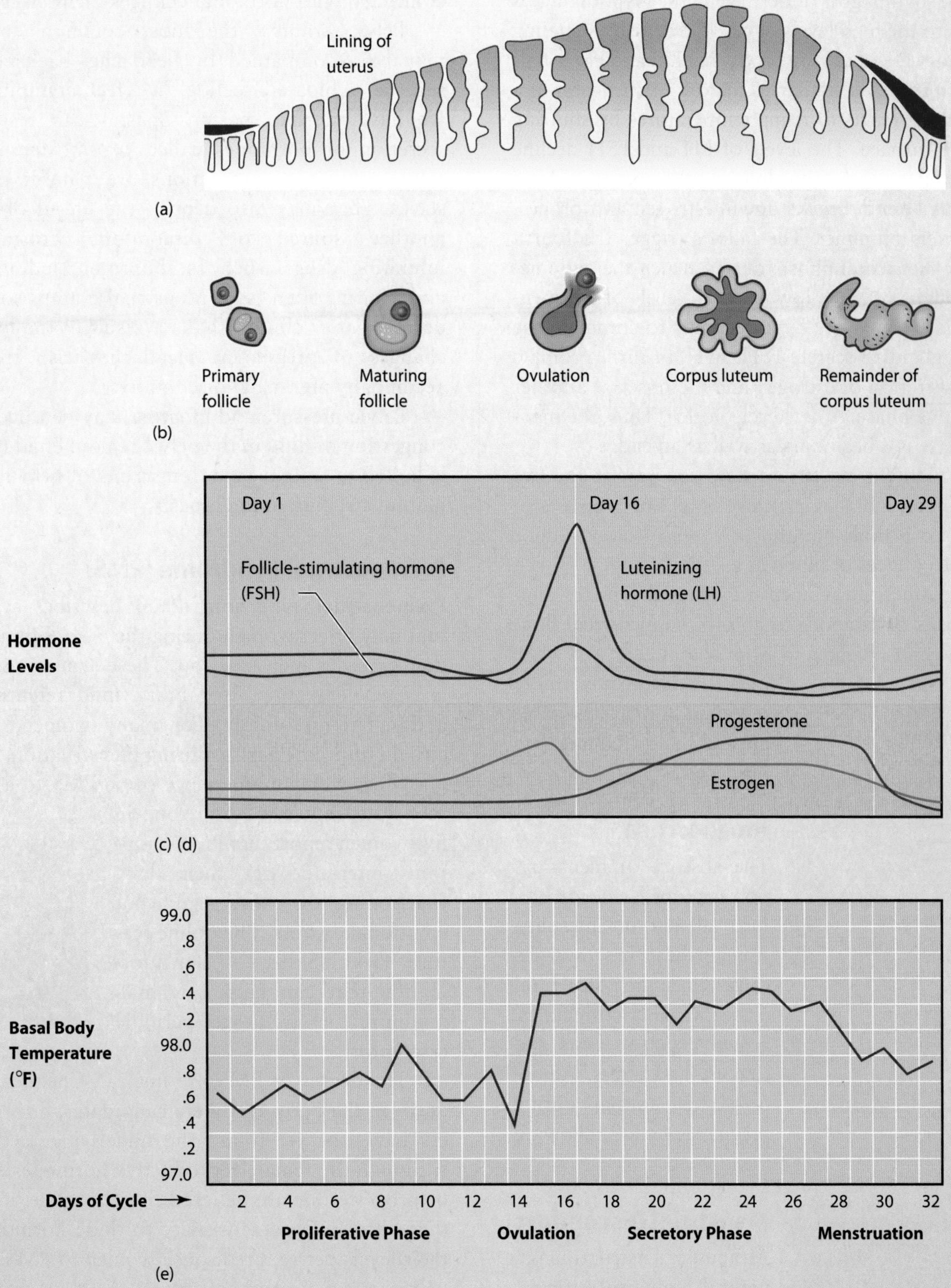

releases the ovum, which is called the **corpus luteum**. LH signals the corpus luteum to produce large amounts of progesterone and estrogen. Progesterone causes the endometrium to thicken to support an embryo. Levels of these hormones peak at around day 20 or 21 of the cycle.

If the ovum goes unfertilized, the hypothalamus responds to the high levels of progesterone by signaling the pituitary gland to stop producing LH and FSH. This feedback process is similar to that of a thermostat in a house, which reacts to rising temperatures by shutting down the furnace. The levels of LH and FSH decline rapidly, causing the corpus luteum to decompose. After the corpus luteum breaks down, estrogen and progesterone levels plummet. The falloffs trigger the fourth phase, or **menstrual phase**, during which the endometrium sloughs off. The low estrogen levels of the menstrual phase signal the hypothalamus to stimulate the pituitary gland to secrete FSH. FSH, in turn, prompts ovarian secretion of estrogen and the onset of another proliferative phase. A new cycle begins. Thus, the menstrual phase is a beginning as well as an end.

Although the menstrual flow can persist for five days or more, most women lose only 2 or 3 ounces of blood (4 to 6 tablespoonfuls). A typical blood donor donates 16 ounces of blood at a sitting.

Most American women use external sanitary napkins or pads or tampons to absorb the menstrual flow. Tampons enable women to swim without concern while menstruating, to wear more revealing or comfortable apparel, and to feel less burdened.

corpus luteum
The follicle that has released an ovum and then produces copious amounts of progesterone and estrogen during the luteal phase of a woman's cycle. (From Latin roots meaning "yellow body.")

menstrual phase
The fourth phase of the menstrual cycle, during which the endometrium is sloughed off in the menstrual flow.

premenstrual syndrome (PMS)
A combination of physical and psychological symptoms (e.g., anxiety, depression, irritability, weight gain from fluid retention, and abdominal discomfort) that regularly afflicts many women during the 4- to 6-day interval that precedes their menses each month.

Amenorrhea

The absence of menstruation is termed *amenorrhea*. It is a sign of infertility. Amenorrhea has various causes, including structural or hormonal abnormalities, growths such as cysts and tumors, and stress. Amenorrhea is normal during pregnancy and following menopause.

Menstrual Discomfort

Although menstruation is a natural biological process, the majority of women experience at least occasional mild discomfort prior to or during menstruation. Pain or discomfort during menstruation, called *dysmenorrhea*, is the most common menstrual problem. Dysmenorrhea may be caused by such problems as endometriosis, pelvic inflammatory disease, and ovarian cysts. Some discomfort is connected with hormonal changes themselves.

Pelvic cramps, the most common complaint, may be accompanied by headache, backache, nausea, or a bloated feeling. We feel cramping when we have uterine spasms. Spasms can result from secretion of hormones called *prostaglandins*. Powerful, persistent contractions are painful in themselves. They may also deprive the uterus of oxygen, another source of discomfort. Prostaglandin-inhibiting drugs, such as ibuprofen, indomethacin, and aspirin, often help. Menstrual cramps sometimes decrease after childbirth, as a result of the hormonal changes of pregnancy. Headaches also frequently accompany menstrual discomfort.

Pelvic pressure and bloating may be traced to the congestion of fluid in the pelvic region. Fluid retention is linked to weight gain, sensations of heaviness, and painful swelling of the breasts.

Premenstrual Syndrome (PMS)

Premenstrual syndrome (PMS) describes symptoms that may affect women during the 4- to 6-day interval that precedes menstruation. These symptoms include anxiety, depression, irritability, fluid retention, and abdominal discomfort. For many women, premenstrual symptoms persist during menstruation.

Most women experience some PMS to a mild to moderate degree.[21] About one in five women report that PMS symptoms interfere with their daily functioning or cause significant emotional distress. The online feature "Health Skills 4-4" has information that can help a woman minimize or eradicate periodic discomfort.

health skills

Access CourseMate for HLTH at www.cengagebrain.com.

The causes of PMS are unclear. Chemical imbalances in the body are likely candidates, but researchers have not yet found the underlying mechanism. Although the female reproductive hormones estrogen or progesterone are believed to play a role, it may be that differences in sensitivity to these hormones, not their levels per se, predispose women to PMS.[22] Irregularities in how the brain uses the neurotransmitter serotonin may also be involved.

Menopause

As women age, their menstrual cycles shorten and become irregular. **Menopause**, or the "change of life," is the cessation of menstruation. Menopause most commonly occurs in the 50s, plus or minus a few years. The ovaries no longer ripen egg cells or secrete estrogen and progesterone.

Perimenopause refers to the beginning of menopause and is usually characterized by 3 to 11 months of amenorrhea (lack of menstruation) or irregular periods. Perimenopause ends with menopause. Menopause is a specific event in a longer-term process known as the *climacteric* (critical period), which generally refers to the gradual decline in the reproductive capacity of the ovaries. The climacteric lasts for about 15 years, from ages 45 to 60 or so. After the age of 35 or so, the menstrual cycles of many women shorten. By the end of her 40s, a woman's cycles often become erratic, with some periods close together and others missed.

Low estrogen levels may cause unpleasant symptoms, such as night sweats, hot flashes (suddenly feeling hot), and hot flushes (suddenly looking reddened). Hot flashes and flushes may alternate with cold sweats, in which a woman suddenly feels cold and clammy. Hot flashes and flushes stem largely from "waves" of dilation of blood vessels across the face and upper body. Other signs of estrogen deficiency include dizziness, headaches, pains in the joints, tingling in the hands or feet, burning or itchy skin, and heart palpitations. The skin also becomes drier. There is some loss of breast tissue, and vaginal lubrication decreases. Women may also awaken more frequently at night and have difficulty returning to sleep.

Long-term estrogen deficiency leads to porosity and brittleness of the bones, a condition called *osteoporosis*. Bones break more easily, and some women develop a so-called dowager's hump. The risk of serious fractures, especially of the hip, increases. Many older women never recover from these fractures. Estrogen deficiency also can impair mental functioning and feelings of well-being.

Some women who experience severe physical symptoms have been helped by *hormone-replacement therapy (HRT)*. HRT typically consists of synthetic estrogen and progesterone that offset the losses of their natural counterparts. HRT may help reduce hot flushes and other symptoms of menopause.

The use of HRT is controversial. Although it has helped many menopausal women, a large-scale study of more than 16,000 postmenopausal women ages 50 to 79 reported that exposure to a combination of estrogen and progestin appeared to increase the risk of breast cancer.[23] (Progestin is used along with estrogen because estrogen alone exposes women to the risk of uterine cancer.) Consequently, the number of women using HRT has dropped sharply.

Progestin alone appears to prevent or lessen the severity of hot flashes in many women. Selective serotonin reuptake inhibitors (SSRIs), such as Effexor, Paxil, and Prozac, which are drugs used to treat depression, may also help control hot flashes.

Did You Know That... The penis contains neither bone nor muscle.

Male Sexual Anatomy

The external male reproductive organs include the penis and the scrotum (see Figure 4-6 on the next page). The penis, like the vagina, is the sex organ used in sexual intercourse. Unlike the vagina, however, urine also passes through the penis. Both semen and urine pass out of the penis through the urethral opening.

In many mammals, including dogs, bones stiffen the penis to facilitate copulation. But despite the slang term "boner," the human penis contains no bones. Nor, despite another slang term "muscle," does the penis contain muscle tissue. Instead, the penis contains spongy material that fills with blood and stiffens, resulting in erection. The urethra is connected to the bladder, which is unrelated to reproduction, and to those parts of the reproductive system that transport semen.

The glans of the penis, like the clitoral glans, is extremely sensitive to sexual stimulation. So is the corona, or coronal ridge, that separates the glans (tip) from the body of the penis.

The body of the penis is called the penile *shaft*. Some skin of the penis folds over to partially cover the glans. This covering is the foreskin. It covers part or all of the penile glans just as the clitoral prepuce (hood) covers the clitoral shaft. In the male, as in the female, a gritty substance called *smegma* may accumulate below the prepuce, causing the foreskin to adhere to the glans.

Men, like women, are subject to bladder and urethral inflammations, which are generally referred to

menopause
The cessation of menstruation.

perimenopause
The beginning of menopause, as characterized by 3 to 11 months of amenorrhea or irregular periods.

Figure 4-6 The Male Reproductive System

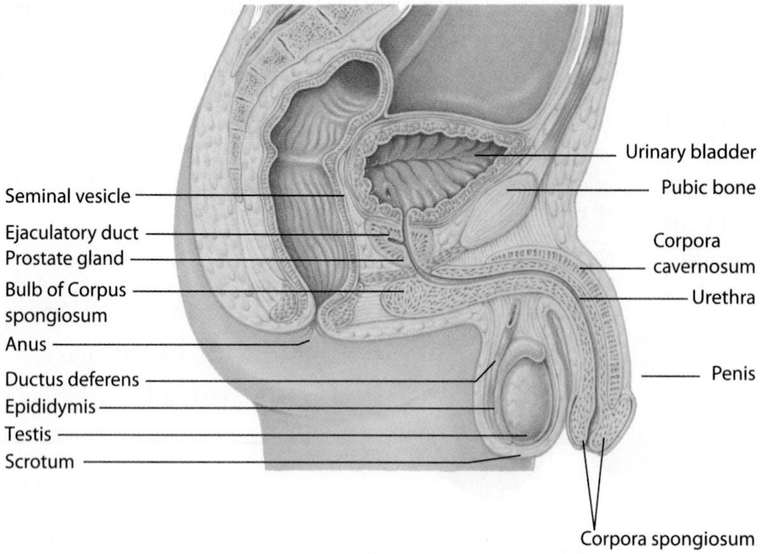

prevention

Access CourseMate for HLTH at www.cengagebrain.com.

as *urethritis*. Symptoms include frequent urination (urinary frequency), a strong need to urinate (urinary urgency), burning urination, and a discharge from the penis. The discharge may dry on the urethral opening so that it must be wiped away before urinating. The urethra also may become constricted when it is inflamed, slowing or halting urination. Preventive measures for urethritis parallel those suggested for cystitis (see online "Prevention 4-1").

The scrotum is a pouch of loose skin consisting of two compartments that hold the testes. Sperm production is optimal at a temperature slightly cooler than the 98.6° F that is desirable for most of the body. Typical scrotal temperature is 5° to 6° lower than body temperature. Thus, the scrotum permits the testes to escape the higher body heat, especially in warm weather.

epididymis
A tube that lies against the back wall of each testicle and serves as a storage facility for sperm. (From Greek roots meaning "upon testicles.")

vas deferens
A tube that conducts sperm from the testicle to the ejaculatory duct of the penis. (From Latin roots meaning "a vessel" that "carries down.")

prostate gland
The gland that lies beneath the bladder and secretes prostatic fluid, which gives semen its characteristic odor and texture.

The testes (also called *testicles*) are analogous to the ovaries. They secrete sex hormones and produce *germ cells*. The sex hormones are androgens, and the germ cells are sperm. The most important androgen is testosterone, which stimulates prenatal differentiation of male sex organs, sperm production, and development of secondary sex characteristics, such as the beard, the deepened voice, and the muscle mass. In contrast to the dramatic changes in hormone levels that occur in women during the phases of the menstrual cycle, in men the hypothalamus, pituitary gland, and testes keep blood testosterone levels at a more or less even level.

The same pituitary hormones that regulate the ovaries—FSH and LH—also regulate the testes. FSH regulates the production of sperm, and LH stimulates the secretion of testosterone. Low testosterone levels signal the hypothalamus to secrete a releasing hormone. Like dominoes falling in line, the releasing hormone causes the pituitary gland to secrete LH, which in turn stimulates the testes (see Figure 4-7).

The forerunners of sperm cells contain 46 chromosomes, including one X and one Y sex chromosome. Each of these divides into two cells with 23 chromosomes. Half have X sex chromosomes, and half have Y sex chromosomes. All ova have X sex chromosomes. Whereas ova are almost visible, sperm cells are about 1/5,000 of an inch long, one of the smallest cells in the body. The testes churn out some 1,000 sperm per second—several billion a year.

Sperm proceed through a maze of ducts that converge in a single tube called the **epididymis**. The epididymis lies against the back wall of each testis and serves as a storage facility. Sperm continue to mature in the epididymis. Each epididymis empties into a **vas deferens**, a thin tube about 16 inches long. The tube leaves the scrotum, follows a path up into the abdominal cavity, and then loops back along the surface of the bladder.

At the base of the bladder, each vas deferens joins a seminal vesicle to form a short ejaculatory duct that runs through the prostate gland. In the prostate, the ejaculatory duct opens into the urethra, which leads to the tip of the penis. The urethra carries sperm and urine out through the penis, but normally not at the same time.

The **prostate gland** lies beneath the bladder and is chestnut-like in shape and size. The prostate gland secretes prostatic fluid, which combines with sperm

Figure 4-7 Hormonal Control of the Testes

Several glands—the hypothalamus, the pituitary gland, and the testes—keep blood testosterone levels at a more or less constant level. Low testosterone levels signal the hypothalamus to secrete LH-releasing hormone (LH-RH). Like dominoes falling in line, LH-RH causes the pituitary gland to secrete LH, which in turn stimulates the testes to release testosterone into the blood. Follicle-stimulating hormone releasing hormone (FSH-RH) from the hypothalamus causes the pituitary to secrete FSH, which in turn causes the testes to produce sperm cells.

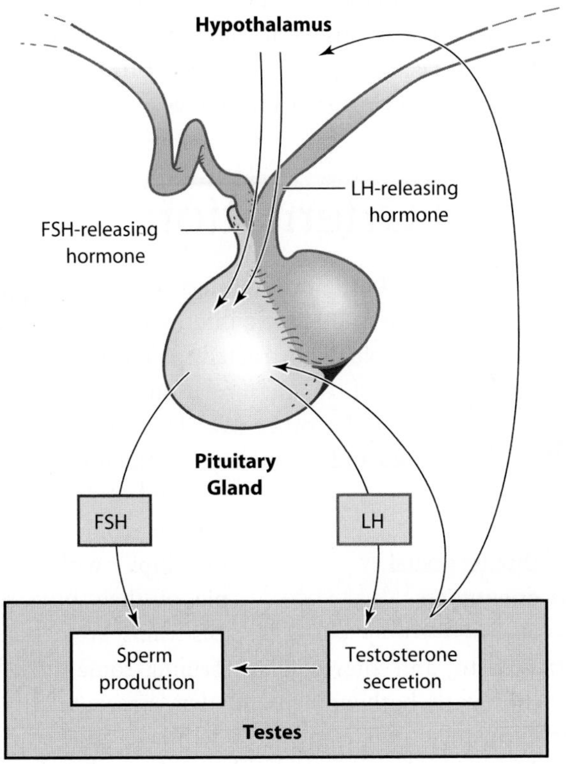

and the fluids contributed by the seminal vesicles, the prostate gland, and other glands to make up **semen**, the whitish fluid that is expelled during ejaculation.

Hormonal changes connected with aging usually enlarge the prostate gland after the age of 50. Because the prostate surrounds the upper part of the urethra, it constricts the urethra as it enlarges. An enlarged prostate causes such symptoms as urinary frequency (including increased frequency of nocturnal urination), urinary urgency, and difficulty starting the flow of urine. Medication is available to help regulate the flow of urine. If necessary, surgical removal of a part of the prostate can help relieve the pressure on the urethra.

Circumcision

Surgical removal of the foreskin of the penis is termed **circumcision**. Advocates of circumcision believe it is healthful because it eliminates a site where bacteria might grow. Opponents believe that regular cleaning is sufficient to reduce the risk. Male circumcision has a long history as a religious rite. Jews traditionally carry out male circumcision shortly after a baby is born as a sign of the covenant between God and the people of Abraham. Muslims also perform ritual circumcisions for religious reasons, often at the age of seven. Medical research indicates that male circumcision helps lessens the risk of infection by the human papilloma virus (the virus that causes genital warts) and HIV (the virus that causes AIDS).[24]

Sexual Response

What happens to our bodies when we are sexually aroused? How are men and women alike in their sexual responses? How do they differ? The changes that take place as people become more sexually aroused are referred to, collectively, as the sexual response cycle. The sexual response cycle is divided into four phases: *excitement*, *plateau*, *orgasm*, and *resolution*.[25]

The response cycles of males and females are characterized by *vasocongestion* and *myotonia*. **Vasocongestion** is the swelling of the genital tissues with blood. It causes erection of the penis and engorgement of the area surrounding the vaginal opening. The testes, nipples, and even the earlobes become engorged as blood vessels in these areas dilate. Myotonia, or muscle tension, is associated with facial grimaces, spasms in the hands and feet, and also spasms of orgasm.

Vasocongestion during the **excitement phase** produces erection in men. In women, vaginal lubrication may start 10 to 30 seconds after stimulation begins. Vasocongestion swells the clitoris, flattens and spreads the labia majora, and expands the labia minora.

semen
The whitish fluid that constitutes the ejaculate, consisting of sperm and secretions from the seminal vesicles, prostate, and Cowper's glands.

circumcision
Surgical removal of the foreskin of the penis. (From the Latin circumcidere, *meaning "to cut around.")*

vasocongestion
The swelling of the genital tissues with blood, which causes erection of the penis and engorgement of the area surrounding the vaginal opening.

excitement phase
The first phase of the sexual response cycle, which is characterized by erection in the male, vaginal lubrication in the female, and muscle tension and increases in heart rate in both males and females.

The inner two-thirds of the vagina expand, and the vaginal walls thicken. The nipples may become erect in both sexes, especially in response to direct stimulation. Men and women show increase in heart rate and blood pressure. Erection and vaginal lubrication are reflexes. People set the stage for these reflexes with erotic thoughts and situations. But erection and lubrication are involuntary. They cannot be forced or willed.

During the **plateau phase**, the level of sexual arousal remains more or less constant. The plateau phase precedes orgasm. The tip of the penis turns a purplish hue, a sign of vasocongestion. The testes are elevated into position for ejaculation. Droplets of seminal fluid are secreted and found at the tip of the penis. In women, vasocongestion swells the tissues of the outer third of the vagina. The inner part of the vagina expands fully. Breathing becomes rapid, like panting. The heart rate may increase to 100 to 160 beats a minute.

In the male, the **orgasmic phase** has two stages of muscular contractions. In the first stage, contractions of the vas deferens, the prostate gland, and other structures cause seminal fluid to collect at the base of the penis. Muscles close off the urinary bladder to prevent urine from mixing with semen. Contraction of muscles at the base of the penis then propel the ejaculate through the urethra and out of the body. Sensations of pleasure tend to be related to the strength of the contractions and the amount of semen. In the female, orgasm is manifested by contractions of the pelvic muscles that surround the vaginal barrel. The contractions release sexual tension and produce pleasure. The first few contractions are most intense for both sexes.

Orgasm, like erection and lubrication, is a reflex. We can set the stage for orgasm through erotic stimulation, but orgasm cannot be forced or willed. In both sexes, orgasm is accompanied by muscle spasms throughout the body. Blood pressure and heart rate peak. The heart beats up to 180 times a minute.

plateau phase
The second phase of the sexual response cycle, which is characterized by increases in vasocongestion, muscle tension, heart rate, and blood pressure in preparation for orgasm.

orgasmic phase
The third phase of the sexual response cycle, characterized by the rhythmic contractions of orgasm.

resolution phase
The fourth phase of the sexual response cycle, during which the body gradually returns to its prearoused state.

refractory period
A period of time following a response (e.g., orgasm) during which an individual is no longer responsive to stimulation (e.g., sexual stimulation).

sexual orientation
The directionality of one's sexual interests—toward members of the same gender, the opposite gender, or both genders.

In the **resolution phase**, the body returns to its prearoused state. The man loses his erection. In women, blood is released from engorged areas. The nipples return to normal size. The clitoris, vaginal barrel, uterus, and labia gradually shrink to their prearoused sizes. Muscle tension (myotonia) dissipates and blood pressure, heart rate, and respiration all return to normal within a few minutes. Both men and women may feel relaxed and satisfied.

During the resolution phase, men but not women enter a **refractory period** during which they cannot experience another orgasm or ejaculation. The refractory period in adolescent males may last only minutes. In men age 50 and above it may last hours or a day. Women can become quickly rearoused to the point of repeated (multiple) orgasms if they wish.

Sexual Orientation

Sexual orientation refers to the directionality of one's erotic interests. *Heterosexuals* are sexually attracted to, and interested in forming romantic relationships with, people of the other sex. *Homosexuals*—gay males and lesbians—are sexually attracted to, and interested in forming romantic relationships with, people of their own sex. *Bisexuals* are sexually attracted to, and interested in forming romantic relationships with, both women and men. A recent national survey of men and women age 18 to 44 showed that 4% of men and women considered themselves homosexual or bisexual.[26]

LEARNING OUTCOME 5

Discuss sexual orientation

Origins of Sexual Orientation

The origins of sexual orientation remain unclear, but heredity may well have something to do with it. Researchers find that when one male twin has a gay sexual orientation, the chances that his co-twin shares the same orientation is greater in identical (MZ) twins (52%) than in fraternal (DZ) twins (22%).[27] Since MZ twins share 100% of their genes in common, as compared to a 50% overlap among fraternal twins, the higher concordance rates among MZ twins support the belief that genes play a role.

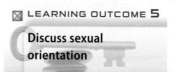

We also know that prenatal sex hormones can masculinize or feminize the brains of laboratory animals by directing the development of certain brain structures. It is conceivable that prenatal sex hormones affect sexual orientation prior to birth by sculpting the developing brain in ways that influence later sexual orientation. Yet researchers believe that sexual orientation does not result from any single factor, but from an interaction of genetics, hormonal factors (likely prenatal), and environmental influences, the intricacies of which remain to be determined.[28]

Whatever the underlying causal influences might be, people do not choose their sexual orientation—either heterosexual or homosexual. We may choose which career to pursue or which person to date, but sexual orientation does not entail a conscious choice. Moreover, there is no evidence that having gay or lesbian parents is linked to a greater incidence of homosexuality among the children.

Sexual Orientation and Psychological Health

Research suggests that people with a gay male or lesbian sexual orientation are more likely than heterosexuals to be anxious and depressed, and that they are more prone to suicide.[29] Does this mean that they are less psychologically healthy than heterosexuals? Perhaps so, but let us remember that there are social and cultural contributors to psychological health—or to psychological pain. Gay males and lesbians have suffered from a history of prejudice and discrimination. When children discover that their sexual orientation is not mainstream, they are likely to question their own normality.

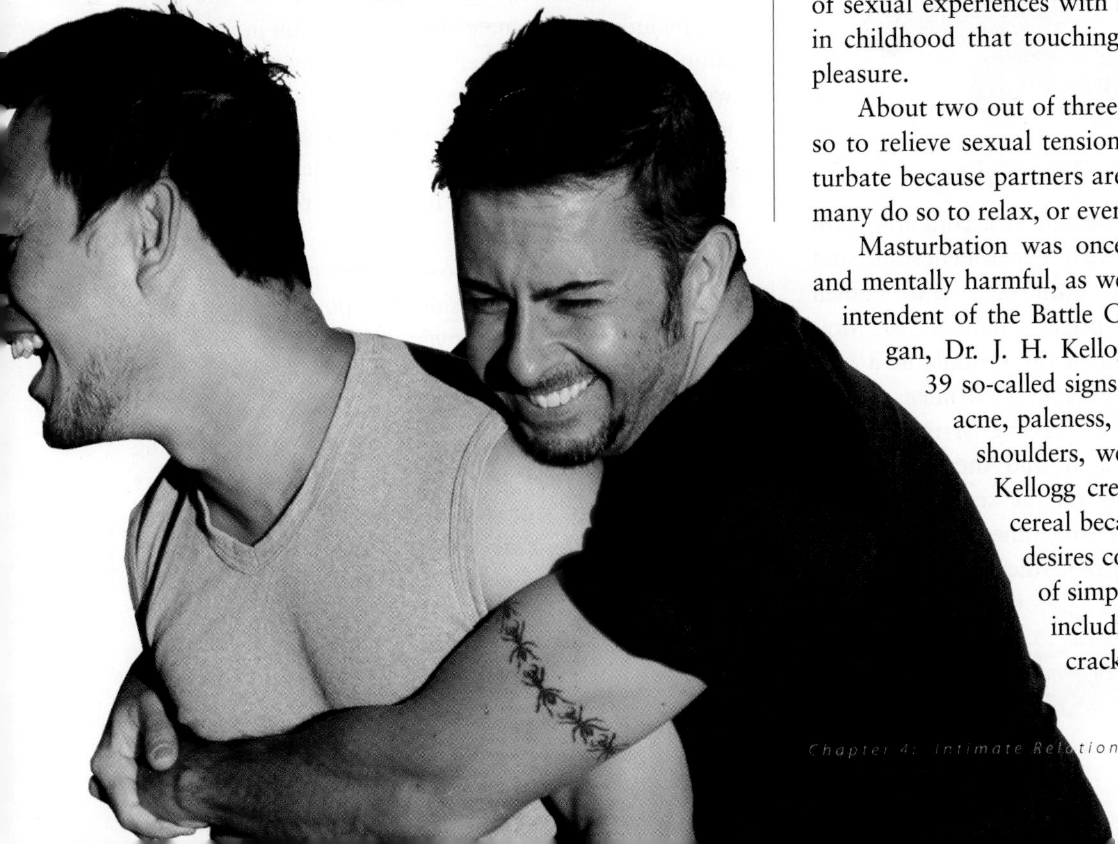

© iStockphoto.com/Anne Clark

Varieties of Sexual Experience

There is great variety in human sexual expression. Our aims here are to describe the diversity of sexual expression and to note some behavior patterns that are unhealthful.

LEARNING OUTCOME 6

Discuss different types of sexual behaviors

The human body is sensitive to many forms of sexual stimulation. Yet biology is not destiny. Cultural expectations, personal values, knowledge of health, and individual experience—in addition to our biological capacities—influence our sexual behavior. What is right for you is right for you, but not necessarily right for your neighbor.

Masturbation

Masturbation may be practiced by manual stimulation of the genitals, perhaps with the aid of artificial stimulation, such as a vibrator. Even before we conceive of sexual experiences with others, we may learn early in childhood that touching our genitals can produce pleasure.

About two out of three adults who masturbate do so to relieve sexual tension. About one in three masturbate because partners are unavailable, and about as many do so to relax, or even to get to sleep.[30]

Masturbation was once thought to be physically and mentally harmful, as well as degrading. The superintendent of the Battle Creek Sanatorium in Michigan, Dr. J. H. Kellogg (1852–1943), identified 39 so-called signs of masturbation, including acne, paleness, heart palpitations, rounded shoulders, weak back, and convulsions. Kellogg created the modern breakfast cereal because he believed that sexual desires could be controlled by a diet of simple foods, especially grains—including cornflakes. (The graham cracker has a similar origin.)

However, there is no scientific evidence that masturbation is harmful to a person's health, save for rare injuries to the genitals from rough stimulation. Even though people who consider masturbation wrong, harmful, or sinful may experience anxiety or guilt if they masturbate or think about doing it, these feelings reflect their attitudes toward masturbation, not masturbation per se. Masturbation is common among adults but more common among men.[31]

Kissing

Kissing is a nearly universal form of foreplay. Other forms of foreplay include cuddling, petting, and oral sex. Women usually prefer longer periods of foreplay (and "afterplay") than men do. Kissing, genital touching, and oral sex may also be experienced as ends in themselves, not as preludes to intercourse.

Kissing is not limited to the partner's mouth. Most women enjoy having their breasts kissed. Women usually prefer several minutes of body contact and gentle caresses before desiring to have their partner kiss their breasts, or lick or suck their nipples.

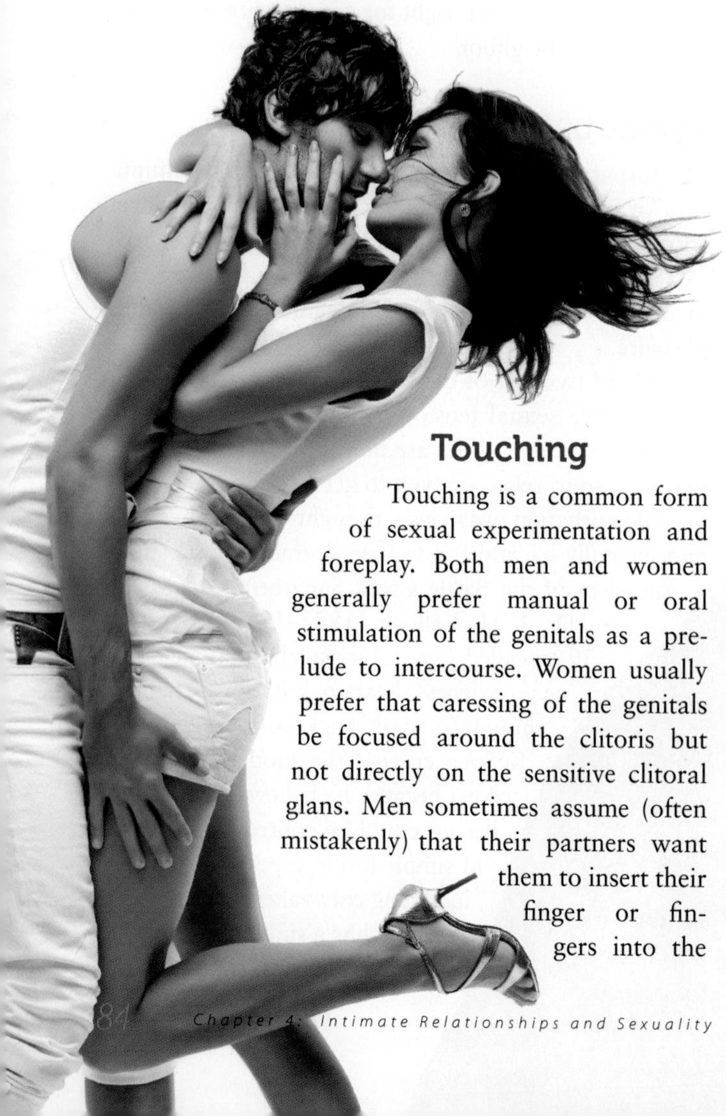

© iStockphoto.com/Lóránd Gelner

Touching

Touching is a common form of sexual experimentation and foreplay. Both men and women generally prefer manual or oral stimulation of the genitals as a prelude to intercourse. Women usually prefer that caressing of the genitals be focused around the clitoris but not directly on the sensitive clitoral glans. Men sometimes assume (often mistakenly) that their partners want them to insert their finger or fingers into the vagina as a form of foreplay, but many women do not enjoy this form of stimulation.

If a finger is to be inserted into the vagina, it should be clean and the nail should be trimmed. Inserting fingers that have been in the anus into the vagina presents a health risk. The fingers may transfer microbes from the woman's digestive tract, where they do no harm, to the woman's reproductive system, where they can cause serious infections.

Oral Sex

Oral stimulation of the male genitals is called *fellatio*. Oral stimulation of the female genitals is called *cunnilingus*. Oral sex has become common among couples today, with more than half of the men and women in the 18- to 49-year age range reporting they had engaged in oral sex during the past year.[32]

Sexual Intercourse

The number of positions for sexual intercourse is virtually endless. The most widely used positions are the male-superior (man-on-top) position, the female-superior (woman-on-top) position, the lateral-entry (side-entry) position, and the rear-entry position.

There was a time when many couples limited themselves to the male-superior position ("superior" is used as a descriptor of body position, but it is sometimes interpreted as a symbol of male domination), which is also called the *missionary position*. Today, the bed has become a stage with more varied parts for the players, including the female-superior position in which the couple faces one another with the woman on top. The woman controls the angle of entry and depth of thrusting and may feel more in charge. She can adjust the angle and depth of penetration, and the speed of movement. Many women find it easier to reach orgasm in this position.

In the lateral-entry position, the man and woman face one another, side by side. This position allows each partner relatively free movement. They can easily kiss each other and stroke one another's bodies.

In the rear-entry position, the man faces the woman's rear and supports himself on his knees, entering his partner from behind. The rear-entry position may be highly stimulating for both partners. But some people object to the rear-entry position because it is the mating position used by most nonhuman mammals. Also, the partners do not face one another, which may create emotional distance. But all in all, many couples vary their positions during sexual intercourse

to introduce variety in lovemaking and to heighten sensations.

Anal Sex

Anal intercourse—insertion of the penis into the rectum—can be performed by male–female couples and male–male couples. The rectum is quite sensitive to sexual stimulation. Both women and men may reach orgasm. Unlike the vagina, the rectum does not produce its own lubrication, so couples are advised to use artificial lubrication and thrust carefully. Anal sex is less commonly practiced than other forms of intimate sexual contact, but a recent national survey showed that more than 20% of men aged 25 to 49 and of women aged 20 to 39 said they had engaged in anal sex during the past year.[33]

Some couples kiss or lick the anus in their foreplay. This practice is called *anilingus*. Oral–anal sex carries a significant health risk. Microorganisms causing intestinal diseases and many sexually transmitted infections can spread this way.

Many couples avoid anal sex because of the fear of HIV/AIDS and other sexually transmitted infections (STIs). Many STIs can be spread by anal intercourse if small tears in the rectal tissues allow microbes to enter the recipient's bloodstream. Women incur a greater risk of being infected with HIV, the virus that causes AIDS, from anal intercourse than from vaginal intercourse—just as receptive anal sex among gay men carries a high risk of infection· However, monogamous partners who are both infection-free are at no risk of contracting HIV or other STIs through any sexual act. HIV and other STI-causing organisms can only be transmitted by people who are infected with them. Nevertheless, people who are uncertain whether their partners are infected would be wise to either avoid anal sex or use a latex condom.

Celibacy

Some people remain celibate either by choice or for lack of opportunity. Many single people remain celibate because they view sex outside of marriage as immoral. Nuns and priests practice celibacy for religious reasons. Others believe that celibacy allows them to focus their energies on their work or other pursuits. Still others remain celibate because they lack sexual interest or available partners.

In sum, our bodies respond to many forms of sexual stimulation. Whether we engage in some, many, or all of the techniques described here, or whether we remain celibate, reflects our personal needs, desires, and, importantly, our values.

Sexual Dysfunctions

LEARNING OUTCOME 7

Discuss sexual dysfunctions and sex therapy

Many of us encounter sexual difficulties from time to time. Men occasionally have trouble achieving an erection or ejaculate sooner than they or their partners would like. Most women occasionally have problems lubricating or reaching orgasm. When such problems become persistent and distressing, they are classified as **sexual dysfunctions**, which are diagnosable disorders involving problems with sexual interest, arousal, or response.

Persistent sexual problems are quite common.[34] About one in three women, and about one in seven men suffer from low sex drive or interest. Male erectile disorder affects upwards of one in five men at some point in their lives, and **premature ejaculation** affects upwards of one in three men, especially during young adulthood. About one in four women suffer from difficulty achieving orgasm. Many more people have occasional sexual problems—or have had these problems at some point during their lives but not presently. Health professionals classify sexual dysfunctions within the four categories shown in Table 4-1 on the next page.

As seen in Table 4-1, some sexual dysfunctions reflect biological causes. Others are caused mainly by psychosocial factors such as sexual anxieties and marital dissatisfaction. Still others involve a combination of biological and psychosocial factors.

Sexual desire in men and women is stoked by testosterone, which is produced by men in the testes and by both men and women in the adrenal glands. Low testosterone levels can thus dampen sexual desire and reduce sexual responsiveness. A gradual decline in sexual desire or erectile functioning, at least in men, may be explained in part by the reduction in testosterone levels that occurs in middle and later adulthood. An abrupt loss of sexual desire is more often explained by psychosocial factors—for example, depression, stress, or problems in the relationship.

Sex shouldn't hurt. Painful sex is a sign that something is wrong. The most common cause of

sexual dysfunction *Problems with sexual interest, arousal, or response.*

premature ejaculation *A sexual dysfunction in which ejaculation occurs too rapidly or with minimal sexual stimulation.*

Table 4-1 Sexual Dysfunctions

CATEGORY	DEFINITIONS	ABOUT . . .
Sexual desire disorders	Defined by lack of sexual desire or aversion (repulsion) to sex. Lack of sexual desire is about twice as common in women as in men.	May reflect low testosterone levels, or fatigue, depression, stress, or problems in a relationship.
Sexual arousal disorders	In men, sexual arousal disorders involve problems in achieving or maintaining erections sufficient to engage in sexual intercourse (*male erectile disorder*). In women, these disorders involve problems in becoming adequately lubricated (*female sexual arousal disorder*).	May reflect chronic diseases such as diabetes, cardiovascular disorders, hormonal problems, effects of prescription drugs, alcohol, illicit drugs, or fatigue. May reflect obesity or aging in males.
Orgasmic disorders	Both men and women might have problems reaching orgasm. Or they might reach orgasm sooner than they or their partners would like. *Female or male orgasmic disorder* involves problems reaching orgasm or inability to reach orgasm at all. Women are more likely to have orgasmic disorder. Another orgasm disorder in males, *premature ejaculation*, is the most commonly reported male sexual dysfunction.	Inability to reach orgasm may reflect lack of adequate sexual stimulation, sex-negative attitudes, problems in a relationship, or a history of sexual trauma. Premature ejaculation is often connected with youth and inexperience.
Sexual pain disorders	Both men and women can suffer from *dyspareunia* (painful intercourse). Some women experience *vaginismus*, involuntary contraction of the muscles surrounding the vagina during attempts at penetration.	Dyspareunia in women often stems from inadequate lubrication, gynecological infections, or resultant scarring. Vaginismus is a psychological problem that often stems from a history of sexual trauma, such as rape or child sexual abuse.

pain during sex in women is inadequate lubrication. In such cases, additional foreplay or artificial lubrication may help. Painful sex in men is generally connected with infections of the sex organs, which can cause burning or painful ejaculation.

Health problems can prevent women and men from becoming sexually aroused or reaching orgasm.[35] Diabetes, multiple sclerosis, spinal cord injuries, epilepsy, complications from surgery (such as prostate surgery in men), complications from drug use, and hormonal problems are among the most common biological causes. People with sexual dysfunctions should have physical examinations to learn whether their problems are biologically based.

Children reared in sexually repressive cultures or homes may learn to respond to sexual stimulation with feelings of anxiety and shame, rather than sexual arousal and pleasure. Women are more likely than men to be taught to repress their sexual desires. Women reared with repressive attitudes are less likely to learn about their sexual potentials and to assert their sexual wishes with their partners.

Couples who fail to communicate their sexual preferences or to experiment may find themselves losing interest. A couple usually finds that their sexual relationship is no better than the other facets of their relationship. Couples who harbor resentments toward one another may make sex an arena of combat.

Victims of rape and other sexual trauma may harbor feelings of disgust and revulsion toward sex. Deep-seated fears of sex may make it difficult for them to respond sexually, even with loving partners. These factors may lead to insufficient lubrication or cause vaginismus, making sexual relations painful or impossible.

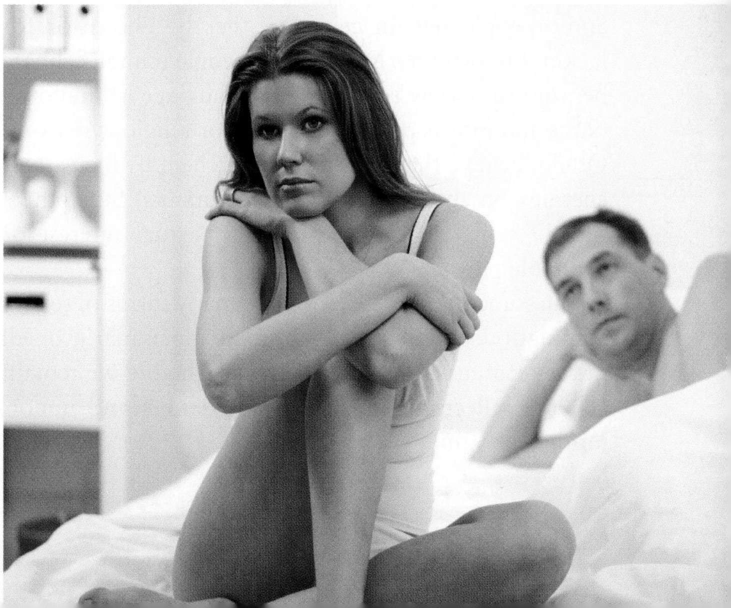

Anxiety—especially *performance anxiety*—plays an important role in sexual dysfunction. Performance anxiety occurs when a person becomes overly concerned with how well he or she is doing. Performance anxiety can inhibit one's sexual response and lead the person to focus on self-doubts and fears rather than erotic sensations. Performance anxiety can set the stage for a vicious cycle in which a sexual failure increases anxiety. Anxiety then leads to repeated failure, and so on.

Sex Therapy

Some forms of sexual dysfunction are treated with therapeutic drugs, such as Viagra and other similar drugs that help men with erectile disorder achieve more reliable erections. Psychological treatment in the form of sex therapy may help couples learn skills and techniques to enhance their sexual satisfaction and counter anxiety that might impede their sexual performance. Sex therapy aims to achieve the following two major goals:

- *Reducing performance anxiety.* Sex therapists break the vicious cycle of performance anxiety and failure by removing the need to perform. Sex becomes pleasurable once more, not anxiety-provoking.
- *Fostering sexual skills or competencies.* Clients are taught about their sexual anatomy and sexual response. They learn how to obtain adequate sexual stimulation and to stimulate their partners sexually. They learn how to relax so that the natural reflexes of erection, lubrication, and orgasm can take place.

HEALTH APPS: YOUR LINK TO ONLINE HEALTH APPLICATIONS

diversity

Sex Differences in Preferences for Mates across 37 Cultures What do men in Nigeria, Japan, Brazil, Canada, and the United States have in common? For one thing, all report that they prefer partners who are younger than themselves. Find out more in "Diversity 4-1".

health skills

Using Small Talk and Opening Lines to Jump-Start Relationships When someone appeals to you, do you shy away or do you steel your courage and say something? If you're not sure what to say, "Health Skills 4-1" has some suggestions.

health skills

Loneliness and Health: "All the Lonely People, Where Do They All Come From?" There are millions of lonely people. Read "Health Skills 4-2" to find out what you can do about it if you're among them.

health skills

Resolving Conflicts in Relationships What do you do to resolve conflicts when they arise? Not sure? We've got tried-and-true methods for you in "Health Skills 4-3."

diversity

Clitoridectomy—Tradition, Mutilation, or Both? Hundreds of millions of women in Africa and the Middle East have undergone ritual removal of the clitoris. Is it tradition, mutilation, or both? Read "Diversity 4-3" and decide for yourself.

prevention

Preventing Cystitis and Vaginitis The urinary tract may become infected with bacteria, leading to a condition called cystitis. Vaginitis might result from an unhealthy level of bacteria in the vagina. Read "Prevention 4-1" to learn how to avert these health problems.

prevention

The Pelvic Exam: What to Expect Women are advised to have an internal pelvic examination at least once a year. "Prevention 4-2" will inform you on what to expect.

health skills

How to Handle Menstrual Discomfort Assess whether or not you have PMS in "Health Skills 4-4," and then learn what you can do to minimize or eradicate the discomfort.

Go to the CourseMate for HLTH at www.cengagebrain.com for additional resources including flashcards, games, self-quizzes, review exercises, web exercises, learning checks, and more.

Reproductive Choices

"Couples today have many reproductive choices. This chapter is about those choices."

The year was 1912. It was a stifling day in July. Margaret Sanger (1879–1966), a nurse practitioner, was called to the home of a woman—a Mrs. Sachs—who was dying from an infection following a bungled self-induced abortion. Her husband had called a doctor, and the doctor sent Sanger. She and the doctor toiled feverishly for several days and nights to save the woman.

Two interminable weeks passed, and finally the woman showed signs of improvement. Her neighbors dropped by to express their joy. But Mrs. Sachs barely acknowledged the positive wishes and continued to look grave and desperate. Three weeks passed and Sanger was preparing to leave, when Mrs. Sachs gave voice to the dread that was still haunting her. Sachs explained that she feared becoming pregnant again. She would again face the choice between attempting another abortion, which might kill her, and bearing a baby whom she could not support. She begged for information about contraception, but Sanger kept silent. In 1912, dispensing information about contraception was a crime. Abortions were also illegal. Sanger offered up some comforting but empty words and promised to return to talk more.

Three months later, Mr. Sachs called Sanger in despair. His wife was feverish once more. The cause was the same. Sanger recalled,

> For a wild moment I thought of sending someone else, but actually, of course, I hurried into my uniform, caught up my bag, and started out. All the way I longed for a subway wreck, an explosion, anything to keep me from having to enter that home again. But nothing happened, even to delay me. I turned into the dingy doorway and climbed

LEARNING OUTCOMES

1. Describe the process of conception
2. Discuss the problem of infertility and alternate methods of having children
3. Discuss the pros and cons of various methods of contraception
4. Discuss methods of abortion
5. Discuss health issues in pregnancy and prenatal development
6. Describe health issues associated with methods of childbirth
7. Discuss health issues in the postpartum period

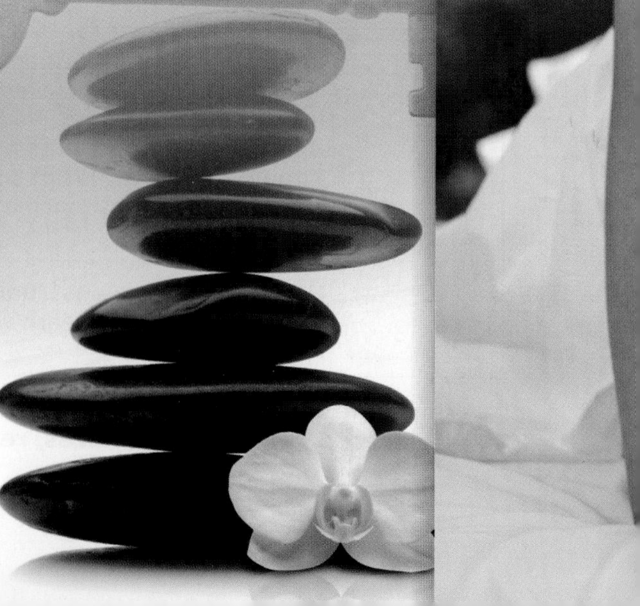

the familiar stairs once more. The children were there, young little things.

Mrs. Sachs was in a coma and died within ten minutes. I folded her still hands across her breast, remembering how they had pleaded with me, begging so humbly for the knowledge which was her right.[1]

Today, partly because of the efforts of Margaret Sanger, who became a major advocate for birth control, information about contraceptives is dispensed freely throughout the United States. Couples today have many reproductive choices. This chapter is about those choices. Let us begin our discussion as all new lives begin, with the process of conception.

Did you know that . . .

- **Conception normally occurs in the fallopian tubes, not in the uterus? [p. 90]**
- **Many birth control pills fool the brain into acting as though the woman is already pregnant? [p. 93]**
- **Most contraceptives do not prevent sexually transmitted infections? [p. 95]**
- **A fertilized egg cell is not attached to its mother's body for the first week or so following conception? [p. 105]**
- **In the United States, about one baby in three is born by cesarean section? [p. 110]**
- **It is normal to experience mood changes in the days or weeks following childbirth? [p. 111]**

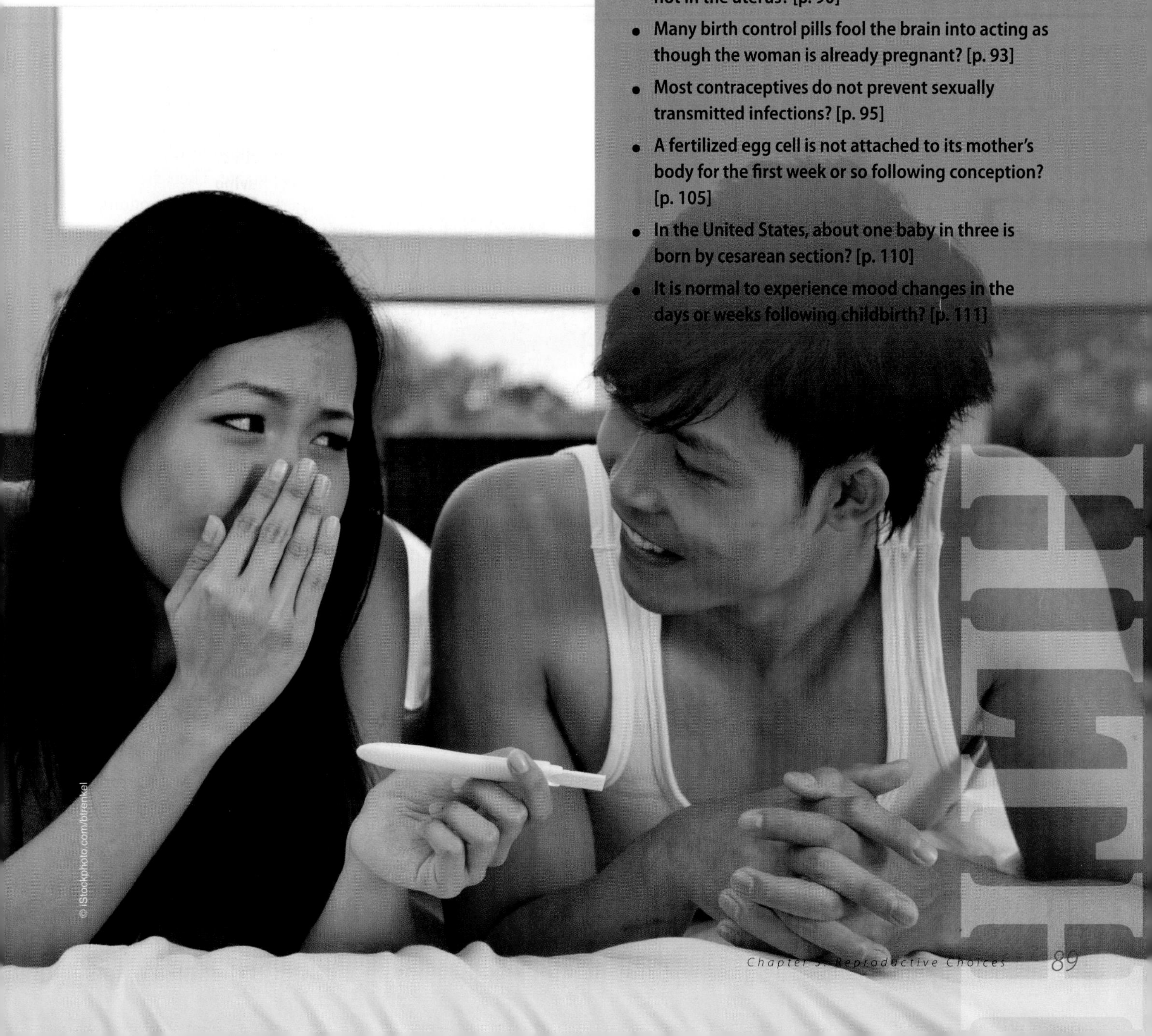

Conception: Against All Odds

Conception is the union of a sperm cell and an egg cell (ovum) into a **zygote**. On one hand, conception is the beginning of a new human life. On the other hand, conception is the end of a fantastic voyage in which an ovum, one of several hundred that will mature and ripen during a woman's lifetime, unites with one of several *hundred million* sperm, the number produced in the average ejaculate.

LEARNING OUTCOME 1

Discuss the process of conception

Ova carry X sex chromosomes. Sperm carry either X or Y sex chromosomes. Girls are conceived from the union of an ovum and an X-bearing sperm, whereas boys are conceived from the union of an ovum and a Y-bearing sperm. Between 120 and 150 boys are conceived for every 100 girls, but male fetuses are more likely to be lost in a *miscarriage*, or **spontaneous abortion**, which usually occurs early in pregnancy. Boys still outnumber girls at birth, but they suffer a higher incidence of infant mortality. Thus, the numbers of boys and girls in the population are further equalized.

The 200 to 400 million sperm in a typical ejaculate may seem excessive, since only one can fertilize an ovum, but millions of sperm flow out of the woman's body because of gravity. Vaginal acidity kills others. Many surviving sperm manage to swim against the current of fluid coming from the cervix, but about half end up in the tube that doesn't contain the ovum.

zygote
A fertilized ovum.

spontaneous abortion
The involuntary expulsion of the embryo or fetus from the uterus before it is capable of independent life. Also called miscarriage.

The majority of parents in the United States would prefer to have a boy—at least as a first child. What happens in a country where the preference for a boy is extreme and there are means to ensure that women bear babies of the sex they want? Check out the online feature "Diversity 5-1" to find out.

diversity

Access CourseMate for HLTH at www.cengagebrain.com.

Fertilization normally occurs in a fallopian tube. Ova are surrounded by a gelatinous layer that must be penetrated if fertilization is to occur. Sperm that have completed their journey secrete an enzyme that briefly thins the layer, enabling one to penetrate. Then the layer thickens, locking out other sperm. The corresponding chromosomes in the sperm and ovum line up across from each other. Conception occurs as the chromosomes from the sperm and ovum combine to form 23 new pairs, which carry a unique set of genetic instructions.

Optimizing the Chances for Conception

Knowledge about fertilization is helpful to couples who wish to optimize their chances of conceiving. The ovum can be fertilized for about 4 to 20 hours after ovulation. Sperm are most active within 48 hours after ejaculation. So, one way to optimize the chances of conception is to have sexual intercourse within a few hours of ovulation. Couples can predict ovulation by consulting a basal body temperature (BBT) chart, checking urine or saliva for luteinizing hormone, or tracking vaginal mucus.

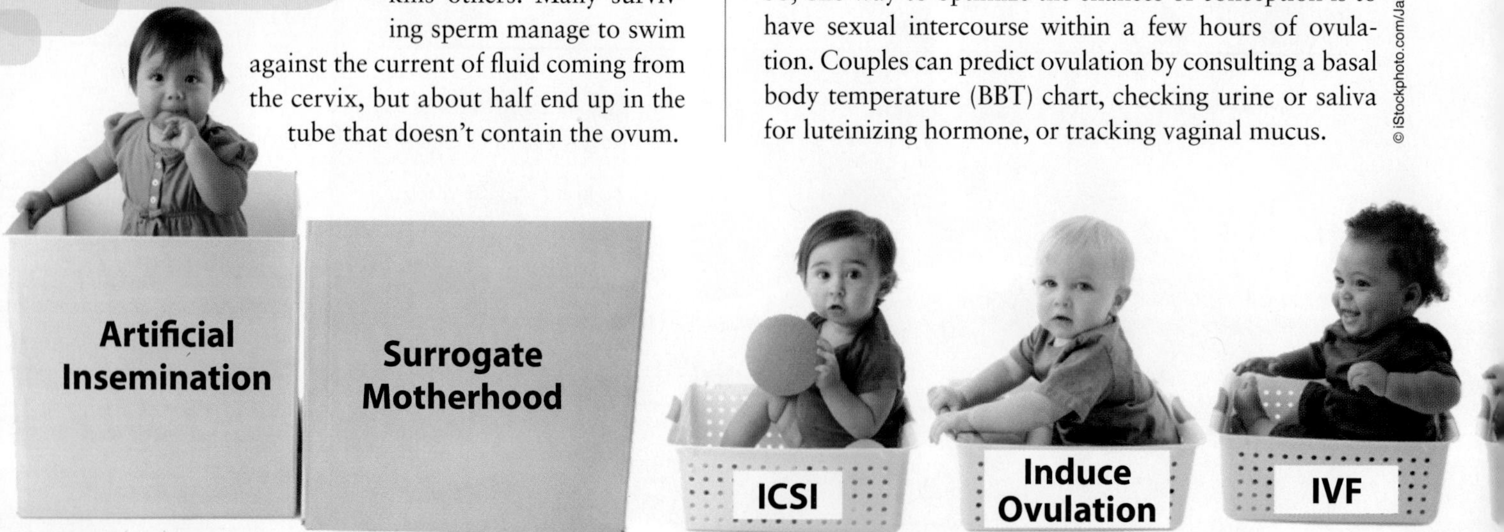

© iStockphoto.com/Jani Bryson

Because the great majority of women do not have perfectly regular menstrual cycles, predicting ovulation is fraught with uncertainty. Use of a BBT chart may provide a more reliable estimate of when a woman is ovulating. Basal body temperature remains fairly stable before ovulation. Just before ovulation, BBT dips slightly. Then, on the day following ovulation, the woman's body temperature tends to rise by about 0.4° to 0.8° F and to remain higher until menstruation. A woman can best detect these changes by taking her temperature first thing in the morning before rising from bed. The woman records her temperature, the day of the cycle, and the day of the month. After charting for six months or so, the woman may be able to more accurately predict ovulation, assuming her cycles are fairly regular.

Over-the-counter kits are more accurate than the BBT method. They predict ovulation by analyzing the woman's urine or saliva for the surge in luteinizing hormone (LH) that precedes ovulation by 12 to 24 hours.

Women can also roll their vaginal mucus between their fingers and note changes in texture. The mucus is thick, white, and cloudy during most phases of the menstrual cycle. It becomes thin, slippery, and clear for a few days before ovulation.

Infertility

For couples who want to have children, few problems are more frustrating and emotionally upsetting than the inability to conceive. Health professionals often advise couples to try to conceive on their own for six months before seeking assistance. The term **infertility** is not usually applied until there is evidence of failure to conceive for more than a year.

LEARNING OUTCOME 2

Discuss the problem of infertility and alternate methods of having children

Because the incidence of infertility increases with age, couples who postpone childbearing until their 30s and 40s run a greater risk. All in all, more than 15% of American couples have a fertility problem.[2] About half of them eventually conceive a child. Many treatment options are available, from drugs that stimulate ovulation to assisted reproductive technologies such as in vitro fertilization.

Male Fertility Problems

About 40% of the time, the fertility problem lies with the man.[3] Male fertility problems include low sperm count, irregularly shaped sperm, low sperm motility, chronic or infectious diseases, injury to the testes, hormonal problems, or an *autoimmune response* in which antibodies produced by the man deactivate his own sperm. Causes of male fertility problems include genetic factors, advanced age, injuries, varicose veins in the scrotum, drugs (alcohol, narcotics, marijuana, tobacco), blood pressure medications, environmental toxins, and stress. Although healthy older men may have viable sperm, male fertility may begin declining as early as age 35.[4]

The most common problem is low or zero sperm count. Frequent ejaculation can reduce the sperm count, as does scrotal temperature that is consistently one or two degrees above the typical temperature of 94° to 95° F. Men may develop fertility problems from tight-fitting underwear, prolonged athletic activity, the pressure from bicycle seats, use of electric blankets, even long, hot baths. In such cases the problem is usually readily corrected. In some cases, sperm count is adequate, but prostate, hormonal, or other factors deprive sperm of motility (movement) or deform them.

Female Fertility Problems

infertility
The inability to conceive a child.

The major causes of infertility in women include irregular ovulation or failure to ovulate, obstructions or malfunctions of the reproductive tract, endometriosis, and age-related decline in levels of female sex hormones.

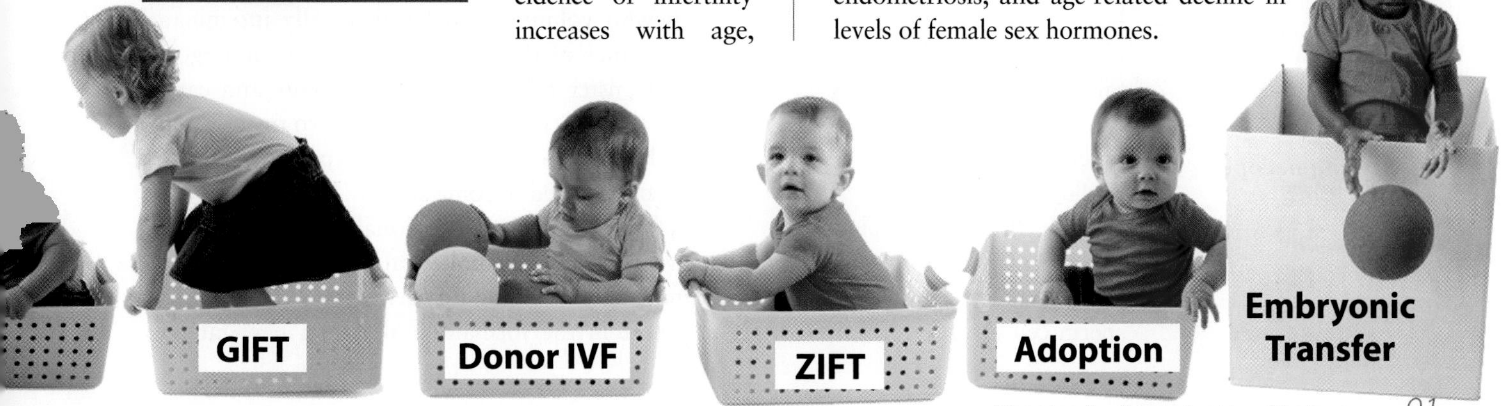

Between 10% and 15% of female infertility problems stem from failure to ovulate. Causes include hormonal irregularities, malnutrition, genetic factors, stress, disease, or abnormally low levels of body fat, as seen in women with eating disorders and athletes.[5]

In *endometriosis*, cells break away from the uterine lining (the endometrium) and implant and grow elsewhere. When they develop on the surface of the ovaries or fallopian tubes, they may block the passage of ova or interfere with conception. About one in six cases of female infertility is believed to be due to endometriosis. Hormone treatments and surgery sometimes reduce the blockage so that women can conceive. Suspected blockage of the fallopian tubes may be checked by a *Rubin test* or a *hysterosalpingogram*. In a Rubin test, carbon dioxide gas is blown through the cervix, and its progress is monitored to determine whether it flows freely. In the hysterosalpingogram, X-rays monitor the movement of an injected dye.

Methods of Increasing Fertility

Various methods have helped many couples with fertility problems conceive and bear children, including the following:

Increasing the Sperm Count. Sperm of men with low sperm counts can be collected and quick-frozen. Sperm from multiple ejaculations can then be combined and injected into a woman's uterus at the time of ovulation. This method is called **artificial insemination**. The sperm of men with low sperm motility can also be injected into their partners' uteruses, so that the sperm begin their journey closer to the fallopian tubes. Sperm from a donor can be used to artificially inseminate a woman whose partner is infertile. A donor can be chosen who resembles the mother's partner.

When circulation in the reproductive system is blocked, sperm counts can be increased by surgery on blood vessels, such as scrotal varicose veins. Surgery can also open blocked passageways that prevent the outflow of sperm.

ICSI. Intracytoplasmic Sperm Injection (ICSI) involves the injection of a sperm cell directly into an ovum. However, children conceived by ICSI may run an increased risk of birth defects such as heart, stomach, kidney, and bladder problems, cleft palate, hernia, and, in boys, malformation of the penis.[6]

Inducing Ovulation. Ovulation may be induced in women who ovulate irregularly by the use of drugs such as *Clomiphene* and *Pergonal*. These drugs may cause the release of two or more ova, resulting in multiple births.

IVF. **In vitro fertilization (IVF)** may be used when women have blocked fallopian tubes. Children conceived in this manner are so-called "test-tube babies," but conception actually occurs in a laboratory dish, and the embryo is placed in the mother's uterus, where it becomes implanted and develops to term. Prior to IVF, fertility drugs stimulate ripening of ova. The ova are surgically removed from an ovary and mixed with the father's sperm in a dish.

GIFT. In **gamete intrafallopian transfer (GIFT)**, sperm and ova are inserted together into one of the woman's fallopian tubes. Unlike IVF, conception occurs in the fallopian tube, not in a laboratory dish.

Donor IVF. Donor IVF represents a variation of IVF. The ovum is first taken from another woman and fertilized, and then injected into the uterus or fallopian tube of the intended mother. The procedure may be used in cases in which the intended mother does not produce ova of her own.

ZIFT. Zygote intrafallopian transfer (ZIFT) involves a combination of IVF and GIFT. Fertilization occurs when sperm and ova are combined in a laboratory dish. Then the resulting zygote is placed in the mother's fallopian tube for its journey to the uterus for implantation.

Embryonic Transfer. Embryonic transfer is also used in cases in which women do not produce ova. First, a woman volunteer is artificially inseminated by the partner of the infertile woman. Five days later, the embryo is removed from the woman and inserted in the uterus of the intended mother.

Surrogate Motherhood. A surrogate mother is a woman who volunteers to be artificially inseminated by the partner of the infertile woman or undergo an embryo transfer from the genetic parents and carries the baby to term. The surrogate agrees to turn the baby over to the intended parents. These types of agreements have been restricted in some states.

Adoption. Despite occasional conflicts between adoptive parents and biological parents who change their minds about giving up their children, most adoptions result in the formation of loving new families.

artificial insemination
The introduction of sperm in the reproductive tract through means other than sexual intercourse.

in vitro fertilization (IVF)
A method of conception in which mature ova are surgically removed from an ovary and placed in a laboratory dish along with sperm.

gamete intrafallopian transfer (GIFT)
A method of conception in which sperm and ova are inserted into a fallopian tube to encourage conception.

Many Americans find it easier to adopt infants who are from other countries or have special needs.

Although many couples do everything they can to conceive children, others are not ready to have children and choose to prevent conception.

Contraception

Broaching the topic of contraception with your partner can be awkward, but not broaching it can be disastrous. The online feature "Health Skills 5-1" has advice on talking with your partner about contraception, and "Health Skills 5-2" has advice on selecting a method of contraception.

LEARNING OUTCOME 3

Discuss the pros and cons of various methods of contraception

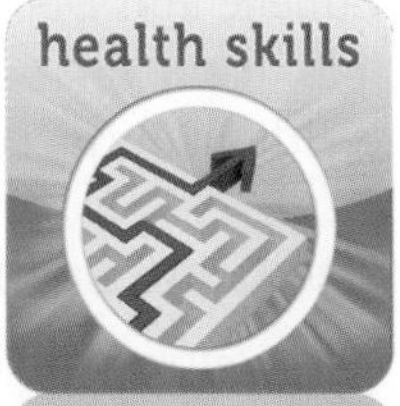

Access CourseMate for HLTH at www.cengagebrain.com.

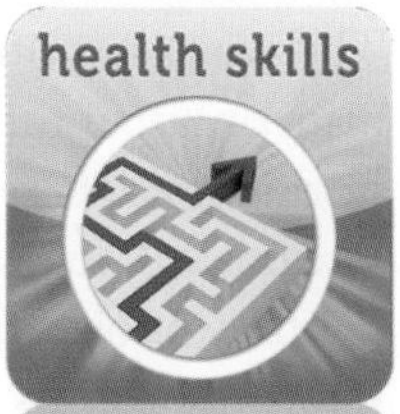

Access CourseMate for HLTH at www.cengagebrain.com.

The safest and most effective method of contraception is also the least popular: abstinence. Short of abstinence, there are many choices available to people seeking to avoid unwanted pregnancies.

Hormonal Methods

Hormonal methods use either a combination of the female hormone estrogen and the male hormone progestin, or progestin alone. Women cannot conceive when they are already pregnant because their bodies suppress the maturation of follicles and ovulation. The combination of estrogen and progestin fools the brain into acting as though the woman is already pregnant. Progestin increases the thickness and acidity of the cervical mucus, making the mucus a more resistant barrier to sperm. It inhibits development of the endometrium. Progestin may also impede the progress of ova through the fallopian tubes and make it more difficult for sperm to penetrate ova.

Figure 5-1 Contraceptive Use

"The pill" is the most popular reversible birth-control method in the United States. Sterilization is highly popular among people who already have all the children they desire.

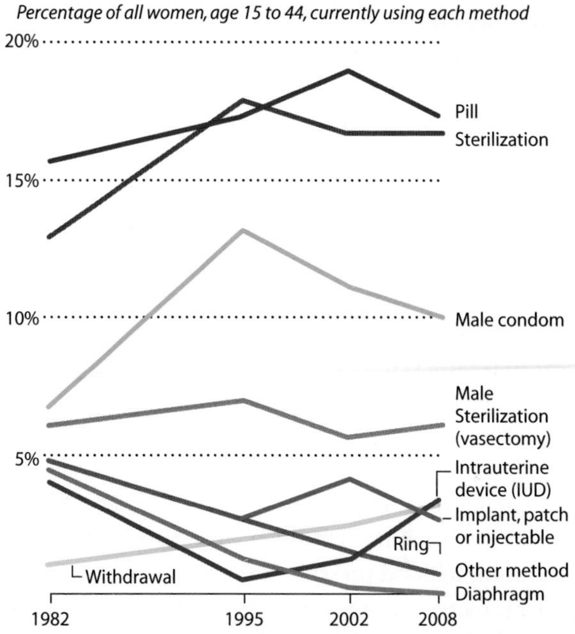

Oral Contraceptives ("The Pill")

Oral contraception is the most commonly used method of reversible contraception (see Figure 5-1). An **oral contraceptive** is also called a *birth control pill* or just simply, "the pill." There are combination pills and minipills, which are available by prescription.

Combination pills contain synthetic forms of the hormones estrogen and progesterone (progestin). The

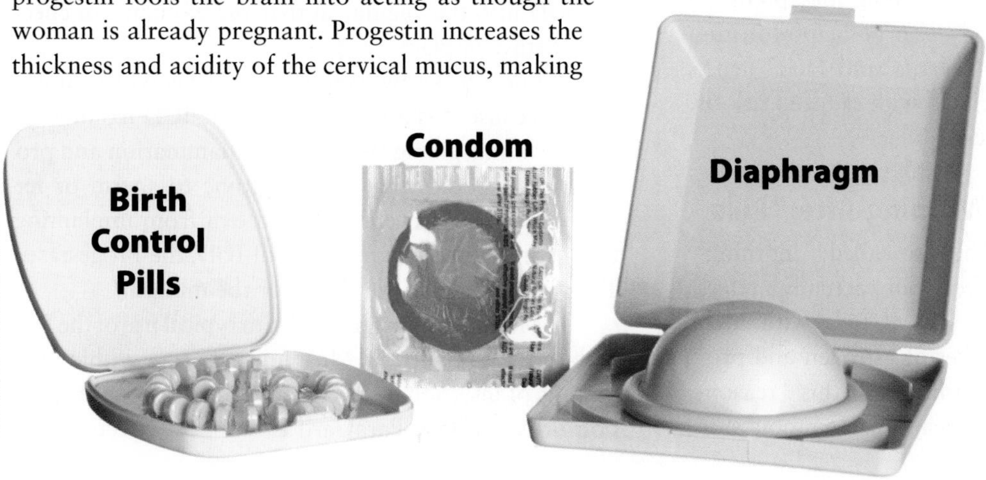

oral contraceptive
A contraceptive, consisting of sex hormones, which is taken by mouth.

the typical 28-day cycle. Then, for 7 days, the woman takes no pill or takes an inert pill to help count days. The sudden drop in hormone levels causes the endometrium to disintegrate and menstruation to follow. This flow contains no ovum.

The *minipill* contains only progestin and is taken on a daily basis throughout the woman's menstrual cycle.

The failure rate of the birth control pill associated with perfect use is very low (see Table 5-1). The failure rate increases with typical use, which takes into account forgetting to take a pill or switching brands.

The pill does not interfere with sexual spontaneity or diminish sexual sensations. Its effects are reversible; a woman simply stops taking it. The pill provides no protection against sexually transmitted infections (STIs) and may reduce the effectiveness of antibiotics used to treat STIs.

The estrogen in combination pills may produce side effects that mimic pregnancy: nausea and vomiting, fluid retention (bloating), increased vaginal discharge, headaches, tenderness in the breasts, and dizziness. Many of these are temporary. Estrogen may also lead to blood clots or high blood pressure. Progestin can cause weight gain by increasing the appetite or developing muscle. Progestin fosters male secondary sex characteristics, so women who take the minipill may develop acne, facial hair, thinning scalp hair, loss of breast tissue, vaginal dryness (making sex painful), missed or shorter periods, and irregular or breakthrough bleeding. Although the pill appears to be safe for healthy women, the American Congress of Obstetricians and Gynecologists (ACOG)[7] suggests caution in women with hypertension or a history of vascular diseases, or women who are older than 35 who smoke or are obese.

Birth control pills may also have *healthful* effects. They appear to reduce the risk of pelvic inflammatory disease (PID), benign ovarian cysts, and fibrocystic (benign) breast growths. The pill regularizes menstrual cycles and reduces menstrual cramping and premenstrual discomfort. The pill may also be helpful in the treatment of iron-deficiency anemia and facial acne. The combination pill is associated with reduced risk of ovarian and endometrial cancer.[8]

"Morning-After" Pills

The so-called morning-after pill actually refers to several pills with high doses of estrogen and progestin. For this reason, nausea is a common side effect but can usually be treated with anti-nausea medication. Morning-after pills prevent fertilization or keep the fertilized ovum from implanting in the uterus. In that respect, some people consider them an early abortion technique.

intrauterine device (IUD)
A small object that is inserted into the uterus and left in place to prevent conception.

Injectable Contraceptives

Lunelle and Depo-Provera are injectable hormone preparations that are available by prescription. Lunelle contains estrogen and progestin and is injected monthly. Depo-Provera contains progestin only and prevents pregnancy for three months. Lunelle's effects are like those of the combination pill. Depo-Provera prevents ovulation. Lunelle, like oral contraceptives, has a failure rate of less than 1% when used properly. Injectable contraceptives are highly effective, permit spontaneous sex, and remain effective without being taken every day. Lunelle and Depo-Provera are considered to be reversible, but ovulation may take a few months to return. Neither contraceptive affords protection against STIs.

The Contraceptive Patch

The contraceptive patch delivers estrogen and progestin to prevent ovulation and implantation. The patch is thin, measuring only about two inches by two inches. The woman wears it on her abdomen, buttocks, upper arm, or upper torso. The patch holds a week's supply of hormones and releases them regularly into the bloodstream. Women who use the patch need not think about contraception daily. Also, like the pill, the patch doesn't interrupt sex. Its side effects and potential hazards are similar to those of the pill.

Intrauterine Device (IUD)

An **intrauterine device (IUD)** is inserted into the uterus by a physician or nurse practitioner, where it remains in place for a year or more. Fine strings hang down from the IUD into the vagina, so that the woman can check that it stays in place.

We do not know exactly how IUDs work. Apparently, because it is a foreign body, the IUD irritates the uterine lining, giving rise to mild inflammation and producing antibodies that may be toxic to sperm or fertilized ova and prevent fertilized ova from implanting. Progestin released by one type of IUD, the Progestasert T, has effects similar to those for the minipill.

The failure rate associated with typical use of the Progestasert T is about 2%. Most failures occur within three months of insertion, often because the device shifts position or is expelled. ParaGard is the most effective IUD.

Table 5-1 Effectiveness of Various Birth-Control Methods

KIND OF METHOD	METHOD	PERCENT OF TYPICAL USERS HAVING AN UNPLANNED PREGNANCY WITHIN A YEAR	PERCENT OF PRECISE USERS* HAVING AN UNPLANNED PREGNANCY WITHIN A YEAR	IS THE METHOD REVERSIBLE?	DOES THE METHOD PROTECT AGAINST SEXUALLY TRANSMITTED INFECTIONS?
Hormonal (using estrogen, progestin, or both)	Combination birth control pills	8	Less than 1	Yes	No; may reduce risk of PID**
	Hormonal implants	Less than 1	Less than 1	Yes	No
	Injection (estrogen & progestin)	Less than 1	Less than 1	Yes	No
	Injections (progestin only)	3	Less than 1	Yes	No
	Transdermal patch	8	Less than 1	Yes	No
	Progestin-only pills (mini-pills)	8	Less than 1	Yes	No
	Vaginal ring	8	Less than 1	Yes	No
Intrauterine device (IUD)	IUD with progestin	Less than 1	Less than 1	Yes, unless fertility is impaired	No; may increase risk of PID
	Copper IUD	Less than 1	Less than 1	Yes, unless fertility is impaired	No; may increase risk of PID
Barrier methods	Male condom	15	2	Yes	Yes
	Female condom	21	5	Yes	(Scarce information)
	Diaphragm with spermicide	16	6	Yes	Somewhat
	Spermicide alone	29	18	Yes	No
	Sponge with spermicide (no previous vaginal childbirth)	16	9	Yes	No
	Sponge with spermicide (after vaginal childbirth)	32	20	Yes	No
	Cervical cap (no previous vaginal childbirth)	16	9	Yes	No
	Cervical cap (after vaginal childbirth)	32	26	Yes	No
Fertility awareness	Periodic abstinence	25	5	Yes	No
Sterilization	Vasectomy	Less than 1	Less than 1	Questionable	No
	Tubal ligation or tubal implants	Less than 1	Less than 1	Questionable	No
Non-Methods	Douching	High	High	Not applicable	No
	Withdrawal	27	4	Yes	No

*Users who follow instructions exactly.
**Pelvic inflammatory disease.
Sources: Cates, W., & Raymond, E. (2007). Vaginal barriers and spermicides. In R. A. Hatcher, et al. (Eds.), *Contraceptive technology* (19th ed.). New York: Ardent Media Inc.; Healthwise staff. (2010). Effectiveness rate of birth control methods. Retrieved from http://monroe.pa.networkofcare.org/mh/library/hwdetail.cfm?hwid=tw9416&cat=search; Trussell, J. (2007). Contraceptive efficacy. In R. A. Hatcher, et al. (Eds.), *Contraceptive technology* (19th rev. ed.). New York: Ardent Media.

IUDs are removed by professionals. Nine out of 10 former IUD users who wish to do so become pregnant within a year.

The IUD is highly effective and does not diminish sexual spontaneity or sexual sensations, and once in place, the woman need not do anything more to prevent pregnancy. If the IUD is so effective and relatively maintenance free, why is it not very popular? One reason is that insertion can be painful. Another reason is side effects—menstrual cramping, spotting, and heavy menstrual bleeding. Women who use the IUD may have an increased risk of PID. The IUD may also perforate (tear) the uterine or cervical walls, which can cause bleeding, pain, and adhesions and become life threatening.

Barrier Methods

Barrier methods include condoms, diaphragms, sponges, and cervical caps.

Condoms

Condoms, the only contraceptive device used by men, are also called "rubbers," "safes," "**prophylactics**" (from Greek roots meaning "on guard" because latex condoms protect against STIs), and "skins" (referring to condoms made from animal intestines). They have several drawbacks: they are less effective than the pill or the IUD and may disrupt spontaneity during lovemaking, and can reduce sexual sensations because the penis does not directly touch the vaginal wall. But they also have a major advantage: latex condoms can help prevent the spread of HIV/AIDS and other STIs, including HPV, chlamydia, and gonorrhea. Condoms (skins) made from the intestinal membranes of lambs may allow greater sexual sensations but do not protect as well against STIs.

The condom is rolled onto the penis following erection (see Figure 5-2). Between 1% and 2% of condoms break or fall off during intercourse or when withdrawing the penis. The following guidelines help ensure a condom is used effectively:

- Use a new condom with each sex act.
- Avoid damaging the condom with fingernails, teeth, or sharp objects.
- Apply the condom after the penis is erect and before any genital, oral, or anal contact with the partner.
- Use only water-based lubricants (e.g., K-Y Jelly, Astroglide, Aqua Lube, and glycerin) with latex condoms.
- Ensure adequate lubrication.
- Withdraw while the penis remains erect and hold the condom firmly against the base of the penis.

The Diaphragm

The **diaphragm** is a shallow latex cup or dome. The rim is a flexible ring. A diaphragm must be fitted to the contour of the vagina by a health professional. Women need to practice insertion in a health professional's office (see Figure 5-3).

When fitted properly, the diaphragm forms a barrier against sperm. But it should be used with a spermicidal cream or jelly to ensure greater protection. The

Figure 5-2 Applying a Condom

Condoms are placed on the head of the penis and then rolled down the shaft. This figure shows a condom with a reservoir for catching the ejaculate.

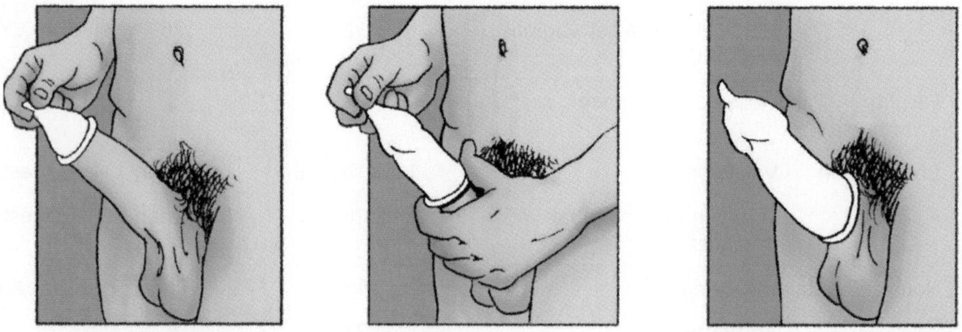

Place condom over head of the erect penis. If condom does not have reservoir tip, pinch the top of the condom to leave room for semen.

While holding the top, unroll the condom.

Continue unrolling the condom to the base of the penis.

prophylactic
An agent that protects against disease.

diaphragm
A shallow rubber cup or dome, fitted to the contour of a woman's vagina, that is coated with a spermicide and inserted prior to coitus to prevent conception.

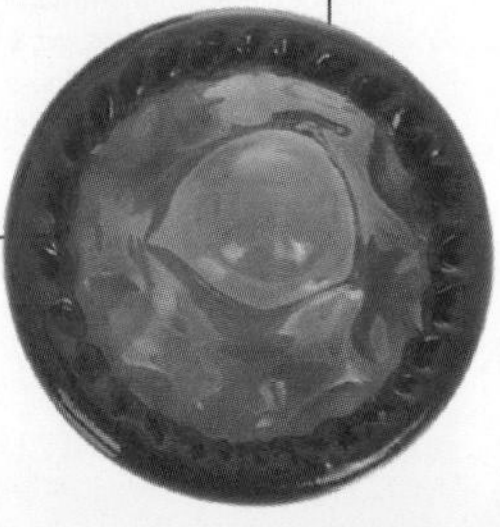

Figure 5-3 Insertion of a Diaphragm.
The diaphragm forms a barrier against sperm but is best used with a spermicidal cream or jelly.

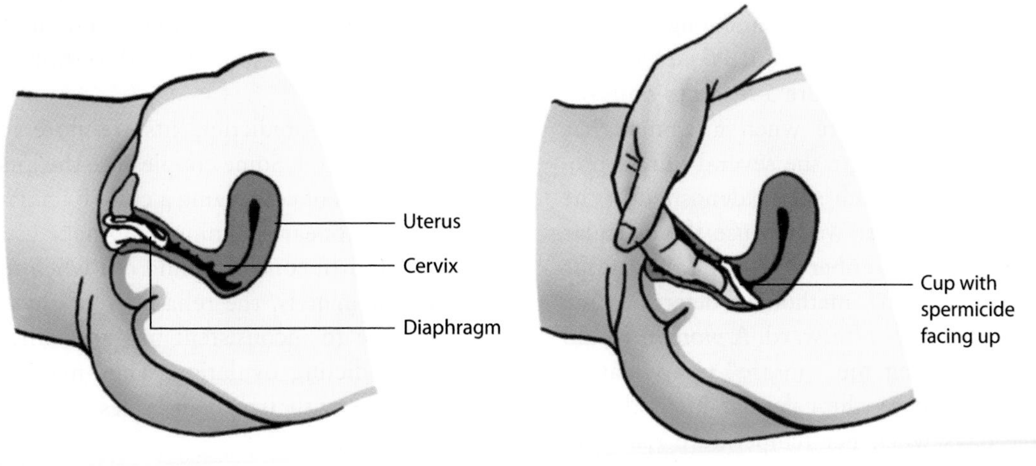

diaphragm and spermicide should be inserted no more than a few hours before sex and should be left in place *at least six hours* afterward to allow the spermicide to work. It should be removed within 24 hours to guard against infection.

The diaphragm does not alter the woman's hormone production or reproductive cycle. The major drawback is the high pregnancy rate associated with typical use.

Spermicides

Spermicides are sperm-killing chemical agents. They include jellies, creams, suppositories, aerosol foam, and contraceptive film. They should be left in place (no douching) for several hours after sex. Spermicides coat the cervical opening, blocking and killing sperm. With typical use, the yearly failure rate of spermicides is high. But if used correctly and consistently, the failure rate drops. Spermicides containing nonoxynol-9 do *not* provide protection against STIs such as HIV/AIDS.

The Contraceptive Sponge

The contraceptive sponge (brand name: Today) contains nonoxynol-9 and provides contraceptive protection for up to 24 hours. It is a soft, disposable device, that provides a barrier against sperm and which holds spermicide. It also absorbs sperm.

The Cervical Cap

The cervical cap, like the diaphragm, is a dome-shaped rubber cup, smaller than a diaphragm, that is fitted by a health professional snugly over the cervical opening. Like the diaphragm, the cap is to be used with a spermicide. It should be left in place for at least eight hours after sex. The cap provides continuous protection for upwards of 48 hours without the need for additional spermicide. The failure rate with typical use is estimated to be high, often due to being dislodged or to changes in the cervix during the menstrual cycle.

Fertility Awareness (Rhythm) Methods

Rhythm methods (also called *natural birth control* or *natural family planning*) rely on fertility awareness—that is, awareness of the fertile segments of the woman's menstrual cycle. These methods are based on predicting ovulation so that the couple can *abstain* when the woman is fertile. Since rhythm methods do not use artificial devices, they have been judged acceptable to the Roman Catholic Church. Many non-Catholics also use rhythm methods because they carry no side effects. As we see next, there are several methods used to predict ovulation.

The *calendar method* assumes that ovulation occurs 14 days prior to menstruation. The couple abstains during the period that begins 3 days prior to day 13 (because sperm are unlikely to survive for more than 72 hours in the female reproductive tract) and ends 2 days after day 15 (because an unfertilized ovum is unlikely to remain receptive to fertilization for longer than 48 hours). The period of abstention thus covers days 10 to 17 of the woman's cycle.

When a woman has regular 28-day cycles, predicting the period of abstention is relatively easy. Women

sterilization
Surgical procedures that render people incapable of reproduction without affecting sexual activity.

with irregular cycles are generally advised to chart their cycles for 10 to 12 months to determine their shortest and longest cycles.

The *BBT method* (see Figure 5-4) relies on basal body temperature to indicate when a woman has ovulated. It does not indicate the several *unsafe* pre-ovulatory days during which sperm deposited in the vagina may remain viable. Women use the calendar method to predict the number of "safe" days prior to ovulation and the BBT method to determine the number of "unsafe" days afterward. A woman would abstain from sex during the "unsafe" pre-ovulatory period (as determined by the calendar method) and then for three days when her temperature rises and remains high.

The *ovulation method* tracks changes in the viscosity of the cervical mucus. Following menstruation, the vagina feels rather dry. These dry days are relatively safe. Then a mucous discharge appears in the vagina that is first thick and sticky and white or cloudy in color. Sex should be avoided at the first sign of mucus. As the cycle progresses, the mucous discharge thins and clears, becoming slippery or stringy. These are the *peak days*. This mucous discharge, called the *ovulatory mucus*, may be accompanied by a feeling of vaginal lubrication or wetness. Ovulation takes place about a day after the last peak day (about four days after this ovulatory mucus first appears). Then the mucus becomes cloudy and tacky once more. Intercourse may resume four days following the last peak day.

Ovulation-prediction kits are more accurate than the BBT method. Some couples use the kits to enhance their chances of conceiving a child by having sex when ovulation appears imminent. Others use them as a means of birth control to find out when to abstain.

Unfortunately, the reliability of rhythm methods is low due to inconsistent use and difficulties accurately predicting ovulation. They may be unsuitable for women with irregular cycles, and they offer no protection from STIs.

Sterilization

Sterilization is used to permanently end fertility and is second to abstinence as the most effective form of contraception. More than a million sterilizations are performed in the United States each year. It is the most widely used form of birth control among couples aged 30 and above in committed relationships.

The male sterilization procedure is the *vasectomy*, which is generally performed in a doctor's office under

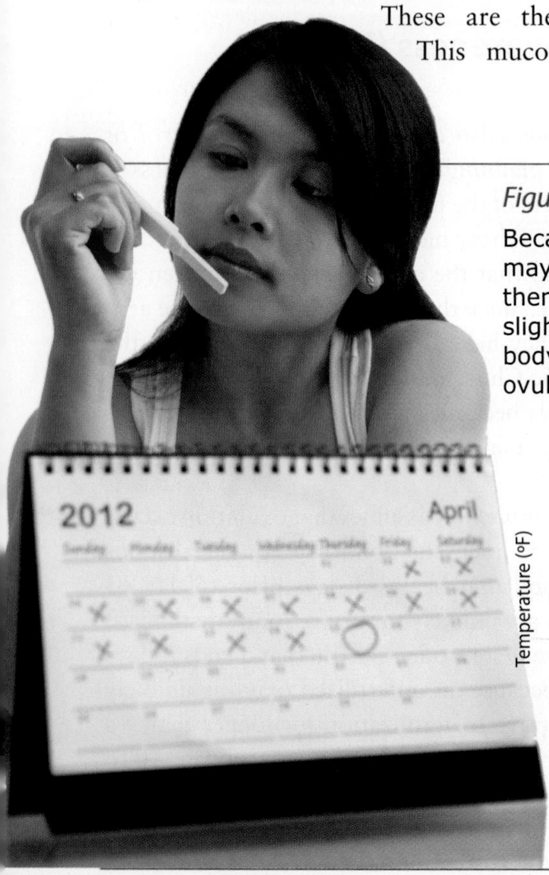

Figure 5-4 A Basal Body Temperature (BBT) Chart

Because most women have somewhat irregular menstrual cycles, they may not be able to predict ovulation perfectly. The BBT chart helps them to do so. Body temperature is fairly even before ovulation but dips slightly just before ovulation. On the day after ovulation, a woman's body temperature increases about 0.4 to 0.8ºF above the level before ovulation.

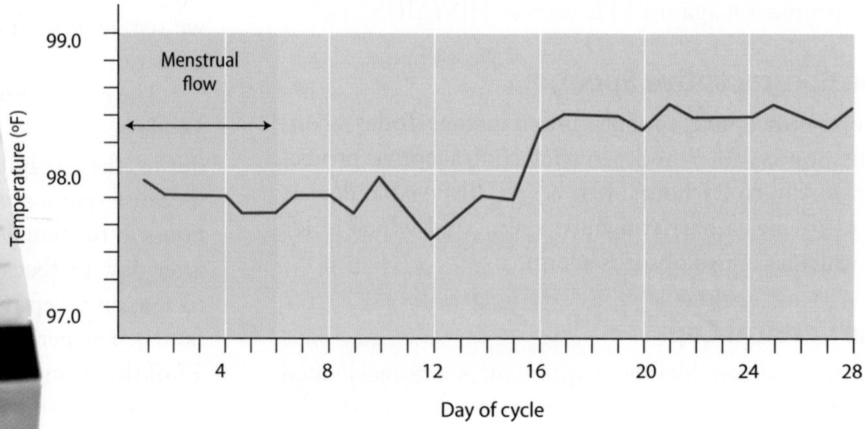

local anesthesia. Incisions are made in the scrotum. Each vas deferens is cut, a segment is removed, and the ends are tied off or cauterized to prevent them from rejoining (see Figure 5-5). Sperm are reabsorbed by the body.

Vasectomy does not diminish the man's sex drive or change his sexual response or the sensations of orgasm. No differences are found in sexual satisfaction, marital satisfaction, communication, and frequency of sexual intercourse in men before and after vasectomy.[9]

Vasectomy should be considered permanent, as the success of surgical reversal (tying the ends of each vas deferens back together) vary wildly—from 16% to 79%![10]

Nearly four in 10 women in committed relationships under the age of 45 have been surgically sterilized. **Tubal sterilization**, also called *tubal ligation*, is the most common method. Tubal sterilization prevents ova and sperm from passing through the fallopian tubes.

Figure 5-5 Vasectomy

In this male sterilization procedure, incisions are made in the scrotum. Each vas deferens is cut, and the ends are tied off or cauterized to prevent sperm from reaching the urethra. Sperm are then harmlessly reabsorbed by the body.

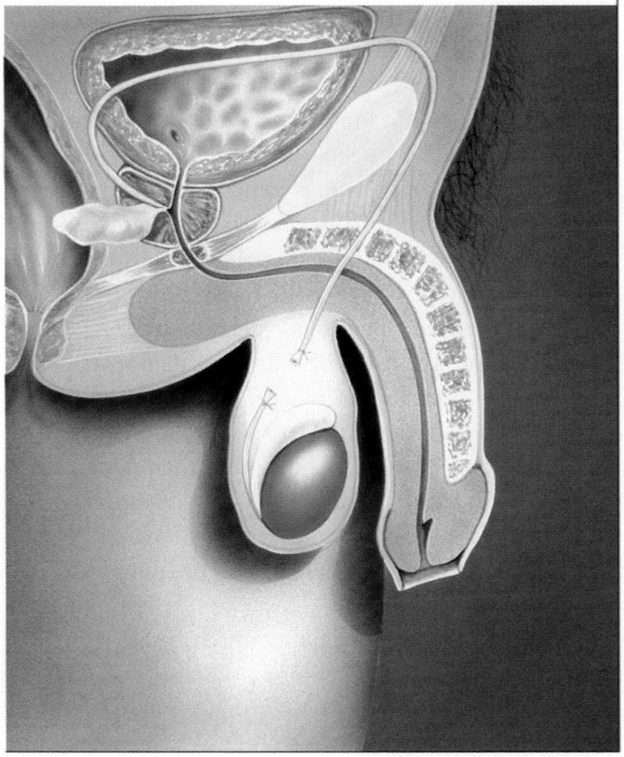

The most commonly used surgical procedures for tubal sterilization are *minilaparotomy* and *laparoscopy.* In a minilaparotomy, the surgeon makes a small incision in the abdomen, just above the pubic hairline, to be able to access the fallopian tubes. The surgeon then cuts and ties back each tube or clamps them with a clip. In a laparoscopy (see Figure 5-6 on the next page), which is sometimes referred to as "belly button surgery," the surgeon accesses the fallopian tubes by making a small incision just below the navel. The surgeon locates the tubes with a narrow, lighted viewing instrument called a *laparoscope.* A section of each tube is cauterized, cut, or clamped. In a *culpotomy*, the fallopian tubes are accessed through an incision in the back wall of the vagina.

Female sterilization methods do not disrupt the woman's sex drive, sexual response, production of sex hormones, or the menstrual cycle. Unfertilized ovum is reabsorbed by the body, rather than sloughed off in the menstrual flow.

Tubal sterilization, like vasectomy, should be considered irreversible, although reversals are successful in 43% to 88% of cases.[11] Surgical sterilization can lead to complications such as abdominal infections, bleeding, inadvertent punctures of nearby organs, and scarring.

A *hysterectomy*—surgical removal of the uterus—also results in sterilization. A hysterectomy is a major operation performed because of cancer or other diseases of the reproductive tract; it is not an appropriate means of sterilization.

"Non-Methods" of Birth Control

Douching and withdrawal are considered "non-methods" of birth control. Translation: they don't work. Douching is ineffective because large numbers of sperm move beyond the range of the douche seconds after ejaculation. In fact, squirting a liquid into the vagina may propel sperm *toward* the uterus. Withdrawal means that the man removes his penis from the vagina before ejaculating. Withdrawal has a high failure rate because the man may not withdraw in time, some ejaculate may fall on the vaginal lips and find their way to the fallopian tubes, and sperm may be present in *pre*-ejaculatory secretions.

tubal sterilization
The most common method of female sterilization, in which the fallopian tubes are surgically severed to prevent the meeting of sperm and ova.

Figure 5-6 Tubal Sterilization Using Laparoscopy

In this female sterilization procedure, an incision is made in the abdomen below the navel. A laparoscope is inserted and used to cut, cauterize, or clamp a section of each fallopian tube to prevent ova from joining with sperm.

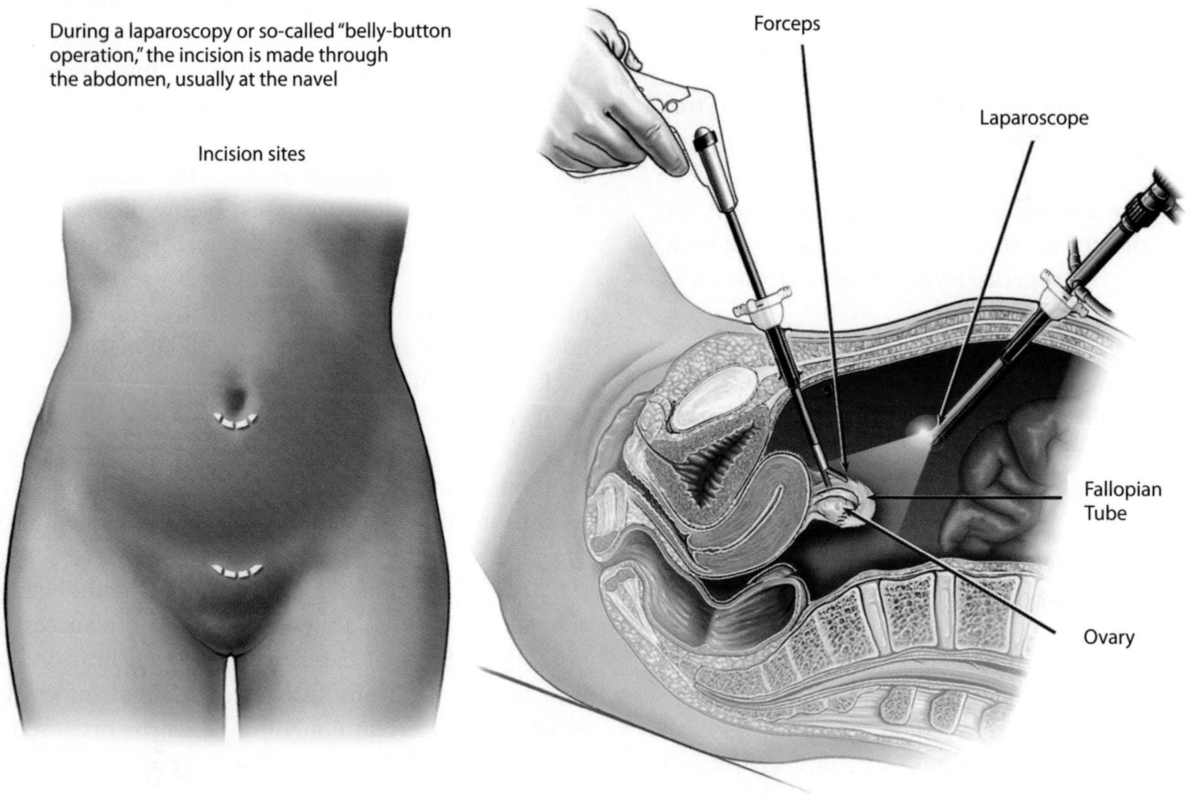
During a laparoscopy or so-called "belly-button operation," the incision is made through the abdomen, usually at the navel
Incision sites
Forceps
Laparoscope
Fallopian Tube
Ovary

Abortion

The term *abortion* usually refers to an *induced abortion* (in contrast to a spontaneous abortion, or miscarriage). It is the purposeful termination of a pregnancy. Although the abortion rate in the United States has been slowly declining over the past 20 years, about one of out of five pregnancies is terminated by abortion.[12] Nearly 90% of abortions in the United States are performed during the first trimester, when they are safest for the woman and least costly. Abortions are most common among women in their 20s, but some 18% of U.S. women obtaining abortions are teenagers. Most women who obtain abortions (61%) have one or more children.

LEARNING OUTCOME 4

Discuss methods of abortion

Most Americans support a woman's right to have a legal abortion, but the majority believe that abortion should be legal only under some circumstances (see Figure 5-7). Those who believe that abortion should always be legal or should never be legal are about evenly split.

The continuing national debate over abortion has played out against a backdrop of demonstrations, marches, and occasional violence. Many in the right-to-life (pro-life) movement assert that human life begins at conception and thus view abortion as the murder of an unborn child. Some in the pro-life movement allow no exceptions, but others would permit abortion to save the mother's life or in cases when pregnancy results from rape or incest.

The pro-choice movement contends that abortion is a matter of personal choice and that the government has no right to interfere with a woman's control over her own body, and over what happens within

Figure 5-7 "Do You Think that Abortion Should Be Legal under Any Circumstances, Legal Only under Certain Circumstances, or Illegal in All Circumstances?"

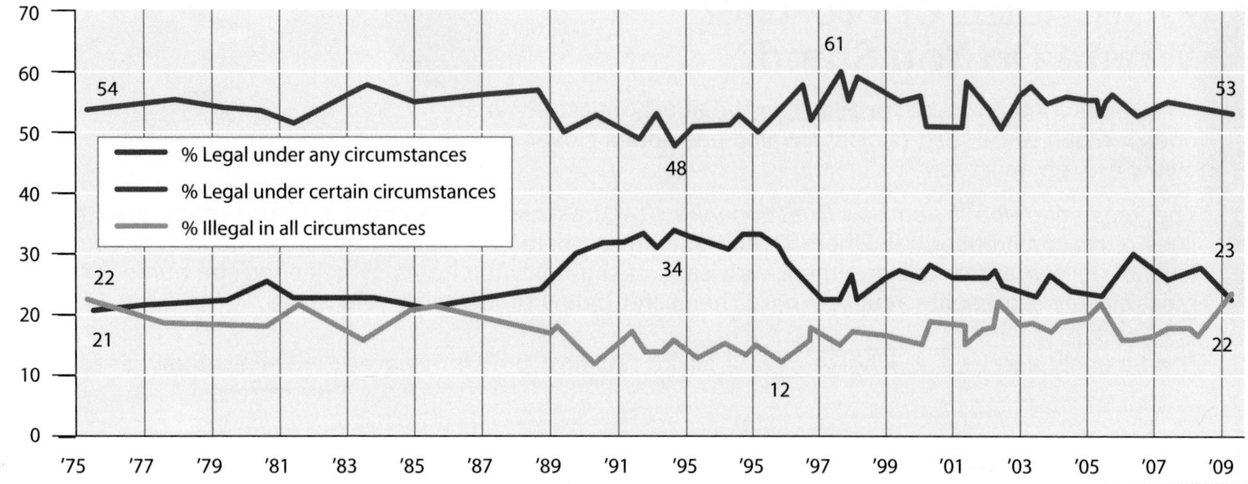

Source: Gallup Poll, http://www.gallup.com/poll/147734/americans-split-along-pro-choice-pro-life-lines.aspx, Copyright © 2011 Gallup, Inc. Used with permission.

her body, including pregnancy. "Health Check 5-1," which begins on page 102, assesses your agreement with pro-life or pro-choice lines of reasoning about abortion.

In 1973, the U.S. Supreme Court in effect legalized abortion in the landmark *Roe v. Wade* decision. *Roe v. Wade* held that a woman's right to an abortion was protected under the Constitution's right to privacy clause. The decision legalized abortions for any reason during the first trimester. The Court ruled that states may regulate a woman's right to have an abortion during the second trimester to protect her health, as in requiring her to obtain an abortion in a hospital rather than a doctor's office. The Court also held that when a fetus becomes capable of independent life (or "viable") its rights outweigh the mother's right to privacy. Because the fetus may become viable early in the third trimester, states may prohibit third-trimester abortions, except when an abortion is necessary to protect a woman's health.

Methods of Abortion

There are many methods of abortion. **Vacuum aspiration**, or *suction curettage*, is the safest and most common method of abortion. It accounts for more than 90% of abortions in the United States. The procedure can be performed with little or no anesthesia in a medical office or clinic, but only during the first trimester. The cervix is usually dilated by insertion of progressively larger curved metal rods (or "dilators") or by insertion, hours earlier, of a stick of seaweed called *Laminaria digitata*. *Laminaria* expands as it absorbs cervical moisture, providing a gentler means of opening the cervix. Then a tube connected to an aspirator (suction machine) is inserted through the cervix into the uterus. The uterine contents are evacuated (emptied) by suction (see Figure 5-8 on page 104). Possible complications include perforation of the uterus, infection, cervical lacerations, and hemorrhaging, but these are rare.

The **D&C**, which stands for **dilation and curettage**, is usually performed 8 to 20 weeks following the last menstrual period (LMP). Once the cervix has been dilated, the uterine contents are scraped from the uterine lining. D&Cs are carried out in a hospital, usually under general anesthesia. The scraping increases the chances of hemorrhaging, infection, and perforation. Because of these risks, D&Cs have largely been replaced by vacuum aspiration. But D&Cs are still used to treat various gynecological problems.

The **D&E (dilation and evacuation)** is used most commonly during the second trimester, when vacuum aspiration alone would be too risky. The D&E combines suction and

vacuum aspiration
Removal of the uterine contents by suction. An abortion method used early in pregnancy.

dilation and curetage (D&C)
An operation in which the cervix is dilated and uterine contents are scraped away.

dilation and evacuation (D&E)
An abortion method in which the cervix is dilated prior to vacuum aspiration.

HEALTH CHECK 5-1

health check

Pro-Choice or Pro-Life? Where Do You Stand?

What does it mean to be "pro-life" on the abortion issue? What does it mean to be "pro-choice"? Which position is closer to your own views on abortion?

The *Reasoning about Abortion Questionnaire (RAQ)* assesses agreement with pro-life or pro-choice lines of reasoning about abortion. To find out which position is closer to your own, indicate your level of agreement or disagreement with each of the following items by selecting the number that most closely represents your feelings. Then refer below to interpret your score.

5 = Strongly agree   4 = Agree   3 = Mixed feelings   2 = Disagree   1 = Strongly disagree

1. Abortion is a matter of personal choice.	5 4 3 2 1
2. Abortion is a threat to our society.	5 4 3 2 1
3. A woman should have control over what is happening to her own body by having the option to choose abortion.	5 4 3 2 1
4. Only God, not people, can decide if a fetus should live.	5 4 3 2 1
5. Even if one believes that there may be some exceptions, abortion is still basically wrong.	5 4 3 2 1
6. Abortion violates an unborn person's fundamental right to life.	5 4 3 2 1
7. A woman should be able to exercise her rights to self-determination by choosing to have an abortion.	5 4 3 2 1
8. Outlawing abortion could take away a woman's sense of self and personal autonomy.	5 4 3 2 1
9. Outlawing abortion violates a woman's civil rights.	5 4 3 2 1
10. Abortion is morally unacceptable and unjustified.	5 4 3 2 1
11. In my reasoning, the notion that an unborn fetus may be a human life is not a deciding issue in considering abortion.	5 4 3 2 1

continued

the D&C. First the cervix is dilated. Then a suction tube removes some of the contents of the uterus. The remaining contents are removed with forceps. A scraper may also be used to scrape the uterine wall. Like the D&C, the D&E is usually performed in the hospital under general anesthesia. Most women recover quickly and relatively painlessly. In rare instances, however, complications can arise, including bleeding, infection, and perforation of the uterine lining.

intra-amniotic infusion
An abortion method in which a substance is injected into the amniotic sac to induce premature labor. Also called instillation.

Second-trimester abortions are sometimes performed by chemically inducing premature labor and delivery. The procedure is called *instillation*, or **intra-amniotic infusion.** A solution of salt or of prostaglandins (hormones that stimulate uterine contractions during labor) is injected into the amniotic sac. Prostaglandins may also be administered by vaginal suppository. Uterine contractions (labor) begin within a few hours. The fetus and placenta are expelled within 24 to 48 hours. Medical complications, risks, and costs are greater with intra-amniotic infusion than with other methods of abortion.

Many Americans express concerns over the late-term surgical abortion method generally known as "partial-birth abortion" and referred to medically as an

12. Abortion can be described as taking a life unjustly. 5 4 3 2 1
13. A woman should have the right to decide to have an abortion based on her own life circumstances. 5 4 3 2 1
14. If a woman feels that having a child might ruin her life, she should consider an abortion. 5 4 3 2 1
15. Abortion could destroy the sanctity of motherhood. 5 4 3 2 1
16. An unborn fetus is a viable human being with rights. 5 4 3 2 1
17. If a woman feels she can't care for a baby, she should be able to have an abortion. 5 4 3 2 1
18. Abortion is the destruction of one life for the convenience of another. 5 4 3 2 1
19. Abortion is the same as murder. 5 4 3 2 1
20. Even if one believes that there are times when abortion is immoral, it is still basically the woman's own choice. 5 4 3 2 1

Scoring Key

First tally your scores for the following items: 1, 3, 7, 8, 9, 11, 13, 14, 17, and 20. This score represents your support for a *pro-choice* point of view: ________

Now tally your scores for the remaining items: 2, 4, 5, 6, 10, 12, 15, 16, 18, and 19. This score represents your support for a *pro-life* point of view: ________

Now subtract your pro-choice score from you pro-life score. Write the difference, including the sign (+ or –) here: ________

A positive score indicates agreement with a pro-life philosophy. A negative score indicates agreement with a pro-choice philosophy. The higher your score, the more strongly you agree with the philosophy you endorsed. Scores may range from –40 to +40. One sample of 230 undergraduate students (115 of each sex) obtained a mean score of –7.48 and a median score of –13.33. This indicates that the students tended to be pro-choice in their attitudes. Another sample of 38 graduate students (31 women and 7 men) obtained mean scores of –11 to –12 and median scores of –17 to –18 on two separate occasions. Scores for other samples may vary.

Source: Reprinted from *Journal of Counseling Psychology*, Volume 37 (1), Parsons, N. K., Richards, H. C., and Kanter, G. D., Validation of a Scale to Measure Reasoning About Abortion, pp. 107-112. © 1990, with permission from Elsevier.

intact dilation and extraction, or "intact D and X." The intact D and X is usually performed after 21 weeks of gestation. The cervix is dilated, and a fetus that may be as much as 10 inches long is extracted from the mother through the birth canal. Brain tissue is destroyed by suctioning to terminate life functions. Pro-choice advocates argue that intact D and X may be necessary to save the life of the mother. Pro-life advocates argue that birth methods such as cesarean section provide workable alternatives.

The procedure called a *hysterotomy* is, in effect, a cesarean section, in which the fetus and uterine contents are surgically removed. It may be performed during the late second trimester, between the 16th and 24th weeks LMP. This procedure involves major surgery and is performed rarely, usually only when intra-amniotic infusion is not advised.

The abortion drug RU-486 (*mifepristone*) induces early abortion by blocking the effects of progesterone. Progesterone is the hormone that stimulates proliferation of the endometrium, allowing implantation of the fertilized ovum and, subsequently, development of the placenta. RU-486 can only be used within 49 days of the beginning of the woman's last menstrual period. The typical course is for the woman to take three mifepristone pills, frequently in the doctor's office. Two

Figure 5-8 Vacuum Aspiration

In this common early-stage abortion method, a tube is inserted through the cervix into the uterus, and the uterine contents are evacuated by suction.

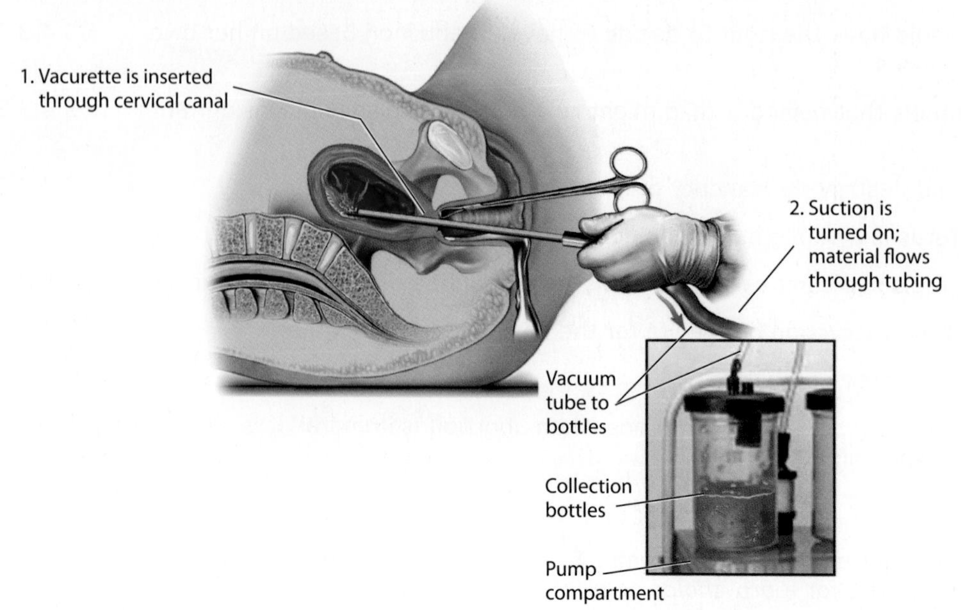
1. Vacuurette is inserted through cervical canal
2. Suction is turned on; material flows through tubing
Vacuum tube to bottles
Collection bottles
Pump compartment

days later, she is given a second oral drug, *misoprostol*, which causes uterine contractions that expel the embryo. There is also usually a follow-up visit within a couple of weeks to make sure the abortion is complete and the woman is well.

Pregnancy

We can date pregnancy from the onset of the last menstrual cycle before conception, which makes the normal gestation period 280 days. We can also date pregnancy from the date at which fertilization was assumed to have taken place, which normally corresponds to two weeks after the beginning of the woman's last menstrual cycle. In this case, the normal gestation period is 266 days.

human chorionic gonadotropin (HCG)
A hormone produced by women shortly after conception, which stimulates the corpus luteum to continue to produce progesterone. The presence of HCG in a woman's urine indicates that she is pregnant.

LEARNING OUTCOME 5

Discuss health issues in pregnancy and prenatal development

Once pregnancy has been confirmed, the delivery date may be calculated by *Naegele's rule*:

1. Jot down the date of the first day of the last menstrual period.
2. Add seven days.
3. Subtract three months.
4. Add one year.

If the last period began on November 12, 2013, adding seven days yields November 19, 2013. Subtracting three months yields August 19, 2013. Adding one year gives a "due date" of August 19, 2014. Most babies are delivered during a 10-day period that spans this date.

Early Days of Pregnancy

Shortly after conception, a woman's body produces the hormone **human chorionic gonadotropin (HCG)**. Pregnancy can be confirmed by tests that detect HCG in the urine or blood a few days into the pregnancy. Over-the-counter home pregnancy tests test the woman's urine for HCG. Women are advised to consult their physicians if they suspect that they are pregnant or wish to confirm a home test result.

A few days after conception, a woman may note tenderness in her breasts. Hormonal stimulation of the mammary glands may make the breasts more sensitive and cause sensations of tingling and fullness.

"Morning sickness"—which may linger all day!—refers to the nausea, food aversions, and vomiting that many women experience during pregnancy. Women carrying more than one child usually experience more nausea. Although the condition is called *morning sickness*, nausea and vomiting during pregnancy are normal and not a "sickness" at all. Biologists reviewed records of some 20,000 pregnancies and reported that morning sickness was associated with a healthy outcome, including lower incidences of miscarriage and stillbirth as compared with women who experienced less severe morning sickness or no morning sickness.[13]

Morning sickness can be so severe that the woman cannot eat regularly. Having small amounts of food in the stomach throughout the day is sometimes of help. Eating a few crackers at bedtime and before getting out of bed in the morning may also help. Other women benefit from medication. Women are advised to discuss their condition with their obstetricians. Morning sickness usually—but not always—subsides by about the 12th week of pregnancy.

Pregnant women may experience greater-than-normal fatigue during the early weeks, so that they sleep longer and fall asleep more readily than usual. The expanding uterus may place pressure on the bladder and cause frequent urination.

Most health professionals agree that sex is safe throughout pregnancy, provided that the pregnancy is developing normally and the woman has no history of miscarriage. Women who experience bleeding or cramps may be advised by their obstetricians to avoid sexual intercourse.

To help ensure a healthy pregnancy, obtain adequate prenatal health care. The online feature "Health Skills 5-3" has advice on how to find an obstetrician who is best for your needs.

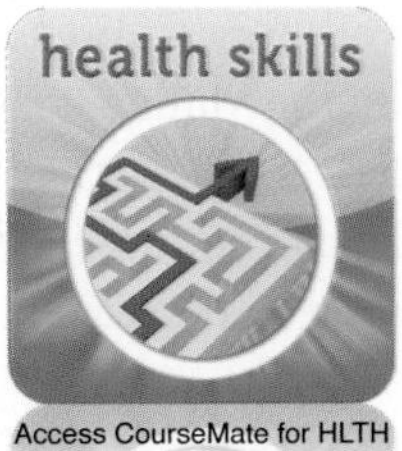

Access CourseMate for HLTH at www.cengagebrain.com.

Stages of Prenatal Development

Shortly after conception, the single cell that results from the union of sperm and ovum begins to multiply—becoming two cells, then four, then eight, and so on. During the weeks and months that follow, tissues, structures, and organs begin to form, and the fetus gradually takes on the shape of a human being (see Figure 5-9). By the time the fetus is born, it consists of hundreds of billions of cells—more cells than there are stars in the Milky Way galaxy. Prenatal development can be divided into three periods: the *germinal stage*, which corresponds to about the first two weeks; the *embryonic stage*, which spans the first two months; and the *fetal stage*, which comprises the final seven months of a nine month pregnancy. We generally speak of pregnancy in terms of three trimesters of three months each.

Figure 5-9 A Human Fetus at 12 Weeks

By the end of the first trimester, the formation of all major organ systems is complete. Fingers and toes are fully formed, and the sex of the fetus can be determined visually.

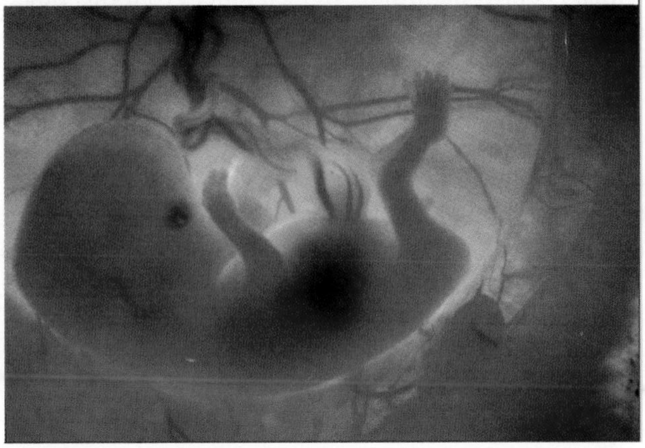

The Germinal Stage

Within 36 hours after conception, the zygote divides into two cells. It then divides repeatedly as it completes a three- or four-day journey to the uterus. The mass of dividing cells "wanders" about the uterus for another three or four days before beginning to implant itself in the uterine wall. Implantation takes about another week. The period from conception to implantation is termed the **germinal stage**.

Implantation may be accompanied by some bleeding resulting from the rupture of small blood vessels that line the uterus. Bleeding can be a sign of a miscarriage, but most women who have implantation bleeding have normal pregnancies.

The Embryonic Stage

The period from implantation to about the eighth week of development is the **embryonic stage**, during which the major organ systems of the body differentiate. By about three weeks after conception, two ridges appear in the embryo. The

germinal stage
The period of prenatal development prior to implantation in the uterus.

embryonic stage
The stage of prenatal development that lasts from implantation through the eighth week, and which is characterized by the differentiation of the major organ systems.

ridges fold together to form the **neural tube**. This tube develops into the nervous system.

During the third week of development, the head and blood vessels begin to form. By the fourth week, the heart begins to beat and pump blood in the embryo, which is only one-fifth of an inch long. From this time, the heart normally continues to beat without rest every minute of every day for the better part of a century. By the end of the first month of development, we observe the beginnings of the arms and legs, called "arm buds" and "leg buds." The mouth, eyes, ears, and nose take shape. The brain and other parts of the nervous system develop.

By six to eight weeks, in an embryo that is about one inch long and weighs one-thirtieth of an ounce, facial features are visible. During the second month, nervous impulses begin to travel through the nervous system.

The embryo—and later, the fetus—develop within a protective environment in the mother's uterus called the **amniotic sac**. The embryo and fetus are suspended in fluids in the sac, which acts as a shock absorber, cushioning the embryo from the mother's movements. The fluid also helps maintain a steady temperature.

Nutrients and waste products pass between the mother and embryo (or fetus) through the **placenta**. The **umbilical cord** connects the fetus to the placenta. The umbilical cord serves as a conduit for nutrients to pass from the mother's blood stream and for fetal waste products to be passed back to the mother.

The two circulatory systems (mother and embryo or fetus) do not mix. Only certain substances pass through the placenta, such as oxygen (from the mother to the fetus); carbon dioxide and other wastes (from the embryo or fetus to the mother, to be eliminated by the mother's lungs and kidneys); nutrients; some microscopic disease-causing organisms; and some drugs, including aspirin, narcotics, alcohol, and tranquilizers.

neural tube
A hollow area in the blastocyst from which the nervous system will develop.

amniotic sac
The sac containing the fetus.

placenta
An organ connected to the fetus by the umbilical cord. The placenta serves as a relay station between mother and fetus, allowing the exchange of nutrients and wastes.

umbilical cord
A tube that connects the fetus to the placenta.

The placenta also secretes hormones, including estrogen and progesterone, that preserve the pregnancy, stimulate the uterine contractions that induce childbirth, and help prepare the breasts for nursing. Some of these hormones may also cause the signs of pregnancy. Eventually, the placenta passes from the woman's body after delivery. Thus, it is also called the "afterbirth."

The Fetal Stage

The fetal stage, which begins by the ninth week of pregnancy, continues until birth. By the end of the first trimester, the major organ systems, the fingers and toes, and the external genitals have been formed. During the second trimester, the fetus grows dramatically in size, and its organ systems mature. The fetus increases in weight more than thirty-fold, from one *ounce* to two *pounds*, and grows from about 4 inches to 14 inches in length.

During the fourth month, the mother can feel fetal movements. The fetus opens and shuts its eyes, sucks its thumb, alternates between periods of wakefulness and sleep, and responds to light and sounds. Some even do somersaults.

During the third trimester, the organs continue to mature and enlarge. Typically, during the seventh month the fetus turns upside down in the uterus so that it will be born headfirst. If birth occurs late during the eighth month, the odds overwhelmingly favor survival.

Although the embryo and fetus are suspended in a protective environment within the mother's uterus, various factors can affect its health and development. These include drugs taken by the mother, X-rays, environmental contaminants such as lead and mercury, and infectious organisms capable of passing through the placenta to the embryo or fetus. More information about specific prenatal risks and how to prevent them is found in the online feature "Prevention 5-1." Read "Health Skills 5-4" to learn about medical procedures used to detect fetal abnormalities.

prevention

Access CourseMate for HLTH at www.cengagebrain.com.

Childbirth

Labor begins with the onset of regular uterine contractions. Signs of impending labor include indigestion, diarrhea, cramping, and an ache in the small of the back. About a day or so before labor begins, blood may appear in the woman's vaginal secretions because fetal pressure on the woman's pelvis causes small blood vessels to rupture in the birth canal. Also, tissue that had plugged the cervix, possibly

HEALTH SKILLS 5-4

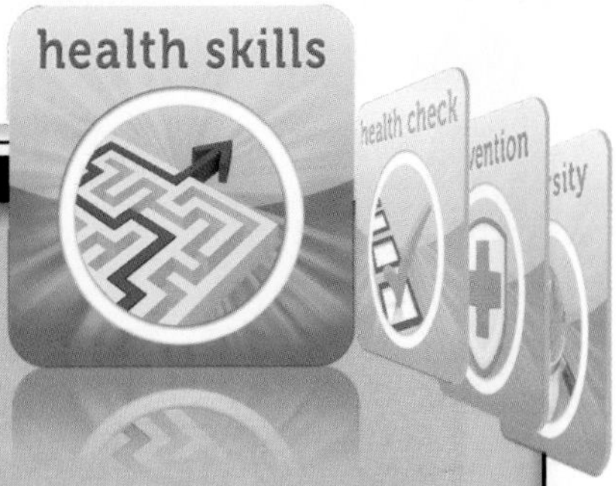

Detecting Chromosomal and Genetic Abnormalities

Genetic counselors help couples evaluate the risks of passing along genetic defects to their children based on information about their medical background, their family history, and tests. Some couples who face a high risk of passing along genetic defects to their children adopt instead.

Various medical procedures are used to detect the presence of genetic disorders in the fetus. *Amniocentesis* is usually performed about four months into pregnancy but is sometimes done earlier. Fluid is drawn from the amniotic sac with a syringe. Fetal cells in the fluid are grown in a culture and examined for abnormalities. *Chorionic villus sampling (CVS)* is performed at about 10 weeks. A narrow tube is used to snip off material from the chorion, the membrane that contains the amniotic sac and fetus. The material is then analyzed. The risks in undergoing amniocentesis and CVS are similar. The tests detect Down syndrome, sickle-cell anemia, Tay-Sachs disease, spina bifida, muscular dystrophy, Rh incompatibility, and other conditions. They also reveal the sex of the fetus.

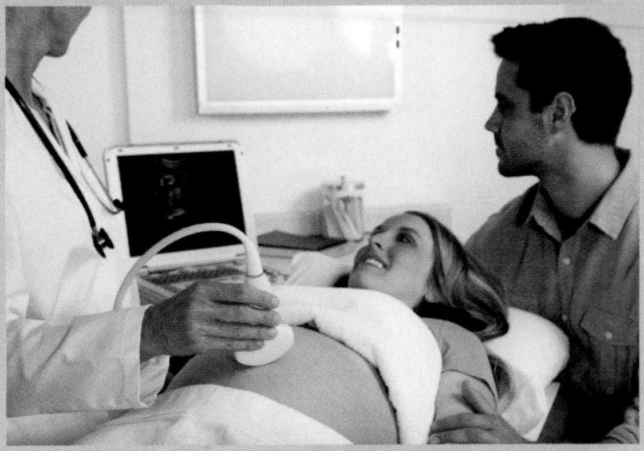

In ultrasound, high-pitched sound waves are bounced off the fetus, like radar, creating a picture of the fetus and allowing the physician to detect certain abnormalities. Parental blood tests can also suggest conditions such as sickle-cell anemia, Tay-Sachs disease, and neural tube defects. Examination of fetal DNA can indicate the presence of Huntington's chorea, cystic fibrosis, and other disorders. Blood tests also allow early detection of Down syndrome.

LEARNING OUTCOME 6

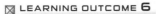

Describe health issues associated with methods of childbirth

preventing entry of infectious agents from the vagina, becomes dislodged, resulting in a discharge of bloody mucus. About one in ten women experience a rush of warm fluid from the amniotic sac and out through the vagina. This means that the amniotic sac (or "bag of waters") has burst. Labor usually begins within a day after rupture of the sac. However, for most women, the amniotic sac does not burst until the end of the first stage of childbirth.

Women typically experience relatively painless false labor contractions, before they experience contractions that widen the cervix or advance the baby through the birth canal. The initiation of labor may involve the secretion of hormones by the fetus that stimulate the mother's glands to secrete **prostaglandins**. Prostaglandins stimulate uterine muscles to contract. Later in labor, the mother's pituitary gland releases **oxytocin**, a hormone that stimulates contractions strong enough to expel the baby.

Stages of Childbirth

Childbirth begins with the onset of labor and involves three stages (see Figure 5-10 on the next page). During the first stage, uterine contractions **efface** and **dilate** the woman's cervix to about four inches (10 cm) in diameter, preparing the way for the baby to pass. Most of the pain experienced in childbirth results from the stretching of the cervix. The first stage may continue for several hours to more than a day. Twelve to 24 hours of labor is considered typical for a first pregnancy. In later pregnancies, labor becomes quicker.

The initial contractions are usually mild and spaced at intervals of 10 to 20 minutes. They may last 20 to 40 seconds. As time passes, contractions become more frequent, long, strong, and regular.

prostaglandins
Uterine hormones that stimulate uterine contractions.

oxytocin
A pituitary hormone that stimulates uterine contractions.

efface
To become thin.

dilate
To open or widen.

Figure 5-10 Stages of Childbirth

In stage 1, uterine contractions efface and dilate the cervix to about four inches so that the baby may pass through. Stage 2 begins with the movement of the baby into the birth canal (vagina) and ends with the birth of the baby. During stage 3, the placenta separates from the uterine wall and is expelled through the birth canal.

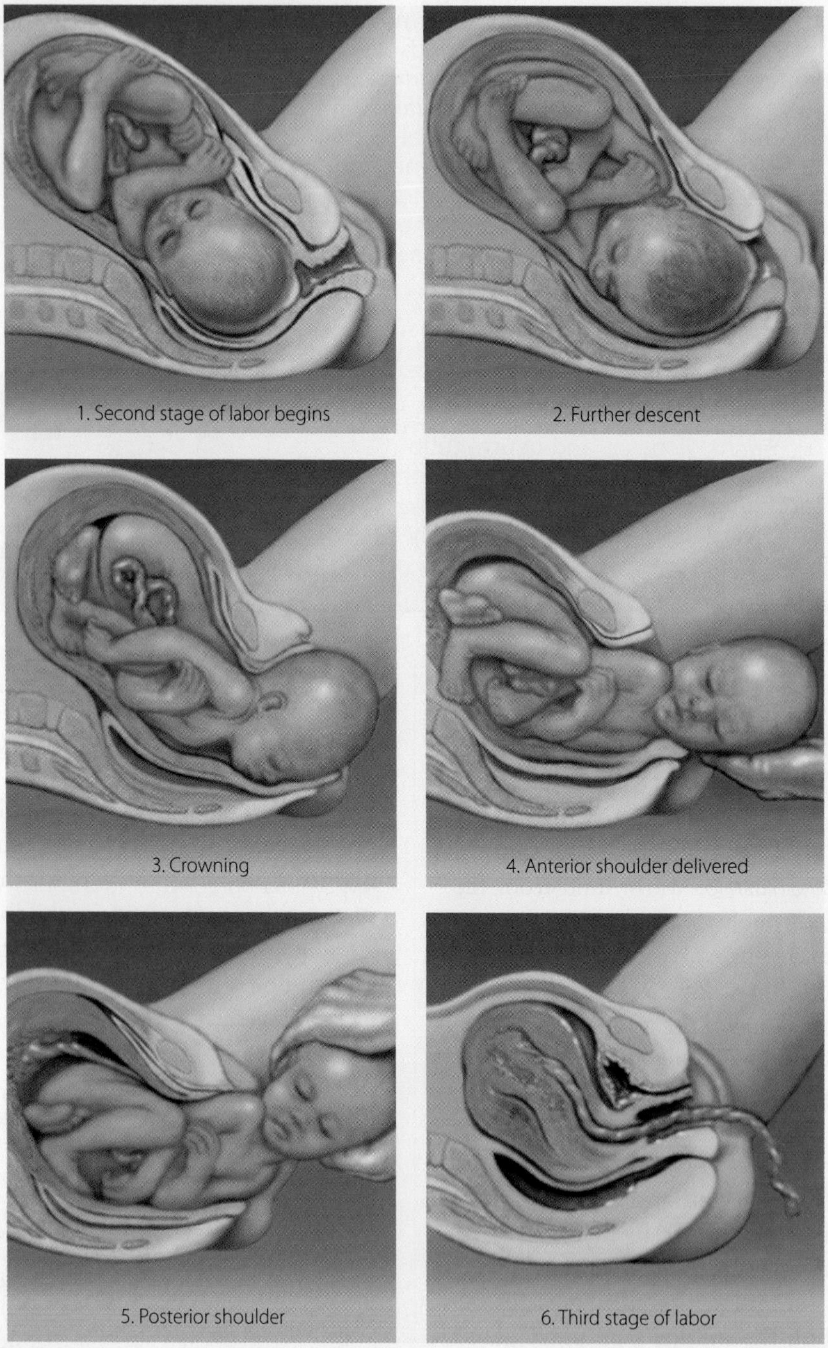

Transition occurs when the cervix becomes nearly fully dilated and the baby's head begins to move into the vagina, or birth canal. Contractions usually come quickly during transition. Transition usually lasts about 30 minutes or less and is often accompanied by feelings of nausea, chills, and intense pain.

The second stage of childbirth begins following transition, when the cervix becomes fully dilated and the baby begins to move into the vagina and first appears at the opening of the birth canal. The second stage is shorter than the first, typically lasting from a few minutes to a few hours and ending with the delivery of the newborn.

Each contraction of the second stage propels the baby farther along the birth canal (vagina). When the baby's head becomes visible at the vaginal opening, it is said to have *crowned*. The baby typically emerges fully a few minutes after crowning.

Once the baby's head has crowned, an **episiotomy** may be performed on the mother to prevent random tearing of the **perineum**, which can occur if it becomes extremely effaced. Episiotomies are controversial because the incision can cause infection and pain, and create discomfort and itching as it heals. As a result of these concerns, rates of episiotomies have dropped sharply. With or without an episiotomy, the baby's passageway to the external world is a tight fit, and the baby's facial features and the shape of its head may be temporarily distended.

The third, or placental, stage of childbirth may last from a few minutes to an hour or more. During this stage, the placenta is expelled. The uterus begins contracting to a smaller size. The physician sews up the episiotomy or any tears in the perineum.

Methods of Childbirth

Before the twentieth century, most women gave birth in their homes, perhaps attended to by a midwife, family, and friends. Today, most women in the United States and Canada give birth in hospitals, attended by obstetricians who use techniques of modern medicine, including anesthetics, to protect mothers and children from infection, complications, and pain.

Anesthetized Childbirth

Advances in science and medicine during the past two centuries have led to the expectation that women should experience minimal discomfort during childbirth. Today, the great majority of women use some form of anesthesia during childbirth.

General anesthesia induces a state of unconsciousness. The drug sodium pentothal, a barbiturate, induces general anesthesia when it is injected into a vein. Barbiturates, tranquilizers, and even narcotics such as Demerol may be given to reduce anxiety and discomfort while the woman remains awake.

Anesthetic drugs, as well as tranquilizers and narcotics, decrease the strength of uterine contractions during delivery. Thus, they may prolong cervical dilation and labor. They also weaken the woman's ability to push the baby through the birth canal. Furthermore, because they cross the placental membrane, they lower the newborn's overall responsiveness.

Regional or **local anesthetics** block pain in parts of the body without generally depressing the mother's alertness or putting her to sleep. In a *pudendal block*, the external genitals are numbed by local injection. In an *epidural block* and a *spinal block*, an anesthetic is injected into the spinal canal, which temporarily numbs the mother's body below the waist. Although local anesthesia decreases the responsiveness of the newborn baby, there is little evidence that anesthetized childbirth has serious long-term effects on children.

Prepared Childbirth: The Lamaze Method

The **Lamaze method** helps women conserve energy during childbirth and reduce pain by associating uterine contractions with other responses, such as pleasant mental images or breathing and relaxation exercises. A woman typically attends Lamaze classes with a "coach"—usually the father—who will aid her in the delivery room by timing contractions, offering emotional support, and coaching her in breathing and relaxation.

The Lamaze method is flexible about the use of anesthetics. Some women forgo anesthetics entirely. Others request them. However, the Lamaze method appears to help women gain a sense of control over the delivery process.

transition
The process during which the cervix becomes nearly fully dilated and the head of the fetus begins to move into the birth canal.

episiotomy
A surgical incision in the perineum that widens the birth canal, preventing random tearing during childbirth.

perineum
The area between the vulva and the anus.

general anesthesia
The use of drugs to put people to sleep and eliminate pain, as during childbirth.

local anesthetic
Anesthetic that eliminates pain in a specific area of the body, as during childbirth.

Lamaze method
A childbirth method in which women learn about childbirth, learn to relax and to breathe in patterns that conserve energy and lessen pain, and have a coach (usually the father) present at childbirth. Also termed prepared childbirth.

Women rightfully stand in the spotlight when it comes to pregnancy and childbirth, but fathers also matter. The online feature "Diversity 5-2" has some useful advice for expectant fathers.

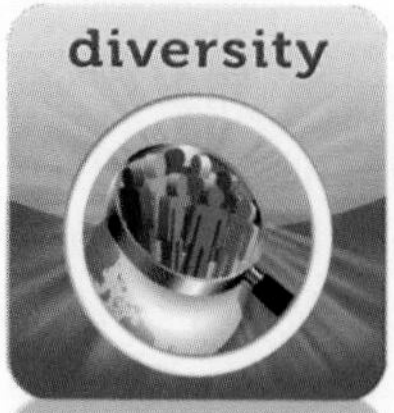

Access CourseMate for HLTH at www.cengagebrain.com.

Cesarean Section

A **cesarean section** delivers the baby by abdominal surgery rather than naturally through the vagina. Legend has it that the Roman emperor Julius Caesar was delivered by this method—hence, its name—but health professionals believe this is unlikely. In a cesarean section (C-section for short), the woman is anesthetized, and incisions are made in the abdomen and uterus. The surgeon removes the baby and sews the incisions. The mother often begins walking on the day of surgery, perhaps with some discomfort. While most C-sections have no complications, some cause urinary tract infections, inflammation of the wall of the uterus, blood clots, or hemorrhaging.

C-sections are most likely to be advised when normal delivery is difficult or threatening to the health of the mother or the child. Vaginal deliveries can become difficult if the baby is large, the mother's pelvis is small or misshapen, or the mother is tired, weakened, or aging. C-sections are also performed to protect babies from herpes and HIV infections that may be present in the birth canal. C-sections are also likely to be performed if the baby presents for delivery feet downward or sideways, or if the baby is in distress.

Use of the C-section has mushroomed. Nearly one-third of births in the United States today are by C-section.[14] Compare this figure to 1 in 20 births in 1965. Much of the increase in the rate of C-sections reflects advances in medical technology, such as the use of fetal monitors that allow doctors to detect fetal distress, fear of malpractice suits, financial incentives for hospitals and physicians, and simply current patterns of medical practice. Yet, some women request C-sections to avoid the discomforts of vaginal delivery or to control the timing of delivery. Critics claim that many of the C-sections being performed are unnecessary. Health professionals express concern that women who have had a C-section should not attempt vaginal deliveries afterward, for fear of rupture of the uterus. Only 10% of women who have had C-sections attempt vaginal deliveries subsequently.

cesarean section
A method of childbirth in which the fetus is delivered through a surgical incision in the abdomen. (Formerly spelled Caeserean.*)*

preterm
Born prior to 37 weeks of gestation.

Birth Problems

Most deliveries are uncomplicated, or "unremarkable" in the medical sense, yet problems can and do occur. Among the most common are oxygen deprivation and the birth of preterm and low-birthweight babies.

Oxygen Deprivation

Two terms describe degrees of oxygen deprivation: *anoxia* means "without oxygen," and *hypoxia* comes from roots meaning "less" and "oxygen." Hypoxia denotes that the baby is not receiving enough oxygen. Prenatal oxygen deprivation can impair development of the central nervous system, causing cognitive and motor problems as well as psychological disorders.[15] Prolonged oxygen cutoff during delivery can cause cerebral palsy; further deprivation is lethal. Fetal monitoring can help detect oxygen deprivation, and a C-section can rescue a fetus in distress.

Oxygen deprivation may result from maternal health problems, immaturity of the baby's respiratory system, or pressure against the umbilical cord during birth. Slight oxygen deprivation at birth is normal because the baby's transition from receiving oxygen through the umbilical cord to breathing on its own may take a bit of time after delivery.

Preterm and Low-Birthweight Children

A neonate born before 37 weeks of gestation is considered premature, or **preterm**. Normal gestation lasts 40 weeks. Prematurity is associated with low birthweight, since the fetus normally makes dramatic gains in weight during the last weeks of pregnancy. A newborn baby is considered to have a low birthweight if it weighs less than 5 pounds (about 2,500 grams). Neonates weighing between 3.3 and 5.2 pounds are seven times more likely to die than infants of normal birthweight, while those weighing less than 3.3 pounds are nearly 100 times as likely to die from causes ranging from asphyxia and infections to SIDS.[16] The lower a child's birthweight, the more poorly he or she is likely to fare in neurological development and cognitive functioning through the school years.[17]

Twins and other babies from multiple births have a greater risk of low birthweight than individual newborns do. Women who have babies less than 18 months or more than 59 months apart show the highest risk of premature infants.[18]

The muscles of premature babies are immature, weakening their sucking and breathing reflexes. Preterm babies are also thin relative to full-term babies, because they have not yet formed the layer of fat that accounts for the round, robust appearance of most full-term babies. During the last weeks of pregnancy, normally developing fetuses secrete a complex substance that prevents the walls of their airways from sticking together. A combination of muscle weakness and incomplete lining of the neonate's airways with this natural substance may result in **respiratory distress syndrome**, which is a cause of many neonatal deaths. Fortunately, advances in medical care have increased the survival rate in preterm infants. Preterm babies may also have underdeveloped immune systems, which leave them vulnerable to infections. Although advances are being made in our ability to help preterm babies survive, developmental disabilities continue to be likely in babies who are born at 25 weeks of gestation or sooner. Online feature "Diversity 5-3" reveals where in the world it's safest to have babies, both for the mother and the child, and why.

diversity

Access CourseMate for HLTH at www.cengagebrain.com.

The "baby blues" are normal, but persistent depression is not.

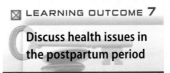

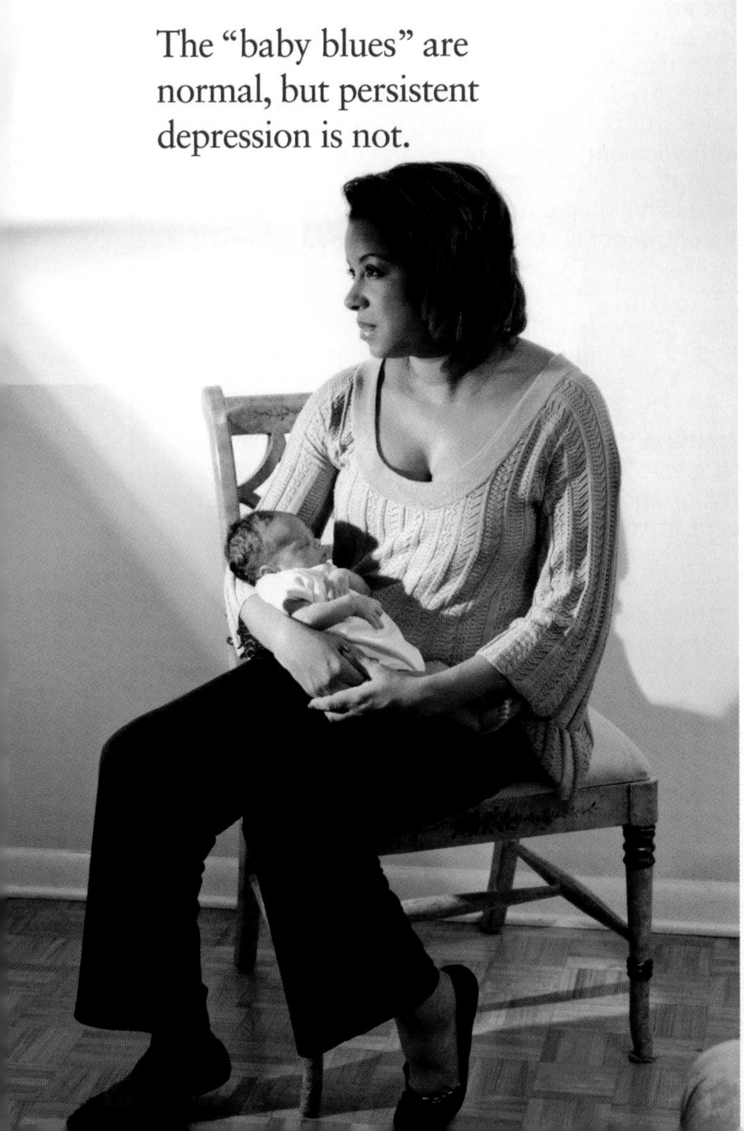

© iStockphoto.com/Kai Chiang

The Postpartum Period

The weeks after delivery are called the **postpartum** period. For parents who desire children, the first days postpartum are usually happy ones. The long wait is over as are any concerns about childbirth. However, many new mothers, perhaps as many as 80%, experience mood changes ("baby blues") shortly after delivery.

LEARNING OUTCOME 7

Discuss health issues in the postpartum period

Postpartum Depression

The "baby blues" reflect hormonal fluctuations around the time of childbirth and generally last a week or two; because of their prevalence they are to be considered normal. However, some new mothers, estimated at between 10% and 15%, develop more serious and persistent mood changes referred to as **postpartum depression (PPD).**[19]

PPD generally begins a few weeks after delivery and may linger for weeks. Symptoms include sadness, feelings of hopelessness and helplessness, feelings of worthlessness, difficulty concentrating, and major changes in appetite (usually loss of appetite) and sleep patterns (frequently insomnia). Severe fluctuations in mood may occur, with intermittent elation. Some women show obsessive concern about the well-being of their babies. PPD is likely caused by a dramatic decline in estrogen,[20] but it may be

respiratory distress syndrome
A cluster of breathing problems, including weak and irregular breathing, to which preterm babies are especially prone.

postpartum
Following birth.

postpartum depression (PPD)
Persistent and severe mood changes during the postpartum period, involving feelings of despair and apathy and characterized by changes in appetite and sleep, low self-esteem, and difficulty concentrating.

worsened by concerns about the responsibilities of motherhood, marital problems, or having a sick baby. For women with serious postpartum depression, drugs that increase estrogen levels or antidepressants may help. Perhaps 1 woman in 500 or 1,000 has so-called psychotic symptoms, which involve a break with reality.

Breast-Feeding Versus Bottle-Feeding

The majority of mothers in the United States today—about three in five—breast-feed their children.[21] However, only about one woman in five continues to breast-feed after 6 months, while the American Academy of Pediatrics recommends a year or more.

Women choose to bottle-feed their babies for several reasons, one being the need to return to work soon after childbirth. Some choose to share feeding with the father, who is equally equipped to prepare and hold a bottle but not to breast-feed.

One disadvantage of breast-feeding is that HIV can be transmitted to infants by breast milk. On the other hand, breast-feeding has several benefits. It reduces the general risk of infections to the baby by transmitting the mother's antibodies to the baby. Breast-feeding also reduces the incidence of allergies in babies.

Should a woman breast-feed her baby? Much of the literature on breast-feeding has little to do with the advantages of breast milk or formula, but with occupational and domestic arrangements, day care, mother-infant bonding, and the politics of domestic decision making. Although breast-feeding can benefit both mother and infant, each woman must make the decision for herself.

HEALTH APPS: YOUR LINK TO ONLINE HEALTH APPLICATIONS

Where Are the Millions of Missing Chinese Girls? What happens in a country where the preference for a boy is extreme and there are means to ensure that women bear babies of the sex they want? Learn more by reading "Diversity 5-1."

Talking with Your Partner about Contraception When is the right time to discuss contraception? Broaching the topic can be awkward, but not broaching it can be disastrous. "Health Skills 5-1" offers advice on talking with your partner about contraception.

Selecting a Method of Contraception There is no simple answer, but "Health Skills 5-2" offers some advice on selecting a method of contraception that is right for you and your partner.

Selecting an Obstetrician One way to help ensure a healthy pregnancy is to obtain adequate prenatal health care. "Health Skills 5-3" can advise you on how to find an obstetrician who is best for your needs.

Safeguarding Your Baby Against Low Birthweight, Stillbirth, Birth Defects, and Disease Are you concerned about whether it's safe for your baby for you to have a glass of wine in the evening when you're pregnant? What about cigarette smoking? If you fear you have an infection or a disease, can you prevent it from being transmitted to the baby? Learn more by reading "Prevention 5-1."

Advice for Expectant Fathers Women rightfully stand in the spotlight when it comes to pregnancy and childbirth, but fathers also matter, as you'll read in "Diversity 5-2."

Maternal and Child Mortality around the World Modern medicine has made vast strides, but the advances may as well not exist for millions of women and their babies in many parts of the world. If you read "Diversity 5-3," you will find out where it's safest to have babies, both for the mother and the child, and why.

Go to the CourseMate for HLTH at www.cengagebrain.com for additional resources including flashcards, games, self-quizzes, review exercises, web exercises, learning checks, and more.

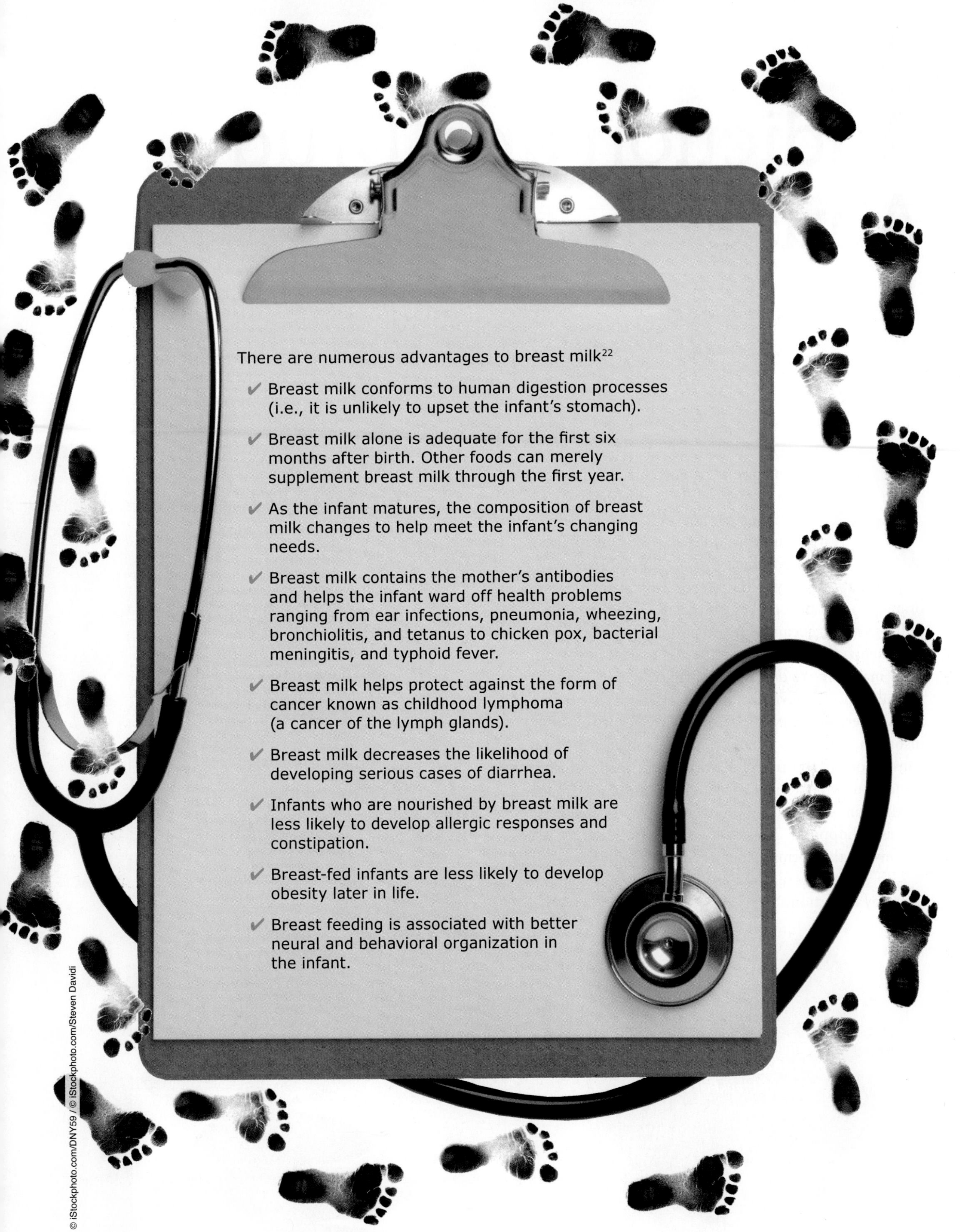

There are numerous advantages to breast milk[22]

- ✔ Breast milk conforms to human digestion processes (i.e., it is unlikely to upset the infant's stomach).
- ✔ Breast milk alone is adequate for the first six months after birth. Other foods can merely supplement breast milk through the first year.
- ✔ As the infant matures, the composition of breast milk changes to help meet the infant's changing needs.
- ✔ Breast milk contains the mother's antibodies and helps the infant ward off health problems ranging from ear infections, pneumonia, wheezing, bronchiolitis, and tetanus to chicken pox, bacterial meningitis, and typhoid fever.
- ✔ Breast milk helps protect against the form of cancer known as childhood lymphoma (a cancer of the lymph glands).
- ✔ Breast milk decreases the likelihood of developing serious cases of diarrhea.
- ✔ Infants who are nourished by breast milk are less likely to develop allergic responses and constipation.
- ✔ Breast-fed infants are less likely to develop obesity later in life.
- ✔ Breast feeding is associated with better neural and behavioral organization in the infant.

Addiction and Drug Abuse

"Excessive video game playing, social networking, and gambling may stimulate release of some of the same chemicals in the brain that follow the use of highly addictive drugs."

Are you addicted to Facebook? How about bridge or pinochle? Online solitaire or Scrabble? Or video games? Or gambling? Or how about buying shoes? Or are you addicted to alcohol, tobacco, or cocaine? Or watching sports?

Wait a minute, you think. We're mixing apples and oranges, or avocadoes. Yes, you can be addicted to alcohol, cigarettes, cocaine, and other drugs. After all, these are chemical substances, and with regular use, your body may come to depend on having a steady supply of the substance(s) in your bloodstream. In that event, you may experience anxiety, tension, sweating, agitation, insomnia, relentless cravings, and in some cases, even convulsions if you try to go without the addictive substance. But what about "Facebooking" and card games? Betting on sports or even watching sports? Online games? Shopping? These activities may be appealing and even habit forming, but are they *addictive*?

To some degree, the answer depends on what we mean by addiction.

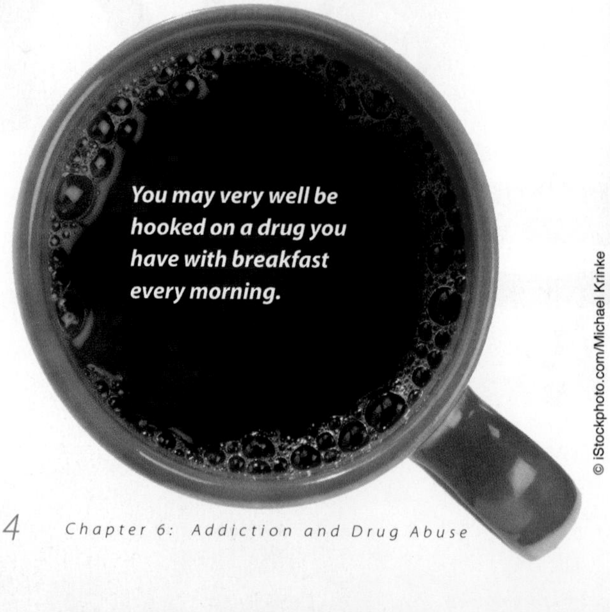

You may very well be hooked on a drug you have with breakfast every morning.

© iStockphoto.com/Michael Krinke

LEARNING OUTCOMES

1 Discuss the concept of addiction and describe various addictive behaviors

2 Discuss various kinds of drugs, including prescription and over-the-counter drugs

3 Discuss different types of psychoactive drugs and their effects

4 Discuss who uses psychoactive drugs

5 Explain how people respond to drugs in different ways

6 Describe pathways to drug abuse and dependence

7 Discuss ways of becoming and remaining drug free

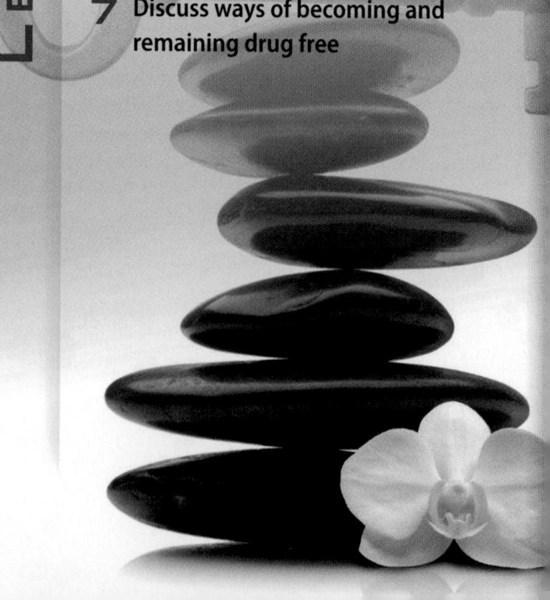

CHAPTER 6

Addictive Behaviors

The term *addiction* has different meanings. **Psychological addiction** is dependence on a chemical substance or an activity—such as visiting a social networking site, throwing away money on shoes or other purchases that are not needed or ever used, or gambling—such that people become dependent on engaging in these behaviors to meet their psychological needs. These substances and activities may fill a void in their lives, and people may become so absorbed with them that they neglect their other responsibilities or personal needs. They may repeatedly turn to using a substance or shopping or the Internet to counter anxiety or depression or to cope with stress. They

LEARNING OUTCOME 1

Discuss the concept of addiction and describe various addictive behaviors

psychological addiction
A pattern of compulsive behavior or habitual use of a drug indicating impaired control but without physiological signs of dependence.

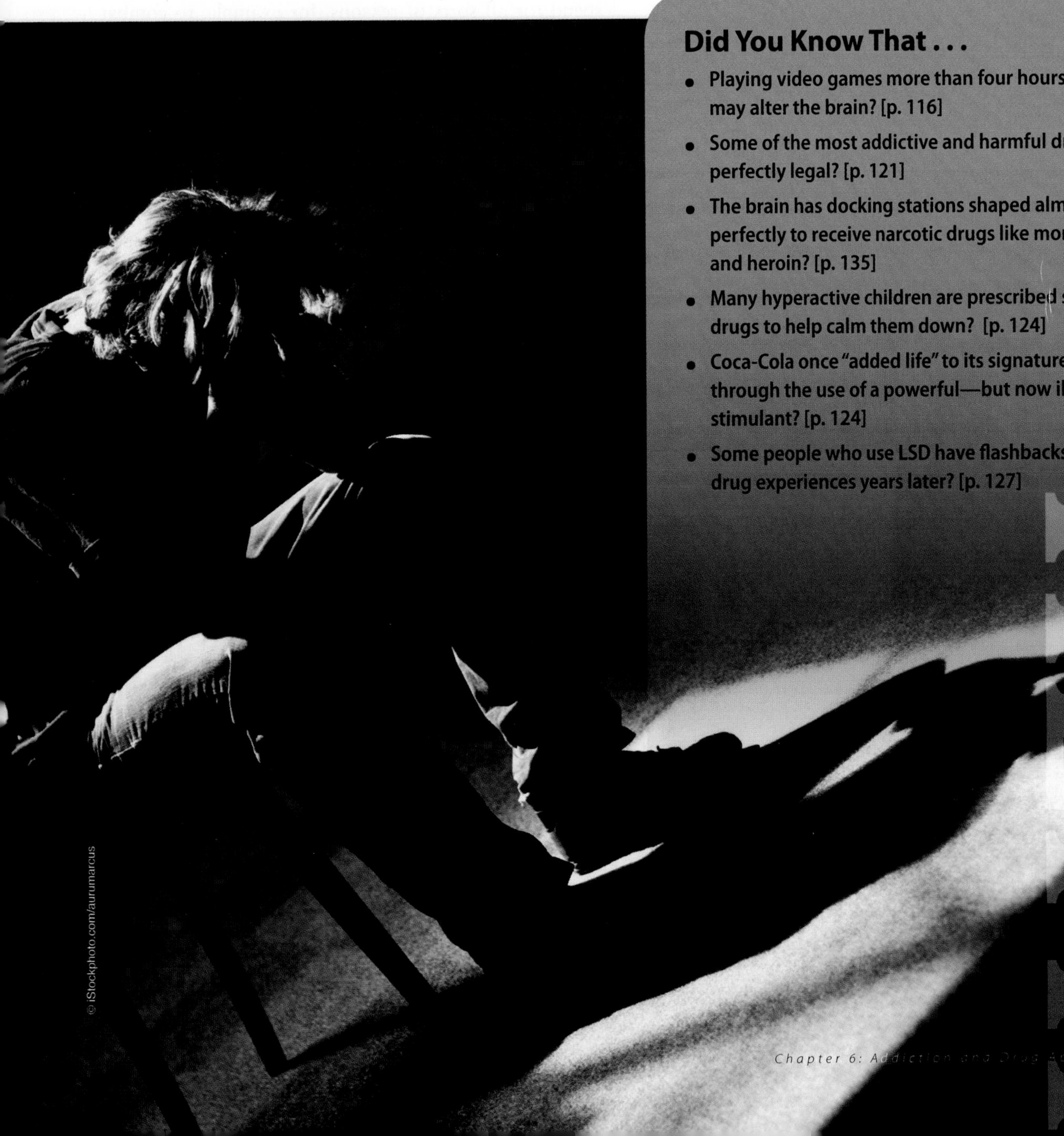

Did You Know That . . .

- Playing video games more than four hours a day may alter the brain? [p. 116]
- Some of the most addictive and harmful drugs are perfectly legal? [p. 121]
- The brain has docking stations shaped almost perfectly to receive narcotic drugs like morphine and heroin? [p. 135]
- Many hyperactive children are prescribed stimulant drugs to help calm them down? [p. 124]
- Coca-Cola once "added life" to its signature drink through the use of a powerful—but now illegal—stimulant? [p. 124]
- Some people who use LSD have flashbacks of their drug experiences years later? [p. 127]

may lose control over their addictive behaviors and orient their lives around these behaviors, even though they suspect—or know—that they are doing themselves more harm than good.

With **physiological addiction**, the person's body chemistry changes as the result of repeated use of a chemical substance, such that it comes to depend on having a steady supply of the drug. If you're chemically addicted to a drug, and you abruptly stop using it (you go "cold turkey") or cut back sharply on it, you are likely to experience an **abstinence syndrome**, which is a cluster of unpleasant and possibly dangerous withdrawal symptoms. You are also likely to lose control over your use of the drug. The tendency to return to using a drug to relieve withdrawal symptoms is a major reason why chemical addiction is so difficult to defeat. Another feature of physiological dependence is **tolerance**. Tolerance develops when your biological responsivity to a drug changes so that you need more and more of it to achieve the same effects.

Both forms of addiction, psychological and physiological, may directly alter brain functioning. Even video game players who average more than four hours of game playing a day may show withdrawal symptoms when they go without playing.[1] Excessive video game playing, social networking, gambling, and other psychologically addictive behaviors may stimulate release of the same pleasure-inducing chemical in the brain (the neurotransmitter *dopamine*) that occurs when people use drugs like cocaine, heroin, and even alcohol and tobacco.[2]

This chapter is about various forms of drug use and abuse and about psychological addictions that can damage our well-being and ability to function effectively in meeting our daily responsibilities. We begin with addictive behaviors and then move on to drug use and abuse.

Compulsive Spending

Some people are compulsive spenders—in effect, addicted to squandering money. It has been estimated that from 6% to 16% of college students are compulsive spenders,[3] which is a high number given most students' limited resources. They spend (waste, really) money on clothing, gadgets, and other items they really don't need, but the very act of shopping provides a source of pleasure or gratification they crave—much like a drug.

Compulsive spending often begins when the student leaves home, especially if he or she has credit cards. They spend for all sorts of reasons, for example, to combat feelings of depression or anxiety. They often get trapped in a vicious circle: They spend to cope with these emotions, but the spending causes feelings of guilt and shame, which then turbo boosts these feelings. Compulsive spenders often have a family background of depression, alcoholism, or substance abuse, so you could say that the problem is often at least partly in their genes. They may also have other problems with compulsive behavior, such as eating disorders and substance abuse.

Pathological Gambling

Most people who gamble can control their wagering and stop if they want to. But some people develop a psychological disorder called *compulsive* or *pathologi-*

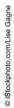

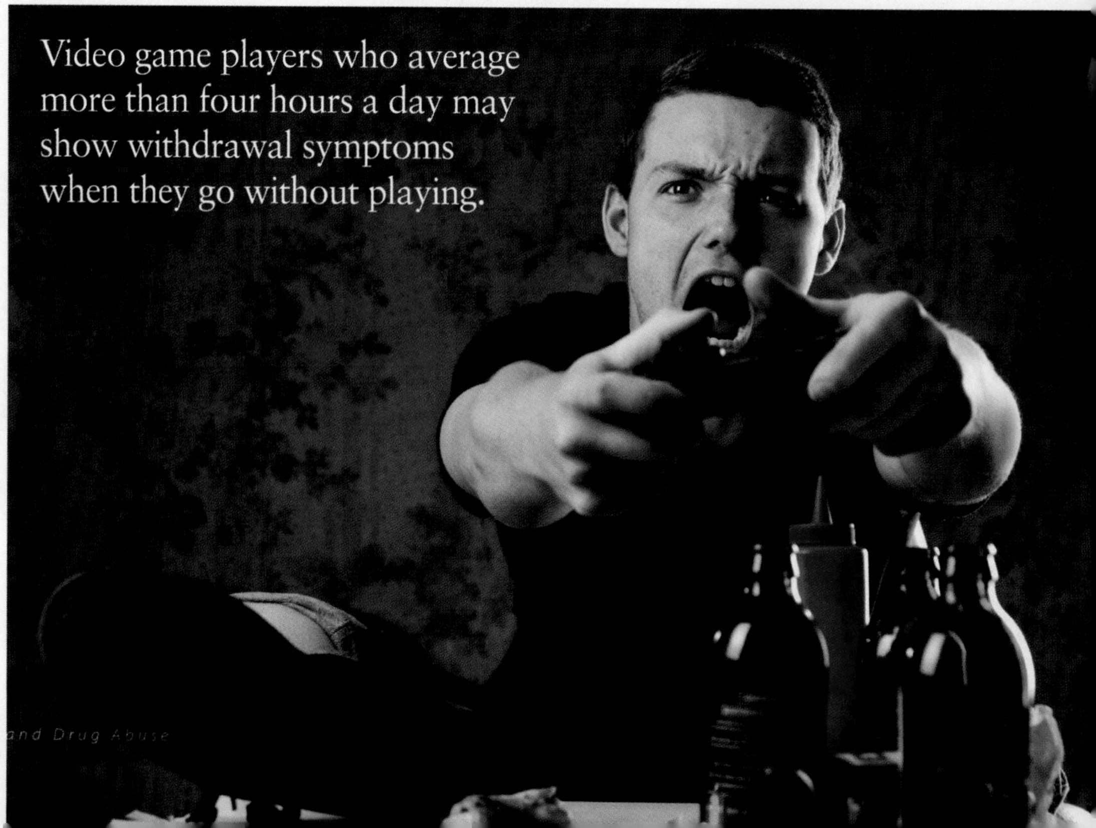

Video game players who average more than four hours a day may show withdrawal symptoms when they go without playing.

© iStockphoto.com/Lise Gagne

physiological addiction
A state of physical need for a drug, characterized by the development of a withdrawal syndrome following abrupt cessation of the use of the substance.

abstinence syndrome
A cluster of withdrawal symptoms that is characteristic of abrupt cessation of use of a particular drug.

tolerance
A feature of drug dependence in which the user comes to need larger amounts or doses of the drug to achieve the same effect.

Signs of Compulsive Spending

health skills

Access CourseMate for HLTH at www.cengagebrain.com.

- Shopping or spending when you feel sad, angry, anxious, or lonely
- Arguing with other people about your spending habits
- Feeling lost without your credit cards
- Buying on credit
- Feeling a rush when shopping
- Feeling guilty or embarrassed after a shopping spree
- Lying about what things cost
- Thinking, thinking, thinking about money

Showing a few or more of these signs suggest that you might be a compulsive spender. To learn more, check out the online feature "Health Skills 6-1."

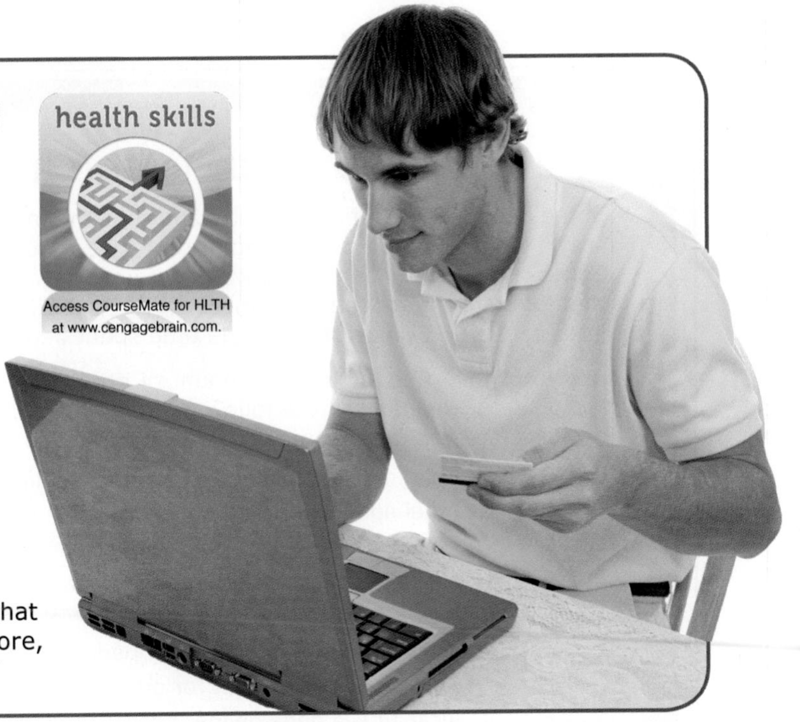

© iStockphoto.com/Lisa F. Young

cal gambling. These individuals experience a lack of control over their gambling, intense pleasure or excitement when gambling, and withdrawal symptoms such as headaches, insomnia, and loss of appetite when the they stop gambling or cut back on it. Pathological gambling is also associated with greater risk of alcohol and substance abuse, which underscores the close relationship between different forms of addiction. Many pathological gamblers suffer from low self-esteem and turn to gambling to prove to themselves (and others) that they are "winners." However, winnings tend to be elusive and losses begin to mount, leading to depression and a vicious cycle of more gambling to win back losses and score the "big payoff."

Pathological gambling is estimated to affect some 5% of college students.[4] It is more common among college males than females, and among members of fraternities. Fraternity men are four times more likely than other college men to wind up in debt because of gambling.[5] Does the social environment of some fraternities encourage risky behavior and poor decision making?

Many pathological gamblers only seek help during a crisis, as when they run out of money or are rejected by their families. Treatment of pathological gambling is challenging. There have been some promising results from the use of antidepressant drugs and mood stabilizing drugs.[6] There are also peer support programs, like Gamblers Anonymous (GA), which is similar to Alcoholics Anonymous. Gamblers are encouraged to take personal responsibility for their behavior within a supportive group setting. They gain insight into their own behavior as group members share experiences and confront them.

Internet Addiction

Internet addiction is a self-defeating behavior pattern involving preoccupation with being online to the extent that it disrupts one's functioning. As with drug addiction, people who are addicted to the Internet may neglect their studies or work and their real (unlike virtual) social lives.[7] The prevalence of Internet addiction among college students has been estimated at anywhere between 1% and 10%.[8]

Some forms of Internet addiction involve gaming and competition, whereas others involve absorption in Internet porn. Still others involve efforts to use social networking and chat rooms to fulfill unmet social needs or combat loneliness or boredom in the real world. Other forms of Internet addiction include a compulsive pattern of participation in virtual communities that provide a diversion from problems in the real world, and status gained by creating fictional assets in the form of avatars as alter-egos that allow one to make up for perceived deficits—to become taller or more attractive than one really is. Like other forms of psychological addiction—pathological gambling and compulsive shopping, for example—Internet addiction is linked to emotional problems of anxiety and depression, impulsivity, and substance abuse.[9] "Health Check 6-1" on the next page will afford you insight as to whether you are "addicted" to the Internet. If you are concerned about your responses to the self-assessment, "Health Skills 6-2" on page 119 may be of use.

HEALTH CHECK 6-1

Are You "Addicted" to the Internet?

Some people have difficulty controlling the amount of time they spend online. Some are emailing or texting everyone they know. Some of them are hopping from news item to news item. Some of them are surfing for the best prices on DVDs, airline fares, whatever. Some are gambling; some are into "cybersex." Unfortunately, the time spent detracts from the completion of college assignments.

Are you concerned about the amount of time you spend online or the nature of the websites you are visiting? Respond to the following items by circling the *T* if an item is true or mostly true for you or *F* if an item is false or mostly false for you.

T F 1. I find myself needing to spend more time online to enjoy it as much.
T F 2. I feel uptight, depressed, or nervous when I can't go online.
T F 3. I find myself spending more time online than I planned to do.
T F 4. I take great pride in the Internet navigational skills I have acquired.
T F 5. I have a desire to cut down or control the amount of time I am spending online.
T F 6. I'd rather email or text most people than talk to them on the phone or see them in person.
T F 7. I find myself impatient for others to leave so I can go online.
T F 8. After I have gone online, I carefully delete my online history and unwanted temporary Internet files.
T F 9. I would rather shop online than go to a "bricks and mortar" store.
T F 10. I am a completely different person when I am online.
T F 11. I sometimes experience a feeling of great satisfaction when I use my user name and my password to log in to a website.
T F 12. I spend a good deal of time in activities directed toward going online.
T F 13. I have lost track of time while online.
T F 14. Shopping online sometimes gives me a sense of power.
T F 15. The fact is that I have reduced social, educational, or recreational activities so that I can spend more time online.
T F 16. I have continued to spend a great deal of time online despite evidence of persistent or recurrent emotional or social problems caused or exacerbated by its use.
T F 17. I sometimes feel that my virtual community is more important to me than my flesh-and-blood community.
T F 18. Spending the same amount of time online is less satisfying than it was.
T F 19. The challenges of finding new things and going new places on the Internet excite me as much as a real outing or trip.
T F 20. Going online for long periods of time has become a habit.
T F 21. I find myself hiding or lying about the amount of time I spend online or the nature of the websites I visit.
T F 22. When I'm online, I sometimes feel as though I'm connected with the computer or the Internet in a way that is hard to put into words.
T F 23. When I cannot find a way to go online, I feel a great sense of loss.
T F 24. I find myself unable to exercise self-control over how much time I spend online.

Key: *T* answers are in the direction of being addicted to the Internet. The term *addiction* implies habitual behavior that is difficult to control and tends to be reserved by the American Psychiatric Association for abuse of substances, including alcohol, cigarettes, heroin, and cocaine. However, the term may be used to refer to any habitual self-destructive behavior that involves cravings.

There are no norms for this self-assessment. Instead, be honest with yourself as you review the items. Is your use of the Internet interfering with your academic or social life? Does it seem to be out of control? Do you find yourself "in a fever" to get online? If any of these are true, you may find it helpful to check out "Health Skills 6-2."

HEALTH SKILLS 6-2

health skills

Combating Internet Addiction

Some students are concerned that they go online too often, they spend too much time online, or the urge to go online is too strong. Here are some suggestions you can use if you are concerned about becoming addicted to the Internet:

- *Give yourself strict limits on the amount of time you allow yourself to spend online for recreational use.* Reward yourself for sticking to the limit by putting money toward something you really want.
- *Shut your computer off (don't just let it go to sleep) after you have spent your allotted amount of time online or finished with your legitimate purposes.*
- *Engage in a competing activity.* Read a book, go for a walk, check your assignments, or chat (offline!) with a friend.
- *Limit Internet use to public places.* For example, use the library, the student center, or the cafeteria.
- *Develop relationships in the real world.* Join clubs and campus organizations, and expand your friendships rather than substitute virtual relationships.

Drug Use, Misuse, and Abuse

A **drug** is a chemical substance that can affect your health, your feelings, or your behavior. Although use of the word *drugs* might convey an image of people shooting up an addictive substance in a darkened alleyway, drugs can be healthful as well as harmful. Using the right drug at the right time can relieve a health problem or save a life. Drug *misuse* can create a health problem or take a life. **Drug misuse** is the use of a drug for the wrong reason, or in the wrong way, or by the wrong person. Using sleeping pills or tranquilizers prescribed for a friend is drug misuse. The drugs might be harmful for you. Popping antibiotics for a cough without consulting the doctor is also misuse. Antibiotics combat bacteria, but the drug is useless to fight a cough caused by a viral infection. A prescription cough syrup with codeine is misused if you use it to get high rather than to relieve a cough or if you take higher doses than prescribed.

LEARNING OUTCOME 2

Discuss various kinds of drugs, including prescription and over-the-counter drugs

The scientific study of drugs and their role in health is called **pharmacology. Pharmacy** is the preparation and dispensing of drugs. *Pharmacologists* work in laboratories and develop new drugs to fight disease. *Pharmacists* are licensed professionals who dispense prescription drugs and usually work in pharmacies. Pharmacists are knowledgeable about the effects and interactions of drugs and can offer useful information on whether a medicine is right for you.

Over-the-Counter (OTC) versus Prescription Drugs

Over-the-counter (OTC) drugs are available without prescription. You decide whether to use a drug on your own or with the help of a pharmacist. If you think it is perfectly safe to use OTC drugs on your own because they are harmless, think again. Many vitamin pills can be bought over-the-counter, but excessive use of certain vitamins can cause health problems such as jaundice and kidney stones. Aspirin can be bought OTC, and it is surely one of the wonder drugs of the day. Not only can aspirin relieve many headaches

drug
Chemical agent that affects biological functions.

drug misuse
The use of a drug for a purpose for which it was not intended, or in ways that deviate from the correct use of the drug.

pharmacology
The study of drugs and their role in medicine.

pharmacy
The discipline relating to the preparation and dispensing of drugs.

over-the-counter (OTC) drug
A drug available for sale without a prescription.

Table 6-1 Over-the-Counter Pain Relievers

	ACETAMINOPHEN	ASPIRIN	IBUPROFEN	NAPROXEN SODIUM
Brand names	Tylenol, Panadol	Anacin, Bayer, Bufferin, Ecotrin	Advil, Motrin, Nuprin	Aleve
Useful for . . .	Aches and pains, fever	Aches and pains, inflammation, fever, arthritic pain	Aches and pains, inflammation, fever, arthritic pain, sports injuries	Aches and pains, menstrual cramps, arthritic pain
Reduces pain and fever?	Yes	Yes	Yes	Yes
Reduces inflammation?	No	Yes	Yes	Yes
Possible side effects	Unlikely if used as directed but overuse may harm the kidneys or the liver	Bleeding in digestive tract, stomach upset, ulceration	Bleeding in digestive tract, stomach upset, ulceration	Bleeding in digestive tract, stomach upset, ulceration
Comments	Especially useful when other pain relievers are not tolerated	Ask pharmacist about coated versions that are less likely to upset the stomach	Should not be taken by people who are allergic to aspirin, have asthma, or have heart or kidney problems	Should not be taken by people who are allergic to aspirin, have asthma, or have heart or kidney problems

and other aches and pains, but it may also reduce the risks of heart attacks in people in higher risk categories for heart disease (see Chapter 11). Yet aspirin can upset the stomach and cause bleeding and ulcers in the digestive tract. Aspirin can also cause *Reye's syndrome* in children with chicken pox. (Reye's syndrome can be deadly and involves kidney damage, swelling of the brain, and convulsions.) Table 6-1 describes the uses and side effects of the most widely used over-the-counter pain relievers, including aspirin.

When in doubt about an OTC drug, ask your health care provider or pharmacist. OTC medications are best used when recommended by a physician.

Prescription drugs are only available if they are prescribed by a physician because their use needs to be monitored by a medical doctor to be safe and effective. In later chapters we examine the use of different kinds of prescription drugs in treating microbial infections and combating chronic diseases such as heart disease and cancer. Confused about the codes doctors use when writing prescriptions? Figure 6-1 helps you decipher their meaning.

psychoactive drugs
Drugs that act on the brain to affect mental processes.

Many drugs are available OTC. However, you should not attempt to diagnose or medicate yourself. For one thing, you might *mis*diagnose yourself and fail to identify a serious illness that requires medical attention. For another, you might medicate yourself with a drug that is ineffective against the particular disease-causing organism. Learn more about the wise use of medications in the online feature "Prevention 6-1."

prevention

Access CourseMate for HLTH at www.cengagebrain.com.

Psychoactive Drugs

LEARNING OUTCOME 3

Discuss different types of psychoactive drugs and their effects

The world is a supermarket of **psychoactive drugs**—drugs that distort your perceptions and change your mood, drugs that take you up, let you down, and move you across town. Some of them are legal, others illegal. Some are used recreationally, others medically. Some are safe if used correctly and dangerous if they are not. Some people use drugs because their friends do or because their parents tell them not

to. Some are seeking pleasure; others are seeking inner truth.

Psychoactive drugs act on the brain to affect your mental state. They alter mood, thought processes, perceptions, and behavior. They may also affect judgment and ability to operate an automobile or perform other complex motor skills. Some psychoactive drugs have legitimate medical uses to relieve pain, induce sleep, or treat psychological disorders. Others are used or abused by people seeking to alter their mental states—to get high or to feel relaxed or more alert. Some of these drugs induce a rush of euphoric pleasure that washes away awareness of the struggles and stresses of daily life.

Some psychoactive drugs are addictive. Some are illegal. You might think that only addictive drugs are illegal, yet some of the most strongly addictive drugs—including nicotine (the psychoactive chemical in tobacco) and alcohol—are legal, although the sale of tobacco and alcohol to minors is prohibited. Nicotine, alcohol, and caffeine (yes, caffeine) are so widely used that many people don't realize that they are psychoactive drugs. Caffeine, the psychoactive ingredient in coffee and tea, is a mild stimulant. Nicotine, also a mild stimulant, is found in tobacco products such as cigarettes, pipe tobacco, and cigars.

Illegal (or *illicit*) drugs include opiates such as morphine, opium, and heroin; stimulants such as methamphethamine and cocaine; and hallucinogens such as LSD, mescaline, marijuana, and hashish. Some drugs used illegally, such as morphine, also have legitimate medical uses and can be used legally but only under the direction of a physician. Are legal drugs less harmful to one's health than illicit drugs? Not necessarily. Despite the attention focused on illicit drugs, two legally available drugs, alcohol and tobacco, account for more deaths, disease, and health costs than do all other drugs combined. Because of their effects on health, we devote the following chapter to them.

Table 6-2 on the next page shows the major types of drugs, their potential for psychological and physiological dependence, their psychoactive effects, and the major risks they pose.

The remainder of this chapter focuses on the uses and misuses of psychoactive drugs. We discuss several types of psychoactive drugs, their effects on health, and how you can avoid problems associated with drug misuse and abuse. The uses of alcohol and nicotine (found in tobacco) are so widespread that we discuss them separately in Chapter 7.

Figure 6-1 How to Read a Prescription

This prescription is for 30 pills of ampicillin, each in a strength of 250 mg (ampicillin 250 mg DISP #30). One pill is to be taken by mouth three times a day for 10 days (1PO TID × 10D).

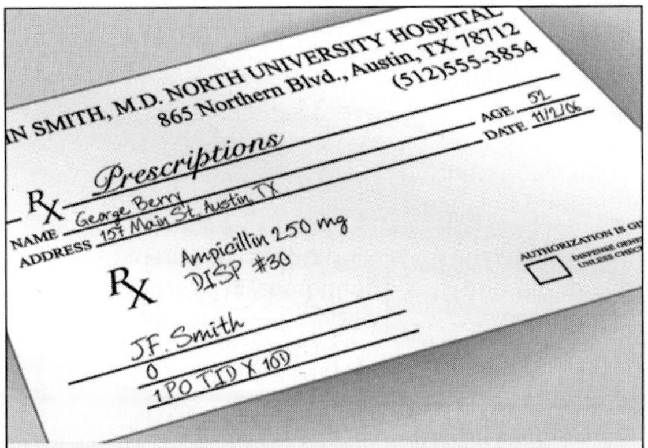

The following are some of the abbreviations doctors use when writing prescriptions.

ABBREVIATION	MEANING
AA	Of each
AC	Before meals
AM	Morning
BID	Twice a day
C	With
CAP	Capsule
CC	Cubic centimeter
D	Days
DISP	Dispense
GT	Drop
GTT	Drops
H	Hour
HS	At bedtime
ML	Milliliter
OD	Right eye
OS	Left eye
PC	After meals
PM	Evening
PO	By mouth
PRN	As needed
Q	Every
QD	Once a day every day
QID	Four times a day
S	Without
SIG	Label as follows
STAT	Immediately
TAB	Tablet
TID	Three times a day
X	Times

Table 6-2 Major Classes of Psychoactive Drugs

	DRUG	POTENTIAL FOR PSYCHOLOGICAL/ PHYSIOLOGICAL DEPENDENCE	MAJOR PSYCHOLOGICAL EFFECTS	MAJOR RISKS
Depressants	Alcohol	Yes/Yes	Induces relaxation, mild euphoria, and intoxication; relieves anxiety; reduces mental alertness and inhibitions; impairs concentration, judgment, coordination, and balance	With heavy use, can cause liver disorders and other physical problems; in overdose, can cause coma or death
	Barbiturates and tranquilizers	Yes/Yes	Reduces mental alertness; induces relaxation and calm; may produce pleasurable rush (barbiturates)	High addictive potential; dangerous in overdose and when mixed with alcohol and other drugs
	Opiates	Yes/Yes	Induces relaxation and a euphoric rush; may temporarily blot out awareness of personal problems	High addictive potential; in overdose, may cause sudden death
Stimulants	Amphetamines	Yes/Yes	Boosts mental alertness; reduces need for sleep; induces pleasurable rush; causes loss of appetite	In high doses, can induce psychotic symptoms and cardiovascular irregularities that may lead to coma or death
	Cocaine	Yes/Yes	Effects similar to those of amphetamines but shorter-lived	High addictive potential; risk of sudden death from overdose; in high doses, can have psychotic effects; risk of nasal defects from snorting
	MDMA ("Ecstasy")	Yes/Yes	Mild euphoria and hallucinogenic effects	High doses can be lethal; may lead to depression or other psychological effects; may impair learning, attention, and memory
	Nicotine	Yes/Yes	Increases mental alertness; produces mild rush but paradoxically may have relaxing and calming effects	Strong addictive potential; implicated in various cancers, cardiovascular disease, and other physical disorders
	Caffeine	Yes/Yes	Increases mental alertness and wakefulness	In high doses, can cause jitteriness and sleeplessness; may increase risk of miscarriage during pregnancy; stimulates release of stress hormones
Hallucinogens	LSD	Yes/No	Produces hallucinations and other sensory distortions	Intense anxiety, panic, or psychotic reactions associated with "bad trips"; flashbacks
	Marijuana	Yes/Probable	Induces relaxation and mild euphoria; can produce hallucinations	In high doses, can cause nausea, vomiting, disorientation, panic, and paranoia; regular smoking of the drug also poses health risks

Depressants

Depressants dampen the activity of the central nervous system. They produce feelings of relaxation and provide relief from anxiety and tension. Tranquilizers are depressants that have widespread use in treating anxiety disorders. Some depressants, notably opiates, produce a rush of pleasure. In high doses, depressants arrest vital body functions, such as breathing, and are lethal.

Barbiturates

Barbiturates are depressant drugs that have sedating effects and help relieve anxiety. They are used medically to block pain during surgery, regulate high blood pressure, and prevent epileptic seizures. Commonly used barbiturates include *amobarbital*, *pentobarbital*, *phenobarbital*, and *secobarbital*. Barbiturates have a high addictive potential, which is why they are not used to treat anxiety or insomnia. *Methaqualone* (called *Quaalude*, or "ludes," and *Sopor*, or "sopors") is a **sedative** that is similar in effect to barbiturates. It also holds similar dangers and potential for dependence.

Barbiturates and sedatives induce states of mild euphoria and relaxation that can last for hours. They also cause drowsiness, slurred speech, irritability, and impaired motor functioning and judgment—making them deadly behind the wheel. Overdoses can cause convulsions, coma, and death. Mixing barbiturates and methaqualone with alcohol is extremely dangerous. People addicted to barbiturates and methaqualone should undergo withdrawal under medical supervision, as abrupt withdrawal can cause convulsions and death.

Opiates

Naturally-occurring opiates are **narcotic** drugs derived from the poppy plant—*opium, morphine, heroin,* and *codeine*. A narcotic is an addictive drug that has pain-relieving and sleep-inducing properties. Synthetic opiates, such as Demerol and Darvon, are synthesized in the laboratory and are similar to natural opiates in chemical structure and effects.

Opiates are often given to postsurgical patients to deaden pain. Because of their high potential for addiction, their medical use is carefully regulated. However, narcotic pain relievers, such as the drugs Vicodin and OxyContin, are used illicitly as street drugs. Abuse of these drugs is associated with many fatal overdoses and accidents.

Opiates produce feelings of pleasure or a rush of pleasurable excitement, which is a primary reason for their popularity as street drugs. They also dampen awareness of problems, which is attractive to people who seek to escape the stresses of everyday life.

Opiates act on the neurotransmitters that stimulate the brain's pleasure circuits—the brain networks responsible for feelings of sexual pleasure or pleasure from eating a satisfying meal.[10]

Heroin ("horse," "junk," "smack") accounts for most cases of opiate addiction. Heroin stimulates brain centers responsible for pleasure and development of physical dependence. Heroin is a white crystalline powder that can be snorted, smoked, or most commonly, injected. It may be injected under the skin (skin popping) or directly into a vein (mainlining). Nearly 1 million Americans are believed to be addicted.[11] Unlike most other drugs, heroin use occurs more commonly among people over age 35 than among younger people. About one-third of heroin users are women, and about a third of these women are prostitutes. They are especially vulnerable to contracting HIV because of sexual activity with multiple partners and sharing needles when injecting heroin.

When injected into a vein, heroin produces a euphoric rush that can last from 5 to 15 minutes. It is so intense and pleasurable that some compare it with the pleasure of orgasm. A second phase of prolonged relaxation, lasting three to five hours, follows, with feelings of satisfaction, mild euphoria, drowsiness, and well-being. Under the influence of heroin, worries and cares evaporate. Drives for sex or food become blunted. Once this carefree state begins to wear off, users may seek their next "fix" to return to the drugged state. Heroin addicts begin to organize their lives around pursuit and use of the drug, often turning to crime or prostitution to support their habits.

Addicts develop tolerance (need for higher doses to achieve the same effects). An unpleasant and potentially severe abstinence syndrome—including rapid pulse and respiration, increased blood pressure, profuse sweating, muscle cramps, tremors, watery eyes, runny nose, loss of appetite, nausea, hot and cold flashes, panic, vomiting, insomnia, diarrhea, and strong cravings—discourages addicted people from attempting to quit. However, withdrawal symptoms can be managed under medical supervision and often relieved through use of prescribed drugs.

depressants
Drugs such as barbiturates, tranquilizers, opiates, and alcohol that lower the rate of nervous system activity.

sedative
A central nervous system depressant that has calming and relaxing effects.

narcotics
Drugs, primarily opiates, that have sleep-inducing and pain-relieving effects with a high potential for addiction.

Heroin overdoses, characterized by shallow breathing, clammy skin, convulsions, and coma, can be deadly. The risk of complications and overdoses is accentuated when heroin is used in combination with other drugs such as alcohol or cocaine.

The sharing of hypodermic needles among heroin addicts is a principal means of transmission of HIV, the virus that causes AIDS. The issue of whether public health officials should distribute clean needles to addicts continues to be debated.

Stimulants

Stimulants heighten the activity of the nervous system. They include amphetamines, cocaine, and the most widely used psychoactive drug of all, caffeine. Some stimulants have medical uses, such as the drugs Ritalin, Concerta, and Adderall, which are used to treat attention deficit hyperactivity disorder. Cocaine is sometimes used as an anesthetic.

Amphetamines

The most common **amphetamines** are *amphetamine sulfate* (trade name Benzedrine), *methamphetamine* (Methedrine), and *dextroamphetamine* (Dexedrine). Amphetamines are known on the street as "speed" or "meth" (for Methedrine), "uppers" or "bennies" (for Benzedrine), and "dexies" (for Dexedrine). They are synthetic compounds not found in nature.

Amphetamines activate the autonomic nervous system, increasing heart rate and respiration rate and raising blood pressure. They also stimulate reward pathways in the brain that control feelings of pleasure. In low doses, they increase mental alertness and concentration, and lessen fatigue. In high doses, they can produce a euphoric rush. Because they also suppress the appetite, they are used by some dieters. High doses can induce restlessness, irritability, anxiety, insomnia, and heart irregularities.

Amphetamines can be taken in pill form or smoked in a relatively pure form of methamphetamine called "ice" or "crystal meth." Ice heightens alertness and excitability and can produce a euphoric high. Prolonged use can cause lung and kidney damage and lead to psychological disorders. The most potent form of amphetamine, liquid methamphetamine, is injected into the veins, producing an intense rush. Some users repeatedly inject "meth" for days on end, maintaining an extended high. All highs eventually come to an end. Users may "crash"—fall into deep sleep or stupor, or experience deep, prolonged depression. Some people commit suicide on the way down.

Tolerance and physiological dependence can develop quickly. Some people overdose—fatally—as they take more and more to try to reach highs similar to those they achieved when they first started using amphetamines. Methamphetamine can cause serious cardiovascular problems, including rapid heart rate, irregular heartbeat, heightened blood pressure, damage to small blood vessels in the brain that can lead to stroke, even death.[12] Methamphetamine abuse can lead to aggressive behavior and depression and cause brain damage, producing deficits in learning and memory.[13] Users may also develop **amphetamine psychosis**, a psychotic state that resembles paranoid schizophrenia. Symptoms include hallucinations (seeing, hearing, or feeling things that are not there) and delusions of persecution (believing people are talking about you or are out to get you when they are not).

stimulant
Psychoactive drug that increases the level of activity of the central nervous system.
amphetamines
A class of synthetic stimulants.
amphetamine psychosis
An acute psychotic reaction induced by the ingestion of amphetamines that mimics acute episodes of paranoid schizophrenia.

Cocaine

Did you know that the original formula for Coca-Cola contained an extract of the drug *cocaine*? In 1906, however, cocaine ("coke") was removed from the brew. The name Coca-Cola still reflects its original sources—the coca plant, from which a cocaine extract was derived and added to the original formula for the drink, and the cola nut, which was used for flavoring. Cocaine is a natural stimulant that is derived from the leaves of the coca plant.

Although cocaine remains a major drug of abuse in the United States, overall use of the drug, as well as use among college students, has been declining. Still, many hardcore users continue to battle cocaine addiction. Cocaine exerts such powerfully rewarding effects that users may not be able to predict or control their use of the drug. Occasional use can quickly lead to habitual use, even among people who want to stop.

Cocaine can be snorted in powder form or smoked in the form of *crack*, a hardened form of the drug that produces a more immediate rush. Cocaine can also be injected in liquid form or ingested as a tea brewed from coca leaves. *Freebase cocaine* is derived from a chemical process that intensifies the effects of the drug. Cocaine is heated with ether, which frees the psychoactive base of the drug, and then smoked. Ether, however, is highly flammable.

Like other stimulants, cocaine increases mental clarity and alertness, and heightens arousal. Like amphetamines, cocaine stimulates reward pathways in the brain, producing states of euphoria. Smoking crack transports the drug almost immediately to the brain, producing an intense and sudden high. The rush wears off in a few minutes, leaving the user wanting more. The high from snorting powder cocaine lasts perhaps 15 to 30 minutes; the high from smoking crack, only 5 to 10 minutes. The user needs to take the drug at frequent intervals to maintain the crack high. Repetition can lead to compulsive use as the user seeks to maintain "highs" and avoid the "lows" of withdrawal. Cocaine abusers typically fall into a cycle of binges lasting 12 to 36 hours, followed by days of abstinence during which cravings increase to the point where they prompt another binge.

Prolonged use of cocaine can lead to psychological disturbances, including anxiety, irritability, and depression. Cocaine-induced depression is sometimes severe enough to prompt a suicide attempt. High doses or chronic use can trigger a **cocaine psychosis** that is characterized by hallucinations and delusions of persecution.

Cocaine is highly addictive. The abstinence syndrome involves intense cravings for the drug, depression, and inability to experience pleasure. Addicts often resume using the drug to relieve withdrawal symptoms. Tolerance develops quickly with repeated use. Severe psychological dependence may also occur. Cocaine becomes the focus of the addict's life.

Cocaine causes an abrupt rise in blood pressure, constricts blood vessels (which limits the supply of oxygen to the heart), and accelerates the heart rate. During cocaine binges, users attempt to maintain the high by taking more and more of the drug, which can lead to irregular heartbeats, heart stoppage, and strokes caused by spasms of blood vessels in the brain. Overdoses can also disrupt breathing, causing gasping and leading in some cases to respiratory arrest and death.

Occasional snorting of cocaine can lead to nasal congestion and a chronic runny nose. Chronic heavy snorting can cause more damage to the nasal cavity, ulcerating the mucous membrane and causing the nasal septum to collapse. Habitual smoking of crack cocaine or freebase cocaine can damage the mouth, throat, and lungs, and lead to lung cancer.

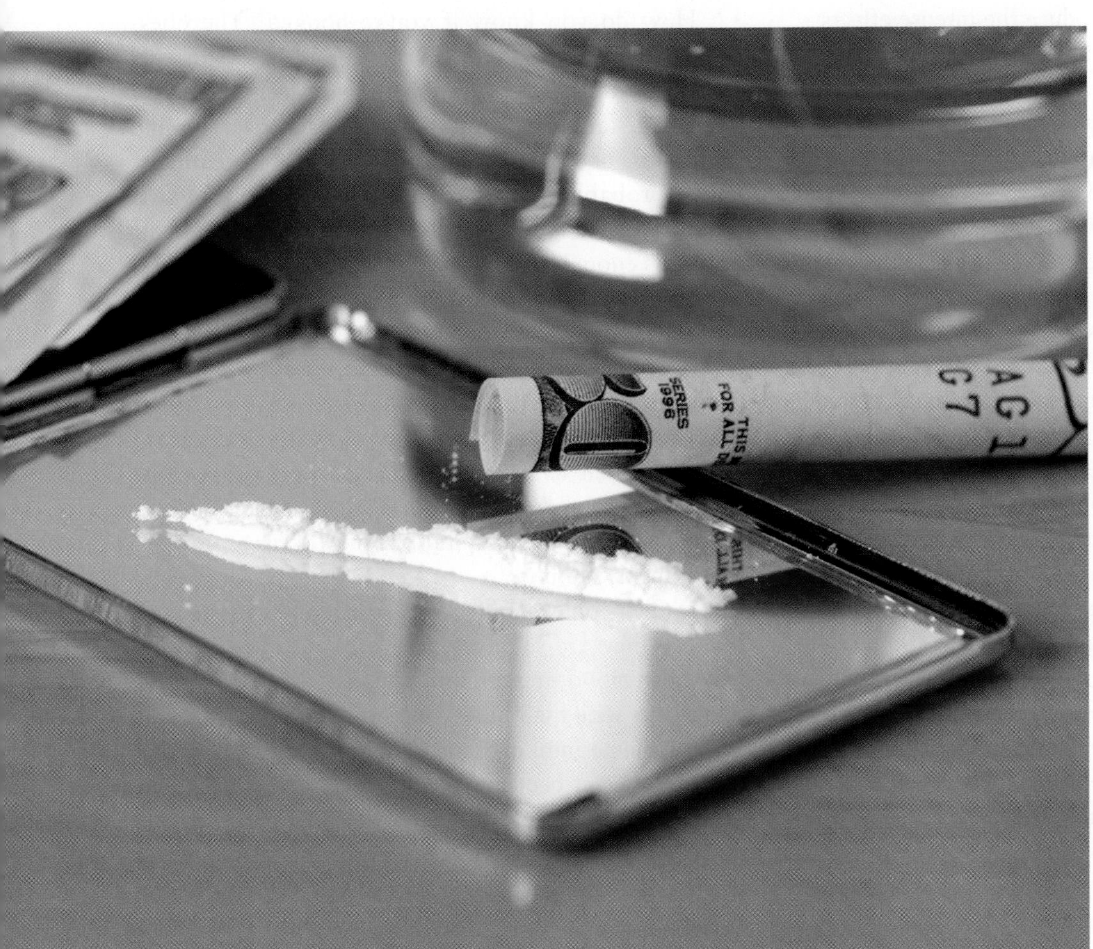

Caffeine

Would it surprise you to learn that many, perhaps most, people who live perfectly normal lives never realize that they are hooked on a mind-altering drug? That drug is available in any supermarket and is probably sitting in your room or kitchen cabinet right now.

cocaine psychosis
An acute psychotic reaction induced by the use of cocaine, often involving paranoid delusions.

Table 6-3 Amount of Caffeine in Coffee and Tea Products[14]

TYPE OF COFFEE	CAFFEINE (MILLIGRAMS)
Dunkin' Donuts, brewed, 16 oz (480 mL)	143–206
Generic brewed, 8 oz (240 mL)	95–200
Generic brewed, decaffeinated, 8 oz (240 mL)	2–12
Generic instant, 8 oz (240 mL)	27–173
Generic instant, decaffeinated, 8 oz (240 mL)	2–12
Starbucks Vanilla Latte, 16 oz (480 mL)	150
TYPE OF TEA	**CAFFEINE (MILLIGRAMS)**
Black tea, brewed, 8 oz (240 mL)	40–120
Black tea, decaffeinated, brewed, 8 oz (240 mL)	2–10
Starbucks Tazo Chai Tea Latte, 16 oz (480 mL)	100
Stash Premium Green, brewed, 6 oz (180 mL)	26

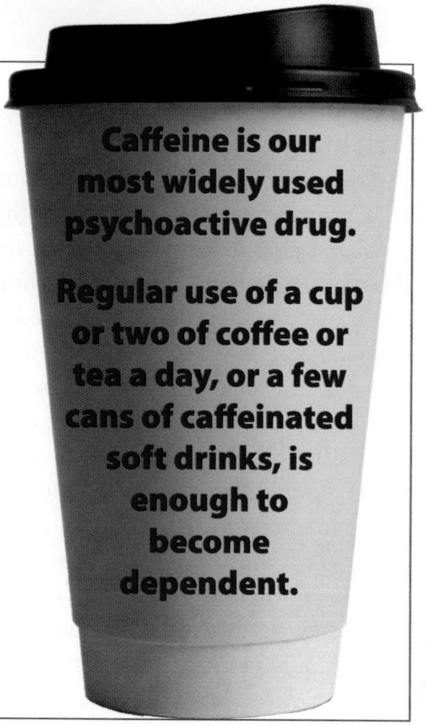
Caffeine is our most widely used psychoactive drug.
Regular use of a cup or two of coffee or tea a day, or a few cans of caffeinated soft drinks, is enough to become dependent.

© iStockphoto.com/Chris Hutchison

It is **caffeine**, the mild stimulant found in coffee, tea, cola beverages, and chocolate (see Table 6-3). As a mild stimulant, caffeine does not produce the intense effects or euphoric highs of stronger stimulants like cocaine and methamphetamine ("ice").

Caffeine is our most widely used psychoactive drug. More than half of American adults drink coffee, averaging more than three cups a day.

If you regularly drink caffeinated beverages, you are probably hooked. Caffeine may be the least harmful of addictive substances, but it still carries some risks. Pregnant women stand an increased risk of giving birth to underweight babies if they drink coffee during pregnancy (or consume other sources of caffeine).[15] Low birthweight increases the risk of infant mortality and some developmental problems.

For most healthy and nonpregnant adults, moderate caffeine intake (200 to 300 mg per day, or about two to three cups of coffee daily) poses no significant health problems.[16] Yet, recent evidence suggests that heavy consumption of coffee can increase the risk of heart attacks in some genetically predisposed people.[17] Though caffeine causes short-term increases in blood pressure, evidence fails to show any clear connection between caffeine intake and the risk of developing hypertension.[18] Caffeine does have some benefits, such as enhancing wakefulness and mental alertness, which is why many of us start the day with coffee or tea.

caffeine
A mild stimulant found in coffee beans, tea, cola beverages, and chocolate.

How do you know if you're hooked? The question is whether you can skip caffeine for a day or two without withdrawal symptoms. If you feel "on-edge," depressed, fatigued, edgy, have headaches or flu-like symptoms, or experience strong cravings for caffeine, you're probably hooked. Regular use of a cup or two of coffee or tea a day, or a few cans of caffeinated soft drinks, is enough to become dependent.

The effects of caffeine are dose related. At 100 milligrams (about the amount in in an average six-ounce cup of coffee), people tend to report feeling stimulated, energetic, and talkative. As the dosage rises from about 250 to 700 milligrams a day, more negative effects are reported, such as feelings of headaches, nausea, jitteriness, nervousness, and difficulty sleeping. Heart irregularities such as palpitations may occur at dosages exceeding 1,000 mg.[19]

Some people should avoid or limit caffeine use because they are highly sensitive to it. Since caffeine may raise blood pressure, physicians often recommend to patients with high blood pressure that they reduce or avoid caffeine intake. Some people can down a strong cup of coffee at bedtime and still sleep like a baby, but others toss and turn for hours if they have had even one cup of coffee or tea after noon. For some people, a cup or two of coffee or tea causes side effects such as nervousness, headaches, trembling, even diarrhea. Decaffeinated coffees and teas allow people to enjoy these beverages without suffering side effects.

If you decide to quit caffeine cold turkey, withdrawal symptoms usually taper off within 48 hours and are gone in a week or so. Cutting down gradually reduces or eliminates withdrawal symptoms. One way to cut down is to brew mixtures of caffeinated and decaffeinated coffee or tea. Gradually reduce the caffeinated proportion. (Don't substitute a six-pack of cola for a cup of caffeinated coffee.)

Hallucinogenic Drugs

Also known as *psychedelics* ("mind-revealing"), **hallucinogenic** drugs or *hallucinogens* alter sensory perceptions, distorting reality and producing hallucinations. Hallucinogens also produce feelings of relaxation or euphoria in some cases, or paranoia or panic in others.

Hallucinogens can produce strong psychological dependence, especially when people turn to them to distract themselves from stress. Most are not known to be addictive, however. The most widely used hallucinogens are *lysergic acid diethylamide (LSD)*, *mescaline*, and *psilocybin*. Other drugs that are sometimes grouped with the hallucinogens because of similar hallucinogenic effects include *phencyclidine (PCP)* and *marijuana*.

LSD

LSD (lysergic acid diethylamide; street name, "acid") is a synthetic hallucinogenic drug that can produce vivid hallucinations and sensory distortions. The experience of taking the drug is called a "trip." LSD trips may last as long as 12 hours. Nearly 23 million Americans report having used LSD in their lifetimes, but under a million use it with any regularity.[20]

LSD causes dilation of the pupils; increased body temperature, heart rate, and blood pressure; sweating; loss of appetite; sleeplessness; dry mouth; and tremors. The psychological effects of LSD are variable and unpredictable. Some users report vivid displays of colors, other visual distortions, and hallucinations, especially with larger doses. Emotions may shift rapidly. There may be changes in the sense of time and of self. Sensations may "cross over"; users may feel that they hear colors or see sounds. Some users report that the drug expands consciousness, helping them discover a deeper reality or acquire new insights. These discoveries are usually fleeting and do not lead to constructive life changes.

Some users have "bad trips" with feelings of intense fear or panic. They may fear death, or loss of control or sanity. There have been fatal accidents during LSD trips. The user's experience with the drug plays a role. Users who have learned to handle the effects of the drug may have better "trips."

Flashbacks—recurrences of perceptual distortions—may take place weeks or years after trips. Flashbacks tend to occur suddenly and without warning. There are occasional psychotic reactions.

Mescaline and Psilocybin

Used for centuries through the present day in religious rites by Indian tribes in the Southwestern United States, Mexico, and Central America, *mescaline* ("mesc") is derived from the peyote cactus. Like LSD, it can produce hallucinations, vivid lights, and visual distortions that can last more than 12 hours. *Psilocybin* is derived from certain mushrooms. These "magic mushrooms" have long been used in religious practices among Native Americans. Although less potent than LSD, psilocybin can produce colorful images and hallucinations that last four to six hours. However, the effects of the drug are not predictable, and people may have negative experiences or "bad trips," with panic attacks or frightening hallucinations. Flashbacks may occur days or weeks afterwards.

Phencyclidine (PCP)

Phencyclidine (PCP) or "angel dust" achieved popularity as a street drug in the 1970s because it could be cheaply and quickly synthesized in basement or garage-type laboratories. Its popularity has since waned, in large part because of its unpredictable effects.

PCP is a **deliriant**, a drug that produces *delirium*—a state of extreme confusion, excitement, disorientation, and difficulty focusing attention. There can be distortions in the perception of time and space, feelings of unreality, distorted body image, and vivid, sometimes frightening, hallucinations. It may seem that an invisible barrier separates the self from the world. This separation can be pleasant and engrossing or frightening.

Physical effects of the drug include increased heart rate and blood pressure, profuse sweating, and flushing. Users may stagger. Their speech may become garbled. They may become relatively

hallucinogenic
A drug that produces hallucinations.

deliriant
A substance that induces delirium, or a state of gross mental confusion, excitability, and disorientation.

insensitive to touch and pain—a phenomenon that can lead to injury, as the person may not perceive threats.

Users sometimes report that the drug makes them feel stronger, more powerful, and even invulnerable. Yet it may also lead to paranoia, blind rage, and blotting out of unpleasant memories. People under the drug's influence have committed shootings, stabbings, or self-inflicted injuries. Bizarre behavior, such as lying down in the middle of busy thoroughfares, is not uncommon. Accidents occur—drownings, falls, and automobile crashes. PCP is toxic in high doses and can result in convulsion, coma, even death.

Marijuana

Marijuana ("pot," "weed," "grass," "reefer," "dope") is derived from the *cannabis sativa* plant. The major psychoactive ingredient in marijuana is *delta-9-tetrahydrocannabinol*, or THC. It is found in the leaves and branches of cannabis but is most concentrated in the resin of the plant, from which the most potent form of the drug, *hashish* ("hash"), is derived. Smoking is the most common form of ingestion. The dried leaves may be rolled into "joints" and then smoked. A pipe may be used to smoke the crunched-up leaves or resin.

Marijuana is the most widely used illegal drug, with nearly 17 million Americans age 12 and older reporting use of the drug during the past month.[21] Marijuana alters perceptions and sometimes produces mild hallucinations. Lower doses can induce relaxation and a mild euphoric high. Users may experience time as passing more slowly and become more aware of body sensations, such as the beating of the heart. This can lead to feelings of anxiety or even panic in users who perceive that the heart is racing out of control. High doses can cause nausea and vomiting, feelings of disorientation, panic attacks, paranoia, and hallucinations.

People use marijuana for a variety of reasons. Some find it relaxing, similar in low doses to drinking a highball of liquor. Some users report that the drug makes them more comfortable in social gatherings. Higher doses, however, may lead users to withdraw into themselves. Some users believe that the drug increases their capacity for self-insight or creative thinking, although the insights achieved under its influence may not seem as deep when the drug has worn off. People may turn to marijuana, as to other drugs, to help them cope with stress. Of course, marijuana and other drugs provide only a temporary escape.

Regular use of marijuana may lead to physiological dependence, as denoted by the development of a withdrawal syndrome among long-term heavy users who abruptly stop using the drug.[22] Regular marijuana use can also lead to psychological dependence, as users come to rely on having a "joint" to deal with stress or to function socially. Marijuana use can impair coordination and motor skills, making it dangerous to operate an automobile. In high doses, it can cause perceptual distortions and induce paranoia. Long-term use of the drug is linked to impaired learning and memory.[23] Smoking marijuana also introduces cancer-causing chemicals into the body, which can damage the body's DNA and increase the risk of various cancers including lung cancer.[24] Marijuana can raise the heart rate to 140 to 150 beats per minute and, in some people, raise blood pressure, posing a risk to people with cardiovascular conditions.

marijuana
Derived from the cannabis sativa *plant, a drug with relaxant and mild hallucinogenic effects.*

club drugs (designer drugs)
Synthetic drugs manufactured in illicit labs that are chemical analogues (drugs having similar properties and effects) of illegal drugs.

inhalants
Chemical fumes that are inhaled for their psychoactive effects.

Club Drugs

Club drugs (also called **designer drugs**) are widely used at late-night dance parties or raves, nightclubs, and musical festivals. They are used to increase the effects of sensory stimulation such as music and light shows and to enhance feelings of connectedness or intimacy with others. The most commonly used club drugs include *MDMA* (commonly called *ecstasy*), GHB, Rohypnol, ketamine, and herbal ecstasy.

These drugs tend to be popular among adolescents and young adults, in large part because they are relatively inexpensive and can be taken conveniently in pill or powdered form or mixed with other beverages, such as alcohol. Many young partygoers and clubbers believe these drugs to be relatively harmless. But they carry significant health risks, as we see in Table 6-4.

Inhalants

Inhalants are chemicals that emit fumes that users inhale to get high. Common inhalants include glues and

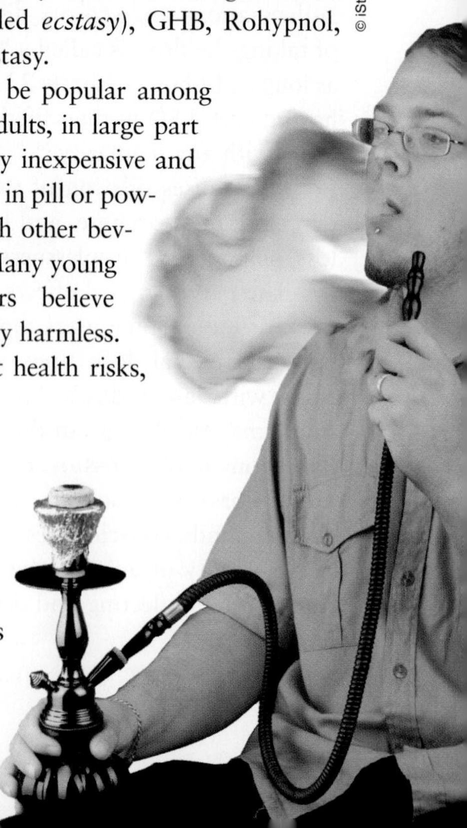
© iStockphoto.com/István Csák

Table 6-4 Club Drugs

CLUB DRUG	STREET NAMES	ABOUT . . .
MDMA (3,4-methylene-dioxymethamphetamine)	Ecstasy, E, X, XTC, X, X-TC, hug drug, Adam	Chemically similar to amphetamines; produces pleasurable sensations and mild hallucinations; can have negative emotional effects, impair learning, concentration, and memory[25]; increases heart rate and blood pressure; can lead to loss of consciousness and seizures
GHB (9 gamma-hydroxybutyrate)	Liquid ecstasy, G, grievous bodily harm, scoop, nitro, Georgia home boy, harm, gamma G, somatomax, growth hormone booster	Produces mild euphoria, relaxation, drowsiness; can cause dizziness, amnesia, blackouts, seizures and respiratory failure; may lower sexual inhibitions and increase sexual feelings; has been used as a "date rape" drug because it is odorless and tasteless and can be slipped into a victim's drink
Ketamine	Special K, K, super K, vitamin K, kit-kat, cat valium, kit-kat, keets, super acid, jet	An anesthetic used by veterinarians; snorted or smoked as a powder; chemically similar to PCP with similar effects; used as a date rape drug; can cause convulsions and respiratory failure
Rohypnol (flunitrazepam)	Roofies, roach-2, roofenol, la rocha, rope, Mexican valium, rib, roopies, ruffies	A strong tranquilizer used before surgery for anesthesia and sedation[26]; used as a date rape drug because it can be dissolved in a victim's drink; has calming and relaxing effects; can induce sleep; can induce memory loss
Herbal ecstasy	Cloud 9, rave energy, ultimate xphoria	A combination of legally available herbs, touted as a safe and natural alternative to ecstasy; can be swallowed, snorted, or smoked; contains ephedrine, a stimulant that can harm people with high blood pressure or heart conditions; can cause stroke, liver failure, heart attacks

rubber cements, gases from aerosol cans, paint thinners, spot removers, lighter fluids, gasoline and other fuels, and nitrous oxide ("laughing gas"). Unlike other drugs, use of inhalants is more common among younger adolescents than older adolescents. They appeal to young people because they are found in common household products and provide a quick "hit." Like PCP, inhalants are deliriants. They produce disorientation, dizziness, and impaired judgment. They also have depressant effects on the nervous system.

Inhalants can be dangerous, even deadly. Inhaled chemicals are quickly absorbed in the bloodstream. They travel throughout the body, damaging various organs, especially the kidneys, liver, lungs, and brain. Overdoses can cause unconsciousness and coma. Sustained inhalation may cause death by suffocation.

Anabolic Steroids

Anabolic steroids are not used for their psychoactive effects (to get high), but rather for their ability to foster muscle development. Anabolic steroids are synthetic versions of the male sex hormone testosterone. They have several medical uses, such as in the treatment of osteoporosis and anemia. They are also used illicitly by bodybuilders, football players, competitive runners, and others bent on building up their muscle mass. Steroid use became a national issue in the early 2000s with widely publicized claims that a number of baseball's best-known power hitters had used steroids. However, the typical user is not a professional athlete, but a young man of about 18 years of age who uses steroids to give himself an edge in athletic competition or to build up his physique in the belief that a "pumped-up" look will attract women. Young people who use steroids typically do not recognize or heed the consequences of their use.

Anabolic steroids also carry serious risks. They can damage various body organs and systems, especially the liver, the organ

anabolic steroid
Synthetic version of the male sex hormone testosterone.

responsible for steroid metabolism. Anabolic steroid use is linked to cancers of the liver, testes, and abdomen, and to impaired reproductive functioning. Steroids also reduce blood levels of "good cholesterol" (HDL), increasing the risk of cardiovascular problems. They can also lead to acne, impotence in men, and breast reduction and beard growth in women.

Anabolic steroids have psychoactive effects, such as boosting self-confidence. They can also have disturbing behavioral effects, the most troubling of which is increasing anger and aggression ("roid rage"). Some cases of homicide are connected with use of anabolic steroids. Psychotic symptoms and mood disturbances have also been observed among some steroid users. Withdrawal from anabolic steroids can cause sleep problems, mood swings, and depression severe enough to lead to thoughts of suicide.

Medical Uses of Psychoactive Drugs

Opiates are used medically for relief of pain, most often to deaden postsurgical pain or to treat severe pain arising from some medical conditions. The opiate codeine is often used as a cough suppressant. Other opiates are used to control post-operative pain. Researchers are also exploring medical uses of marijuana. The drug has been used to reduce fluid pressure in the eyes of glaucoma patients and to lessen pain and muscle spasms in patients with epilepsy and multiple sclerosis.

Some psychoactive drugs, called *psychotherapeutic drugs* or *psychotropics*, are used to treat psychological disorders. They include antidepressants (like Prozac), antianxiety agents (like Xanax), stimulants (like Ritalin), and antipsychotic drugs (like Risperdal).

Many drugs with psychoactive properties are available over the counter. Sleep aids such as Nytol and Sominex contain **antihistamines** that have sedating effects on the central nervous system and make you feel sleepy. Antihistamines are also used in allergy and cold medications such as NyQuil and Dimetapp Cold and Allergy Elixir to dry up runny noses and combat hay fever or other allergic reactions. This is why cold medications containing antihistamines carry warnings that they may cause drowsiness. Antihistamines may also have adverse reactions when combined with alcohol.

Although OTC sleep medications may provide temporary relief from insomnia, they have their drawbacks. For one thing, their effectiveness tends to diminish over time. For another, they may interfere with natural sleep cycles and make it difficult to achieve a truly deep, restful sleep. People may also become unable to sleep without them.

antihistamine
A drug that blocks the actions of histamine, a substance released in the body during an allergic reaction.

Other OTC drugs with psychoactive properties include decongestants. Sudafed, for example, is a decongestant used to relieve nasal congestion that often accompanies colds or allergies. It's active ingredient, *pseudoephedrine*, has a mild stimulant effect. The drug should not be used by people with certain medical conditions, such as high blood pressure and heart disease, unless they are directed to do so by a physician.

Who Uses Psychoactive Drugs?

The short answer is nearly all of us, at some time or another. Many begin using drugs such as alcohol or caffeine at an early age. About one in two young people begin using alcohol before the legal age of 21.[27] Cigarette smoking, which introduces the stimulant drug nicotine into the body, has been rising among young people in recent years; nearly three of 10 high school students (28%) are now lighting up. Nearly one in 11 Americans (8.7% according to the latest available statistics) age 12 and older reports using illicit drugs during the past month.[28] Marijuana is the most commonly used illicit drug, used by about 6%–7% of Americans age 12 and older during the previous month.

LEARNING OUTCOME 4

Discuss who uses psychoactive drugs

More than one in six people of college age smokes marijuana regularly. Many college students take depressants to get to sleep at night and stimulants to get going in the morning or to stay awake while studying. But it is alcohol, as we see in Chapter 7, that is the BDOC—the biggest (most popular) drug on campus.

There are troubling signs on the horizon, as the numbers of teenagers using marijuana has been rising in recent years.[29] Ecstasy, which had fallen out of favor, also appears to be making a comeback. But illicit drug use is dwarfed by the use of two substances that are legally available to adults: alcohol and tobacco. Alcohol, not illicit drugs like heroin or cocaine, remains the most popular drug on campus. Figure 6-2 shows the prevalences of drug use for adults in the United States, as indicated by percentages of people reporting cur-

Figure 6-2 Prevalence of Drug Use in the United States[30]

Nearly half of adult Americans admit to having used an illicit (illegal) drug at some point in their lives. About one in 12 is a current (past-month) user. But illicit drug use pales in comparison to use of two psychoactive substances that adults may use legally—alcohol and tobacco.

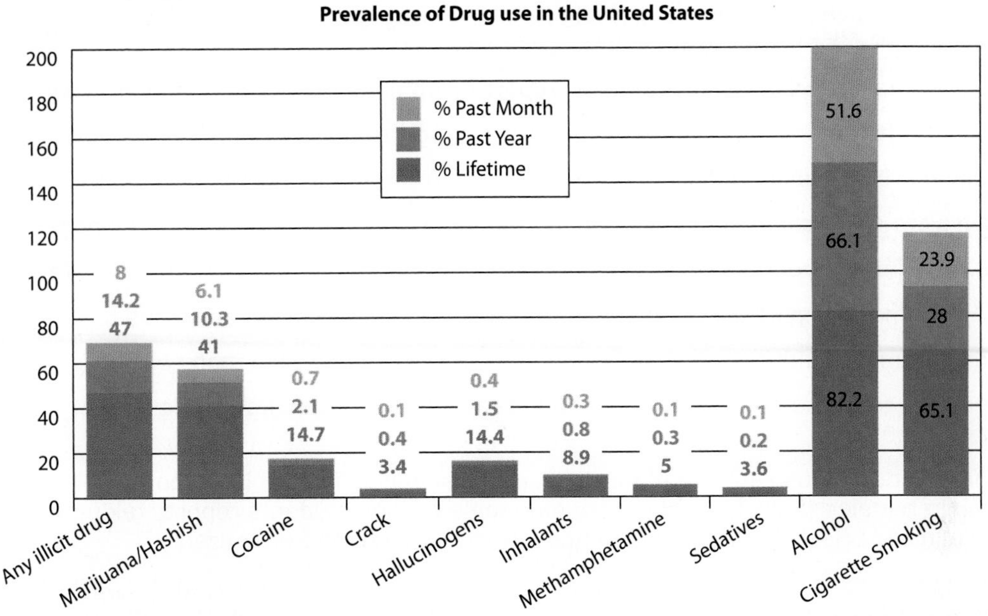

rent (past month) use, past year use, and lifetime use. "Diversity 6-1" on the next page summarizes gender differences in the use of psychoactive drugs among college students.

Response to Drugs

The response to drugs varies with the type of drug, how it is administered, the user's biological response to the drug, the user's frame of mind, the presence of other drugs, and the social setting.

LEARNING OUTCOME 5

Explain how people respond to drugs in different ways

Routes of Administration

Drugs enter the body in different ways. Alcohol, barbiturates, and amphetamines are taken orally in liquid or pill form and pass into the bloodstream through the digestive system. Other drugs enter the body through the lungs, either by smoking the drug or, as in the case of powder cocaine, inhaling or snorting. Chemical fumes are inhaled, usually by drawing the fumes into the nose or mouth. Smoking is the usual route of administration for cigarette and pipe tobacco and for such illegal drugs as marijuana, hashish, and crack cocaine. Chewing tobacco is typically placed between the cheek and gum, where the juices are absorbed through the mucosal lining of the mouth. Snuff, a powder form of smokeless tobacco, may be inhaled through the nostrils or placed inside the cheek and sucked.

Drugs may be injected *intravenously* (into a vein), *intramuscularly* (into a muscle), or *intracutaneously* (just under the skin). An *injecting drug user (IDU)* injects drugs in any of these ways. An *intravenous drug user* (*IVDU* or *IV-drug user*) injects a drug into a vein. Injection of a drug typically produces stronger reactions than swallowing it. Drugs injected into a vein enter the bloodstream directly and may travel to the brain relatively intact. Drugs that enter the body through the stomach may be partially digested before they reach the bloodstream. Drugs that are injected, smoked, or snorted may reach the brain in a matter of seconds, whereas drugs taken orally may take 30 minutes or longer to reach the brain. Intravenous injection delivers more immediate effects than injection into skin or muscle because the drug is deposited directly into the bloodstream.

DIVERSITY 6-1

Drugs on Campus: Gender Differences in Prevalence of Use[31]

College males have higher annual prevalence rates of usage than college females for most drugs:

- 38% of males versus 35% of females report using any illicit drug in the past year.
- 35% of males versus 31% of females report using marijuana in the past year.
- Daily marijuana use is significantly higher among male college students (6.9% vs. 3.6%).
- Males are significantly more likely than females to report use of most hallucinogens.
- 10.5% of males report using the narcotic Vicodin in the past year versus 7.0% for females.
- 9.1% of males report using the narcotic OxyContin in the past year versus 6.1% of females.
- Annual amphetamine use is higher among college males (8.5%) than college females (6.8%).
- Annual Ritalin use among college students is a bit higher among females (2.1%) than among males (1.0%).
- Annual Adderall use outside of medical supervision is twice as high among males (11.3%) as among females (5.7%). One in every nine male college students reports taking Adderall at least once in the prior 12 months, presumably to stay awake and energized.
- College males are slightly more likely to report getting drunk (48%) in the past 30 days than females (39%). Male students report higher rates of occasional binge drinking (45%) than female students (31%).
- More extreme levels of binge drinking show a large gender difference. Among college students, the prevalence of having 10 or more drinks in a row in the prior two weeks was 7% for college females versus 25% for college males. The prevalence of having 15 or more drinks in a row was 1.4% for college females versus 11% for college males.
- Flavored alcoholic beverages are consumed by more college females (68%) than males (63%).
- Daily smoking is reported by a slightly higher proportion of college males than college females (8.6% vs. 7.7%). Rates of smoking a half pack or more per day are 4.1% and 3.7%, respectively, for male and female college students.

The nicotine in tobacco smoke reaches the brain within 10 seconds after a puff of a cigarette. This is a few seconds sooner than it takes heroin to reach the brain when it is injected into a vein.[32]

People who inject opiates like morphine or heroin intravenously typically experience an initial rush of pleasure followed by a second, longer phase of a tranquil, dreamlike state in which they feel emotionally disconnected from reality. Injecting the drug under the skin, however, does not produce the early high concentrations of the drug in the brain that causes the initial euphoric rush. The predominant effect is the tranquility associated with the second phase.

dose-response relationship
The relationship between the dosage level of a drug and its effects on the individual, usually expressed in the form of a graph showing the drug's effects at specific dosage levels.

Dosage: More Is More

The relationship between the dosage level of a drug and its effects is called the **dose-response relationship**. The dose-response relationship is not necessarily a straight line. The difference between your second and third alcoholic drink, for instance, will likely be greater than that between your eighth and ninth drink. For some drugs, such as LSD, the effects of the drug plateau with increasing dosage, so that higher doses do not intensify the effect.

Dosage level is an important determinant of the risk of overdose ("OD"). The amounts of a drug needed to induce an overdose, even a fatal overdose, also vary among individuals. People with certain heart conditions can suffer deadly cardiac irregularities from relatively small amounts of cocaine.

Biological Responsivity

People vary in their responsiveness to drugs. The same amount of a given drug affects different people in different ways. The effects depend on such factors as the user's weight and gender. A heavier person may be less responsive than a lighter person. Women tend to become intoxicated at lower doses of certain drugs, such as alcohol, than men do. Regular use of a drug may lead to tolerance so that higher dosages are needed to achieve the same effect.

Frame of Mind

A cheerful user may experience greater euphoria from amphetamines or heroin than a gloomy user. A user's expectations play a role in determining a drug's effects. If you expect that a drug will make you feel high, you may feel high even if the drug is a sugar pill (placebo). If you believe that alcohol is a sexual stimulant, you may feel sexually aroused after a few drinks. If you hold negative expectations about LSD, you are more likely to have a "bad trip."

Drug Interactions

Drugs can interact in ways that increase their **toxicity**. Mixing drugs is a dangerous practice. Mixing alcohol and barbiturates reportedly led to fatal overdoses in the deaths of famed entertainers Marilyn Monroe and Judy Garland. People who abuse more than one drug at a time are called *polyabusers*.

In some cases the psychoactive effects of combining drugs are *cumulative* or *additive*, meaning that the overall effect is equal to the sum of the effects of each drug. Other drug combinations (as with alcohol and barbiturates) have a **synergistic effect**. Their combined effect is multiplied—many times greater than their additive effects. Combining alcohol and barbiturates creates effects four times as powerful as those caused by either drug alone. A given drug may also **potentiate** the effects of another drug: The second drug intensifies the effects of the first drug. Alcohol, for instance, can potentiate the effects of marijuana.

Some drugs block the effects of other drugs. These drugs, called **antagonists**, are useful in the treatment of drug addictions because they block the rewarding effects of addictive drugs. *Naltrexone* is an antagonist for opiates like heroin and morphine. So long as the opiate user takes naltrexone, the pleasurable effects of heroin or morphine are blocked.

Social Factors

The social setting can affect users' responses to drugs. Drinking might make you feel mellow and drowsy at home alone, but giddy and bubbly with friends. Marijuana use may induce paranoia if it is smoked in an abandoned building in a crime-ravaged neighborhood but not when it is used in the suburbs.

Pathways to Drug Abuse and Dependence

Drug abuse is repeated use of a drug even when use harms the user's health, impairs the user's ability to meet academic, occupational, or family responsibilities, or exposes the user or other people to danger, as in driving under the influence. If you are missing school or work because you are drunk or "sleeping it off," you are abusing alcohol. Even prescription drugs, such as prescription pain killers, can become drugs of abuse when they are misused.[33] It is not so much the amount of the drug taken or its legality that matters as much as its effects on the lives of the user and other people. From a legal perspective, however, *any* use of an illicit drug is abuse. So, too, is use of alcohol or nicotine by a minor.

Why and how do people make the transition between drug use and drug

LEARNING OUTCOME 6

Describe pathways to drug abuse and dependence

toxicity
The quality or degree of being poisonous.

synergistic effect
As applied to drug interactions, the action of two or more drugs operating together to enhance the overall effect to a level greater than the sum of the effects of each drug operating by itself.

potentiate
Relating to drugs, to enhance a drug's effects or potency.

antagonist
A drug that blocks or neutralizes the effects of another.

drug abuse
Persistent use of a drug despite the fact that use of the drug is harmful to the user's health, impairs the user's ability to function, or exposes the user or others to dangerous situations.

abuse and dependence? The answer may lie in multiple factors, including environmental, psychological, and genetic factors.

Environmental Factors

Peer pressure and exposure to family members and friends who use drugs can encourage young people to experiment with drugs. Continued use can become reinforced by the pleasurable effects of the drugs (the "rush" or "high") as well as by the approval of drug-using friends. Some young people who feel alienated from the mainstream culture come to identify with subcultures in which drug use is sanctioned or encouraged, such as gangs. Unemployment often figures into drug abuse. The relationship can work both ways: Drug abuse can contribute to unemployment, and unemployment, in turn, can contribute to drug abuse.

Psychological Factors

People use and abuse drugs for psychological reasons such as feelings of hopelessness, relief from troubling emotions, and a need for stimulation or physical sensations. Young people whose hopes for a successful future are dashed early on may turn to drugs out of hopelessness and despair. If the future doesn't hold promise, why not live for the pleasurable moment that drugs can provide? People who cannot cope with feelings like anxiety, tension, and depression, and who have nowhere to turn for help, may seek relief from alcohol and other drugs. People with high needs for sensation (excitement) may come to rely on drugs to provide the stimulation they seek.

Genetic Factors

Some people claim they were addicted to a substance, such as alcohol, the first time they tried it. The claim may be an exaggeration, but genetic factors are linked to increased risk of abuse and dependence on alcohol, opiates, and even tobacco in the form of cigarette smoking.[34] Though we don't inherit alcoholism or other forms of drug dependence directly, people may inherit a genetic predisposition that makes them more sensitive to the rewarding or stimulating effects of drugs. People may also inherit a predisposition for greater tolerance of the negative effects (such as nausea and dizziness) of alcohol, which can make it more difficult for them to learn when to say when.

Biochemical Factors

Many psychoactive drugs, including cocaine, alcohol, amphetamines, heroin, marijuana and even nicotine, produce pleasurable effects through a common pathway. They increase the availability in the brain of the chemical dopamine, a neurotransmitter that carries signals in the brain's pleasure or reward circuits—the brain cells responsible for the pleasurable feelings we experience from sex, winning a sporting event, or eating a delicious meal.[35] To varying degrees, these drugs flood the brain with dopamine and increase activity of other neurotransmitters involved in regulating mood states (norepinephrine and serotonin), producing changes in mental states ranging mild happiness to a euphoric high. Figure 6-3 illustrates the molecular underpinnings explaining why cocaine users experience altered mood states such as euphoria and why they crash when the drug effects wear off or they go without using the drug.

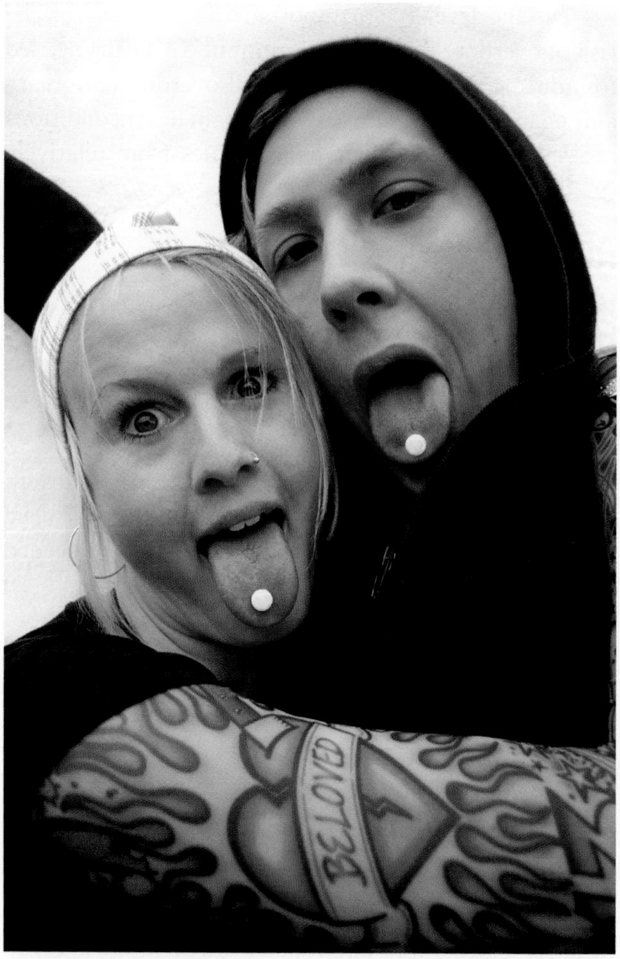

People use drugs to achieve pleasurable effects, but with regular use the table is turned. Chronic drug use damages brain circuits that produce feelings of pleasure and may even impair the brain's ability to manufacture dopamine and other neurotransmitters.[36] As a result, the ability to reap pleasure from ordinary activities of

Figure 6-3 How Cocaine Produces Euphoria and Why People "Crash"

A. In the normal functioning of the nervous system, neurotransmitters are released into the synaptic cleft by vesicles in terminal buttons of sending neurons. Many are taken up by receptor sites in receiving neurons.

B. In the process called reuptake, sending neurons typically reabsorb excess molecules of neurotransmitters.

C. Molecules of cocaine bind to the sites on sending neurons that normally reuptake molecules of neurotransmitters. As a result, molecules of norepinephrine, dopamine, and serotonin remain longer in the synaptic cleft, increasing their typical mood-altering effects and providing a euphoric rush. Over time, the brain comes to rely on the drug to maintain feelings of pleasure, leading to a "crash" in mood when the person stops using cocaine.

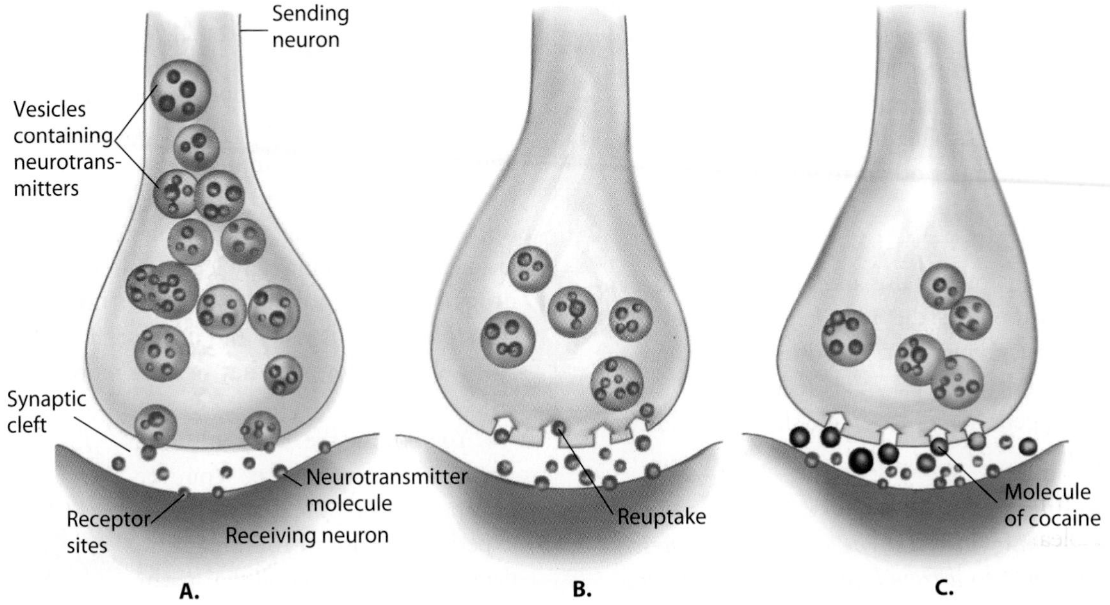

daily life, from a good meal to social activities, begins to wane. The drug abuser comes to depend on the drug for feelings of pleasure that no longer occur naturally, as well as to ward off unpleasant emotions such as depression and anxiety. Without drugs, life seems drab and unfulfilling. Changes in the brain's reward system help explain the intense cravings that may accompany drug withdrawal and difficulties in abstaining.

We also know that opiates such as heroin mimic the actions of neurotransmitters called **endorphins** (for *endogenous*, or built-in, *morphine*). Endorphins block pain and produce pleasure in a manner similar to opiates. Endorphins and opiates dock at the same receptor sites in the brain. Opiates fit into them like keys fit into locks. Normally, the brain produces enough endorphins to maintain a steady state of comfort and the potential to experience pleasure. But with continued use of opiates, the brain may stop producing endorphins, making the user dependent on opiates. If the habitual user then stops using opiates, feelings of discomfort and little aches and pains may be magnified until the body resumes adequate production of endorphins.

Stages in Drug Dependence

People do not become drug addicts overnight. A progression of steps leads from occasional use to addiction. For some, the slide into addiction is rapid; for others, gradual. While the particular steps to addiction may vary among addicts and from one drug to another, there are some common pathways.[37]

Stage 1: Experimentation

Experimentation involves occasional use of a drug—perhaps on weekends, perhaps monthly. The drug produces pleasant, even euphoric feelings. The user feels in control and capable of stopping at any time. Experimentation typically lasts a short time, perhaps weeks or months, before giving way to routine use.

Stage 2: Routine Use

The user begins taking the drug more often, eventually daily. More time is spent obtaining and using drugs.

endorphins
Naturally occurring chemicals in the body that are similar in their effects to opiates.

Appointments are rescheduled as the need to obtain drugs takes precedence. Users may deny the effects of the drugs on their lives. Values shift. What was formerly important—school, work, or a child's recital or baseball game—now pales in comparison with the need for the drug.

Problems mount with routine drug use. Family possessions, even heirlooms, are pawned for a fraction of their worth. A woman claims to have been robbed of her wedding ring at gunpoint. A man claims that a burglar made off with the large-screen TV. Lying and manipulation become staples of everyday life. Family relationships are strained. Days are lost from work, and family finances become depleted. Mortgage and car payments are skipped. The drug abuser may even steal from family members or others to feed the habit.

Stage 3: Addiction

The line between routine use and addiction or dependence is crossed when the user begins to feel powerless to resist cravings for the drug and when the physical signs of dependence—tolerance and withdrawal symptoms—appear. With heroin, the slide into addiction can be rapid:

> *One morning you awaken with what seems to be a cold—running nose, a slight feeling of chilliness. You mention it to a friend, who says: "That's no cold. Try some heroin and see how fast it goes away. You're hooked!"*[38]

Pursuit and use of the drug dominate virtually everything else in life, becoming more important than family relationships.

Codependence

A **codependent** helps the drug-dependent person remain dependent, perhaps unintentionally. The codependent is an *enabler* who remains silent about the abuser's behavior, makes excuses for it, or minimizes its impact—as by calling in sick for an abuser on a binge and telling the boss the abuser is out with the flu. Abusers in codependent relationships may never have to face the full consequences of their behavior and therefore may be less motivated to change. Codependents may realize that the abuser has a problem with drugs but mistakenly believe the best way to deal with it is to shower the person with love and support. Codependents may choose drug-dependent people as partners because it serves their own needs to have someone dependent on them. The online feature "Health Check 6-2" can help you evaluate whether you are a codependent.

codependent
A person involved in a close relationship with a drug-dependent person who plays a part in enabling or maintaining the other person's chemical dependency.

gateway drug
A drug serving as a "stepping-stone" or gateway to use of other, usually "harder," drugs.

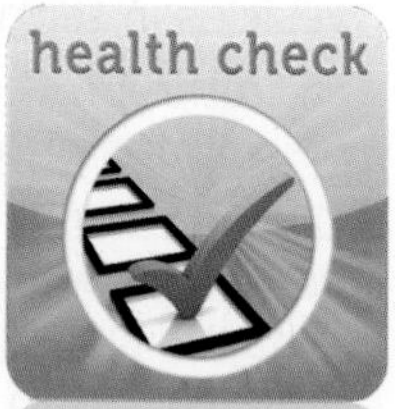

Access CourseMate for HLTH at www.cengagebrain.com.

Gateway Drugs

A **gateway drug** is a stepping-stone drug to "harder" drugs. Many users of so-called hard drugs like cocaine and heroin began their illicit drug career with marijuana. Alcohol and tobacco may become gateway drugs for harder drug use among adolescents.[39] Regular cigarette smoking may lead adolescents to use hard drugs because smoking has come to be viewed, even by adolescents, as risky and deviant. If adolescents see themselves as deviant, they may be more likely to take risks.

You know the costs of drug abuse and dependence. You see how people walk the pathway from experimental use to routine use to dependence. Are you on that path? To find out, complete the online feature "Health Check 6-3."

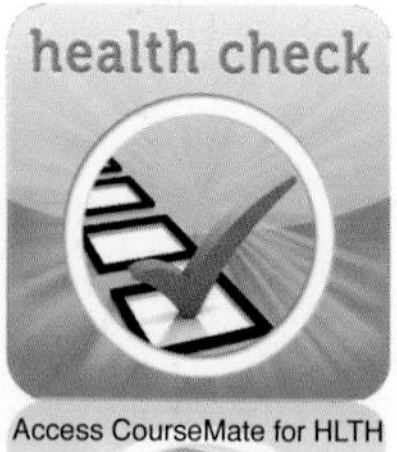

Access CourseMate for HLTH at www.cengagebrain.com.

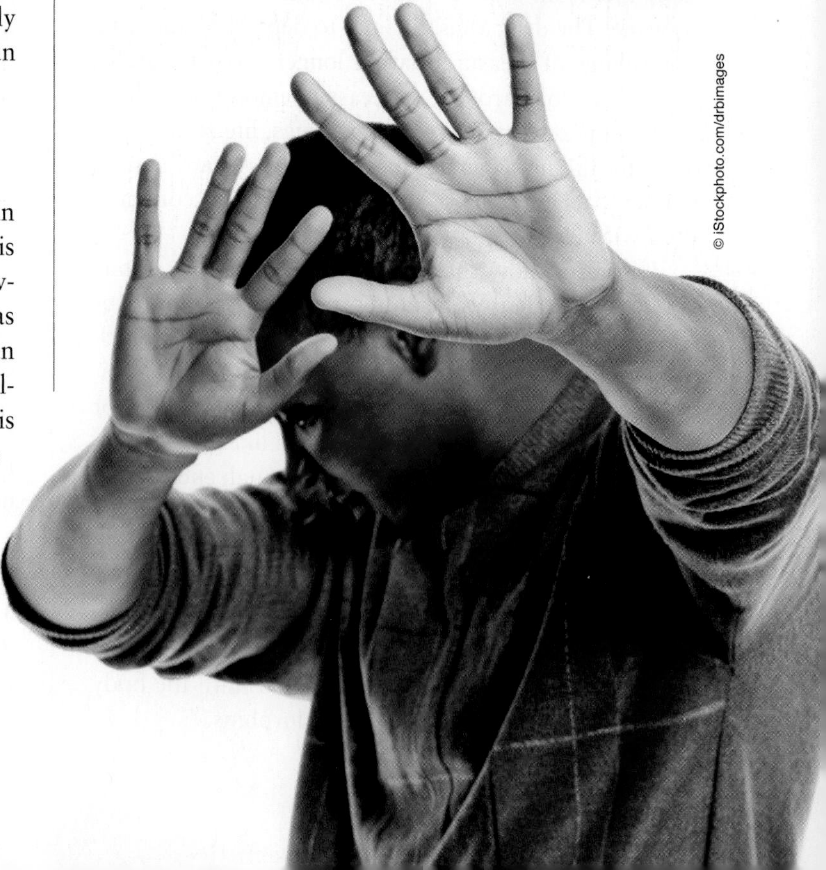

© iStockphoto.com/drbimages

Becoming Drug Free, Remaining Drug Free

There are many ways of helping people with drug abuse or dependence problems live free of drugs. They include clinic or hospital-based inpatient and outpatient treatment programs, and residential and community-based rehabilitation centers. Yet the great majority of drug abusers do not receive treatment. Most addicts do not seek help, although that may change if they hit "rock-bottom" or are brought to an emergency room because of an overdose or adverse drug reaction. Then, too, many addicts who *want* help find no openings in drug treatment centers. A Canadian study put the lack of treatment into perspective; only one in three applicants received treatment.[40]

LEARNING OUTCOME 7

Discuss ways of becoming and remaining drug free

Although drug treatment programs can help drug abusers turn their lives around, the truth is that treatment often fails to break the cycle of addiction. There's no doubt that the best "treatment" for drug abuse and dependence is preventing them from developing in the first place. How can we do that? Go to the online feature "Prevention 6-2" for advice.

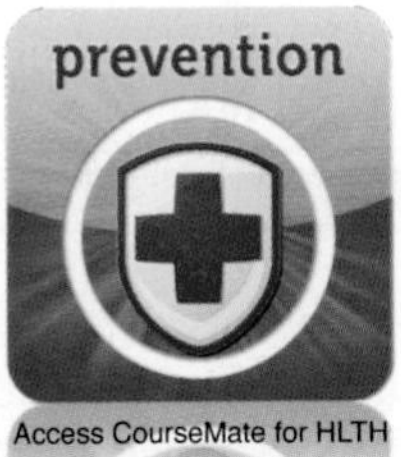

Access CourseMate for HLTH at www.cengagebrain.com.

Detoxification

For those who are addicted to drugs, the first step in treatment may be detoxification. **Detoxification** is the ridding of the body of drugs. "Detox" may take place in a hospital so that people with chemical dependencies can be medically supervised while they withdraw from drugs. The typical program is 28 days, during which recovering addicts work with counselors to prepare them for remaining drug-free upon discharge. Counselors attempt to break through the chemical haze and the layers of denial that prevent drug abusers from coming to grips with the consequences of their addictions. Detox may also take place on an outpatient basis, when it is deemed safe to withdraw addicts while they continue with their daily lives.

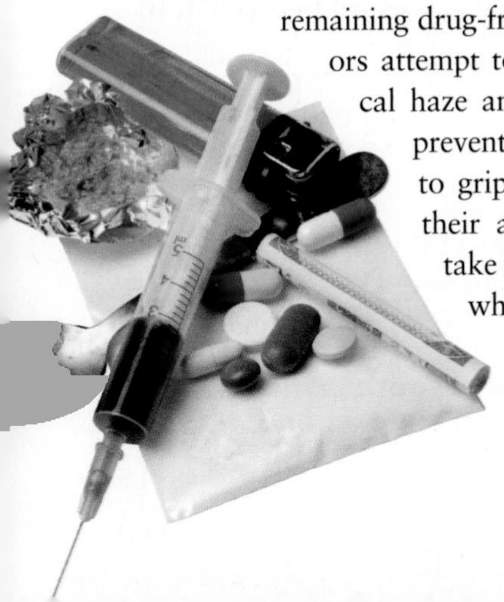
© iStockphoto.com/mark wragg

Detox is only the start. Outpatient programs following detox help recovering addicts to live drug free. The recovering addict may also be referred for additional help to Narcotics Anonymous, a peer-support, self-help organization fashioned after Alcoholics Anonymous (AA).

Therapeutic Communities

Therapeutic communities are drug-free residential treatment facilities in which recovering addicts live under strict rules. They make their own beds, prepare their own meals, and participate in daily group therapy sessions in which they are confronted with their denial of responsibility for their behavior. The treatment philosophy is that addicts will not break the bonds of addiction until they accept responsibility for their behavior and admit the damage they have done. Counseling and job training are often part of the program, which may extend beyond a year. While therapeutic communities have their successes, they suffer from high dropout rates. At least 75% of newly admitted patients leave prematurely. There is also a lack of evidence as to how many recovering addicts are able to maintain abstinence after they have returned to the larger community.

Methadone Maintenance

Methadone is a synthetic opiate that blocks the heroin high but prevents addicts from developing withdrawal symptoms. An estimated 200,000 heroin addicts in the United States participate in methadone programs. However, methadone, like heroin, is addictive. Methadone is taken orally in a single daily dose. Addicts on methadone maintenance can hold jobs or attend training programs after receiving their daily dose in a clinic. Methadone programs are subject to strict monitoring because overdoses can be lethal and the drug can become abused as a street drug.[41]

Critics of methadone maintenance contend that it is a game of musical addictions. It substitutes one addiction for another. Methadone can be taken indefinitely, but individuals can also be weaned from it without returning to heroin. Methadone maintenance eliminates the need for addicts to resort to crime to support their habits and permits them to lead more functional lives. Deaths from opiate overdoses declined

detoxification
The process of eliminating drugs from a person's body, usually taking place under supervised conditions where withdrawal symptoms can be monitored and controlled.

methadone
A synthetic opiate that is used as a substitute for heroin in the treatment of heroin addiction.

about 33% following the introduction of methadone maintenance,[42] but critics point out that methadone maintenance programs suffer from high rates of early dropouts and relapses. Results are better when methadone maintenance is combined with counseling.

Psychological Interventions

Psychotherapy can help addicts understand the roots of their addictive behavior and learn more adaptive ways of handling stress and interpersonal problems. Family therapy and marital therapy can be used to deal with family stresses and issues of codependence. Part of marital therapy may involve the use of a signed behavioral contract between the drug abuser and his or her partner. The contract might stipulate that so long as the drug abuser remains drug-free, the partner agrees to refrain from negative comments about the patient's drug use or potential for relapse.

Pharmacotherapeutic Approaches: Using Drugs to Combat Drugs

Some drugs are used to treat addictions to other drugs. The nonaddictive drug naltrexone blocks the high produced by alcohol and opiates. Thus, naltrexone can help blunt cravings for these drugs.[43] The problem with naltrexone, as with other therapeutic drugs, is that addicts who are bent on resuming their use of addictive substances can simply stop taking it.

Certain antidepressant drugs are helpful in treating cocaine addiction. The antidepressant *desipramine* (brand name Norpramin) increases neurotransmitters in the brain that make it possible for addicts to derive more pleasure from ordinary experiences of life. They thus may become less reliant on cocaine to experience pleasure.

Many self-help organizations in the alcohol and drug abuse field offer assistance to addicts and their families. For information about the services provided by self-help organizations, such as Alcoholics Anonymous (AA) (discussed in Chapter 7), Narcotics Anonymous (NA), and Cocaine Anonymous (CA), consult the online feature "Health Skills 6-3." In the following chapter, we discuss alcohol and nicotine in greater depth.

health skills

Access CourseMate for HLTH at www.cengagebrain.com.

HEALTH APPS: YOUR LINK TO ONLINE HEALTH APPLICATIONS

What To Do about Compulsive Spending Do you shop alone? Do you get into arguments with family members about what you spend? Do you feel lost without your credit card? If this sounds like you, get some guidance from "Health Skills 6-1."

Using Medications Wisely Prescription and OTC medications can cause serious problems if they are used inappropriately. You and your family should learn about the drugs you take and their possible side effects. Read "Prevention 6-1" to learn how to reap the benefits of drugs and avoid pitfalls.

Are You a Codependent? Are you involved in a relationship with a drug-dependent person? If so, do you recognize any of the following signs of codependence in yourself? Learn more by reading "Health Check 6-2."

Warning Signs of Drug Dependence You know the costs of drug abuse and dependence. You see how people walk the pathway from experimental use to routine use to dependence. Are you on that path? To find out, complete "Health Check 6-3."

Preventing Drug Abuse There's no doubt that the best "treatment" for drug abuse and dependence is preventing them from developing in the first place. How can we do that? Go to "Prevention 6-2" for advice.

Self-Help Organizations Many self-help organizations in the alcohol and drug abuse field offer assistance to addicts and their families. For information about the services provided by self-help organizations, consult "Health Skills 6-3."

Go to the CourseMate for HLTH at www.cengagebrain.com for additional resources including flashcards, games, self-quizzes, review exercises, web exercises, learning checks, and more.

Alcohol and Tobacco

"Two of the most harmful psychoactive substances known to humans are perfectly legal—at least for adults."

Two of the most harmful psychoactive substances known to humans are perfectly legal—at least for adults. But even children and adolescents find them available nearly anywhere and everywhere. One of them kills more than a thousand college students each year. The other is the only known substance that is harmful—potentially lethal, in fact—when used exactly as directed. It kills many times as many college students each year, but it takes decades to do so, and the process of dying, when it arrives, can be torturously prolonged.

You know what these substances are. The first one is alcohol. The second one is tobacco, which contains a highly addictive stimulant drug, nicotine.

LEARNING OUTCOMES

1 Explain what alcohol is

2 Explain which segments of the population are most likely to drink

3 Describe the effects of alcohol

4 Define *alcohol abuse* and *dependence*

5 Discuss the causes of alcoholism

6 Describe various methods of treating alcoholism

7 Explain which segments of the population are most likely to smoke

8 Explain why people smoke

9 Describe the effects of smoking on health

10 Discuss the health benefits of quitting smoking

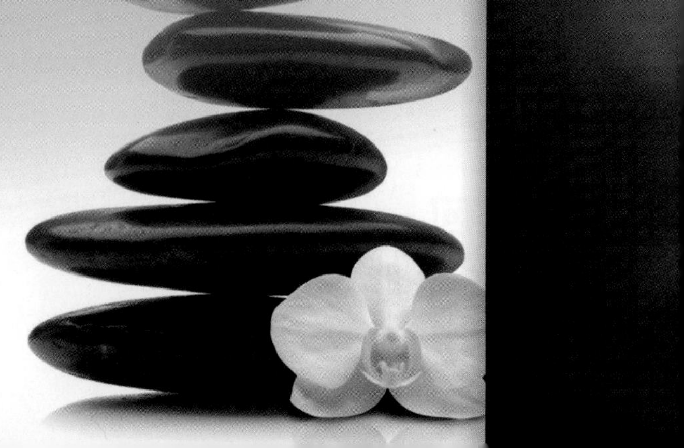

What Is Alcohol?

LEARNING OUTCOME 1
Explain what alcohol is

Alcohol is a colorless, flammable liquid. The psychoactive chemical in alcohol is *ethyl alcohol*—**ethanol**, for short. Ethyl alcohol is considered safe to drink in moderate amounts. Other kinds of alcohol have different household or medicinal uses but are toxic if drunk. Among these are isopropyl (*rubbing alcohol*) and methyl (wood) alcohol.

Alcoholic beverages are manufactured by **fermentation**, from which beer and

ethanol
Another term for ethyl alcohol.

fermentation
As applied to the making of alcoholic beverages, a process by which yeast plants are used to convert sugar in grains into ethyl alcohol and carbon dioxide.

wine are derived, and **distillation**, which yields hard liquors such as vodka, gin, and whiskey. Yeast used in fermentation converts sugars into ethyl alcohol and carbon dioxide. The chemical process is self-halting because an alcohol concentration of about 14% destroys the yeast. Thus, wine cannot have a greater alcohol concentration unless it is "fortified" by adding distilled alcohol, as in the preparation of ports and sherries. Distillation is the boiling out of alcohol from the fermentation process and condensing the vapors back into liquid form.

The alcohol content of beverages is graded in terms of **proof**. The proof value of an alcoholic beverage is two times the alcohol concentration of the beverage. A beverage containing 50% alcohol is 100 proof. Hard liquors generally vary from 80 to 100 proof (40% to 50% alcohol). Wines are typically 18 to 28 proof (9% to 14% alcohol). Most beers are 3% to 6% alcohol (6 to 12 proof). Heavier, darker beers, such as stout, are 6% to 7% alcohol. Malt liquor beers contain as much as 8% or 9% alcohol.

distillation
As applied to the making of distilled spirits, a process of boiling out the alcohol from the fermentation process and then condensing the vapors back into a liquid form.

proof
The alcoholic strength of a beverage, expressed by a number that is twice the percentage of alcohol in the beverage.

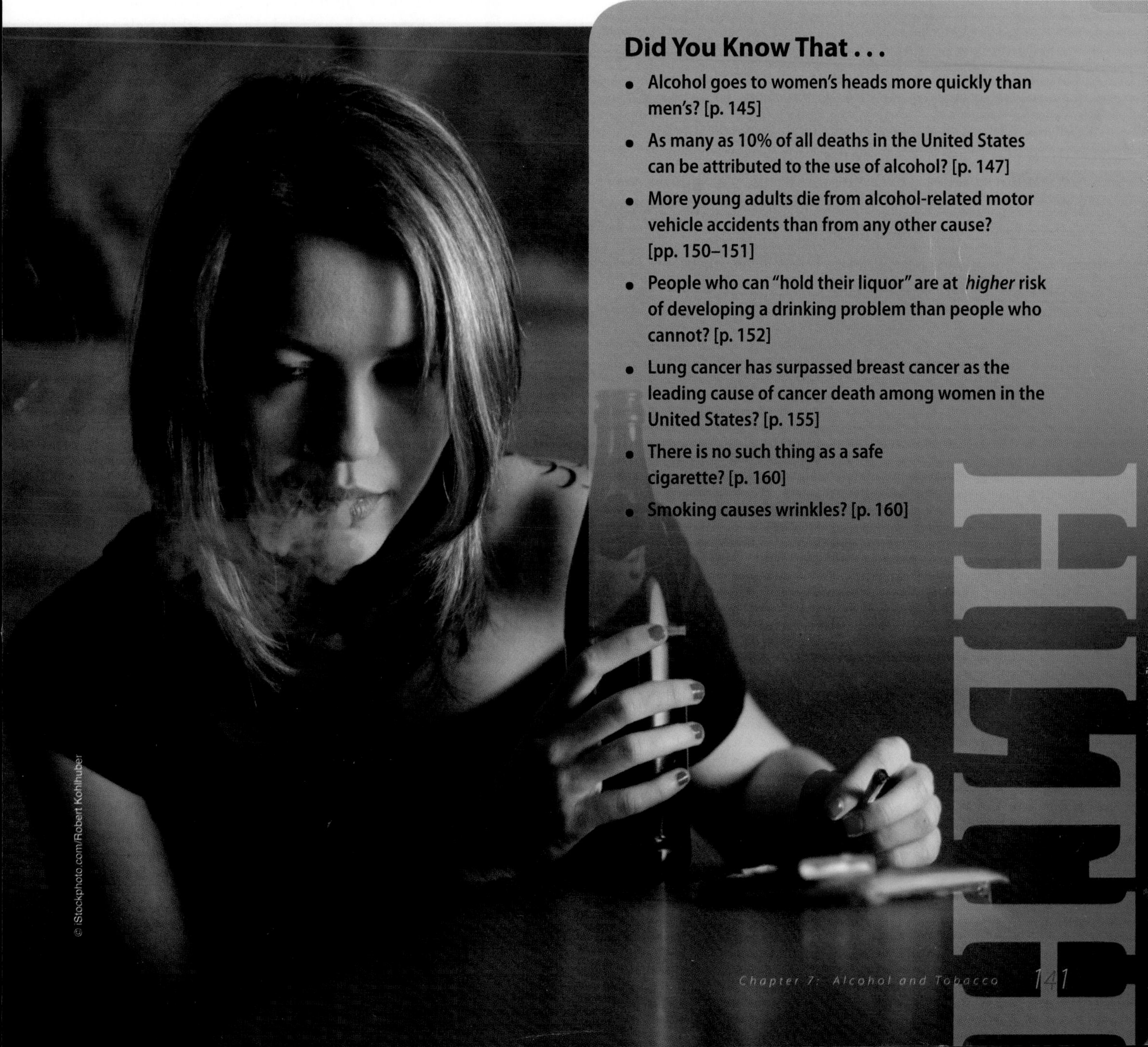

© iStockphoto.com/Robert Kohlhuber

Did You Know That . . .

- Alcohol goes to women's heads more quickly than men's? [p. 145]
- As many as 10% of all deaths in the United States can be attributed to the use of alcohol? [p. 147]
- More young adults die from alcohol-related motor vehicle accidents than from any other cause? [pp. 150–151]
- People who can "hold their liquor" are at *higher* risk of developing a drinking problem than people who cannot? [p. 152]
- Lung cancer has surpassed breast cancer as the leading cause of cancer death among women in the United States? [p. 155]
- There is no such thing as a safe cigarette? [p. 160]
- Smoking causes wrinkles? [p. 160]

Alcohol—The Swiss Army Knife of Drugs

No drug has meant so much to so many as alcohol. Alcohol is our dinnertime relaxant, our bedtime sedative, our cocktail-party social facilitator. We use alcohol to celebrate holy days, applaud our accomplishments, and express joyous wishes. The young assert their maturity with alcohol. Alcohol is used regularly by the majority of college students and adults.[1] Alcohol even kills germs on surface wounds.

Alcohol is the Swiss Army knife of drugs. It does it all. Alcohol is the all-purpose medicine you can buy without prescription. It is the relief from anxiety, depression, or loneliness that you can swallow in public without criticism or stigma. It lubricates social interactions. A man who takes a tranquilizer may look weak. A man who downs a bottle of beer may be seen as "macho."

But the army knife also has a sharp blade. No drug has been so abused as alcohol. Ten to 20 million people in the United States are alcoholics. In contrast, 750,000 to 1 million use heroin regularly and about 800,000 use cocaine regularly.[2] Excessive drinking has been linked to lower productivity, loss of employment, and downward movement in social status.

What about alcohol on campus? A study by the National Institute on Alcohol Abuse and Alcoholism[3] found that nearly four college students die each day from alcohol-related causes, another 1,300 to 1,400 have alcohol-related injuries, and nearly 200 are raped by their dates after drinking. Binge drinking—defined as having five or more drinks in a row for a male or four or more for a female—is connected with aggressive behavior, poor grades, sexual promiscuity, and serious accidents.[4] About 79,000 accidents per year are related to binge drinking.[5] Nevertheless, nearly half of college men and three in 10 college women binge at least twice a month.[6] The media pay more attention to deaths due to heroin and cocaine overdoses, but many more college students die each year from causes related to drinking, including accidents and overdoses.[7] Despite widespread marijuana use, alcohol remains the drug of choice among adolescents and adults.

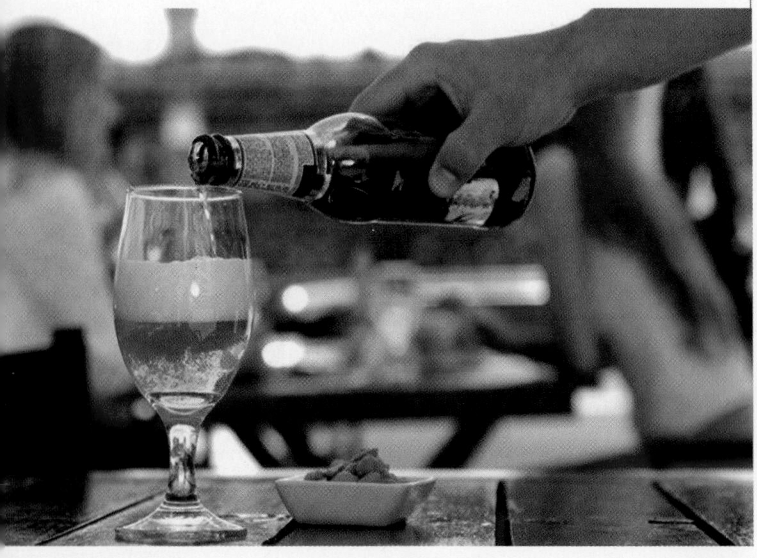

© PhotoAlto Photography/Veer

Who Drinks?

Two of three adults in the United States drink alcoholic beverages. About half of them are light drinkers; the other half are moderate or heavy drinkers. Alcohol use is most prevalent among 21- to 34-year-olds. European Americans are more likely than African Americans, Latin Americans, or Asian Americans to use alcohol. Within each of these groups, men are more likely to drink than women. Although the legal drinking age is 21 in every state, more than half of junior and senior high school students have used alcohol during the past year, and more than a third drink weekly.[8] Young people typically have their first drink by age 12 or 13.

LEARNING OUTCOME 2

Explain which segments of the population are most likely to drink

College Students

Heavy drinking is popular on college campuses. Alcohol, not cocaine, heroin, or marijuana, is the most popular drug on campus.[9] About four of five college students, mostly underage, drink (see Table 7-1). College students drink more than their agemates who do not attend college.[10] Drinking is as much a norm in college life as football or basketball.

The typical college student consumes more than 35 gallons of alcoholic beverages per year—mostly beer. Overall, college students consume more than 4 billion cans of beer annually, which, stacked end to end, would stretch to the moon and 70,000 miles beyond. The typical student spends more on alcohol (and MP3 players and downloads) than on textbooks.

Problem drinking is a major concern on college campuses. Nearly one in three college students reports driving under the influence during the previous year.[11] More

Table 7-1 Snapshot of College Drinking[12]

The consequences of excessive and underage drinking affect virtually all college campuses, college communities, and college students, whether they are younger or older than the minimum legal drinking age and whether or not they choose to drink.

- **Alcohol Consumption** About four in five of all college students drink, including nearly 60 percent of students age 18 to 20.
- **Binge Drinking** Approximately two of every five college students of all ages—more than 40 percent—have reported engaging in binge drinking at least once during the past two weeks.
- **Deaths** About 1,700 college students between the ages of 18 and 24 die each year from alcohol-related unintentional injuries, including motor vehicle crashes (about half among students under 21).
- **Injuries** About 600,000 college students between the ages of 18 and 24 are unintentionally injured under the influence of alcohol each year (about half among students under 21).
- **Assaults** It is estimated that each year more than 696,000 students between the ages of 18 and 24 are assaulted by another student who has been drinking (430,000 of them by a college student under 21).
- **Sexual Abuse** More than 97,000 students between the ages of 18 and 24 are victims of alcohol-related sexual assault or date rape each year (about half among students under 21).
- **Unsafe Sex** Each year more than 400,000 students between the ages of 18 and 24 had unprotected sex as a result of their drinking, and more than 100,000 students between the ages of 18 and 24 report having been too intoxicated to know if they consented to having sex.
- **Academic Problems** About 25% of college students report academic consequences of their drinking including missing class, falling behind, doing poorly on exams or papers, and receiving lower grades overall.
- **Vandalism** About 11 percent of college student drinkers report that they have damaged property while under the influence of alcohol.

than 40% of college students engaged in binge drinking during the past 30 days.[13] More than half report getting drunk at least once a year; between one-quarter and one-half get drunk at least once a month.[14]

Repeated binge drinking can lead to regular heavy drinking and alcoholism. Binge drinkers are also six times more likely to drink and drive than moderate drinkers. Binge drinkers are three times as likely to engage in unplanned or risky sex, increasing the risk of a sexually transmitted infection or an unwanted pregnancy. As one AIDS prevention ad put it, "First you get drunk, then you get stupid, then you get AIDS."

Binge drinkers are also at risk of cutting classes, getting poorer grades, getting into arguments or fights, and having trouble with the law. One reason that heavy drinking hurts grades is that students who do so typically get too little sleep.[15]

Belonging to a fraternity (and, to a lesser extent, a sorority) can be a risk factor for developing alcohol problems. Some "Greeks" drink heavily at parties. If you are rushing a fraternity or sorority, you may want to check out their attitudes toward drinking.

Many colleges have instituted "get tough" policies, prohibiting use of alcohol in college facilities or functions, expelling students who drink underage, and requiring off-campus fraternities and sororities to check IDs and control how much alcohol they serve at social functions.

Effects of Alcohol

Many users report that alcohol helps calm feelings of anxiety and produces feelings of pleasure and well-being. Alcohol can also have negative effects such as nausea, vomiting, and hangovers, especially when one drinks too much or too fast. Unpleasant sensations are a built-in deterrent to excessive drinking

LEARNING OUTCOME 3

Describe the effects of alcohol

intoxication
A state of drunkenness brought on by the use of alcohol or other intoxicating drugs.

for some. But for genetic reasons, some people are more tolerant of alcohol, even when they drink excessively, predisposing them to alcoholism.

For people who are anxious about their jobs or social lives, alcohol may become a form of self-medication. Because long-term heavy drinking can lead to health problems and social problems, people who turn to alcohol to alleviate problems may instead compound them. Positive expectations about alcohol also affect use and abuse. People who believe that alcohol will make them more sexually responsive or sexually alluring, make them more outgoing or assertive, or produce or enhance feelings of pleasure are more likely to drink and to develop problems with alcohol. The online feature "Health Check 7-1" will help you probe the reasons that you drink—if you do.

health check

Access CourseMate for HLTH at www.cengagebrain.com.

Alcohol is considered a depressant drug because it slows the functioning of the body. However, it can initially have stimulating properties because it dilates blood vessels, increasing alertness and even sexual arousal. The more one drinks, the stronger the depressant effects become.

After one or more drinks, the drinker becomes **intoxicated**. The brain mechanisms controlling the sense of balance are disturbed, making it more difficult to walk a straight line or stand still with one's eyes closed. Speech becomes slurred and incoherent. Heavier doses begin to act on the parts of the brain that control vital functions such as heart rate, respiration, and body temperature. In extremely high amounts, the depression of vital functions can induce stupor, unconsciousness, even death, especially if alcohol is combined with other depressants, such as sedatives or tranquilizers. Alcohol also dulls minor aches and pain. Although alcohol may induce sleep, larger amounts can disrupt the normal sleep cycle and lead to a hangover upon awakening.

How much alcohol does it take to intoxicate a person? Intoxication depends on factors such as what is drunk and the person's weight, gender, and ability to metabolize alcohol in the stomach (learn more by reading "Diversity 7-1"). Generally speaking, the more you weigh, the more alcohol it takes to intoxicate you.

You can reduce your chances of intoxication if you drink slowly and limit the alcohol content of your drinks, by diluting them or choosing beverages with lower alcohol content. When you drink slowly, you give your liver, the main metabolizer of alcohol, more time to break it down. The liver can metabolize alcohol at about half an ounce or one standard drink per hour. (A standard drink is a single "shot" of an 80-proof hard liquor, 5 ounces of wine, or 12 ounces of beer.) As you drink more than your liver can metabolize, the percentage of alcohol in your bloodstream—that is, your blood alcohol concentration (BAC)—rises and you become intoxicated. A BAC of .08 or above is the threshold level for drunk driving (8 parts alcohol to 10,000 parts of blood). The average 120-pound woman would reach this level after two drinks; the average 180-pound man, after four drinks. Table 7-2 shows the relationship between various kinds of drinks, the number of drinks it takes to reach a BAC of 0.10, and the caloric content of drinks.

Some people, especially alcoholics, develop a higher *tolerance* for alcohol. They can consume large amounts of alcohol without obvious signs of intoxication, even though their BAC registers 0.15% or more. However,

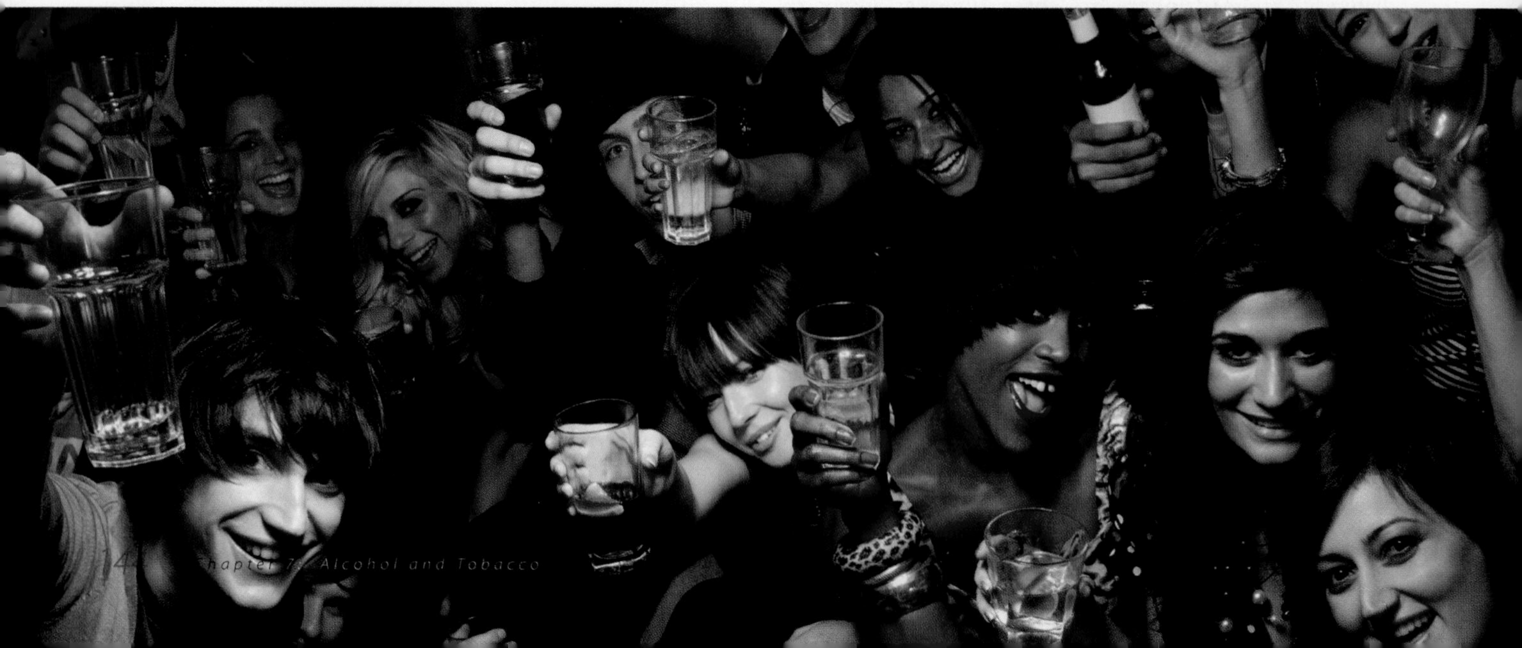

Table 7-2 *Percent Alcohol Content, Number of Drinks to Reach 0.10% Blood Alcohol Concentration, and Caloric Content of Alcoholic Beverages*

ALCOHOLIC BEVERAGE	% ALCOHOL (APPROXIMATE)	APPROPRIATE NUMBER OF DRINKS PER HOUR TO REACH 0.10% BAC (PER SERVING SIZE) FOR 150-POUND PERSON	APPROPRIATE CALORIES (PER SERVING SIZE)
Hard liquors (whiskey, vodka, gin, tequila, rum)	40–50	4 1.5-oz. jiggers	100
Beers (light, regular)	3–6	4 12-oz. cans or bottles	140–150 (regular) 95 (light)
Table wines (red or white, dry)	9–14	4 5-oz. glasses	125
Fortified wines (sherry, port)	18–20	4 3.5-oz. glasses	135

they are not as capable of performing skilled tasks, such as driving, as when they are sober—although they may *believe* they can. For people who have not built up a tolerance for alcohol, intoxication may occur with a BAC as low as 0.03%. People with a greater tolerance may drink to levels that become dangerous, even life-threatening. Death can occur at BACs of .035% or higher.

You've probably heard the expression "beer belly." Beer, which contains 140 to 150 calories per 12-ounce can, can put on the pounds. Some of it does settle in that paunch in the middle called a *beer belly*. A five-ounce glass of wine contains about 125 calories. A jigger (1.5 ounces) of an 80-proof distilled spirit like gin or vodka has about 100 calories, not counting the mixer. Tonic water adds some 72 calories per eight ounces.

But it may not just be the calories in alcoholic beverages that put on the pounds. Habitual use of alcohol slows the body's metabolic rate—the speed at which the body converts food to energy. Fat that is not metabolized and eliminated from the body gets stored in the hips, thighs, and—yes—the belly.

Alcohol enters the bloodstream through the stomach and small intestine. The speed of absorption depends on the amount of food in the stomach and the rate of drinking. The less alcohol that is broken down in the stomach, the more is passed directly into the bloodstream—and the more intoxicated you become. If you down a shot of whiskey on an empty stomach, it will enter your bloodstream and affect you sooner and harder than if you had sipped a cognac after a meal.

DIVERSITY 7-1

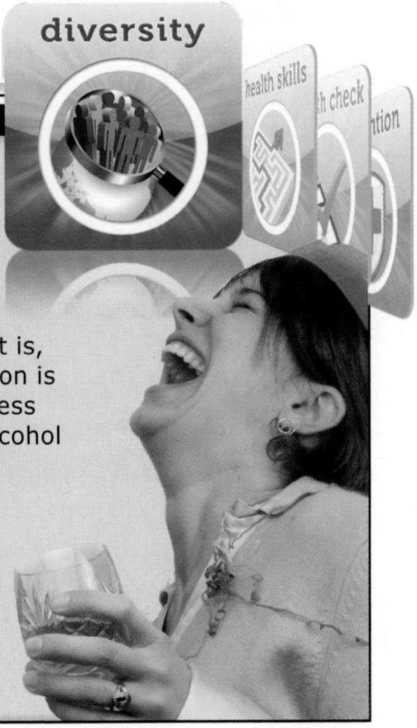

Gender Differences in Sensitivity to Alcohol

Women tend to become intoxicated by less alcohol than men do. That is, alcohol goes to women's heads more quickly than to men's. One reason is that women tend to weigh less than men. Another is that they have less of the stomach enzyme *alcohol dehydrogenase*, which metabolizes alcohol in the stomach. Women thus become about as intoxicated from one drink as men do from two.

American men, including college men, are more likely than women to drink and to drink heavily. Alcoholism is two to five times more common in men than in women. However, the gender gap appears to be narrowing. An increasing percentage of alcoholics are women, especially younger women.

Behavioral Effects

The behavioral effects of alcohol depend on the amount that is drunk. A person with a BAC in the range of 0.01% to 0.05% may feel mildly euphoric or somewhat relaxed (see Table 7-3). A BAC above 0.05% may reduce alertness and social inhibitions. The person may feel cheerful and more self-confident but be less capable of exercising good judgment, which can lead to behavior that the person would ordinarily reject, such as risky sex. Effects of higher blood levels are also shown in Table 7-3.

Alcohol directly affects the brain. It produces feelings of euphoria and elation, but it also clouds judgment and impairs concentration. At higher dosages, alcohol can cause unconsciousness or gross confusion. Some people find that alcohol boosts their self-esteem and drowns out their self-doubts, at least temporarily. But heavy, regular drinking deepens feelings of depression.

Alcohol and Sex

Some people feel that alcohol makes them more sexually responsive. A small or moderate amount of alcohol may produce this effect by dilating blood vessels, which is part of the body's response to sexual stimulation. But some of the effect on sexual responsiveness may reflect the drinker's expectations about alcohol or a loosening of inhibitions. And some drinkers are less able to foresee the consequences of their sexual behavior. Because alcohol is a depressant, larger amounts can dampen sexual response. Men may find it difficult to attain or keep an erection. Women may experience reduced vaginal lubrication and difficulty reaching orgasm.

The effects of alcohol vary from person to person. Different people metabolize alcohol differently. They hold different attitudes toward alcohol. People who expect alcohol to boost their social confidence or sexual responsiveness may enact these roles. They may do things they might not otherwise do, such as approach a stranger at a party. Feelings of elation and euphoria may wash away their inhibitions, self-criticisms, and misgivings. Then, too, alcohol use is associated with a liberated social role. People who engage in questionable behavior while drinking can blame it on the alcohol. ("It was the alcohol that made me do it.")

Alcohol and Violence

Many crimes of violence, including rape, robbery, and assault, are connected with the use of alcohol.[16] More than one in three prison inmates reports drinking heavily before committing his crime. More than half the people convicted of murder and rape, and more than two-thirds of those convicted of manslaughter, were drinking before they committed their crimes. College administrators report that alcohol is involved in more than half of the crimes reported on campus, ranging from assaults to vandalism.[17]

If alcohol dampens central nervous system activity, how do we explain the linkage between alcohol and violence? As with sex, a small amount of alcohol dilates blood vessels, helping mobilize the body for action. Alcohol also apparently reduces inhibitions. People who have been drinking may be less capable of weighing the consequences of their behavior. Then, too, crimes closely linked to the use of alcohol, assault and manslaughter, sometimes involve misunderstandings that escalate in social settings such as bars and athletic arenas. Drinking can also put people at greater risk of being victimized. Criminals choose victims who look

Table 7-3 Behavioral Effects of Blood Alcohol Concentrations

BLOOD ALCOHOL CONCENTRATION	BEHAVIORAL EFFECTS
0.05%	Lowered alertness; usually good feeling; release of inhibitions; impaired judgment
0.10%	Slowed reaction times; impaired motor function; less caution
0.15%	Large, consistent increases in reaction time
0.20%	Marked depression in sensory and motor capability; decidedly intoxicated
0.25%	Severe motor disturbance; staggering; sensory perceptions greatly impaired; smashed!
0.30%	Stuporous but conscious; no comprehension of the world around them
0.35%	Surgical anesthesia; minimal level causing death
0.40%	About half of those at this level die

Source: Based on data from the National Highway Traffic Safety Administration.

vulnerable, and heavy drinkers may appear to be "easy marks" or fail to take precautions.

The link may also reflect a selection factor. People seeking highly stimulating experiences may choose to drink and also engage in criminal conduct. Similarly, drinking heavily and committing acts of violence are both high-risk pursuits; risk takers may choose both paths.

Heavy Drinking and Health

Alcohol abuse and alcoholism account for about 100,000 deaths in the United States each year. This number includes deaths due to alcohol-related diseases and motor vehicle and other accidents. Following tobacco, alcohol is the second cause of premature death in our society. Between 3% and 10% of all deaths in the United States can be attributed to the use of alcohol. Men who drink heavily stand nearly twice the risk of dying before the age of 65 as men who do not drink. Women who drink heavily are more than three times as likely to die before the age of 65.

Chronic, heavy alcohol use affects virtually every organ and body system—either directly or indirectly (see Figure 7-1). The effects of alcohol depend on the amount and duration of use. Heavy alcohol use is linked to cirrhosis of the liver and cancers of the pharynx, larynx, esophagus, pancreas, stomach, colon, and liver. Heavy drinking places women at risk for breast cancer. Adding heavy smoking to heavy drinking is an even deadlier mix, multiplying the risk of cancers of the mouth and pharynx. Chronic alcohol use weakens the

Figure 7-1 Effects of Heavy Drinking

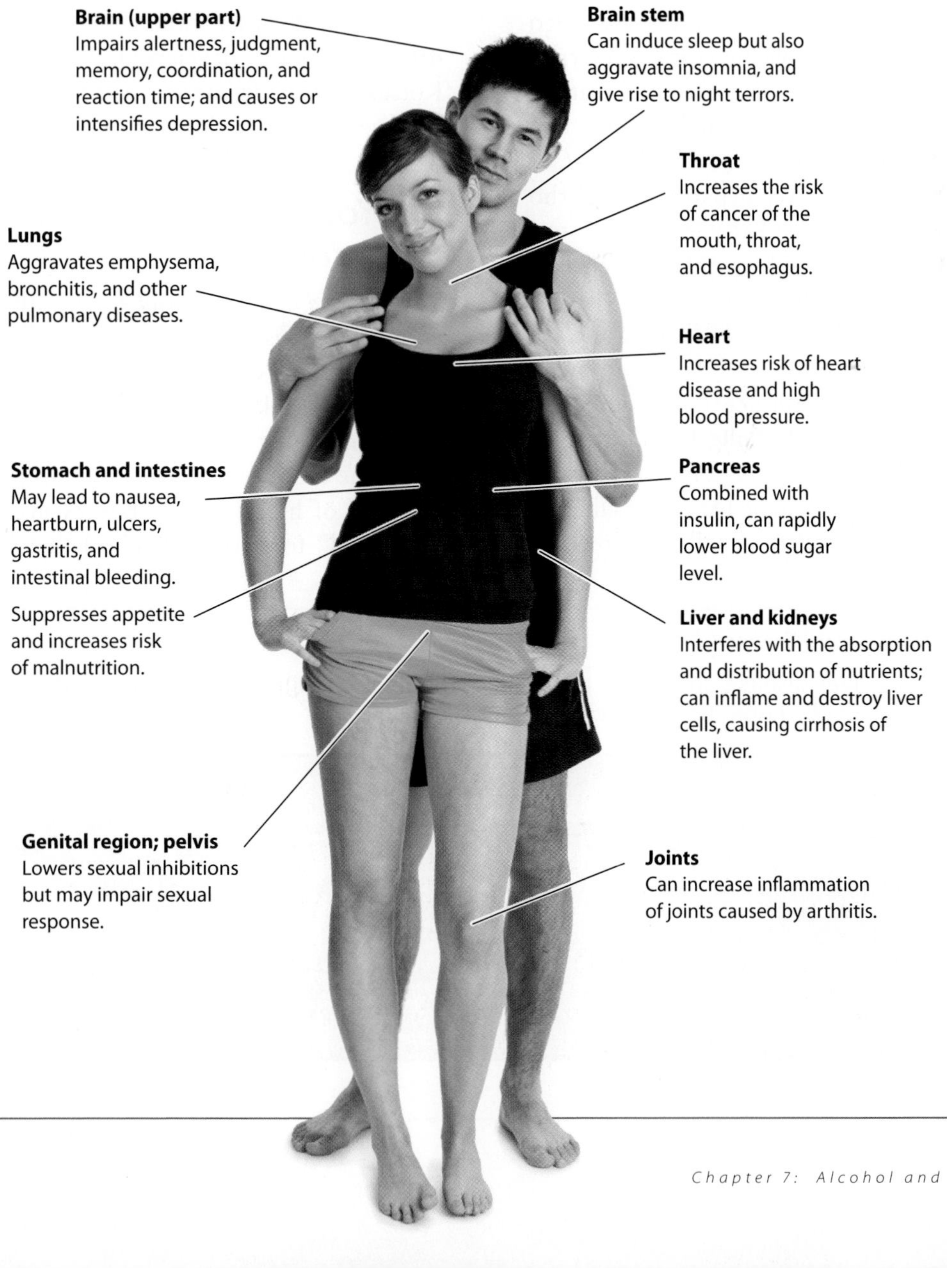

Brain (upper part)
Impairs alertness, judgment, memory, coordination, and reaction time; and causes or intensifies depression.
Brain stem
Can induce sleep but also aggravate insomnia, and give rise to night terrors.
Throat
Increases the risk of cancer of the mouth, throat, and esophagus.
Lungs
Aggravates emphysema, bronchitis, and other pulmonary diseases.
Heart
Increases risk of heart disease and high blood pressure.
Stomach and intestines
May lead to nausea, heartburn, ulcers, gastritis, and intestinal bleeding.
Suppresses appetite and increases risk of malnutrition.
Pancreas
Combined with insulin, can rapidly lower blood sugar level.
Liver and kidneys
Interferes with the absorption and distribution of nutrients; can inflame and destroy liver cells, causing cirrhosis of the liver.
Genital region; pelvis
Lowers sexual inhibitions but may impair sexual response.
Joints
Can increase inflammation of joints caused by arthritis.

immune system, making it less capable of ridding the body of cancerous cells, which then develop into cancerous lesions. Heavy drinking may also directly damage cells and the DNA within them, or make cells more sensitive to chemical carcinogens, such as those found in cigarette smoke.

Chronic, heavy drinking is also linked to coronary heart disease (CHD), ulcers, hypertension, osteoarthritis, and pancreatitis—painful inflammation of the pancreas. Alcohol affects brain cells, can trigger bleeding, and can lead to hormonal changes that dampen the sex drive in men and disrupt the menstrual cycles of women. Heavy consumption of alcohol increases the risk of neurological problems such as seizures and dementia.

Heavy drinking may have its most damaging effects on the liver, the main organ that metabolizes it. Chronic heavy drinking is the single most important cause of illness and death from liver disease (alcoholic hepatitis and cirrhosis) in the United States.

fatty liver
A condition involving an accumulation of fat in the liver, causing enlargement of the organ.

alcoholic hepatitis
An inflammation of the liver caused by viruses, chronic alcoholism, or exposure to toxic materials.

cirrhosis of the liver
A disease of the liver in which scar tissue comes to replace healthy liver tissue.

Wernicke-Korsakoff's syndrome
A form of memory impairment related to chronic alcoholism and deficiencies of the vitamin thiamine.

Alcohol-related liver diseases include fatty liver, hepatitis, and cirrhosis. **Fatty liver** refers to a buildup of fat that enlarges the organ. Fatty liver is relatively benign and can usually be reversed by abstinence (see Figure 7-2). **Alcoholic hepatitis** is inflammation of the liver. It can be life-threatening but can usually be reversed with abstinence, although there may be permanent scarring of the liver. **Cirrhosis of the liver** claims about 30,000 lives in the United States each year, making it the 12th leading cause of death[18] and the third leading *preventable* cause of death.[19] In cirrhosis of the liver, scar tissue replaces healthy liver cells. The more chronic and heavy a person's drinking, the greater the risk of the disease. Most of its victims are in middle adulthood. Although cirrhosis is irreversible, abstinence may prolong life by preventing further damage. Between 10% and 20% of heavy drinkers develop cirrhosis. Ten percent to 35% develop alcoholic hepatitis. Nearly all develop a fatty liver.

Alcohol is high in calories and carbohydrates but lacking in other nutrients. Alcohol makes it more difficult for the body to absorb certain vitamins, such as vitamin B1 (thiamine). As a result, alcoholics are prone to diseases related to vitamin and protein deficiencies, such as cirrhosis of the liver (protein deficiency) and a memory disorder called **Wernicke-Korsakoff's syndrome** (thiamine deficiency). People with Wernicke-Korsakoff's syndrome experience confusion, disorientation, and memory loss for recent events.

"To Your Health"? Is a Drink a Day Good for You?

With all the concern about the health risks associated with heavy consumption of alcohol, it may seem ironic that *moderate* drinking may have healthful effects. Up to two drinks a day for men and one drink a day for women may reduce the risk of heart attacks and lower the death rate.[20] Moderate drinking may elevate the level of high-density lipoproteins (HDL). HDL is the "good" form of cholesterol that lessens blockage

Figure 7-2 Alcoholic Liver Disease[21]

Biopsies of alcoholic liver disease show how the cells of the liver change as a person progresses from (a) fatty liver and (b) alcoholic hepatitis to (c) cirrhosis of the liver.

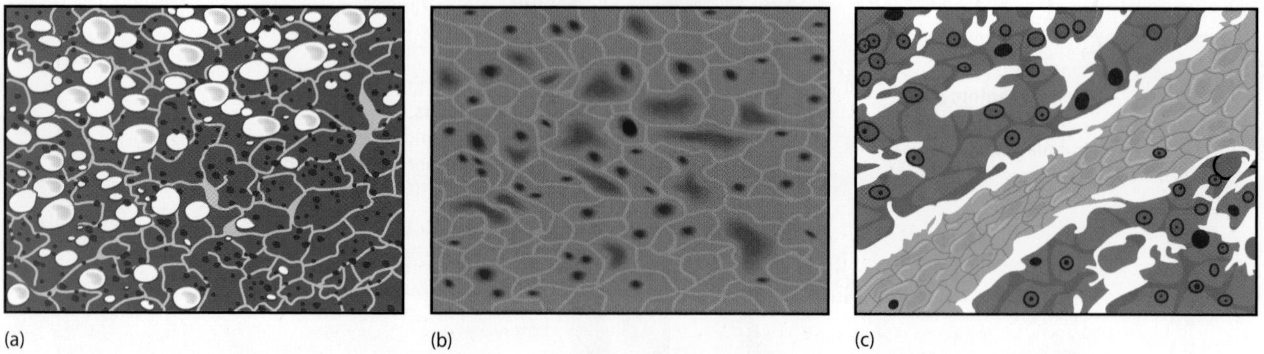

HEALTH CHECK 7-2

health check

Do You Have a Problem with Alcohol?[22]

How can *you* tell whether you have a drinking problem? Answering the following four questions can help you find out:

Yes No Have you ever felt you should cut down on your drinking?

Yes No Have people annoyed you by criticizing your drinking?

Yes No Have you ever felt bad or guilty about your drinking?

Yes No Have you ever had a drink first thing in the morning (as an "eye opener") to steady your nerves or get rid of a hangover?

Just one "yes" answer suggests a possible alcohol problem. If you answered "yes" to more than one question, it is highly likely that a problem exists. In either case, it is important that you see your doctor or other health care provider right away to discuss your answers to these questions. He or she can help you determine whether you have a drinking problem and, if so, recommend the best course of action.

of blood vessels by low-density lipoproteins (LDL, or "bad cholesterol").

Even so, few health officials recommend drinking just to pursue cardiovascular benefits. Some people cannot limit themselves to one or two drinks a day. Connections between moderate drinking and cardiovascular benefits are correlational in nature; thus, it may be that people who choose to drink moderately are healthier than those who abstain or who drink heavily—not because moderate drinking bestows health benefits.[23]

Alcohol Abuse and Dependence

Most people who drink do so responsibly, but use can cross the line into alcohol abuse or alcohol dependence. Not only alcoholics, but also people who drink when they're driving or pregnant or who binge are abusing alcohol.

LEARNING OUTCOME 4

Define *alcohol abuse* and *dependence*

Alcohol Abuse

Alcohol abuse is a pattern of heavy or continued drinking that becomes linked with health problems or impaired social functioning. If your drinking causes you to repeatedly miss school or work, it fits the pattern. You are abusing alcohol if you persist in drinking although you know that it is causing or aggravating a social relationship or a physical problem, such as ulcers. Alcohol abuse also applies to drinking in situations in which it is dangerous, such as driving or boating.

Alcohol Dependence (Alcoholism)

Alcohol dependence, or *alcoholism*, is a state of physical dependence on alcohol that is characterized by loss of control over its use. Despite the popular image of the alcoholic as a skid-row drunk, only perhaps 5% fit that stereotype. The great majority are people you see every day—neighbors, co-workers, friends, and family members. Many have families, hold good jobs, and live comfortably. Yet alcoholism can also wreck careers and marriages and lead to accidents and health problems. If you use alcohol, "Health Check 7-2" offers four important questions to ask yourself.

Physical dependence occurs when the body changes from using a particular drug, as evidenced by the development of tolerance and/or a withdrawal syndrome. The alcoholic is addicted to, or chemically dependent on, alcohol. The alcoholic may crave alcohol

alcohol abuse
A pattern of misuse of alcohol in which heavy or continued drinking becomes associated with health problems and/or impaired social functioning.

alcohol dependence
A physical dependence on, or addiction to, alcohol that is characterized by a loss of control over the use of the substance. Also called alcoholism.

as heroin addicts crave heroin. Tolerance may develop, such that more alcohol is needed to achieve the same effects.

Alcoholics tend to be less sensitive to the effects of alcohol, which allows them to consume larger amounts without immediate ill effects such as an upset stomach and nausea. They can tolerate larger doses without appearing intoxicated or slurring their speech, but they may feel more capable of performing skilled tasks such as driving than they are.

Alcoholism tends to develop in early adulthood, and earlier in men than women. Female alcoholics tend to suffer more serious health consequences than male alcoholics and have higher death rates. These differences may involve biological factors, as more alcohol is directly absorbed into a woman's body.

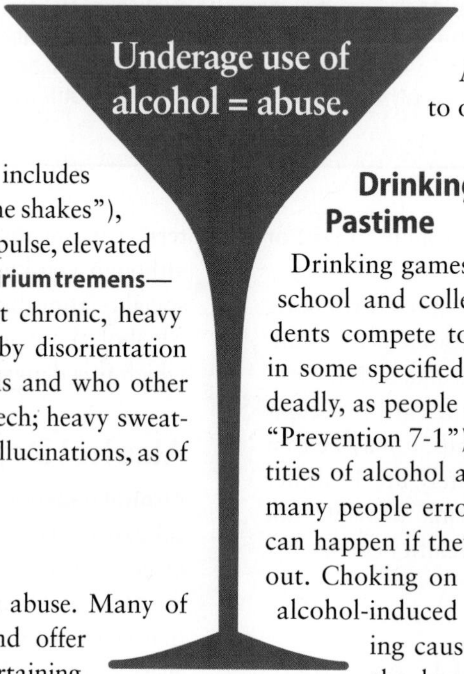
Underage use of alcohol = abuse.

Alcohol Withdrawal Syndrome

The withdrawal syndrome for alcohol includes anxiety, nausea, sweating, shaking ("the shakes"), irritability, agitation, weakness, rapid pulse, elevated blood pressure, and, in some cases, **delirium tremens**—the DTs. The DTs usually only affect chronic, heavy drinkers. The DTs are characterized by disorientation (confusion as to who or where one is and who other people are); incoherent, rambling speech; heavy sweating; rapid heart beat; and terrifying hallucinations, as of insects crawling on the skin.

Patterns of Abuse

Social factors affect alcohol use and abuse. Many of us go out drinking with friends and offer guests alcoholic beverages when entertaining at home. When social activities regularly revolve around alcohol, use may edge into abuse.

Some alcoholics drink heavily every day. Others binge on weekends. Others can abstain for lengthy periods but periodically "fall off the wagon" and binge for weeks or months. Male alcoholics are more likely to alternate between periods of heavy drinking and periods of sobriety. Female alcoholics tend to drink more regularly. Males are somewhat more likely to drink when they are in a good mood; women, to cope with negative feelings.[24]

delirium tremens
A withdrawal syndrome in chronic alcoholics occurring following a sudden reduction or cessation of drinking; denoted by extreme restlessness, sweating, disorientation, and hallucinations.

blackout
Episode involving a loss of consciousness.

seizure
A sudden attack involving a disruption of brain electrical rhythms, as in the type of convulsive seizures occurring during epileptic attacks.

Alcohol use and abuse often begins at a young age. Although every state prohibits alcohol consumption by people under the age of 21, more than 70% of high school seniors have tried alcohol, as have more than one in three (37%) eighth graders.[25] More than half (54%) of 12th graders report having been drunk at least once, as compared with about 37% of 10th graders and 16% of eighth graders.

Teenagers skirt drinking laws by finding alcoholic beverages at home or friends' homes, using fake IDs, or buying alcohol at outlets that don't card them. Most youths who drink do not become alcoholics, but regular youthful drinking foreshadows alcoholism among those who do. Alcohol also often serves as a gateway to other drugs.

Drinking Games: A Potentially Deadly Pastime

Drinking games are gaining popularity among high school and college students. In one variation, students compete to see who can chug the most beers in some specified amount of time. This game can be deadly, as people can die from alcohol overdose (read "Prevention 7-1"). Drinkers who consume large quantities of alcohol also risk **blackouts** and **seizures**. Yet many people erroneously assume that the worst that can happen if they drink too much is that they'll pass out. Choking on one's own vomit is also a cause of alcohol-induced deaths. In such cases, heavy drinking causes a person to vomit reflexively, yet the depressant effects of the drug prevent the person from vomiting properly. The vomit accumulates in the air passages and causes death by asphyxiation.

Costs of Alcohol Abuse and Alcoholism

Between 20% and 40% of people who occupy hospital beds have medical conditions that result from alcohol abuse or alcoholism. The toll includes lost jobs, ruined careers and marriages, severe health problems, reduced productivity, and downward social mobility. Many of the nation's homeless are alcoholics. Alcohol plays a role in nearly one in four suicides.[26]

Because of impaired skills and judgment, death due to alcohol abuse can come early in life, before cirrhosis and other health problems develop. More teenagers and

PREVENTION 7-1

Preventing Death from Alcohol Overdosing

Alcohol overdose is a medical emergency that requires prompt medical attention. Drinkers who have overdosed show symptoms such as the following:

- Failure to respond when talked to or shouted at
- Failure to respond to being pinched, shaken, or poked
- Inability to stand on one's own
- Failure to wake up
- Purplish color or clammy skin
- Rapid pulse rate or irregular heart rhythms, low blood pressure, or difficulty breathing

Here are some things to do if you come across someone who has overdosed on alcohol:

- Don't leave an unresponsive or unconscious person alone. Don't assume he or she will "sleep it off." Stay with the person until you access police or a health professional.
- Place the person on his or her side; if possible, sit the person up with head bowed.
- Do not give the person any food or drink; do not try to induce vomiting.
- If the person is responsive, ask whether he or she has taken other drugs or medication that might have interacted with the alcohol; ask if the person has an illness such as diabetes or epilepsy that might be contributing to the problem.
- Carefully reach into the person's mouth to clear the airway if the person vomits; if you have been trained, provide CPR if necessary.
- Most important, call a physician, hotline, or 911 as soon as possible.

young adults die from alcohol-related motor vehicle accidents than any other cause. More than one-third of alcohol-impaired drivers are between the ages of 21 and 24.[27]

Americans stand a 4 in 10 chance of becoming involved in an alcohol-related traffic accident in their lifetime. Overall, about one in three motor vehicle fatalities involves a driver who has been drinking. Alcohol is implicated in about one in four fatal falls and accidents caused by fire, and in about one in two homicides.

Drivers age 16 to 20 make up only 6% percent of the U.S. driving population, but they are involved in 20% of fatal motor vehicle accidents. According to Russ Rader of the Insurance Institute for Highway Safety, the lack of maturity in teenage drivers is to blame. "They think they're immortal," Rader says, "and they don't recognize the dangers of risky driving."[28] Read the online feature "Prevention 7-2" to see how you can help prevent youthful drinking and driving.

prevention

Access CourseMate for HLTH at www.cengagebrain.com.

Causes of Alcoholism

After a century of research, the causes of alcoholism remain less than clear. However, the most widely held view is that many factors are involved, including genetics.

LEARNING OUTCOME 5

Discuss the causes of alcoholism

The Disease Model of Alcoholism

According to the disease model of alcoholism, alcoholism is a permanent, irreversible condition. That is, "once an alcoholic, always an alcoholic." The view holds that alcoholics cannot drink responsibly, because just one drink creates an irresistible biologically based craving for more. This is why adherents to the disease model, especially Alcoholics Anonymous, maintain that alcoholics must maintain strict sobriety.

Genetic Factors

Genes make an important genetic contribution to alcoholism,[29] at least among males. The sons of alcoholics stand about four times greater chance of becoming alcoholics than do men without a paternal history of alcoholism. However, there is no single gene or group of genes for alcoholism per se. Genes apparently provide a tendency to reap greater pleasure from alcohol or greater tolerance for the negative effects of drinking.

Sons of alcoholics tend to metabolize alcohol more slowly. They can tolerate larger doses of alcohol without unpleasant physical effects, such as upset stomach, dizziness, and headaches, than people whose bodies more quickly metabolize it.[30] Differences in tolerance, which are believed to have a strong genetic component, enable sons of alcoholics to better hold their liquor, which, ironically, put them at greater risk of alcoholism.

Other Factors

Genes don't tell the whole story, because at least one in three alcoholics has no family history of alcoholism. Peer pressure often encourages drinking that can lead to problems. Adolescents who drink heavily are more likely to come from families with lax control and lack of emotional support. Adolescents from single-parent homes tend to drink more heavily than those from two-parent families. Exposure to parents who drink heavily also contributes to problem drinking.

Some people turn to alcohol as "liquid relief" from personal problems. Problem drinking may begin with using alcohol as a form of self-medication. Cultural and ethnic factors may also play roles in development of alcoholism, as the online feature "Diversity 7-2" illustrates.

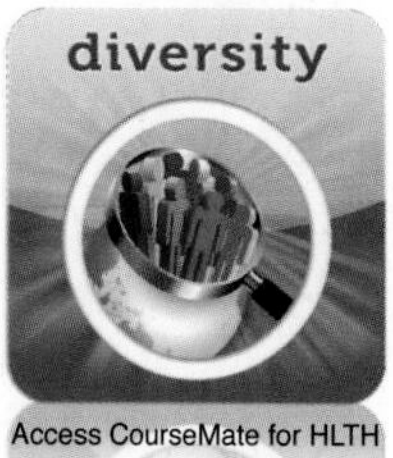

Access CourseMate for HLTH at www.cengagebrain.com.

Treatment of Alcoholism

Some alcoholics recover on their own or with the support of family or friends. Most need some form of help. The first step toward recovery is recognition of the problem. Once the drinker admits to having a problem, a range of treatment options becomes available.

LEARNING OUTCOME 6

Describe various methods of treating alcoholism

Detoxification

Treatment for alcohol-dependent people begins with detoxification. Detoxification, or *detox*, permits addicted people to be medically monitored as they withdraw. Detox often takes place in a hospital or in-patient facility. People undergoing detox are often given tranquilizers to quell anxiety and prevent some physical withdrawal symptoms, such as convulsions, seizures, elevated blood pressure, irregular heart rhythms, and tremors. Detox generally takes about a week, although a "drying out period" of 28 days provides the individual an opportunity to live free of alcohol.

Alcoholics Anonymous

Withdrawing from alcohol is one thing; maintaining abstinence is another. Alcoholics Anonymous (AA) has become so synonymous with alcoholism treatment that following detox, many health care professionals refer alcoholics to AA as a matter of course. AA holds that alcoholism is a lifelong disease: "Once an alcoholic, always an alcoholic." There is no such thing as a cured or "ex-alcoholic"—only a "recovering alcoholic."

The AA approach is part religion, part group therapy. The groups are run by recovering alcoholics and offered without charge. Group participants are encouraged to appeal to a higher power to help them maintain sobriety. AA follows a 12-step program of self-reclamation and recovery. Meetings provide group support. A "buddy system" encourages members to seek support if they feel tempted to drink.

AA does not appeal to everyone. Some are put off by its spiritual approach. Others chafe at the regimentation and rituals.

AA has spawned spin-offs, such as Al-Anon, which supports the spouses, partners, and parents of alcoholics. Another spin-off, Alateen, offers support groups for children of alcoholics. Al-Anon and Alateen help those close to alcoholics understand that they are not to blame for the alcoholic's drinking.

Psychotherapy and Counseling

Psychotherapy and counseling may be used to help people change self-destructive behavior. Family therapy or couple's therapy may deal with the effects of problem drinking on the family or couple.

Cognitive-behavioral therapists use techniques such as social-skills training to help alcoholics learn to fend off social pressures to drink (Just say, "No, thank you"). **Aversive conditioning** pairs painful (aversive) stimuli with alcohol to make alcohol itself aversive. For example, nausea-inducing drugs can be administered when the individual tastes an alcoholic beverage so that the drinker acquires an aversion to alcohol.

Relapse prevention training helps former drinkers resist temptations to drink in high-risk situations. They learn to artfully refuse drinks at social gatherings. They learn to relax without turning to alcohol. One approach focuses on treating a slip as a correctable and isolated problem, not as a sign of ultimate failure ("What's the use? I'm doomed to fail"). It helps people avoid turning a lapse into a relapse.

Pharmacological Treatment

Numerous chemical agents block the pleasurable effects of alcohol or combat cravings. *Disulfiram* (brand name Antabuse) does not quell cravings but rather produces nausea, sweating, flushing, a throbbing headache, pounding of the heart, and vomiting if the person drinks. However, people who are bent on drinking can simply discontinue disulfiram.

Researchers are targeting the possible role of neurotransmitters such as *serotonin* in cravings for alcohol.[31] They are testing whether the appetite for alcohol can be curbed by using *selective serotonin reuptake inhibitors* (SSRIs; Prozac is one) that increase the action of serotonin. Another neurotransmitter, **dopamine**, may help account for the euphoric effects of alcohol. Drugs that mimic dopamine may help block the pleasurable effects of alcohol.

Despite the availability of treatment, many problem drinkers do not seek help. Many others leave treatment prematurely. Still others relapse. These problems underscore the need for prevention. We need to find better ways to cope with stress and challenge than turning to alcohol (see the online feature "Health Skills 7-1").

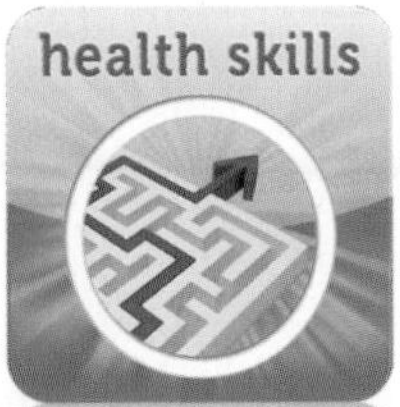

Access CourseMate for HLTH at www.cengagebrain.com.

aversive conditioning
A technique of behavior therapy involving the pairing of noxious stimuli, such as nausea or electric shock, with undesirable behavior, for the purpose of acquiring a conditioned aversion to the stimuli associated with the undesirable behavior.

dopamine
A type of neurotransmitter that is believed to be involved in brain mechanisms regulating states of pleasure as well as other functions.

tobacco
A member of a family of plants containing nicotine whose leaves are prepared for smoking, chewing, or use as snuff.

nicotine
A stimulant drug found naturally in tobacco.

Tobacco—Safe When Used as Directed?

No, it's not. Tobacco is not safe when used as directed, that is, when it is smoked or chewed. Cigarette smoking is the major preventable cause of death in the United States and many other countries.[32]

Tobacco is a plant that contains the stimulant **nicotine**. Nicotine is found in the leaves of the plants and

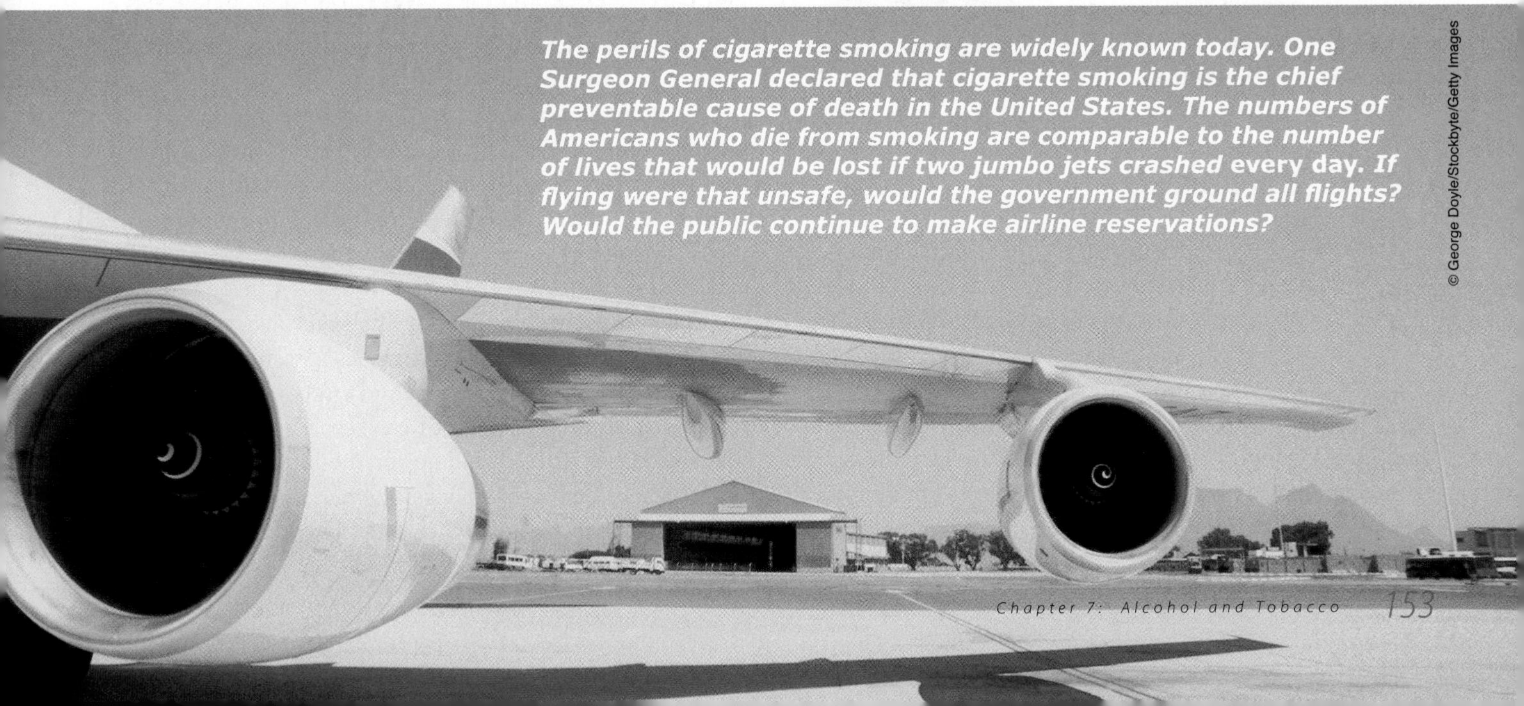

The perils of cigarette smoking are widely known today. One Surgeon General declared that cigarette smoking is the chief preventable cause of death in the United States. The numbers of Americans who die from smoking are comparable to the number of lives that would be lost if two jumbo jets crashed every day. If flying were that unsafe, would the government ground all flights? Would the public continue to make airline reservations?

© George Doyle/Stockbyte/Getty Images

snuff
A powdered form of tobacco that can be inhaled through the nose or sucked when placed inside the cheek.

chewing tobacco
Tobacco leaves that have been prepared for chewing or sucking when lodged between the cheek and gum.

tar
The sticky residue in tobacco smoke, containing many carcinogens and other toxins.

carbon monoxide
An odorless, poisonous flammable gas produced from the burning of carbon with insufficient air.

can be ingested by smoking cigarettes, cigars, or pipe tobacco; inhaling as a powder called **snuff**; or chewed after being ground into **chewing tobacco**.

You already know that smoking is unhealthful, but just how dangerous is it? Very. Nearly eight times as many people die from smoking-related causes as from all types of motor-vehicle accidents. Smoking harms organs throughout the body and kills more than 440,000 Americans each year, accounting for about one of every five deaths in the United States.[33] The number of smoking-related deaths exceeds the losses we would incur if two jumbo jets crashed into each other every day. Worldwide, smoking claims more than 3 million lives a year. Smoking-related deaths are expected to jump to 10 million annually by the year 2020.[34]

Cigarette smoking in the United States peaked in the early 1960s, when about one in two adult men and about one in three adult women smoked. Since then, smoking among adults has fallen off to about 20% today,[35] but further declines have stalled.[36] One in five high school students also smokes. Every day, some 1,000 teenagers begin smoking regularly.[37] One of every three people who tries cigarettes becomes a regular user.[38] (Smoking is highly addictive, so the best way to deal with smoking is to never get started. To learn more about preventing smoking, go online to read "Prevention 7-3.")

prevention
Access CourseMate for HLTH at www.cengagebrain.com.

Who Smokes?

LEARNING OUTCOME 7

Explain which segments of the population are most likely to smoke

Cigarette smoking is not an equal opportunity destroyer. Men are more likely than women to smoke (23.5% vs. 17.9%; see "Diversity 7-3"). Smoking is concentrated among younger and less well-educated segments of society.[39] Smokers who are better educated are more likely to quit than their less well-educated peers. Smoking is more prevalent and rates of quitting lower among people with less education, being highest among people with a GED degree (49.1%) and lowest (5.6%) among those with a graduate degree.[40] Smoking is also more common among people of lower socioeconomic status. Nearly six in 10 (57%) of college-educated people who once smoked no longer do so. Though smoking is still more prevalent among men overall, women under 30 are now the fastest growing group of smokers. Smoking is also more prevalent among some ethnic minorities, especially African American men (see the online feature "Diversity 7-4"). Moreover, the sharpest rise in teenage smoking is among African American males, portending dire health problems in the future.

diversity
Access CourseMate for HLTH at www.cengagebrain.com.

The major constituents of cigarette smoke are nicotine, hydrocarbons—commonly called tars—and carbon monoxide. Nicotine spurs the release of the hormone adrenaline, which increases the heart rate and produces a mild rush or psychological "kick." Adrenaline (epinephrine) causes reserves of sugar to be released into the blood, quelling the appetite. As a stimulant, nicotine acts on nerve cells in the brain to increase alertness and concentration. Although nicotine is a stimulant, cigarette smoking may help smokers relax by prompting the release of *endorphins* in the brain—naturally occurring hormones that function much like opiates, producing pleasure and reducing pain.

The stimulant properties of nicotine can also cause sensations of cold, clammy skin and nausea and vomiting in novice smokers. However, the unpleasant symptoms disappear as the smoker's body becomes accustomed to the drug.

Nicotine is not the most dangerous component of cigarette smoke. That dishonor falls on tars and carbon monoxide. **Tars** are thick, sticky residues that blacken the lungs and prompt cancerous growths. **Carbon monoxide** is the same toxic gas emitted by the exhaust systems of cars. It impairs the transport of oxygen through the circulatory system by plugging the spaces in red blood cells that normally carry oxygen. As a result, smokers experience shortness of breath, and vital organs, including the heart, are deprived of oxygen. Carbon monoxide is at least partly to blame for the increased risk of heart attacks and strokes in smokers. It may precipitate heart attacks in smokers whose supply of oxygen to the

DIVERSITY 7-3

Women and Smoking

Smoking is as much of a health risk for women as for men. Lung cancer deaths in women have more than tripled since 1970—a direct result of increased smoking rates (see Figure 7-3). Lung cancer has surpassed breast cancer as the leading cause of death from cancer among women.

In the early twentieth century, smoking was almost an exclusively male preserve. By the 1930s and 1940s, however, smoking had become more popular among women. Smoking was spurred in large part by the images of glamorous actresses smoking or having their cigarettes lit for them by dashing leading men. Smoking rates among adult women peaked at 34% in the mid-1960s, but has declined to about 18% today. Yet smoking rates are higher among poorer, less well-educated women.

Although men have had higher rates of lung cancer deaths than women over the years, gender differences are fast disappearing. Female smokers also face an increased risk of uterine, cervical, and breast cancers. Female smokers have nearly a four times greater chance of suffering a heart attack than nonsmokers. The relative risk increases with the number of cigarettes smoked daily. Smoking a low-nicotine or low-tar cigarette does not diminish the risk of a heart attack.

Figure 7-3 Rise in Number of Deaths Due to Lung Cancer among U.S. Women[41]

The increased prevalence of smoking among women in the second half of the twentieth century led to a sharp rise in the lung cancer mortality rates among women.

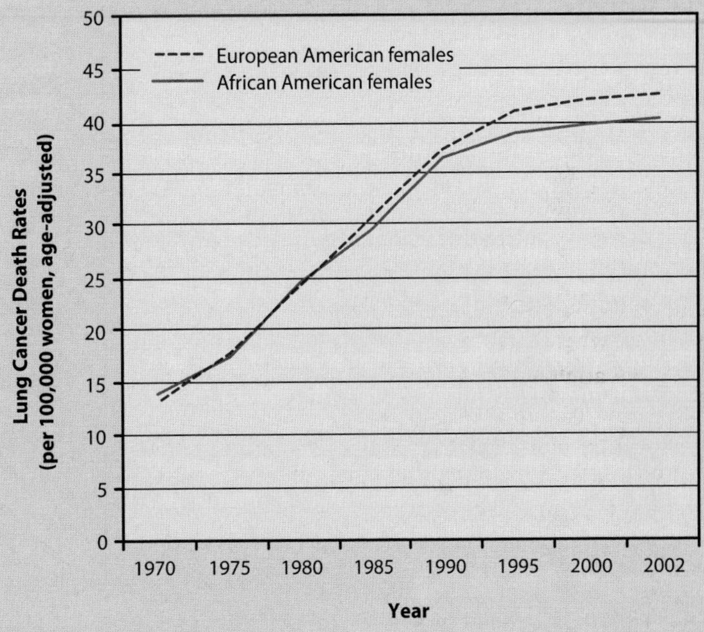

heart is already compromised by a narrowing of the arteries due to build-up of fatty deposits.

We're not letting nicotine off the hook. Nicotine causes users to return and inhale more tars and carbon monoxide. In its role as a stimulant, nicotine can also damage the cardiovascular system, especially in people with heart conditions.

Cigarette smoking is not the only means of ingesting tobacco. Some people smoke pipes or cigars. Others use smokeless tobacco. And then there are those who find themselves in the vicinity of smokers—sometimes trapped.

Pipe and Cigar Smoking

Though pipe and cigar smokers may not inhale or inhale as deeply as cigarette smokers, they still draw carcinogens into their body with each mouthful of tobacco smoke. They face an increased risk of cancer of the lungs, oral cavity, and esophagus, as well as other health problems.[42] Oral cancers are actually more prevalent among pipe and cigar smokers than among cigarette smokers. Sidestream smoke from cigars actually fouls the air with more cancer-causing particles than cigarette smoke inhaled by smoking—something to think about if you should enter a cigar bar.

Smokeless Tobacco

Some people ingest tobacco without lighting up. Snuff is a powdered form of tobacco that can be inhaled through the nose. It may also be placed inside the cheek, where it is sucked. Chewing tobacco, another smokeless tobacco product, is used by lodging a pinch between the cheek and gum and then chewing or sucking. The use of snuff or chewing tobacco allows nicotine to pass through the mucosal membranes of the nose or mouth into the bloodstream.

Many people operate under the false assumption that smokeless tobacco is a safe or relatively harmless substitute for cigarette smoking. The fact is that smokeless tobacco in snuff or chewable form contains some of the most powerful carcinogens in tobacco. Smokeless tobacco contains 28 cancer-causing substances[43] and is responsible for about three of four cases of oral cancer (cancers of the mouth, lips, and pharynx) in the United States. It also causes cancer of the esophagus as well as noncancerous conditions of the oral cavity. Smokeless tobacco delivers about the same levels of nicotine to the user as cigarettes, so it's no surprise that regular use leads to nicotine addiction.

Oral cancers are among the most devastating forms of cancer, not only because of the risk of fatality, but also because of the disfiguring operations of the face and jaw that may be required to halt the spread of the disease. Unlike some slow-forming forms of cancer that don't usually strike until later in life, oral cancers brought on by the use of smokeless tobacco often strike early, at the outset of adulthood.

Sidestream Smoking

How often have you heard a cigarette smoker ask, "Do you mind if I smoke?" Though it was once a matter of social etiquette for nonsmokers to extend permission, mounting evidence of the dangers of inhaling smoke from other people's cigarettes and cigars may well lead people to answer the question with a resounding, "Yes, I do mind." **Sidestream smoking** (also called *second-hand* or *passive smoking*) involves exposure to smoke from other people's cigarettes, cigars, or pipes. Forty percent of non-smoking Americans (88 million people) are exposed to sidestream smoke.[44]

Sidestream smoke contains even greater concentrations of potent carcinogens than the smoke inhaled from the cigarette itself. The amount of exposure to these carcinogens varies with proximity to the smoker and room ventilation, but we can generally assume that people who are close to the smoker will inhale some sidestream smoke.

sidestream smoking
Ingestion of tobacco smoke from other people's lit cigarettes.

Risks of Sidestream Smoking

Sidestream smoking causes heart disease and lung cancer in nonsmokers, as well as risks of respiratory disease and other serious illnesses in nonsmokers.[45] Because of these added health risks, smoking has been banned in most public places, including schools, hospitals, elevators, and airplanes. Sidestream smoke is especially dangerous to people with heart problems or respiratory conditions such as asthma.

Dangers to Children

Children who are repeatedly exposed to cigarette smoke stand an increased risk of asthma and other respiratory diseases in childhood and are at increased risk of developing lung cancer later in life. Exposure to maternal smoking accounts for as many as one in four cases of childhood asthma.[46] There are many steps we can take to protect ourselves and others from the dangers of sidestream smoke (see "Prevention 7-4").

Why Do People Smoke?

Despite the dangers of smoking, millions of people continue to smoke, and millions more start smoking each year. *Why?*

LEARNING OUTCOME 8

Explain why people smoke

There are many reasons. Some young (and some not so young) people remain ignorant of the dangers of smoking. Some young people smoke because their peers smoke and they believe that smoking helps them "fit in"—that smoking is "cool" or sophisticated. Others smoke because they find it pleasurable.

An Addiction, Not Just a Bad Habit

Whatever the initial reasons for smoking, smoking leads to addiction to the stimulant nicotine, which is found in tobacco. Although not every smoker becomes addicted, most do, and do so quickly (see the online feature "Health Check 7-3"). Typically,

health check

Access CourseMate for HLTH at www.cengagebrain.com.

PREVENTION 7-4

prevention

Reducing Exposure to Sidestream Smoke

Despite the restrictions on public smoking, many people are still regularly exposed to sidestream smoke, especially at home. Nonsmokers who live with smokers are at special risk, especially in residences that are not well ventilated. If you live with a smoker or have friends or relatives who smoke when you are around, consider yourself at risk. Here are some ways you can reduce, if not eliminate, your exposure to sidestream smoke:

- Establish no-smoking zones in your home.
- Establish a no-smoking rule in your home. Smokers who wish to smoke can politely be asked to step outside to smoke or to go into another, preferably well-ventilated, room.
- Post no-smoking signs around the house. These cues may prevent arguments.
- If you can't completely prohibit smoking in your residence, restrict it to well-ventilated rooms.
- Avoid being in these rooms when others are smoking.
- Restrict smoking to times when nonsmokers are not present.
- Install fans to remove smoke that may waft through the house.
- When somebody asks you for permission to smoke in your vicinity, "just say no."

casual experimentation—a cigarette every now and then—yields to daily smoking and dependence. The greatest number of addicts in our society don't lurk in alleyways. They hold jobs, pay taxes, and are just like the people next door. In fact, they are the people next door. They give themselves a "fix" of a drug every time they light up. Each puff or "drag" introduces nicotine into their bloodstream. Smoking is the leading form of addiction in our society and accounts for more deaths than all other drugs combined, legal or illegal.

What makes smoking an addiction and not just a bad habit? For one thing, regular smoking is compulsive. Addicted people feel compelled to light up even if they know that smoking is harmful. Smoking is also associated with *tolerance* and a *withdrawal syndrome*. Smokers need more nicotine over time to achieve the same effect, which leads smokers to increase the number of cigarettes they smoke, often to a pack or two a day. With smoking, going "cold turkey" produces characteristic withdrawal symptoms such as nervousness, irritability, lightheadedness, dizziness, restlessness, difficulty concentrating, loss of energy, headaches, fatigue, irregular bowel movements, insomnia, cramps, sweating, palpitations, and intense cravings for cigarettes.

Advertising is an important influence. Although cigarette manufacturers are no longer permitted to advertise their products on TV, they spend more than $3.5 billion annually for advertising in other media, such as magazines and billboards. Many advertising campaigns are directed at the young and minority smokers. Cigarette companies invest a great deal in advertising in African American and Latin American magazines (see the online feature "Diversity 7-4"). Some magazines, such as *Ms.* and *Good Housekeeping*, now refuse cigarette ads. It remains to be seen whether the media at large will refuse them.

diversity

Access CourseMate for HLTH at www.cengagebrain.com.

Some people smoke to control their weight. As a stimulant, nicotine depresses the appetite and raises the metabolic rate. People usually eat more when they stop smoking, which leads some people who have quit to resume. (Note that you would need to gain about 100 pounds for your health to be damaged as much as it is by smoking one pack of cigarettes a day[47]; however, being overweight is often associated with lower perceived attractiveness in our culture.)

Some people smoke to relieve anxiety or depression. Some people smoke for a combination of reasons. Smokers can gain some insight into their own reasons for smoking by completing "Health Check 7-4."

HEALTH CHECK 7-4

Why Do You Smoke?[48]

People smoke for many reasons—for pleasure, for relaxation, for a lift, or simply out of habit. How about you? If you smoke, read each of the following statements and indicate how it applies to you by selecting the appropriate number. Then use the key on the next page to interpret your responses.

IMPORTANT: Answer every question.

1 = never 2 = seldom 3 = occasionally 4 = frequently 5 = always

A. I smoke cigarettes in order to keep myself from slowing down.	1 2 3 4 5
B. Handling a cigarette is part of the enjoyment of smoking it.	1 2 3 4 5
C. Smoking cigarettes is pleasant and relaxing.	1 2 3 4 5
D. I light up a cigarette when I feel angry about something.	1 2 3 4 5
E. When I have run out of cigarettes, I find it almost unbearable until I get more.	1 2 3 4 5
F. I smoke cigarettes automatically, without even being aware of it.	1 2 3 4 5
G. I smoke cigarettes to stimulate me, to perk myself up.	1 2 3 4 5
H. Part of the enjoyment of smoking a cigarette comes from the steps I take to light up.	1 2 3 4 5
I. I find cigarettes pleasurable.	1 2 3 4 5
J. When I feel uncomfortable or upset about something, I light up a cigarette.	1 2 3 4 5
K. I am very much aware of the fact when I am not smoking a cigarette.	1 2 3 4 5
L. I light up a cigarette without realizing I still have one burning in the ashtray.	1 2 3 4 5
M. I smoke cigarettes to give me a "lift."	1 2 3 4 5
N. When I smoke a cigarette, part of the enjoyment is watching the smoke as I exhale it.	1 2 3 4 5
O. I want a cigarette most when I am comfortable and relaxed.	1 2 3 4 5
P. When I feel "blue" or want to take my mind off cares and worries, I smoke cigarettes.	1 2 3 4 5
Q. I get a real gnawing hunger for a cigarette when I haven't smoked for a while.	1 2 3 4 5
R. I've found a cigarette in my mouth and didn't remember putting it there.	1 2 3 4 5

continued

Smoking and Health

LEARNING OUTCOME 9

Describe the effects of smoking on health

The average male smoker's life expectancy is cut by 13.2 years; the average female's, 14.5 years.[49] If you are a chronic smoker, your chances of dying prematurely from a smoking-related cause are about 50%.[50] More than 7,000 chemicals enter your body when you draw smoke into your lungs. More than 40 of them are carcinogens (cancer-causing agents).[51] You probably know that smoking causes lung cancer. It also causes cancers of the bladder, esophagus, mouth, and throat. Men who smoke are 23 times more likely to develop lung cancer than male nonsmokers; women smokers, 13 times more likely.[52] Smoking causes about 90% of lung cancer deaths in men and almost 80% in women.[53]

Scoring Key

1. Enter the number you have selected for each question in the spaces, putting the number you have selected for question A over line A, for question B over line B, and so forth.
2. Add the three scores on each line to get your totals. For example, the sum of your scores over lines A, G, and M gives you your score on Stimulation; lines B, H, and N give the score on Handling, etc.

Scores can vary from 3 to 15. Any score 11 and above is high; any score 7 and below is low.

							Totals
______	+	______	+	______	=		______
A		G		M			Stimulation
______	+	______	+	______	=		______
B		H		N			Handling
______	+	______	+	______	=		______
C		I		O			Pleasurable relaxation
______	+	______	+	______	=		______
D		J		P			Crutch: tension reduction
______	+	______	+	______	=		______
E		K		Q			Craving: psychological addiction
______	+	______	+	______	=		______
F		L		R			Habit

What kind of smoker are you? What do you get out of smoking? This test will help you identify what you use smoking for and what kind of satisfaction you think you get from smoking: a sense of increased energy or stimulation; the satisfaction of handling things; pleasurable feelings and a state of well-being; a decrease of negative feelings such as anxiety, anger, or shame; satisfying a "craving" for a cigarette—the psychological addiction to smoking; or habit—purely automatic smoking.

A score of 11 or above on any factor indicates that this factor is an important source of satisfaction for you. The higher your score (15 being the highest), the more important a particular factor is in your smoking and the more useful the discussion of that factor can be in your efforts to quit.

Smoking accounts for 80% of deaths from **chronic obstructive pulmonary disease (COPD)**, which includes chronic bronchitis and emphysema. COPD is among the leading causes of death in the United States, claiming more than 100,000 lives annually. Smokers are more susceptible to the common cold, coughs, and respiratory infections. Smoking is a recognized cause of coronary heart disease (see Figure 7-4 on the next page). Smoking increases blood cholesterol levels and contributes to hardening of the arteries, both of which increase the risks of heart attacks and strokes.[54]

Smoking in women raises additional concerns. Smoking causes women to enter menopause a year or two earlier than normal. Smoking during pregnancy increases the risks of birth defects, low birthweights, premature births, and miscarriages.[55] About 10% of infant deaths are attributable to maternal smoking.[56]

chronic obstructive pulmonary disease (COPD)
A disease process that results in diminished capacity of the lungs to perform respiration. Chronic bronchitis and emphysema are among the leading causes.

Researchers find increased levels of a cancer-causing substance in the blood of pregnant women, and in the blood of their newborns, when pregnant women are exposed to sidestream or secondhand smoke from other household members. Young children exposed to sidestream smoke stand an increased risk of asthma and sudden infant death syndrome.[57]

Smoking depletes the body of vitamin C, a key antioxidant nutrient. Smokers are more likely to develop dental problems, such as gum disease and tooth loss.

> **carcinogenic**
> *Cancer-causing.*
>
> **smoker's face**
> *A characteristic wrinkling of the face due to smoke, denoted by the appearance of many fine wrinkles emanating in spoke-like projections from the lips and eyes.*

There is no safe cigarette or safe level of smoking. U.S. Surgeon General Regina Benjamin warned that smoking even one cigarette immediately begins to spread toxins throughout the body and can trigger a heart attack in people with coronary heart disease. Benjamin told an interviewer, "That one puff on that cigarette could be the one that causes your heart attack."[58] Filters fail to remove many toxic and **carcinogenic** compounds in cigarette smoke. Many smokers of "light" cigarettes compensate by puffing harder or deeper. A federal law was enacted in 2009 to empower the Food and Drug Administration (FDA) to regulate tobacco products. The law requires more prominent warning labels on tobacco products, prohibits use of misleading terms such as "light" or "mild," prohibits tobacco advertisements in teen-oriented magazines, and bans tobacco sponsorship of sporting or entertainment events.[59]

Smoking and Appearance

Some people who might smoke despite health issues may think twice when they learn that smoking also causes wrinkles. Many smokers develop a **smoker's face**, with fine wrinkles radiating from the lips and eyes. The facial skin takes on a grayish, bloodless look. Smoking also yellows the teeth.

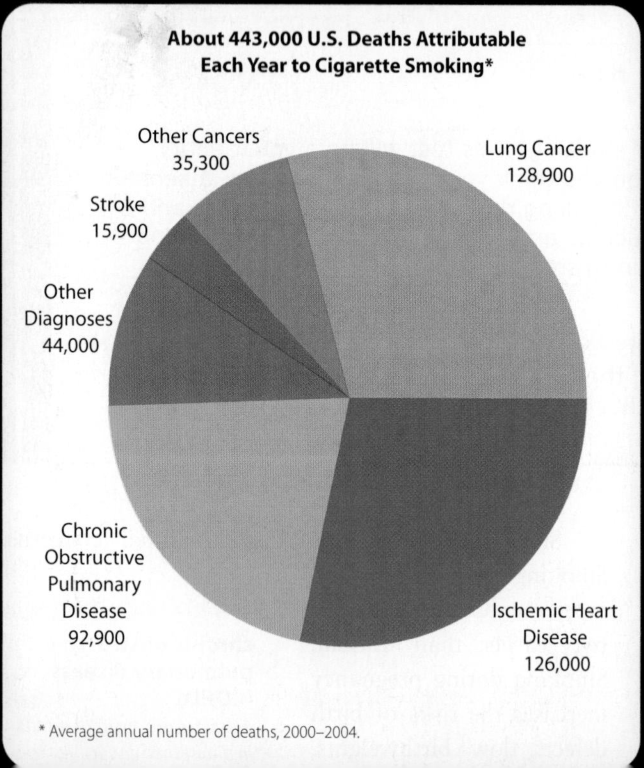

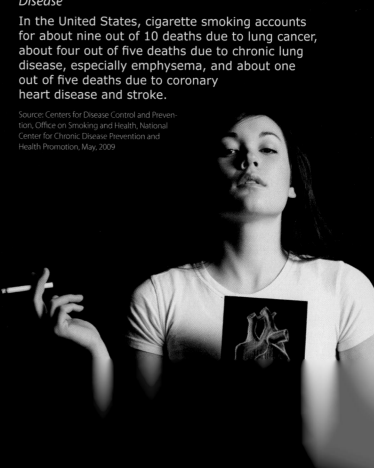

Figure 7-4 Deaths Due to Smoking, by Type of Disease

In the United States, cigarette smoking accounts for about nine out of 10 deaths due to lung cancer, about four out of five deaths due to chronic lung disease, especially emphysema, and about one out of five deaths due to coronary heart disease and stroke.

Source: Centers for Disease Control and Prevention, Office on Smoking and Health, National Center for Chronic Disease Prevention and Health Promotion, May, 2009

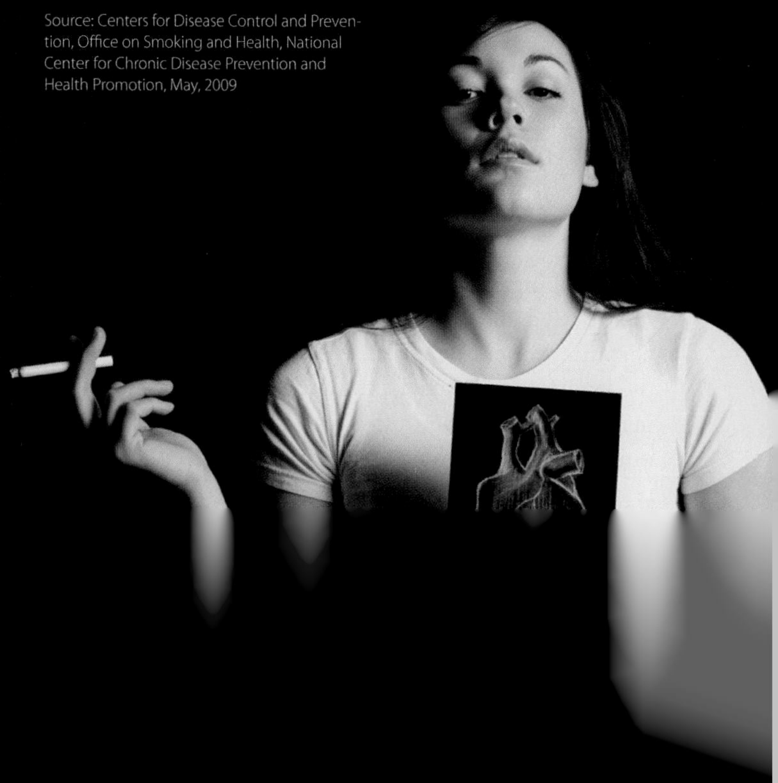

© iStockphoto.com/Rubberball

Becoming an Ex-Smoker

Whether you've smoked for one year or 30, smoke every now and then or have a three-pack-a-day habit, you can achieve substantial health benefits from quitting.[60] The sooner you quit, the sooner you reap them (see Figure 7-5).

LEARNING OUTCOME 10

Discuss the health benefits of quitting smoking

When you quit, your excess risk of heart disease relative to people who continue to smoke is cut in half within a year. Your excess risk of suffering a heart attack disappears within either two or three years (for women) or five years (for men) of quitting. By 10 years after quitting, your risk of suffering lung cancer is reduced by as much as half.

Quitting smoking also cuts in half the risk of cancers of the mouth and esophagus within five years. Greater reductions occur as abstinence continues. The risk of bladder cancer is halved only a few years after quitting. The risks of cervical and pancreatic cancer are reduced. The risk of dying from stroke returns to the level of nonsmokers in 5 to 15 years after quitting. The risk of respiratory diseases like emphysema and chronic bronchitis declines. Whereas smoking accelerates the onset of menopause in women, women who quit smoking enter menopause at an age similar to that of nonsmokers.

Overall, smokers who quit before age 50 lessen their risks of dying within the next 15 years by half as compared to those who continue to smoke. The average male smoker 35 to 39 years of age can expect to add five years to his life by quitting; for the average female smoker in this age range, quitting will add another three years to her life. Figure 7-5 shows the reduction in the increased risk of early death for nonsmokers in relation to amount of time since quitting.

Compared to current smokers, former smokers who quit during their 30s reduce their risk of dying of lung cancer by at least 90%. But smokers who wait until their early 50s to quit have five to six times the risk of dying from lung cancer than people who have never smoked. If you don't smoke, don't start. If you smoke, quit as soon as possible.

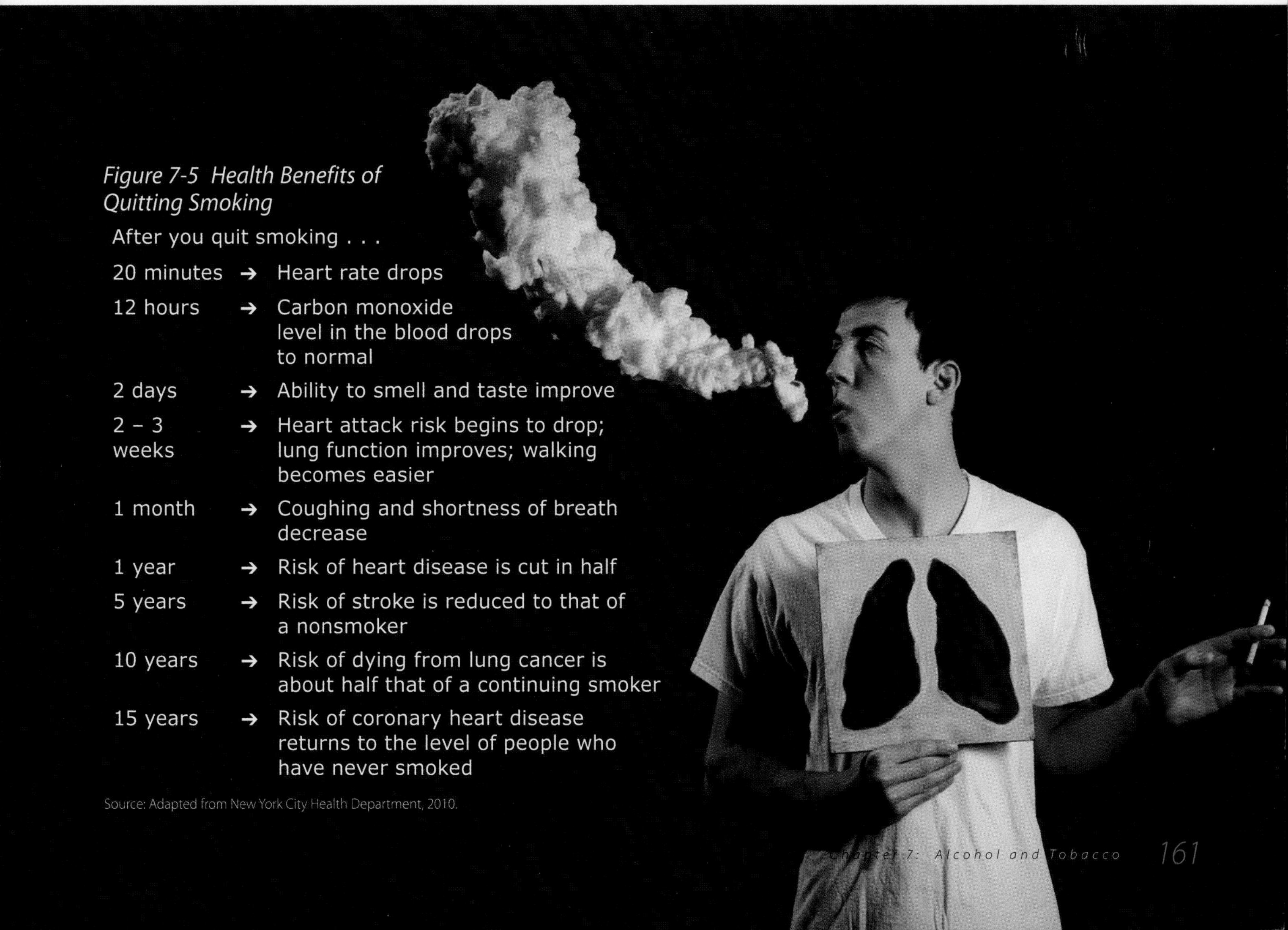

Figure 7-5 Health Benefits of Quitting Smoking

After you quit smoking . . .

20 minutes	→	Heart rate drops
12 hours	→	Carbon monoxide level in the blood drops to normal
2 days	→	Ability to smell and taste improve
2 – 3 weeks	→	Heart attack risk begins to drop; lung function improves; walking becomes easier
1 month	→	Coughing and shortness of breath decrease
1 year	→	Risk of heart disease is cut in half
5 years	→	Risk of stroke is reduced to that of a nonsmoker
10 years	→	Risk of dying from lung cancer is about half that of a continuing smoker
15 years	→	Risk of coronary heart disease returns to the level of people who have never smoked

Source: Adapted from New York City Health Department, 2010.

Mark Twain quipped that quitting smoking was easy—he'd done it at least a dozen times. Why is it so difficult to quit—and quit for good? When you make the commitment to quit, is it better to quit all at once (that is, go "cold turkey") or does it make more sense to cut down gradually? What does it mean if you relapse—give in once or twice and have a cigarette or two? Are you doomed to smoke forever or can you handle the relapse? For answers to these questions and more, read the online feature "Health Skills 7-2."

health skills

Access CourseMate for HLTH at www.cengagebrain.com.

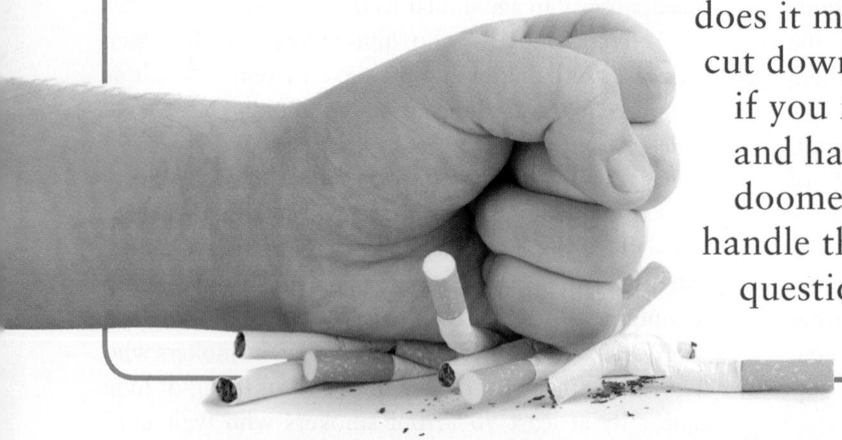

© iStockphoto.com/Ruslan Olinchuk

HEALTH APPS: YOUR LINK TO ONLINE HEALTH APPLICATIONS

health check — **Why Do *You* Drink?** People drink for many reasons. Do you drink? If so, why? To relax? For pleasure? To get high? To increase your awareness of the reasons you drink, go to "Health Check 7-1."

prevention — **Preventing Youthful Drinking and Driving** Drivers age 16 to 20 are involved in 20 percent of fatal motor vehicle accidents. Read "Prevention 7-2" to see how you can help prevent youthful drinking and driving.

diversity — **Ethnicity and Alcoholism** Overall, about one in 13 Americans has a drinking problem. Various ethnic groups have higher rates of alcoholism than others. Learn more about the relationships between culture, ethnicity, and alcohol from "Diversity 7-2."

health skills — **Getting a Handle on the ABCs of Your Drinking** So, sometimes you drink too much? You enjoy drinking and don't want to abstain completely, but you'd like to exert better control over how much you drink? We have just the thing for you: "Health Skills 7-1."

prevention — **Preventing Smoking** Smoking is highly addictive, so the best way to deal with smoking is never to get started. "Prevention 7-3" offers suggestions on how to do that.

diversity — **Smoking and Ethnic Minorities** Why do cigarette companies invest a great deal in advertising in African American and Latin American magazines? Why do Native Americans smoke more than any other ethnic group? To learn more, read "Diversity 7-4."

health check — **Are You Addicted to Nicotine?** Many people who think of their smoking as just a habit are actually addicted to nicotine. For insight as to whether you might be one of them, go to "Health Check 7-3."

health skills — **Becoming an Ex-Smoker** Why is it so difficult to quit smoking? What do you do if you've tried and tried to quit but then have relapses? Are you doomed to smoke forever? For answers to these questions and more, read "Health Skills 7-2."

Go to the CourseMate for HLTH at www.cengagebrain.com for additional resources including flashcards, games, self-quizzes, review exercises, web exercises, learning checks, and more.

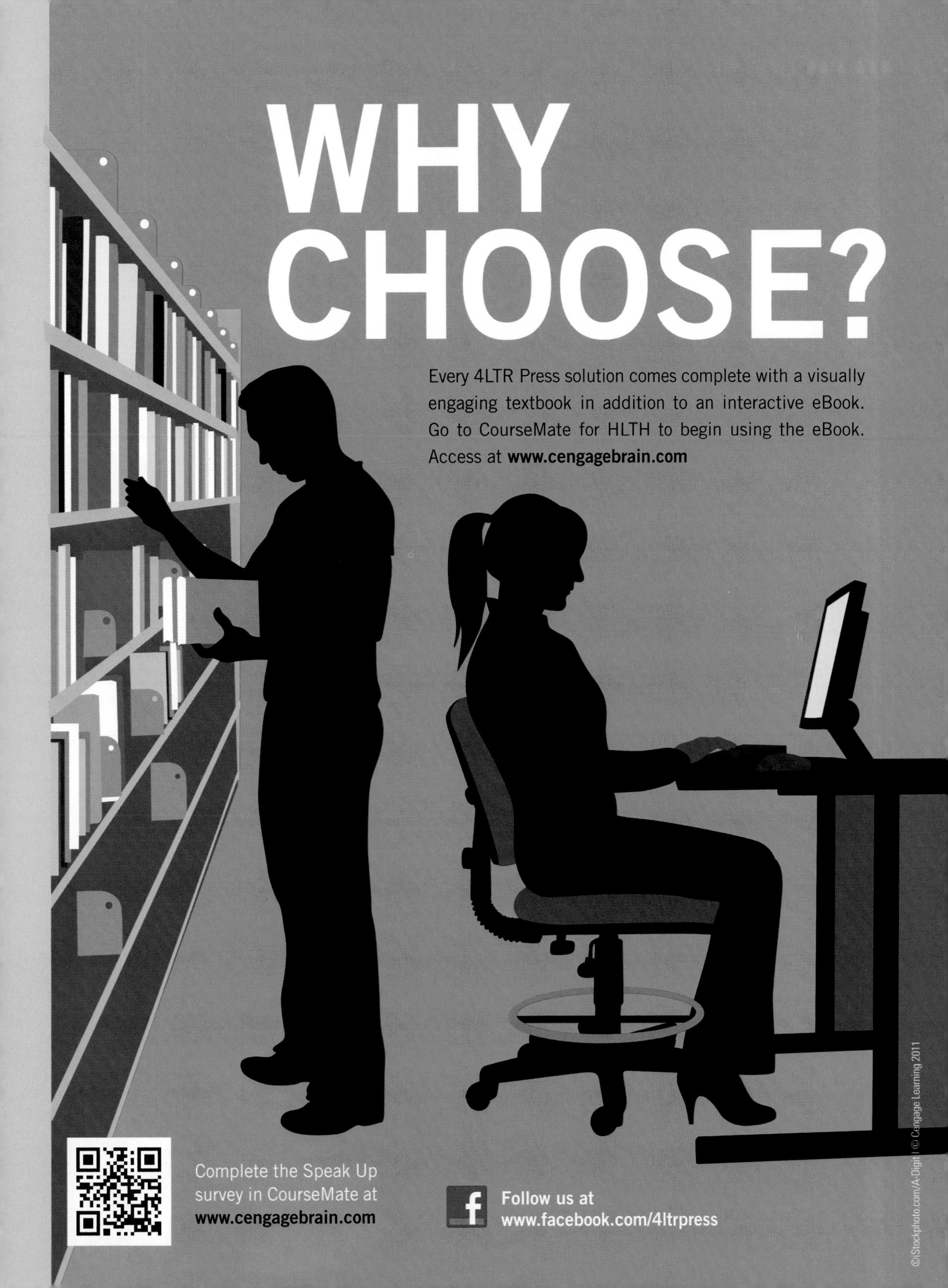
WHY CHOOSE?
Every 4LTR Press solution comes complete with a visually engaging textbook in addition to an interactive eBook. Go to CourseMate for HLTH to begin using the eBook. Access at www.cengagebrain.com
Complete the Speak Up survey in CourseMate at www.cengagebrain.com
Follow us at www.facebook.com/4ltrpress
©iStockphoto.com/A-Digit | © Cengage Learning 2011

Fitness for Life

"No pain, yes—gain!"

We are in the midst of a fitness boom. Health clubs and gyms have sprung up everywhere, dotting the urban and suburban landscapes. Many companies equip their workplaces with fitness centers where employees can work out and ease stress during the workday. Fitness TV channels are offered through most cable television systems. The Boston and New York marathons attract tens of thousands of runners.

In 1970, about 100 runners entered the first New York City Marathon, a 26.2-mile race that sets the standard for endurance racing. By the turn of the twenty-first century, more than 40,000 marathoners were clamoring to enter the race. Among them were nearly 100 wheelchair racers. Participation has also grown in other types of exercise, including walking, weight training, and the use of exercise machines such as stair-climbers and rowing machines.

Bicycle riding has achieved renewed popularity. Millions of Americans stay in shape through *aerobic exercise*—jogging, swimming laps, brisk walking, and aerobic dance classes.

Fitness has become a mainstay of modern culture for good reason: It is an essential component of a healthy lifestyle. Becoming physically fit through regular exercise tones and builds muscles, increases stamina and flexibility, strengthens the heart, improves lung capacity, combats stress, helps relieve depression and anxiety, sheds excess pounds, and reduces the risk of serious health problems, such as coronary heart disease (CHD), diabetes, and even some forms of cancer. Regular exercise may even lengthen life. Whatever goals you set for yourself, from improving your physical appearance

LEARNING OUTCOMES

1. **Describe the physical and psychological health benefits of exercise**
2. **Explain how to begin to get fit**
3. **Describe the uses of aerobic exercise**
4. **Describe the uses of anaerobic exercise**
5. **Discuss the benefits of stretching**
6. **Describe exercise injuries—how to prevent them, how to treat them**

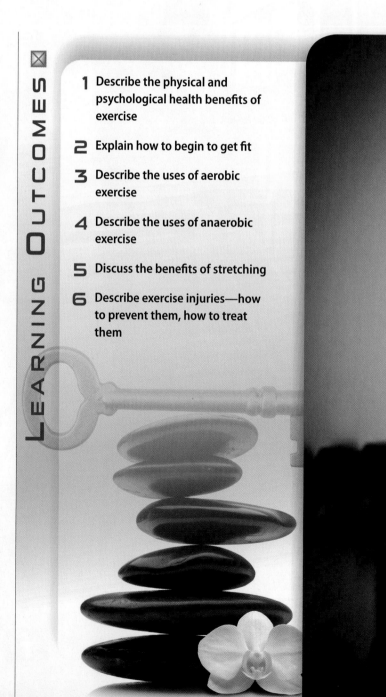

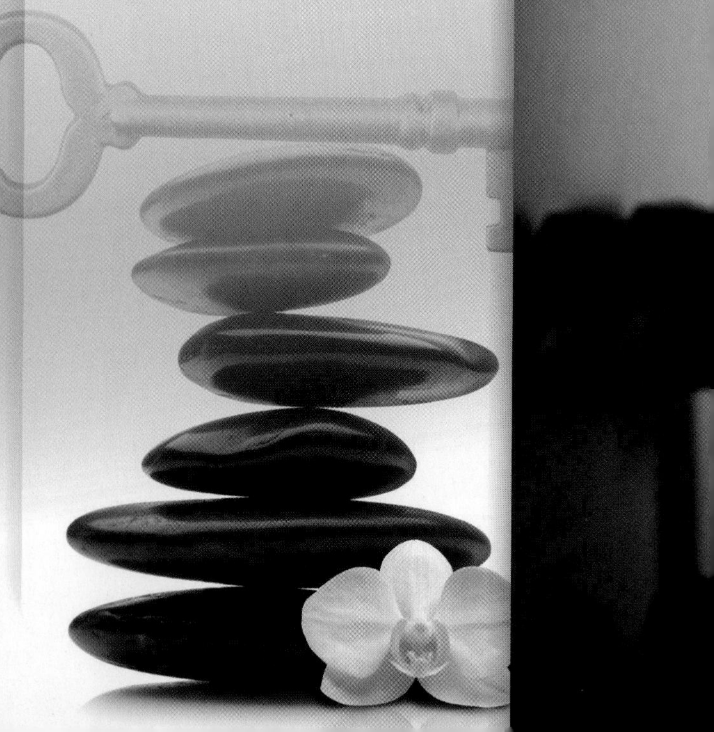

and mental outlook to lowering your risk of heart disease, exercise can help you achieve them. Exercise also gives you the energy and sense of well-being you need to "keep on pushing" and meet the challenges of life.

Yet, although millions of Americans exercise regularly, more than one in three adults (37%) are not at all physically active, and only 3 in 10 adults meet the recommended level of physical activity.[1] Children, older women, and people with lower incomes exercise least.

Among young people age 12 to 21, only about one-half engage in vigorous physical activity regularly. The message is clear: More Americans need to make exercise a part of their lifestyle.[2] Given that high rates of heart disease, obesity, and other health problems are associated with an inactive lifestyle, many Americans are dangerously unfit. But they are not destined to remain unfit. They can improve their fitness by making exercise part of their lifestyle.

Did You Know That . . .

- Regular exercise boosts the level of "good cholesterol" in your blood? [p. 167]
- People who exercise regularly burn more calories than couch potatoes—even when they're watching television? [p. 167]
- Bones are living tissues that need to work in order to remain strong? [p. 168]
- The saying "no pain, no gain" is inaccurate? You can improve your health through exercise without pain. [p. 173]
- Too much exercise can be harmful to your health? [p. 178]
- America's top sport is walking? [p. 180]

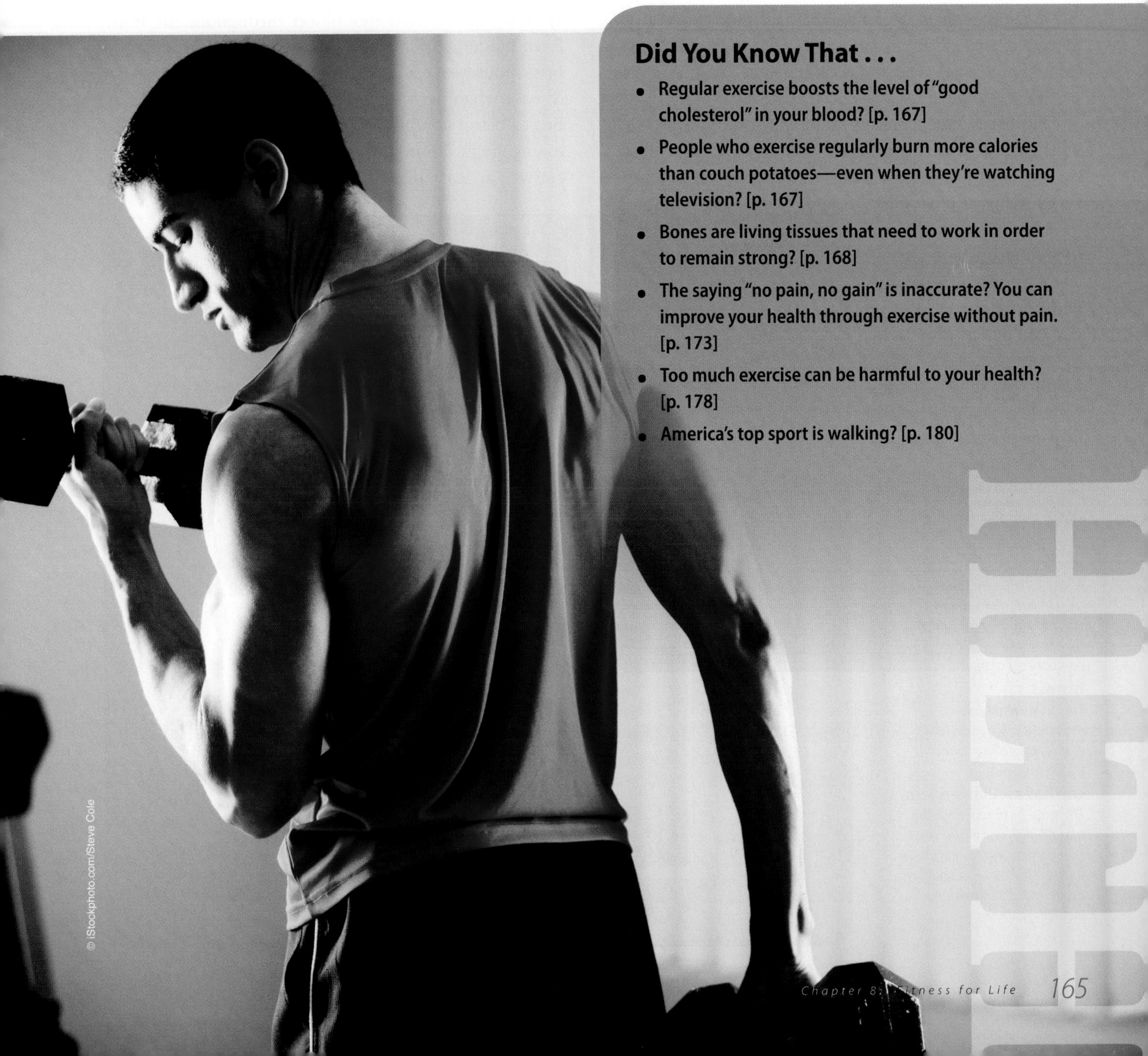

© iStockphoto.com/Steve Cole

Fitness and Health

Regular physical **exercise** can build fitness and improve your lifestyle. You may feel more energetic, sleep better, lose excess weight or maintain a healthy weight, get in shape or keep in shape, and cope better with stress. Regular exercise reduces the risks of many health problems, including high blood pressure (hypertension), diabetes, and stroke. It may even slow down some of the effects of aging.[3] All it takes to begin reaping the healthful benefits of regular exercise is 30 minutes a day of moderate physical activity—such as brisk walking—five or more days a week (see Figure 8-1).

LEARNING OUTCOME 1

Describe the physical and psychological health benefits of exercise

Fitness is not a matter of how strong you are or whether you can run an eight-minute mile. Rather, it is your body's ability to withstand stress and pressure. People who are physically fit are able to perform moderate to vigorous levels of physical activity without undue fatigue. If you can't climb the stairs to your office or walk uphill without losing your breath or exhausting yourself, consider yourself unfit.

exercise
A structured sequence of movements performed consistently over a period of time sufficient to build the components of fitness.

fitness
The ability to perform moderate to vigorous levels of physical activity without undue fatigue.

cardiovascular system
The system composed of the heart, lungs, and blood vessels that carries oxygen-rich blood through the body and delivers oxygen to all body tissues, including muscles.

The Physical Benefits of Exercise

Inactivity is a key risk factor in many chronic diseases that cut lives short, including coronary heart disease (CHD), adult-onset diabetes, and some cancers. Regular exercise, especially vigorous exercise, can increase lung capacity, the amount of air the lungs can hold. Increased lung capacity is associated with greater longevity. And that is only the beginning.

Reduced Risk of Cardiovascular Disease

Inactive people have about double the risk of developing heart disease as their more active peers. By becoming more active, even seasoned couch potatoes can reduce their risk of diseases of the **cardiovascular system**, which circulates blood throughout the body. Even moderately intense activity, such as gardening or brisk housework, can reduce the risk of cardiovascular disease when performed for at least 30 minutes a day. But to better condition your heart and lungs, you need to engage in 20 minutes or more of vigorous (aerobic) activity at least three times a week. Aerobic dancing,

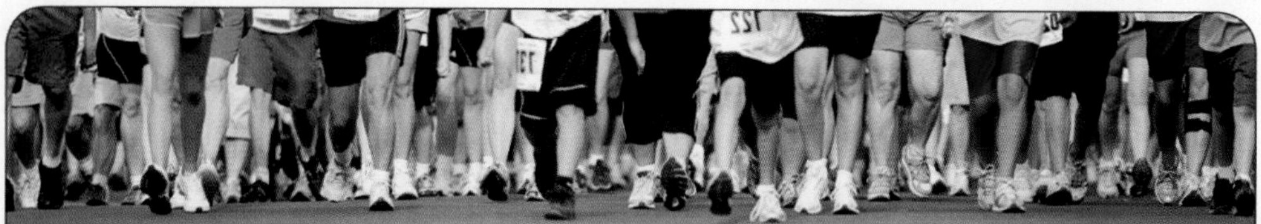

Figure 8-1 America, Let's Get Moving

The figure shows the percentages of Americans in different age groups who are physically active—who engage in light to moderate physical activity for 30 minutes or more a day at least five times a week, or vigorous physical activity for 20 minutes or more at least three times a week. Although the percentage of people who engage in physical activity declines with age, only about 40% of Americans aged 18 to 24 are physically active.

Source: Centers for Disease Control. (September 2008). *Leisure time physical activity*. Retrieved online at http://www.cdc.gov/nchs/data/nhis/earlyrelease/200809_07.pdf

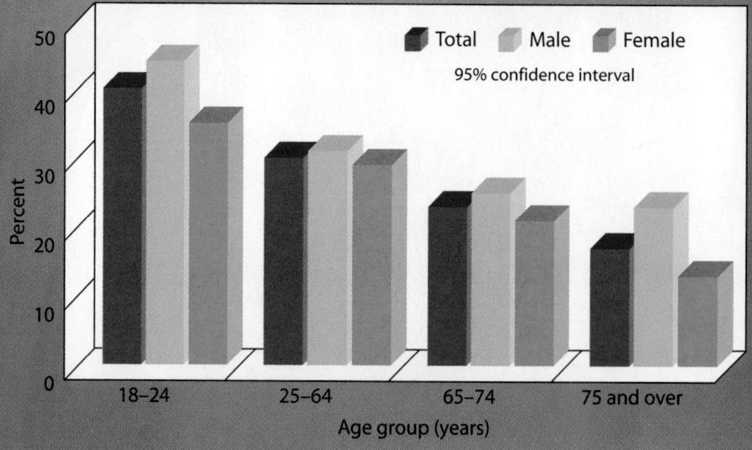

bicycling, cross-country skiing, hiking uphill, running, rowing, stair climbing, and fast walking all fit the bill. **Aerobic exercise**, which requires a sustained increase in the use of oxygen, widens blood vessels, allowing blood to circulate more freely. Better circulation reduces high blood pressure (hypertension), a risk factor for heart disease. Exercise, along with stress management training, even improves the cardiovascular risk profile of patients with established heart disease.[4]

Regular exercise boosts the level of the good form of cholesterol, the *high-density lipoproteins* (HDL), that sweeps away fatty deposits from artery walls. High levels of HDL are associated with lower risk of heart disease. A landmark study of 7,000 male runners showed that the more miles the men ran, the higher were their HDL levels.[5] Even men who logged only seven miles per week showed significantly higher HDL levels than people who did not exercise. Regular exercise also helps lower the blood levels of **triglycerides**, a type of fat associated with increased risk of heart disease, especially in people with low levels of HDL.

Exercise helps maintain an adequate supply of oxygen to the heart, which is vital to health. Regular vigorous (aerobic) exercise also lowers the resting heart rate, enabling the heart to pump with less wear and tear.

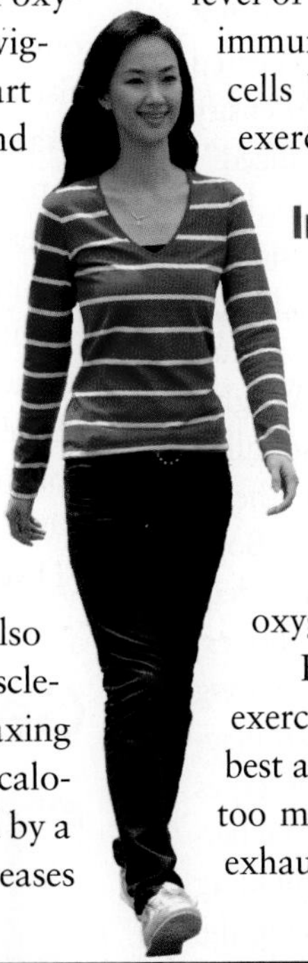

Weight Management and Improved Body Composition

Regular exercise helps people maintain a healthy body weight and avoid obesity—yet another risk factor for cardiovascular disease, as well as for diabetes and other health problems. Exercise takes weight off directly by burning *calories* (units of food energy released during metabolism). It also improves body composition by increasing the muscle-to-fat ratio. At rest—for example, when we're relaxing and watching TV—muscle tissue burns about 75 calories per hour, compared to a mere 2 calories burned by a pound of fat. In other words, regular exercise increases the metabolism, the rate at which the body burns calories.

Improved Immune System Functioning

Regular exercise helps boost the functioning of the **immune system**, the body's line of defense against disease-causing organisms such as bacteria and viruses.[6] People who exercise regularly show higher levels of **natural killer (NK) cells**, a type of white blood cell that renders the death blow to invading pathogens.[7]

Reduced Cancer Risk

A physically active lifestyle reduces the risks of certain types of cancer, especially colorectal cancer and breast cancer.[8] Regular exercise is associated with as much as a 60% reduction in the risk of breast cancer in young women.[9] The sharpest reductions are found in women who run, swim, or play tennis about four hours a week. Even women who exercise two or three hours a week show some reduced risk.

What accounts for the cancer-preventive role of exercise? For colorectal cancer, one possibility deserving further study is that exercise helps speed waste material through the colon, allowing less time for cancer-causing substances to affect the colon lining. We know that breast cancer is linked to length of exposure to the sex hormone estrogen, and exercise lowers the blood level of the estrogen. One of the responsibilities of the immune system is to help rid the body of cancerous cells before they turn into malignant growths, and exercise strengthens the immune system.

Increased Energy

Regular exercise helps boost energy levels and combat fatigue. People often report feeling energized and more alert after a brisk walk, swim, or workout. Why? We're not certain. Exercise may boost energy by inducing changes in brain chemicals or in the brain's electrical output. Exercise also increases the body's utilization of oxygen, which improves stamina and circulation. However, moderate exercise seems to work best as an energy booster; too much exercise can be exhausting.

Did You Know That...

People who exercise regularly burn more calories than couch potatoes—even when they're watching television?

aerobic exercise
Strenuous physical activity that requires a sustained increase in the use of oxygen by the body.

triglycerides
A type of lipid or fatty substance found in the blood.

immune system
The body's system of defense for identifying and eradicating invading bacteria and viruses as well as diseased, mutated, and worn-out cells.

natural killer (NK) cell
A type of white blood cell that kills viruses.

Prevention of Osteoarthritis and Osteoporosis

Muscles are bundles of fibers that contract to move the body. Maintaining strong muscles improves mobility, reduces the likelihood of injury, and helps prevent lower back problems. Muscle strengthening is also important to healthy bones. Bone is living tissue composed of a lacelike matrix of the protein collagen and the mineral calcium. Bones grow in length until about age 21 but continue to change in density or thickness throughout life. Density gives bones their strength; stronger bones are less vulnerable to fractures or breaks. Unless bones are worked, especially through weight-bearing activity, they become thinner and more brittle.

Important physical benefits of muscle strengthening exercise include reduced risks of both osteoarthritis and osteoporosis. **Osteoarthritis** (also called *arthritis*) is a chronic, degenerative disease of the joints. It is linked to wear and tear on the joints and can result in painful and restricted movement. Muscle strengthening and stretching helps keep joints and tendons flexible.

When bones are not stressed through repeated use, they begin to lose density (become "demineralized") due to loss of calcium. Loss of bone density is a sign of **osteoporosis**, a bone disease that makes bones more vulnerable to fractures. Weight-bearing exercise—also called **resistance training**—helps maintain bone density. Bone mass (a measure of the density or strength of bones) is typically greater among regular exercisers than inactive people, but some types of exercise appear to be better than others for building bone mass and reducing the risk of fractures.

osteoarthritis
A chronic, degenerative disease of the joints that produces pain and restricted movement. More commonly called arthritis.

osteoporosis
A degenerative condition of the bones characterized by the loss of bone density, which makes bones more brittle and prone to break.

resistance training
Muscle training involving repeated movement or lifting against an opposing force or weight.

insulin
A hormone produced by the pancreas that plays an essential role in the metabolism of blood sugar (glucose) and the maintenance of a proper level of blood sugar.

cardiorespiratory fitness
The ability of the heart, lungs, and blood vessels to provide muscles with sufficient amounts of oxygen to sustain vigorous activity for an extended period of time. Also called aerobic fitness *or* aerobic endurance.

Increased Sensitivity to Insulin

Regular exercise can also increase insulin sensitivity—the body's ability to utilize insulin. **Insulin** is a hormone produced by the pancreas that stimulates cells to absorb blood sugar (glucose) and other nutrients from the bloodstream. Insulin is essential to maintaining blood sugar at a proper level. By increasing insulin sensitivity, regular exercise helps the body regulate blood sugar levels. In *diabetes mellitus*, either the pancreas produces too little insulin or insulin is not used efficiently. Even people who show early warning signs of diabetes can cut their risk of developing the disease in more than half by engaging in just 30 minutes of moderate physical activity per day and by reducing their body weight by 5% to 10%.[10]

The Psychological Benefits of Exercise

Regular exercise can enhance one's mood, helping people feel less tense, anxious, and depressed, not only during workouts but also afterward. The connection between improved mood and exercise is so strong that mental health professionals often encourage depressed patients to exercise. Regular exercise can help relieve stress and depression.[11] Aerobic exercise helps normalize the levels of the neurotransmitters that play key roles in regulating our moods, thereby helping to combat depression. Exercise can also be enjoyable, providing a break from the strains of everyday life, another reason that it may help combat depression. Furthermore, exercise can give us a sense of mastery and accomplishment, boosting our self-image and self-confidence and helping to combat the sense of helplessness that is often associated with depression. How much exercise do you need? You can figure that out with the help of the online feature "Health Skills 8-1."

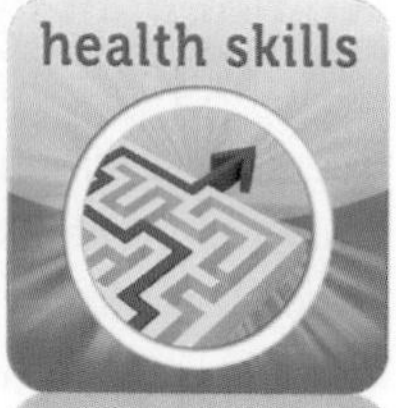

Access CourseMate for HLTH at www.cengagebrain.com.

Getting Fit

The key to becoming fit is to work your body through a program of regular physical exercise. Exercise increases fitness in several ways:

LEARNING OUTCOME 2
Explain how to begin to get fit

- *Regular vigorous exercise strengthens the heart, increases lung capacity, and reduces the risk of cardiovascular disease.* In people with good **cardiorespiratory fitness** (also called *aerobic fitness* or *aerobic endurance*), the heart and lungs are able to supply muscles and body tissues with oxygen-laden blood, thus sustaining vigorous activity. Fit people can perform strenuous activities for extended periods without becoming breathless and exhausted.

- *Regular weight-bearing or resistance exercise builds muscle strength and endurance.* Working with weights or resistance builds both **muscle strength** (the amount of force a muscle can apply when contracted) and **muscle endurance** (the ability of a muscle or muscle group to contract repeatedly or maintain a force against a fixed object, such as holding a weight above the head).
- *Stretching exercises increase the flexibility of joints, making it easier for joints and muscles to work together.* Regular stretching promotes flexibility in our joints and helps keep muscles and their supporting tissues from becoming strained or torn. Stretching improves posture, helps prevent lower back, shoulder, and neck problems, and enables you to achieve a full **range of motion** for physical activities.
- *Exercise burns calories and improves the ratio of muscle-to-fat, and muscle increases the metabolism.* Increased metabolism means that calories are burned faster.

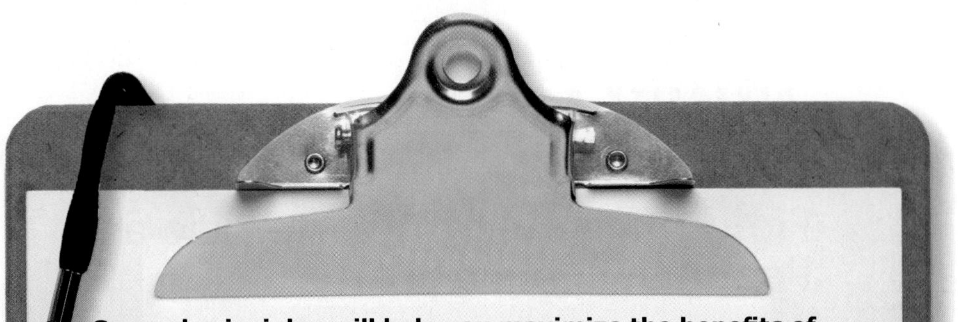

Several principles will help you maximize the benefits of training:

1. *Specificity.* To improve fitness or build endurance, train specifically toward that end. Working on the treadmill won't build stronger upper body muscles, and working solely with weights won't increase your aerobic endurance. Target an area for improvement, such as the arms or abdomen, by selecting exercise that focuses on the area.
2. *Overload.* To achieve your fitness goals, you need to stress or *overload* your body beyond its normal level. **Overloading** means increasing the demands or burdens placed on the body—as in increasing your running speed or the steepness of the incline, the distance you run, or the amount of resistance in weight training. The benefits achieved by overloading are termed a **training effect**.
3. *Progressive overload.* Gradually increase the demands on your body. Allow your body to adapt to progressively heavier workloads without undue stress or strain. If you exercise too hard or too long, you increase the risks of injury.
4. *Warm-ups and cool downs.* Before strenuous exercise, warm up with mild exercise and stretching for 5 to 10 minutes. The warm-up prepares your body for vigorous exercise by raising your body temperature, increasing your respiration and heart rates, and warming up your muscles. It reduces the risks of injuries such as strains and sprains. Stopping vigorous exercise abruptly can lead to dizziness, cramps, and muscle soreness, so cool down for 5 to 10 minutes by slowing the rate of exertion. Walk for five minutes at the end of a jog rather than stopping cold. Follow this by a few minutes of gentle stretching.
5. *Regularity.* Exercise the same muscle groups regularly to produce a training effect. Three workouts a week are good for weight training. When you discontinue exercising for a period of time, your fitness gains begin to fade: "Use it or lose it."

muscle strength
The amount of force, or power, a person can apply with one or more muscles in a single contraction.

muscle endurance
The ability to contract muscles repeatedly over time.

range of motion
The arc of motion of a joint, or the extent to which a joint can be moved through its normal spectrum.

overloading
The process of gradually increasing the stressful burden placed on the body to achieve a training effect.

training effect
The benefits to the heart, lungs, muscles, and bones produced by overloading.

training
The gradual adjustment of the body to increasingly higher demands through a structured sequence of repetitive and progressive movements. Also called conditioning.

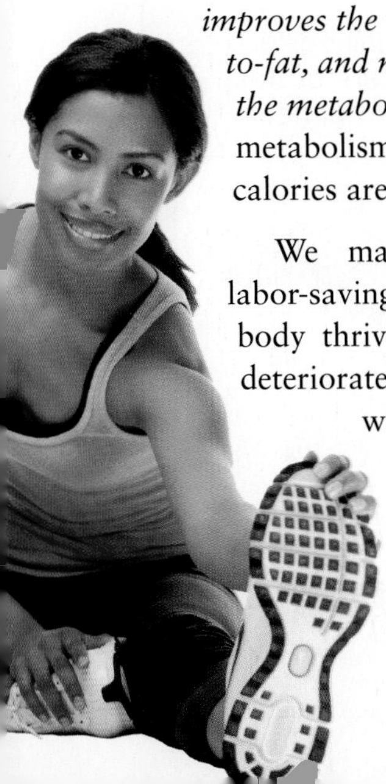

We may benefit from labor-saving devices, but the body thrives on activity. It deteriorates and becomes vulnerable to disease when sedentary. To become fit and help safeguard our health we must compensate for lowered daily activity levels by challenging the body through exercise.

Training (also called *conditioning*) refers to the gradual adjustment the body makes to increasingly higher demands from repetitive movements. Training

DIVERSITY 8-1

diversity

Fitness for Everyone: Exercise and People with Disabilities[12]

Janet Reed's videotape workout is similar in many ways to other exercise videos. She doesn't require special expertise or equipment, and viewers are encouraged to consult with their health-care professionals before participating. It includes warm-up stretches, activities that foster relaxation and range of motion, and exercises that enhance flexibility, strength, balance, and coordination.

However, Reed's workout differs in a very important way: It is aimed at users of wheelchairs.

Reed was thrown from a horse and suffered spinal cord injuries that paralyzed her from the waist down. For many years she had difficulty accepting her limitations. One year, however, a friend asked her to dance during a fund-raiser, and her outlook began to change. The friend manipulated her wheelchair while Reed moved her upper body in time with the music. It was the most fun she'd had since her accident, and eventually led to the idea that she could help other disabled people profit from physical activity. With the assistance of a physical therapist, Reed put together her "Wheelchair Workout" and found that creating it helped her retake charge of her life. Working out regularly "strengthens the body, relaxes the mind, and toughens the spirit," she says. "It can prove to you that you have what it takes to do what is necessary."

Exercise serves similar functions for people with and without disabilities:

- Improved health and fewer medical problems
- Increased self-esteem and self-confidence
- Improved fitness
- Enhanced stamina in daily activities

When people spend their lives in wheelchairs—or on the couch—their cardiovascular functioning suffers, their muscles atrophy, and their joints stiffen. People in wheelchairs can also develop pressure sores. Exercise, of course, does not cure paralysis. However, it helps people with spinal cord injuries improve their upper body strength and flexibility, their cardiovascular condition, their overall outlook on life, and their self-esteem. Exercise may actually be more crucial to the well-being of disabled people than to others.

The benefits of physical activity for disabled people have been known for some time. Physical activities, including tournaments, were organized as therapy for wounded war veterans after World War II. Today, wheelchair athletic organizations encourage disabled people to participate in archery, basketball, bowling, table tennis, racquetball, softball, swimming, weight lifting, and even marathons.

The Special Olympics fosters fitness and independence in people with intellectual deficiency. It provides training and competition in more than 20 sports and sponsors more than 20,000 competitions annually around the world. The Special Olympics works to remove obstacles, change attitudes, and open minds, and on a broader societal level, it helps promote understanding, respect, and acceptance of people with intellectual deficiency. A ranking system—a sort of literal "handicap" ranking—gives everyone a more or less equal chance to win.

Rehabilitation specialists suggest the use of isometric exercises to enhance muscle strength in wheelchair users—for example, by pressing the palms together and making a fist. Isotonic exercises can help increase range of motion and stamina. In "wheelchair sit-ups," participants lock their wheels, grasp the arms of the chair, and straighten the elbows, which lifts them off the seat. They repeat the lift several times.

Swimming is ideal for disabled people. Swimming is a low-impact activity that fosters flexibility, strength, and cardiovascular conditioning. The water helps support the body.

Like other athletes, people with disabilities are encouraged to consult with health-care professionals before undertaking exercise regimens.

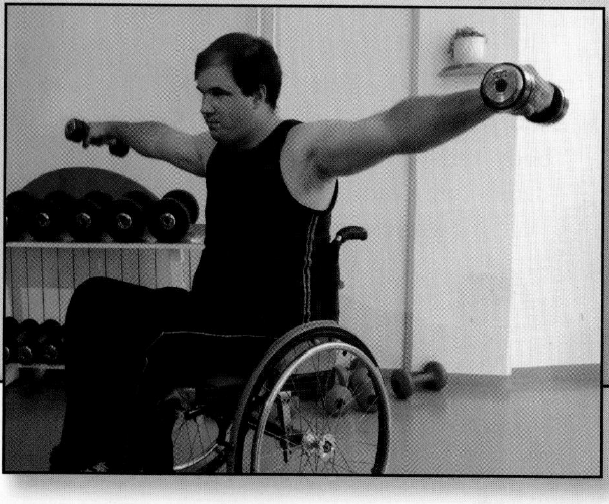

is the key to overall fitness. The amount and type of exercise necessary to train for fitness varies according to the specific amounts of energy and muscle groups required for a given activity. Certain kinds of training build aerobic endurance; others build strength; and still others build flexibility.

Using Aerobic Exercise

When we are physically active, our heart and lungs need to work harder to supply oxygen-rich blood to our muscles. In people with good cardiorespiratory (aerobic) fitness, the heart and lungs are able to sustain vigorous activity for extended periods of time. If you can engage in vigorous whole-body activities, such as swimming, jogging, or walking briskly, for a period of at least 20 minutes without feeling overcome by breathlessness, consider yourself to have at least a moderate level of aerobic fitness.

LEARNING OUTCOME 3

Describe the uses of aerobic exercise

Bagging groceries, stocking store shelves, or waiting tables are physically demanding tasks that may help build muscle strength, but they are not likely to improve aerobic fitness. Exercise needs to be sustained to develop aerobic fitness. The word *aerobic* means "with oxygen," and aerobic exercise involves sustained elevation of your use of oxygen.

Aerobic exercises include running, walking briskly, swimming laps, working out in an aerobics class, or cycling quickly. They use large muscle groups in repetitive, rhythmic body movements. The heart pumps more rapidly to meet the needs of working muscles for increased supplies of oxygen. Many exercise physiologists believe that at least 20 minutes of continued effort is required to obtain the training effect of aerobic exercise—that is, to promote cardiorespiratory fitness.

Muscles engaged in aerobic exercise may require as much as 10 times the amount of oxygen they need at rest. For example, if you are sitting quietly while reading this book, your heart is pumping about 5 quarts of blood through your body each minute, but if you were running around a track, your heart would need to pump at least four times as much blood, or 20 quarts or more, per minute. People in excellent aerobic condition, such as conditioned athletes, have a **cardiac output** (the amount of blood the heart pumps per minute) as high as 30 quarts or more per minute.

People who are aerobically fit have a **resting heart rate** lower than that of their less fit peers. The trained heart works more efficiently, even at rest. It can pump the same amount of blood with fewer beats.

Aerobic exercise has a hidden fat-burning effect: It increases the rate at which the body metabolizes fat. This **afterburner effect** means that people who exercise aerobically burn more calories than those who don't, even when they're watching television.

To improve your aerobic fitness, you need to elevate your heart rate during exercise to the recommended **target heart rate (THR)**. "Health Check 8-1" offers some guidelines for determining your target heart rate.

General Recommendations for Aerobic Exercise

To build aerobic endurance, the American Academy of Sports Medicine (AASM) recommends that you exercise at least three times weekly, at a level intense enough to give your heart and lungs a workout, for at least 20 minutes per session. The workout should raise the heart rate to a target range that is between 60% and 85% of your maximum attainable level (see "Health Check 8-1" on page 172 to compute your target heart rate).

People who are least fit make the most gains—a nice motivating factor for couch potatoes who want to change their ways. People who exercise aerobically less than three days a week may not show much change in aerobic fitness. On the other hand, people who exercise more than five days a week generally do not show greater gains than those who stick to a three- to five-day program.

Take at least one day off each week for aerobic exercise. Most experts advise skipping a day between anaerobic workouts. Older people usually benefit from more time between exercise sessions to recuperate.

Beginners should start at an easy pace. Whether you opt for jogging, bicycling, or an aerobic dance class, remain at the lower end of your target heart range—the 60% level—for several weeks. Don't overdo it by making yourself breathless. Then apply the principles of overload and gradual progression.

cardiac output
The amount of blood the heart pumps per minute.

resting heart rate
The number of times per minute the heart beats while the person is resting.

afterburner effect
The increased rate of metabolism of fat following exercise.

target heart rate (THR)
The recommended range of heartbeats per minute during vigorous exercise intended to improve cardiorespiratory fitness.

health check

prevention

diversity

skills

Determining Your Target Heart Rate

Step 1. Begin by measuring your *resting heart rate.* The best time to measure your resting heart rate is upon awakening in the morning or after sitting quietly in a chair for a few minutes. Your *heart rate* is the number of times your heart beats per minute. You can measure your heart rate (also called the *pulse rate*) by applying your index and middle fingers to the carotid artery in your neck (located just under the jawbone and next to the Adam's apple) or to the radial artery on the thumb side of your wrist (see Figure 8-2). Press lightly and count your resting pulse for 20 seconds, and then multiply by 3. This calculation is your resting heart rate. Before aerobic training, the average resting heart rate for adult males is about 72 beats per minute; for adult females, about 80 beats per minute. After regular aerobic exercise, the resting heart rate typically declines. If you're out of shape to begin with, your resting heart rate should decrease after several months of regular aerobic exercise. Highly trained athletes may have resting heart rates as low as 35 to 40 beats per minute.

Figure 8-2 Measuring Your Heart (Pulse) Rate

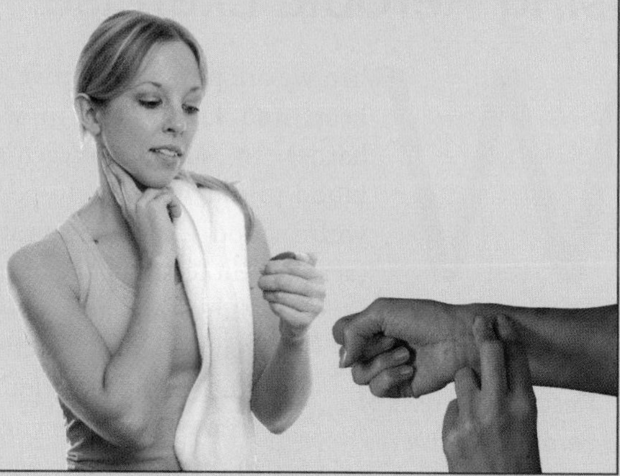

Step 2. Determine your recommended *maximum heart rate,* the fastest rate that your heart should be beating. To calculate this rate, subtract your age from the number 220 as follows:

220 – _______ (your age) = _______ (your maximum heart rate)

If you are 20 years old, your maximum heart rate would then be 200 beats per minute (220 – 20).

Step 3. Compute the lower and upper limits of your *target heart rate*, the desired range for sustained aerobic exercise. To obtain the cardiorespiratory benefits of aerobic exercise, you should achieve a heart rate range of 60% to 85% of your maximum heart rate. To compute the lower limit of your target heart rate range, multiply your maximum heart rate (number calculated above) by 0.60, and enter the result here:

_______ = low end of your target heart rate range

Next, multiply your maximum heart rate by 0.85. Enter the result here:

_______ = high end of your target heart range

As an example, a 30-year-old male with a maximum heart rate of 190 (220 minus 30) has a target heart rate ranging from 114 beats per minute (190 × 0.60) to 162 beats per minute (190 × 0.85, rounded off). He can obtain the cardiorespiratory benefits of sustained activity by exercising intensely enough that his heart beats between 114 and 162 times per minute.

Many people gauge whether they are exercising within their target heart rate range by taking their pulse 10 minutes into an exercise session. To measure your heart rate, count your pulse for 15 seconds, then multiply by 4.

At the beginning of an exercise program, remain near the lower end of the target heart rate range—the 60% range. When you are in good condition, you will be able to sustain heart rates in the higher part of your range. Generally speaking, you benefit more from exercising for a longer period of time at the lower end of your range than from exercising for a shorter time at the higher end.

A simpler test to gauge whether you are in the target heart range during exercise is called the *talk test.* If you can talk a little without gasping while continuing to exercise vigorously for a full 20 minutes, you can safely assume you are in your target heart rate range.

Table 8-1 *Benefits of Selected Aerobic and Anaerobic Exercises*

EXERCISE	TYPE	BENEFITS
Aerobic dancing	Aerobic	Improved cardiorespiratory fitness and whole-body muscle tone
Jogging and running	Aerobic	Improved cardiorespiratory fitness and increased leg muscle strength and endurance
Bicycling	Aerobic	Improved cardiorespiratory fitness and increased thigh muscle strength and endurance
Swimming	Aerobic	Improved cardiorespiratory fitness and improved whole-body muscle tone
Sprinting	Anaerobic	Increased leg muscle strength and endurance
Weight training	Lifting heavier loads for fewer repetitions is generally anaerobic; lifting lighter loads for more repetitions can be aerobic if done long enough within the target heart rate range	Increased muscle strength and endurance
Push-ups	Anaerobic	Increased arm and chest muscle strength and endurance
Sit-ups	Anaerobic	Increased abdomen and lower back muscle strength and endurance

Challenge (overload) yourself to do more—jog another quarter mile, swim another lap, or walk briskly for another 5 minutes. After several weeks of exercising at the lower end of your target heart rate range—between 60% and 70%—for at least 20 minutes, try exercising for 30 minutes in the same range. After several more weeks, increase the intensity of your routine to work out for 20 minutes at 75% of your target heart rate range. Then work gradually toward the upper limit of your target heart rate range. Give your body time to adjust. No pain—yes, gain. (To determine which exercises might be right for you, check out the online feature "Health Skills 8-2.")

health skills

Access CourseMate for HLTH at www.cengagebrain.com.

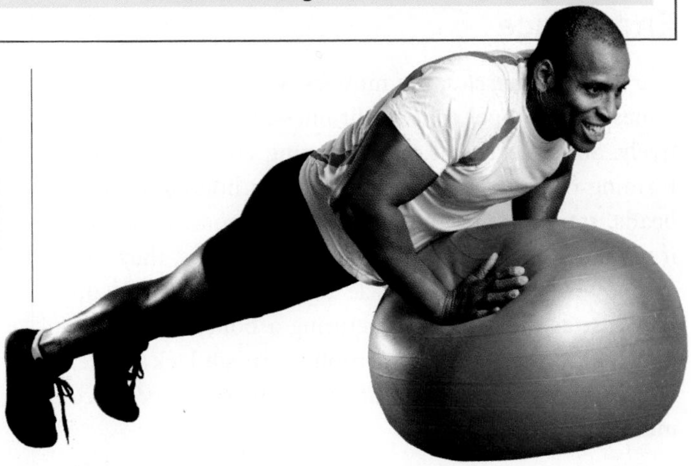

Using Anaerobic Exercise

Anaerobic (or "nonaerobic") **exercise** involves short bursts of muscle activity. We perform anaerobic exercise when we do sit-ups or push-ups, lift weights, or sprint to first base to beat out a throw in baseball. We can only sustain anaerobic exercise for short periods of time, perhaps two or three minutes, before our muscles begin to fatigue.

LEARNING OUTCOME 4

Describe the uses of anaerobic exercise

We need to engage in aerobic exercise to build aerobic or cardiorespiratory fitness, but anaerobic, or muscle strengthening, exercises tone and build muscle. Most health and exercise experts recommend a combination of aerobic and anaerobic exercise to achieve fitness. Table 8-1 compares the benefits of types of aerobic and anaerobic exercises.

anaerobic exercise
Exercise involving short bursts of intense muscle activity.

Figure 8-3 Isometric, Isotonic, and Isokinetic Exercise

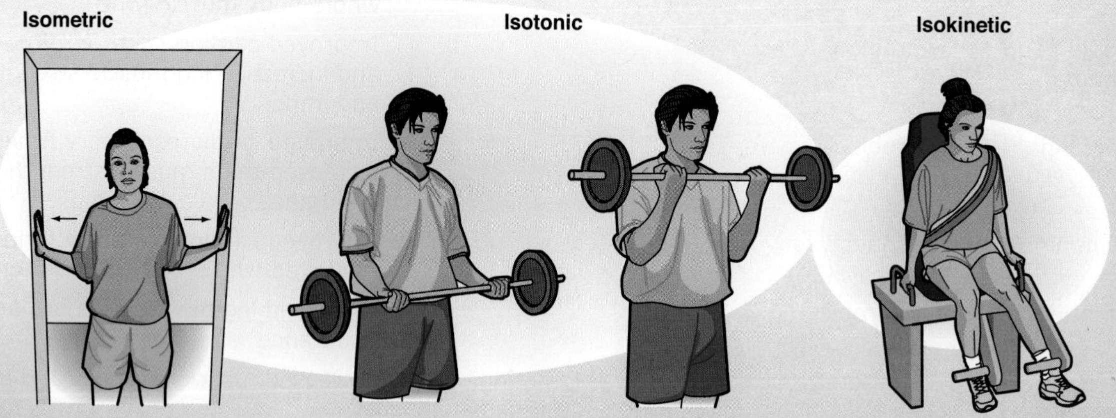

Building Muscle Strength and Endurance

Our *skeletal muscles*, the muscles we use to move our bones, need proper *tone*, or firmness, to perform effectively. Some degree of muscle toning comes from performing ordinary movements, such as holding up our heads, standing upright, and moving about. However, if we fail to adequately exercise our muscles, they can *atrophy*—that is, lose muscle tone. If we are laid up in a cast as the result of fracturing a bone, the muscle attached to the bone may atrophy through lack of use. People who lead sedentary lifestyles can also experience **muscle atrophy.**

Muscular fitness refers to our muscles' capability to perform the contractions needed to accomplish the work required of them. The two components of muscular fitness are muscle strength and muscle endurance. *Muscle strength* is the amount of force (power) a muscle can exert during a single contraction. *Muscle endurance* is our ability to contract our muscles repeatedly to complete tasks.

muscle atrophy
Deterioration or loss of muscle tone.

isometric exercise
Working a muscle by contracting it in a stationary position, such as by pushing against a wall or other immovable object.

isotonic exercise
Exercise in which muscles repeatedly contract under constant resistance throughout the range of motion; most weight-training exercises are of this type.

We build muscle strength and endurance through *resistance training*, a type of exercise in which we apply muscular force repeatedly against an opposing force or weight for a certain number of *repetitions* (called "reps"). A group of reps is called a "set."

We can use three types of exercise—*isometric, isotonic,* and *isokinetic*—to train for strength and endurance (see Figure 8-3). These terms also refer to the different types of muscle contractions.

In **isometric exercise**, your muscles contract or exert pressure against an immovable object, as when you push against a wall or place your palms together and push. Isometric exercise is used to increase muscle strength, but the improvement is limited to the particular joint angle where the contraction occurs. In performing isometric exercises, people exert as much force as they can without risking injury. They hold the contraction for about six seconds before releasing or pausing, then do 5 to 10 repetitions. Isometric exercise is generally not advised for people with cardiovascular problems, including hypertension, because it can lead to a sudden rise in blood pressure.

In **isotonic exercise**, force is applied against constant resistance. Muscle-strengthening equipment, such as traditional free weights (dumbbells or barbells) or Nautilus- or Universal-type equipment, is commonly used for isotonic exercise. Although the resistance remains constant (i.e., the weight of the barbell doesn't change), the amount of muscular force required to perform the task varies throughout the range of motion. Lifting a barbell requires more exertion than lowering it to the floor because gravity helps the lowering. Unlike isometric exercise, in which force is exerted at a specific joint, isotonic exercise requires muscle contractions throughout the full range of motion. Consequently, more muscle fibers are worked.

To build muscle strength, it is best to perform isotonic exercises with high resistance (i.e., heavier weights) and fewer repetitions. To build muscle endurance, use low resistance and a high number of repetitions.

In **isokinetic exercise**, specialized equipment provides resistance that varies with the user's level of exertion through the full range of motion. An isokinetic stationary bicycle, for example, sets a particular number of revolutions per minute, despite how hard or how fast the person pedals. Isokinetic exercise is believed to be the most effective way of overloading muscles to strengthen them. Machines made by Cybex and MiniGym are examples of variable resistance equipment used for isokinetic exercise. For more guidelines to muscle-strengthening exercises, check out the online feature "Health Skills 8-3."

health skills

Access CourseMate for HLTH at www.cengagebrain.com.

It's a Stretch: Staying Static or Going Ballistic?

Training for **flexibility** focuses on achieving and maintaining a full range of motion in the body's joints. We can enhance the flexibility of our joints with regular stretching exercises. The most widely recommended form of stretching is **static stretching**, in which you stretch until you encounter mild resistance, or feelings of tightness, in your muscles. Further stretching may cause pain or risk injury. Before stretching, engage in a warm-up exercise, such as fast walking or slow jogging in place. Figure 8-4 on the next page illustrates some static stretches; use the following suggestions for practicing static stretching.

LEARNING OUTCOME 5

Discuss the benefits of stretching

Getting Started with Static Stretching

- Select the muscle group you'd like to stretch. Gradually stretch it until you feel mild tension or tightness.
- Hold the stretch for 10 to 30 seconds.
- Repeat each stretch three or four times.
- Don't overstretch to the point that you feel pain. (Beginners may encounter some initial soreness.)
- Breathe slowly and normally while stretching. Do not hold your breath.
- Practice stretching exercises at least three or four days per week, or make it part of your daily routine.

Most fitness experts recommend not using *ballistic stretching* (or *bouncing*). Ballistic stretching involves a series of bounces, such as bobbing up and down to touch your toes with your hands. Ballistic stretching can cause injuries and muscle soreness and is less efficient than static stretching. Some forms of stretching involve the use of a partner and are best learned with a qualified trainer. Now that you're warmed up, you can further stretch your legs; read about the benefits of walking in the online feature "Health Skills 8-4."

health skills

Access CourseMate for HLTH at www.cengagebrain.com.

Exercise Injuries: Yes, Pain—Not Necessarily Gain

Exercise has many health benefits, but it can be dangerous if it is not carried

LEARNING OUTCOME 6

Describe exercise injuries—how to prevent them, how to treat them

isokinetic exercise
Exercise in which muscles contract against resistance that varies with the user's level of exertion throughout the range of motion; requires use of exercise machines.

flexibility
The ability of the joints to move through their entire range of motion without undue stress. Flexibility is measured by the length and amount of stretch in the tissues surrounding the joints.

static stretching
Slowly stretching a muscle to an extended stretch and holding it for 10 to 30 seconds.

Figure 8-4 Examples of Static Stretching

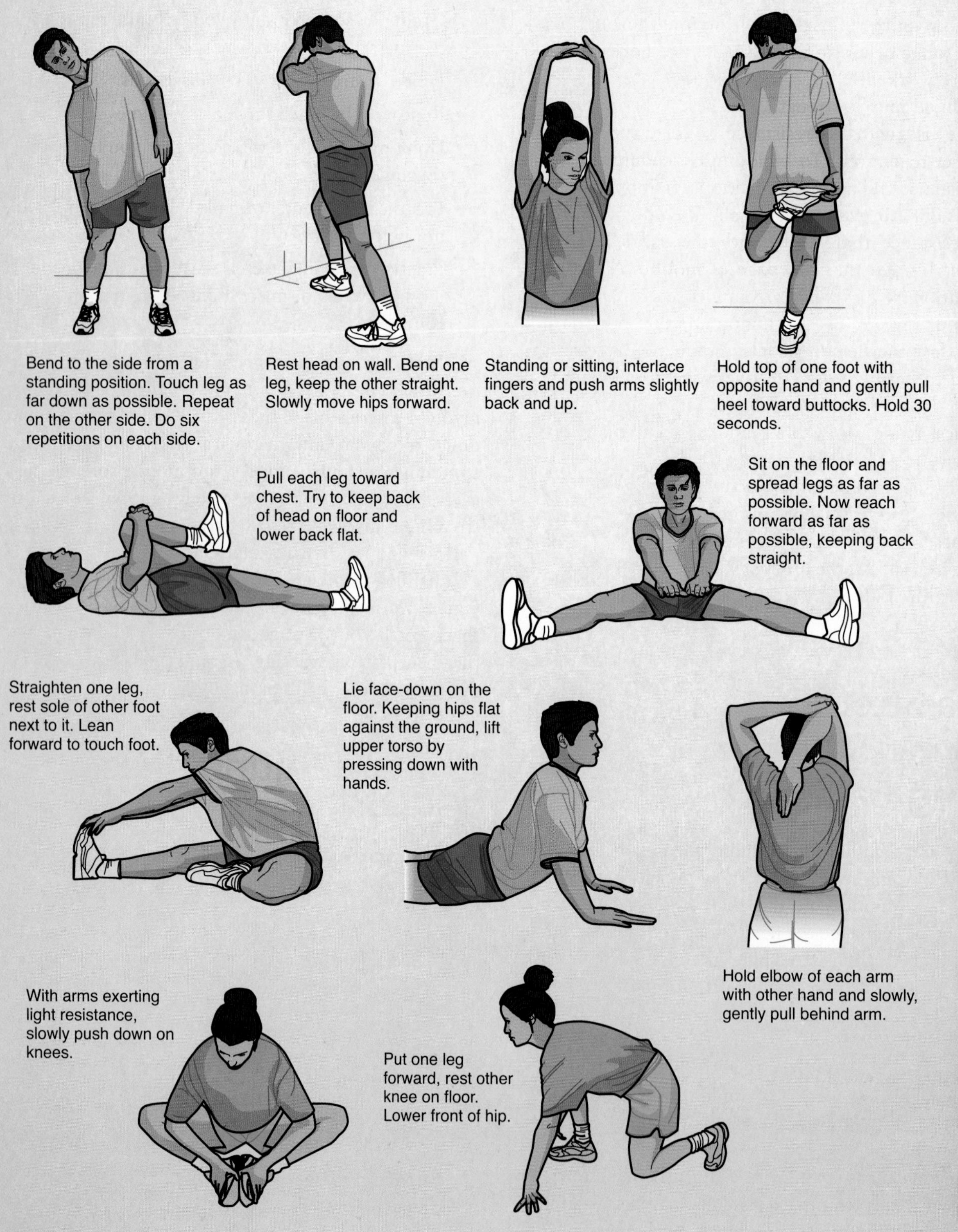

Bend to the side from a standing position. Touch leg as far down as possible. Repeat on the other side. Do six repetitions on each side.
Rest head on wall. Bend one leg, keep the other straight. Slowly move hips forward.
Standing or sitting, interlace fingers and push arms slightly back and up.
Hold top of one foot with opposite hand and gently pull heel toward buttocks. Hold 30 seconds.
Pull each leg toward chest. Try to keep back of head on floor and lower back flat.
Sit on the floor and spread legs as far as possible. Now reach forward as far as possible, keeping back straight.
Straighten one leg, rest sole of other foot next to it. Lean forward to touch foot.
Lie face-down on the floor. Keeping hips flat against the ground, lift upper torso by pressing down with hands.
Hold elbow of each arm with other hand and slowly, gently pull behind arm.
With arms exerting light resistance, slowly push down on knees.
Put one leg forward, rest other knee on floor. Lower front of hip.

out carefully. Vigorous exercise and weight-bearing exercise exert tremendous forces on muscle, bone, tendons, and ligaments. When we begin an exercise program, we should expect some minor muscle soreness afterward, but as muscles adapt and strengthen, soreness following exercise should diminish, although it may not disappear.

Muscle soreness usually lessens and disappears in a few days. We may be able to prevent muscle soreness by increasing loads more gradually. Feelings of excessive soreness should be used as a cue to stop what we're doing and rest our muscles before resuming our exercise routine. Soreness that persists beyond a week, or worsens rather than improves, requires medical attention.

Some people have painful muscle cramps when they exercise. A *cramp* is a muscle spasm that can usually be relieved through rest, replacing depleted fluids, and gently massaging the area. Repeated cramps should be medically evaluated.

Let's consider the two major types of exercise-related injuries: sudden injuries and overuse injuries.

Sudden Injuries

Sudden injuries occur in single, abrupt incidents. They include strains and sprains as well as bone fractures or breaks, torn cartilage, and ruptured tendons. Sudden injuries are more likely to occur in "weekend athletes"—people who generally lead a sedentary lifestyle but try to become instant athletes on the weekends or during vacations. However, even the most seasoned athletes can experience strains, sprains, and other types of sudden injuries.

Muscle Strains

A **strain** (or muscle pull) occurs when a muscle is overstretched to the point that tears occur in muscle fibers or in the surrounding tissue. You may strain a muscle when you try to use it in an unusual way, such as during vigorous exercise. Virtually all of us experience occasional muscle strains. Recovery is usually quick and complete, typically within three to six weeks. Recovery is aided by applying ice packs to reduce swelling and pain, resting the muscle for several days, and perhaps bandaging or strapping it for additional support. You should also avoid exercising the muscle until it has healed (substitute another exercise in the meantime). If the muscle is ruptured or torn, it may require surgery.

Sprains

A **sprain** results from the sudden twisting of a joint that causes tearing of a **ligament**, the band of tough, fibrous tissue that holds two bones together at a joint. The ankles, knees, fingers, and shoulders are most vulnerable to sprains. The severity of a sprain depends on the extent to which the ligament is torn. Minor sprains involve feelings of tenderness and some pain, but major sprains can lead to significant swelling, pain, and loss of function. Pain lasting for more than a few days should be reported to a health-care professional. In some cases, a cast or surgery is needed.

Cardiovascular Problems

Now and then, athletes die suddenly from heart attacks or other cardiovascular problems while exercising or competing. Nearly all exercise-related cardiac fatalities result from preexisting cardiovascular problems, such as *atherosclerosis* (narrowing of the arteries) or heart defects. In people under age 35, sudden death during exercise is typically related to abnormalities such as irregular heart rhythm.

Overall, it is riskier not to exercise than to exercise, especially for people who are at risk of heart disease.

Cardiovascular risks can usually be detected by a stress test. In a **stress test**, medical personnel monitor heart function and blood pressure while the patient engages in vigorous exercise, usually on a treadmill or bicycle. If you're over 40 or lead a sedentary life style, get a medical evaluation before embarking on any exercise regimen. Medical evaluations are especially recommended for people who smoke, are overweight, or have family histories of cardiovascular disorders.

Overall, it is riskier not to exercise than to exercise, especially for people who are at risk of heart disease. Build up your intensity level gradually to allow your body to become accustomed to increased stress.

The following symptoms during exercise are suggestive of heart problems: pain or pressure in the left or mid-chest area or the left neck, shoulder,

strain
A stretch (or muscle pull) or actual tear in muscle fibers or surrounding tissue.

sprain
An injury caused by a sudden joint twist that stretches or tears a ligament.

ligament
Tough, fibrous tissue that connects two bones together at a joint.

stress test
A medical test for determining cardiorespiratory fitness by measuring oxygen consumption and heart functioning during strenuous exercise; commonly involves the use of a treadmill or stationary bicycle.

or arm during or just after exercising, sudden lightheadedness, cold sweat, extreme paleness, or fainting. However, vigorous exercise may produce a side stitch, a pain below your bottom ribs, which is not a sign of a heart problem. Should you experience any of these signs, stop exercising and call your doctor for an evaluation.

Other Sudden Injuries

Other sudden injuries include bone **fractures** (broken bones), torn *cartilage*, and ruptured *tendons*. A fracture results when too much pressure or stress is placed on a bone. Broken bones are uncommon in low-impact physical activity. They occur more often in contact sports, such as football, ice hockey, basketball, and boxing, where fractures involving bones in the hands and nose are especially common. Fractures of bones in the feet are common in runners, especially those who run on hard pavement.

Cartilage acts as padding between the surfaces of a joint. The knee is the usual site of sports-related injuries involving damaged cartilage. Torn cartilage in the knee results from a sudden twisting of the knee joint, which may occur by taking a misstep or making an abrupt change in direction. These injuries, which typically require surgery, are common in running, tennis, football, and basketball.

Tendons are bands of tough, fibrous tissue that connect muscle to bone. They allow your muscles to move the bones in various parts of your body, such as those in your fingers, hands, arms, legs, and feet. A ruptured tendon is a severe, sudden injury in which the tendon is torn away from the bone or actually snaps in half. If you sever a tendon, you lose all or some movement of the bone to which it is connected. Ruptured tendons often produce searing pain (unless nerve damage is present) and demand immediate medical attention.

fracture
A broken bone.

cartilage
Tough, flexible type of connective tissue that covers the surface of a joint, serving as padding or a "shock absorber" for the joint.

tendon
Fibrous connective tissue that attaches muscle to bone in the body.

tendonitis
Inflammation of a tendon.

stress fracture
A microscopic break in a bone (such as in the foot, shin, or thigh) caused by repeated and excessive pressure or pounding.

Overuse Injuries

During vigorous exercise, we may push parts of our bodies beyond their ability to absorb the forces we impose on them. Overuse injuries develop gradually as bone, muscle, or connective tissues are repeatedly stressed beyond their capacity to recover and adapt. Tendonitis, stress fractures, and shin splints are among the most common overuse injuries. A neglected overuse injury, like tendonitis, may result in a sudden injury, such as a ruptured tendon. Overuse injuries often result from overtraining or exercising too much (learn more in the online features "Prevention 8-1" and "Prevention 8-2").

Select the right shoe for the particular type of exercise. Shoes for *jogging* and *running* should provide extra cushioning in the heel (see Figure 8-5). However, this extra cushioning may not help, and may actually be harmful, if you use them during an aerobic dance class. *Aerobics shoes* should provide more lateral support to prevent the kind of side-to-side movement that can lead to stress injuries. *Walking shoes* should have low heels and strong arch supports to provide extra stability.

Fitness magazines evaluate the latest models in athletic footwear. When shopping, ask the salesperson for a shoe specifically designed for the type of exercise you intend to use it for, but don't buy a pair of shoes without first walking around in the store while wearing them for about 10 minutes to make sure they are comfortable.

Tendonitis

When muscles contract, tendons pull on bones to make them work, bearing the brunt of the force that muscles exert. The most common form of tendon injury is inflammation, or **tendonitis**. Tendonitis most often occurs around the joints and can result from overuse of a tendon during repetitive motion. Microscopic tears develop in tendons, causing symptoms such as pain, redness, warmth, and swelling.

"Tennis elbow," a form of tendonitis, is not limited to tennis players. It results from repeated stress on the tendons around the elbow, which can occur following repeated motions during tennis, rowing, and weight lifting. It can even occur in people who repeatedly swing their elbows while carrying briefcases.

Stress Fractures

Stress fractures are tiny breaks in bones that result from repeated and excessive stress or pressure. In its early stages, a stress fracture can lead to a persistent, dull ache

Figure 8-5 Features of a Good Running Shoe

Go to a running store, rather than a fashion-oriented shoe store, to increase the likelihood that you will have a knowledgeable salesperson. When buying a running shoe, *Consumer Reports* suggests shopping late in the day, when your feet are at their largest. Bring along an old pair of running shoes so the salesperson can examine the wear pattern to analyze your running motion. Make sure the shoes are flexible enough to bend easily at their widest point. Wear the socks you normally use when running, and bring along any orthotics or other inserts you regularly use. Jog around in the store to test the comfort and feel.

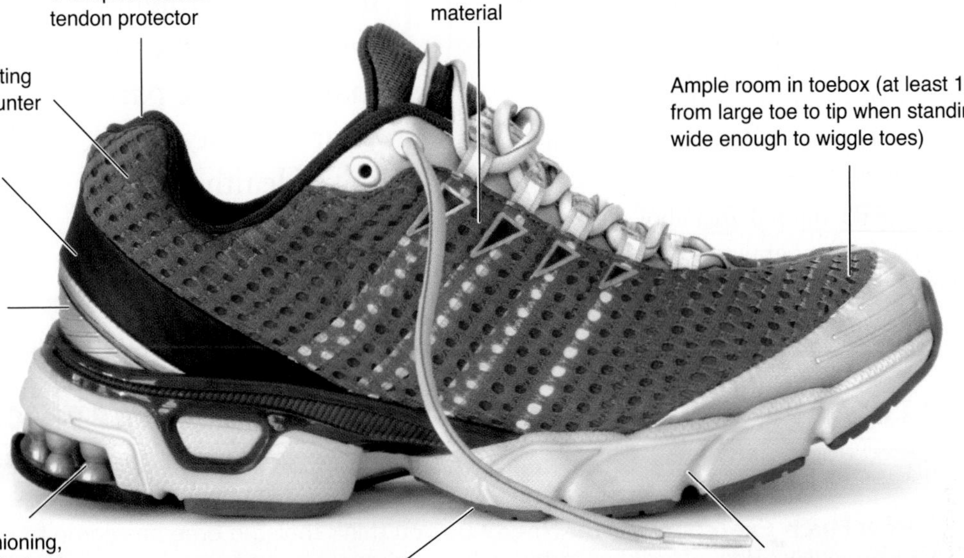

in the area of the broken bone. The pain may become severe if the injury is left untreated. In many cases, rest and application of ice packs allow the bone to heal naturally. However, when pain or inflammation is persistent, medical attention may be needed to align and immobilize the broken pieces so that they heal properly.

Shin Splints

Shin splints are slight tears in the muscles serving the **tibia**, the inner and larger of the two bones in the leg between the knee and the ankle. Shin splints are typically caused by high-impact exercise, such as running, and can cause tenderness and pain. Shin splints usually resolve on their own, but runners should rest until the condition improves, which usually occurs within a couple of weeks. It's also prudent to wear proper shoes for arch support and cushioning.

For many minor injuries, a program of *rest, ice, compression,* and *elevation* (the R.I.C.E. principle) may be sufficient to relieve the problem.

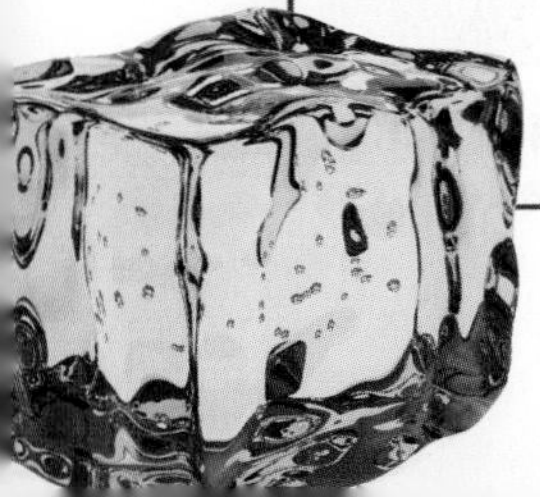

The R.I.C.E. Principle

Any injury that produces sharp pain or persistent swelling should be brought to the attention of a health-care professional. Even minor strains and sprains or muscle soreness should be medically evaluated if they persist. For many minor injuries, a program of *rest, ice, compression,* and *elevation* (the **R.I.C.E. principle**) may be sufficient to relieve the problem.

The R.I.C.E. principle has four steps:

1. *Rest.* Rest the injured area. Avoid exercising the affected area until pain, swelling, and inflammation subside. It

shin splints
Injuries similar to stress fractures but involving tears in muscle fibers rather than tiny breaks in bone.

tibia
The larger of the two bones of the lower leg, extending from the knee to the ankle.

R.I.C.E. principle
A program of rest, ice, compression, and elevation used in the treatment of exercise-related injuries.

may be possible to practice other forms of exercise that don't affect the injured area so you can keep in shape while you heal. Tendonitis in the elbow needn't keep you from exercising your legs.

2. *Ice.* To reduce swelling, periodically apply an ice pack to the injured area for no more than 20 minutes at a time, several times a day.
3. *Compress.* Compress the injured area by wrapping it in a close-fitting bandage. Compression reduces the flow of blood to the injured site, lessening inflammation. Don't wrap the injured area so tightly that you cut off the flow of blood. If possible, seek professional advice on wrapping injuries.
4. *Elevate.* Elevate the injured area above heart level to use the force of gravity to aid in reducing swelling.

Now that you know about the benefits of exercise, can distinguish between aerobic and anaerobic exercise, know to use stretching, and are acquainted with the types of injuries you might encounter, let's see if we can help you make exercise part of your lifestyle. Check out "Health Skills 8-5," and give it a try.

health skills

Access CourseMate for HLTH at www.cengagebrain.com.

HEALTH APPS: YOUR LINK TO ONLINE HEALTH APPLICATIONS

health skills **How Much Exercise Do You Need?** Do you think that the time has come to exercise? How strenuously? How often? For answers to these questions and more, read "Health Skills 8-1."

health skills **Which Kinds of Exercise Are Right for You?** Do you like to exercise alone or with others? Do you prefer indoor activities or outdoor activities? Would you prefer exercising at a health club or at home? What can you afford in the way of exercise equipment, classes, or club memberships? Examine your options in "Health Skills 8-2."

health skills **Guidelines for Muscle-Strengthening Exercises** Getting ready to pump iron? "Health Skills 8-3" will help you prepare.

health skills **Take a Hike! Walking for Fitness** Has anyone ever told you to take a hike? It might not have been meant in a positive way, but taking a hike is one of the best things you can do to become fit. Walking—even brisk walking—is relatively low impact, and there are many health benefits. No wonder it is America's top sport. Learn more in "Health Skills 8-4."

prevention **Overtraining: Are You Doing Too Much of a Good Thing?** Are you concerned that you might be going overboard with exercising? Are you tired much of the time and unsteady on your feet? Perhaps you're overtraining. For some ideas on what you can do about it, read "Prevention 8-1."

prevention **Preventing Exercise-Related Injuries** Exercise-related accidents and injuries can happen to anyone. However, many can be prevented by taking some precautionary measures. Learn more in "Prevention 8-2."

health skills **Making Exercise Part of Your Lifestyle** "Health Skills 8-5" can help you decide what activity is right for you by helping you sort out your exercise goals, needs, and interests.

Go to the CourseMate for HLTH at www.cengagebrain.com for additional resources including flashcards, games, self-quizzes, review exercises, web exercises, learning checks, and more.

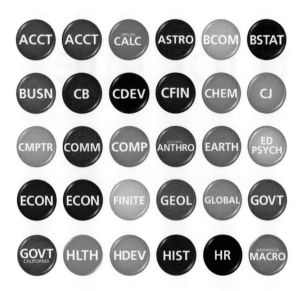

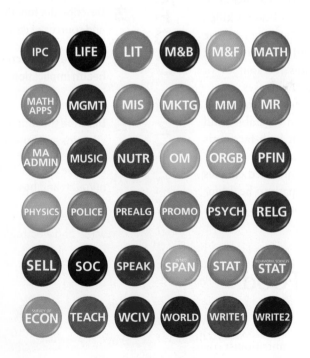

Nutrition for Life

"We really are what we eat. Yet, fewer than one in four Americans follows a healthful diet."

The saying "You are what you eat" contains more than a kernel of truth. We really *are* what we eat: We convert the food we eat into bones, muscles, skin, blood, and other tissues. Diet also plays a vital role in determining our risk of developing diseases such as cancer, cardiovascular disease, and diabetes. As many as one-third of all cancer deaths in the United States and a large proportion of deaths due to heart disease, the nation's leading killer, are linked to consumption of high-fat, high-calorie foods. A sensible diet—low in fat and ample in fruits, vegetables, high-fiber grains, and low-fat sources of protein—helps reduce the risks of these diseases.

Yet fewer than one in four Americans follows a healthful diet. Too many of us skimp on vegetables and whole grain products and load up on high-fat foods such as French fries, tacos, and burgers.

This chapter will help you make informed choices about your diet. To get started on the path to healthier eating, check out "Health Skills 9-1" on page 184.

Learning Outcomes

1 **Describe tips for eating right based on the *Dietary Guidelines for Americans***

2 **Describe the functions and sources of proteins**

3 **Describe the functions, types, and sources of carbohydrates**

4 **Describe the functions of fats and health implications of excess fat intake**

5 **Describe the functions of vitamins and how to obtain them**

6 **Describe the functions of minerals and how to obtain them**

7 **Describe the nutritional roles of water and electrolytes and the risks of excess sodium intake**

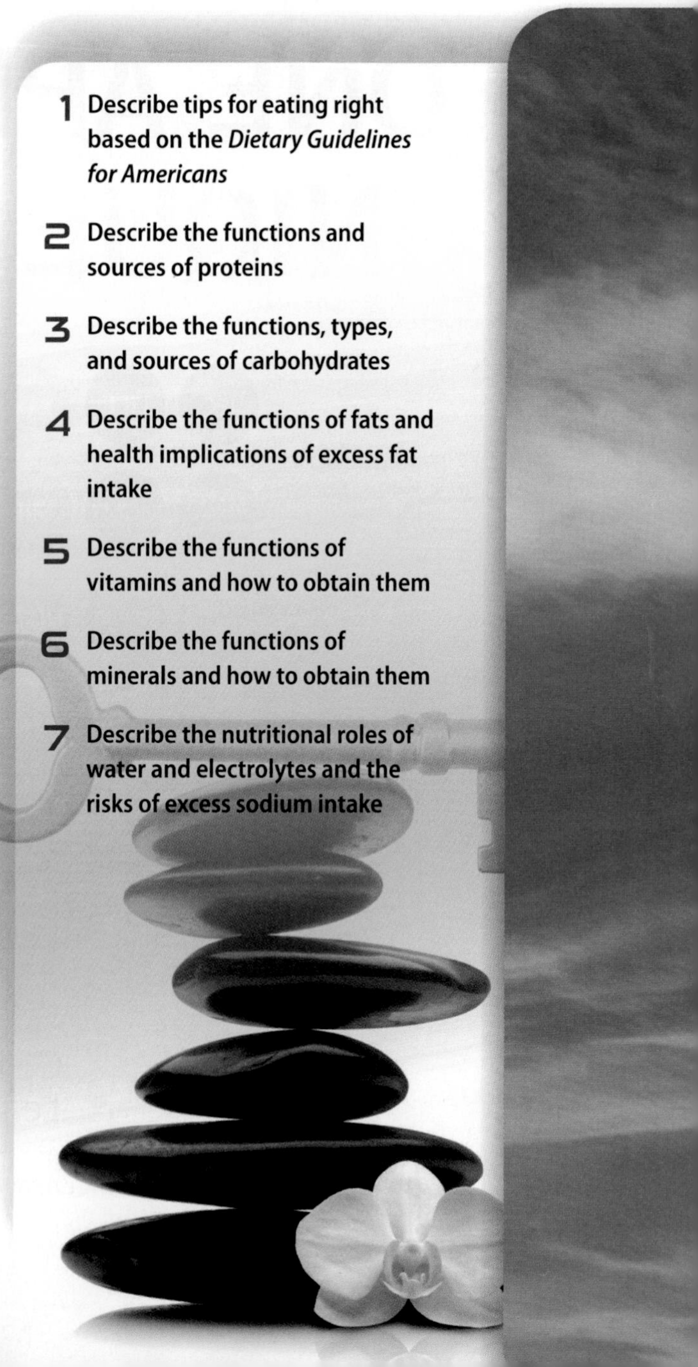

Making Healthier Food Choices

You don't have to be a nutritionist or dietician to eat correctly. Americans are eating too much fat, added sugars, and sodium and too few whole grains, vegetables, fruits, seafood, fiber, and sources of vital nutrients such as potassium, Vitamin D, and calcium. The *2010 Dietary Guidelines*

☒ LEARNING OUTCOME 1

Describe tips for eating right based on the *Dietary Guidelines for Americans*

are intended to help Americans eat right and reduce their risks of overweight, obesity, and chronic diseases. (For more information on the guidelines, go to www.usda.gov and enter "dietary guidelines" in the search box.) The federal government also recently replaced the familiar MyPyramid model for healthy eating with a new image of a healthy plate (see Figure 9-1 on the next page). MyPlate is a visual reminder to Americans to fill their plates with a balance of healthy foods representing five major food groups: fruits, grains, proteins, vegetables, and dairy products.[1]

We'll illustrate steps you can take to make healthier food choices as we discuss the basic nutrients: proteins, carbohydrates, fats, vitamins, minerals, and water and electrolytes.

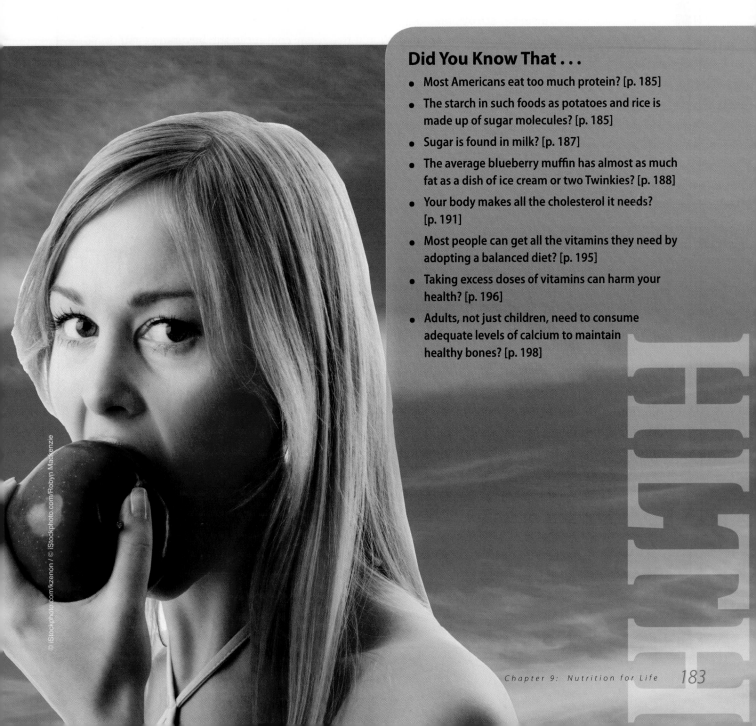

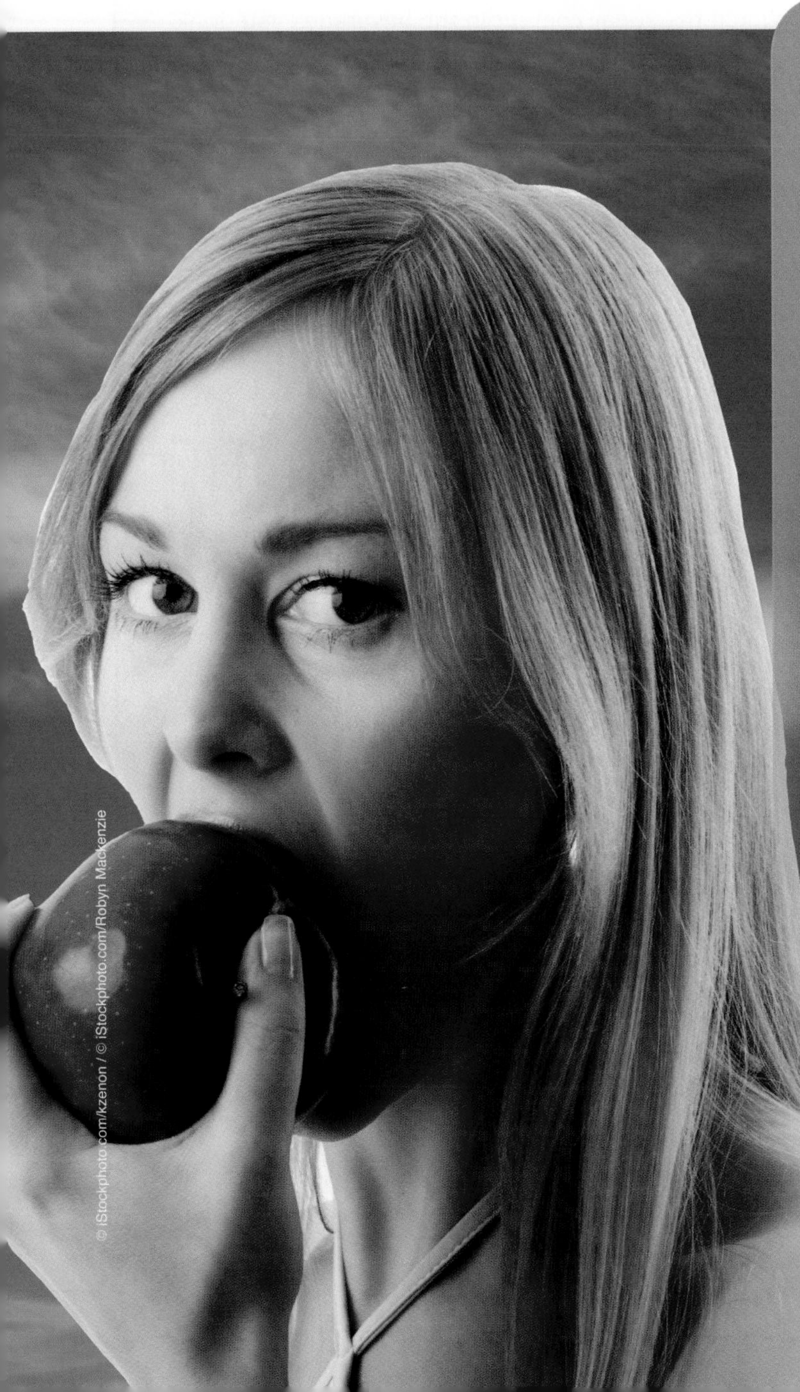

© iStockphoto.com/kzenon / © iStockphoto.com/Robyn Mackenzie

Did You Know That . . .

- **Most Americans eat too much protein? [p. 185]**
- **The starch in such foods as potatoes and rice is made up of sugar molecules? [p. 185]**
- **Sugar is found in milk? [p. 187]**
- **The average blueberry muffin has almost as much fat as a dish of ice cream or two Twinkies? [p. 188]**
- **Your body makes all the cholesterol it needs? [p. 191]**
- **Most people can get all the vitamins they need by adopting a balanced diet? [p. 195]**
- **Taking excess doses of vitamins can harm your health? [p. 196]**
- **Adults, not just children, need to consume adequate levels of calcium to maintain healthy bones? [p. 198]**

health skills

Tips for Eating Right from the *Dietary Guidelines for Americans*

Here are some tips from the guidelines to help Americans adopt healthier eating habits:

- *Enjoy your food, but eat less.* Americans are consuming too many calories, which contributes to the nation's expanding waistline.
- *Avoid oversized portions.* Avoid piling on food or supersizing menu choices.
- *Switch to fat-free or low-fat (1%) milk.* Making the switch can help you keep your fat intake at a healthy level.
- *Compare sodium in foods like soup, bread, and frozen meals—and choose the foods with lower numbers.* Most Americans consume too much sodium, which can raise their risks of cardiovascular disease, stroke, and kidney diseases.
- *Drink water instead of sugary beverages.* Watch the sugar content in the beverages you drink as well as the foods you eat.
- *Cover half your plate with vegetables and fruits at meal time.* Rebalance your portions to increase plant sources of nutrients and whole grains. Whole grains should comprise more than half of all grains consumed.
- *Choose a variety of vegetables, especially dark-green and red and orange vegetables and beans and peas.*
- *Substitute a variety of seafood in place of some meat and poultry choices.*

Sources: *The 2010 dietary guidelines for Americans.* (2011, January 31). U.S. Department of Agriculture; *USDA and HHS announce new dietary guidelines to help Americans make healthier food choices and confront obesity epidemic,* [Press release]. (2011, January 31). USDA Office of Communications; and *Dietary guidelines for Americans 2010: Executive summary.* (2011, January 31). U.S. Department of Agriculture.

Figure 9-1 MyPlate: Are You Filling Your Plate with Healthy Food Choices?

Plan your meals to fill half your plate with fruits and vegetables.

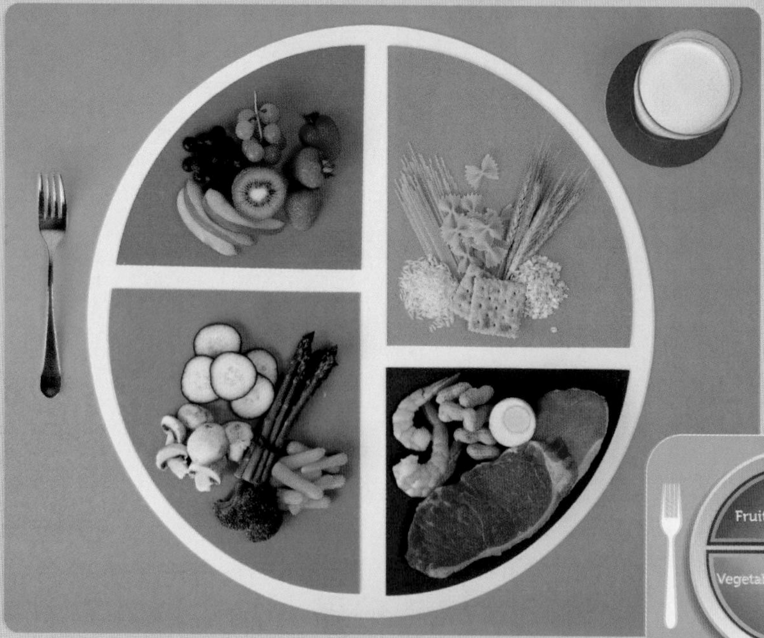

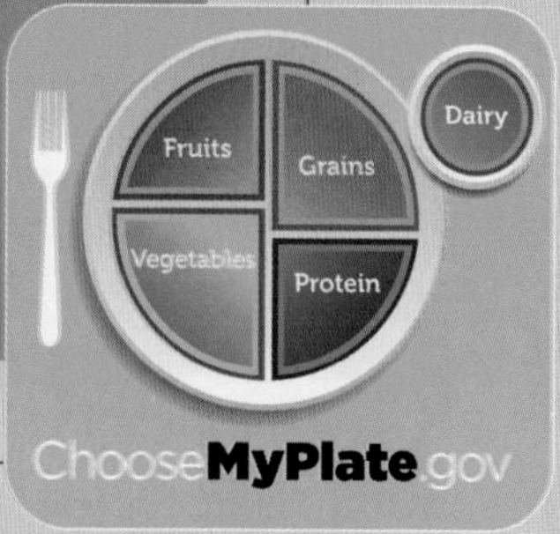

Source: Icon at right reprinted from choosemyplate.gov, U.S. Department of Agriculture, June 2011.

Proteins

Proteins are organic molecules that form the basic building blocks of muscle, bone, hair, blood, fingernails, antibodies, enzymes, hormones, and other body tissues. Proteins are composed of 22 different **amino acids**, 13 of which the body produces by itself. The other nine must be obtained from food or dietary supplements. These nine are called **essential amino acids** because they are vital to our survival.

LEARNING OUTCOME 2

Describe the functions and sources of proteins

With proteins, variety is key. The principal sources of dietary protein are meat (beef, pork, poultry, and fish) and dairy products (eggs, milk, and cheese). Some vegetables, such as legumes (beans, chickpeas, and lentils) and grains, are also rich sources of protein. We get about two-thirds of our protein from animal sources; the rest comes from a combination of grains, beans, and other sources.

Most Americans consume more than enough protein in their diets. Excess protein is converted into body fat. Protein deficiencies are rare in the United States. They are most commonly seen among children in impoverished countries. The physical signs of protein deficiency include stunted growth, poor muscle development, swelling, skin lesions, and thin, fragile hair.

Carbohydrates

Carbohydrates ("carbs") furnish the body with energy and give bulk to food. There are complex and simple carbohydrates. **Complex carbohydrates** include starches and fibers. **Simple carbohydrates** include sugars. They are the major sources of energy in our diet.

LEARNING OUTCOME 3

Describe the functions, types, and sources of carbohydrates

Starches

A **starch** is actually a chain of sugar molecules. Common table sugar, by contrast, is made up of only one or two sugar molecules. Starch is the form in which sugar (glucose) is stored in plant material. Because of its chemical composition, starch provides a steadier flow of energy than dietary sugar, which provides a quick spurt of energy but little else of nutritional value. Starchy vegetables such as potatoes, corn, green peas, and dry beans are abundant sources of energy. They are low in fat and calories. A **calorie** is a measure of the energy content of food. Calories that are not consumed ("burned-off") by the body through bodily processes and physical activity are converted into body fat. It's the sour cream or butter that people spread on baked potatoes and the sauces they ladle over pastas that add excess calories, not the starches themselves. Starches are also rich in vitamins and minerals, and some starches are also good sources of fiber (see Table 9-1 on the next page).

Nutritionists recommend that about half of our daily diet consists of complex carbohydrates. Complex carbohydrates are found in breads and cereals; crucifers such as broccoli, cauliflower, and cabbage; citrus fruits; green leafy vegetables (spinach, romaine lettuce, broccoli); legumes; pasta; root vegetables (potatoes and yams); and orange fruits and vegetables (squash, sweet potatoes, and carrots).

Dietary Fiber

Dietary fiber consists of complex carbohydrates found in the structural parts of plants, such as cellulose and pectin, which cannot be broken down by human digestive enzymes. However, some forms of dietary fiber are broken down by bacteria in the digestive tract and converted into fat that the body absorbs, providing a small amount of energy. But

protein
Organic molecule that forms the basic building blocks of body tissues.

amino acids
Organic compounds that are the building blocks from which proteins are made.

essential amino acids
Amino acids essential to survival that must be obtained from the food we eat since the body is unable to manufacture them on its own.

carbohydrates
Organic compounds forming the structural parts of plants that are important sources of nutrition for animals and humans.

complex carbohydrates
A class of carbohydrates that includes starches and fibers.

simple carbohydrates
A class of carbohydrates consisting of small molecules, including various sugars.

starch
A complex carbohydrate that forms an important part of the structure of plants such as corn, rice, wheat, potatoes, and beans.

calorie
A measure of food energy, which is equivalent to the amount of energy required to raise the temperature of one gram of water by one degree Celsius.

dietary fiber
Complex carbohydrates that form the structural parts of plants, such as cellulose and pectin, that cannot be broken down by human digestive enzymes.

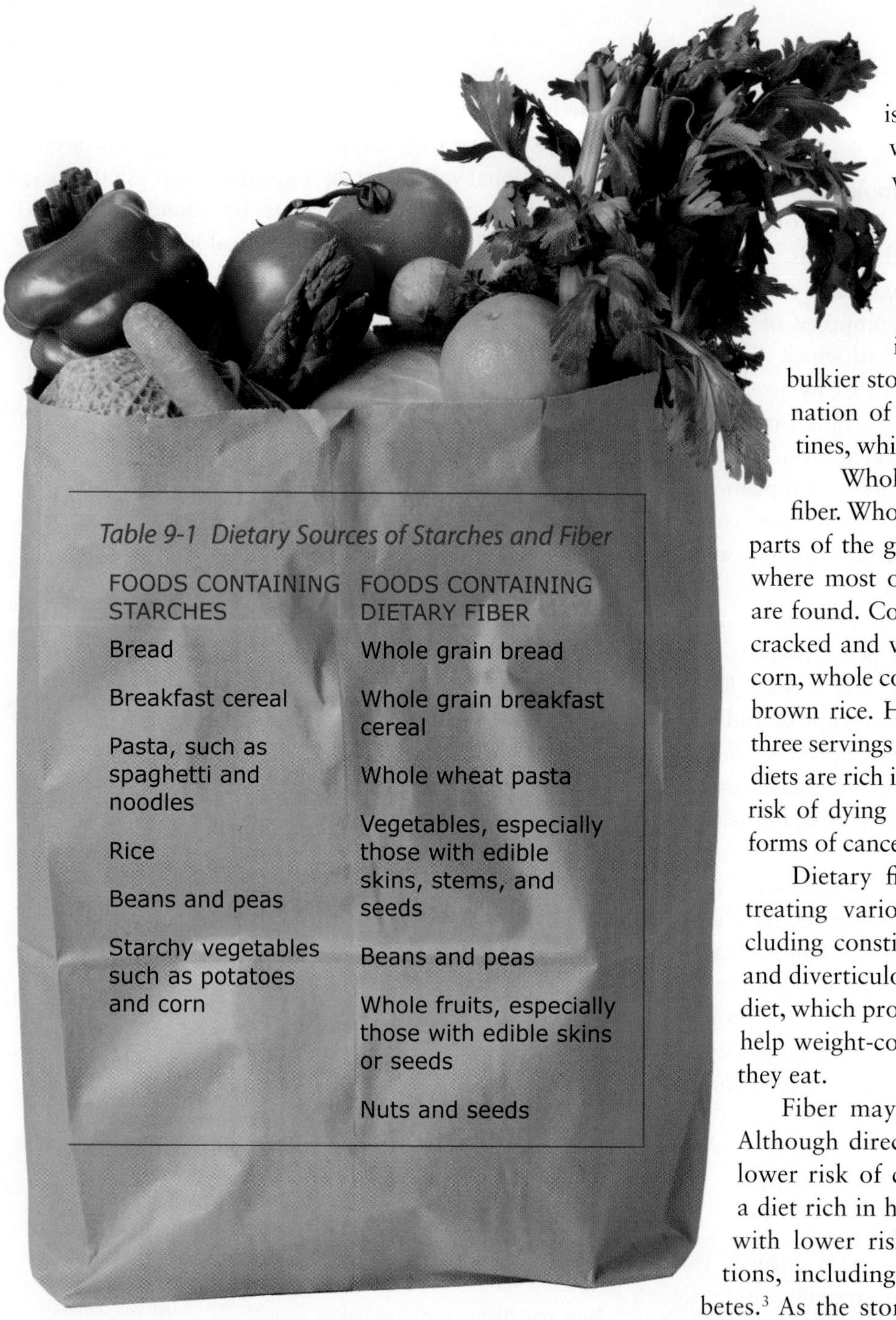

© iStockphoto.com/ginosphotos

Table 9-1 Dietary Sources of Starches and Fiber

FOODS CONTAINING STARCHES	FOODS CONTAINING DIETARY FIBER
Bread	Whole grain bread
Breakfast cereal	Whole grain breakfast cereal
Pasta, such as spaghetti and noodles	Whole wheat pasta
Rice	Vegetables, especially those with edible skins, stems, and seeds
Beans and peas	
Starchy vegetables such as potatoes and corn	Beans and peas
	Whole fruits, especially those with edible skins or seeds
	Nuts and seeds

most fiber passes through the digestive tract unchanged, giving bulk to the stool.

Different types and amounts of dietary fiber are found in various plant foods, such as vegetables and grains. Fibers that are readily dissolvable in water are called **soluble fibers**. Those that are not are called **insoluble fibers**. Soluble fiber is found in many fruits and vegetables, beans, and grains such as oats and barley. Insoluble fiber is found mostly in dark-green leafy vegetables, in the skins of fruits and vegetables, and in the bran (outer layer) of wheat and corn. Different types of fiber have different health benefits. Soluble fiber helps reduce blood cholesterol levels, while insoluble fiber produces softer, bulkier stools and promotes more rapid elimination of waste products through the intestines, which increases regularity.

soluble fiber
A type of dietary fiber that is dissolvable in water.

insoluble fiber
Type of dietary fiber that is not dissolvable in water.

Whole grains are rich sources of dietary fiber. Whole grains consist of the entire edible parts of the grain, including the bran and germ, where most of the fiber, vitamins, and minerals are found. Common sources of whole grains are cracked and whole wheat, bulgur, oatmeal, popcorn, whole cornmeal and ryes, scotch barley, and brown rice. Health officials recommend at least three servings of whole grains daily. People whose diets are rich in whole grains tend to have a lower risk of dying from both heart disease and some forms of cancer.[2]

Dietary fiber is helpful in preventing and treating various gastrointestinal problems, including constipation, irritable bowel syndrome, and diverticulosis. Fiber also provides bulk in the diet, which produces a feeling of fullness that may help weight-conscious people control how much they eat.

Fiber may also have other health benefits. Although direct links between dietary fiber and lower risk of cancer have not been established, a diet rich in high-fiber plant foods is associated with lower risk of other serious health conditions, including cardiovascular disease and diabetes.[3] As the story of the health effects of dietary fiber continues to be written, it makes good health sense to follow a diet with plentiful amounts of fiber-rich foods, such as fruits and vegetables, legumes, and whole grain cereals.

Many health experts recommend that we consume 20 to 35 grams of dietary fiber a day, although only about half of Americans consume more than 10 grams. On the other hand, some eat too much. Excessive dietary fiber can interfere with the absorption of minerals. Note, too, that fiber pills and supplements lack nutritional components found in food sources of fiber, so they are not adequate substitutes. Table 9-2 lists foods that can boost your fiber intake.

Table 9-2 High-Fiber Foods and Grams of Dietary Fiber Provided

FRUITS	BREADS	GRAINS	LEGUMES	VEGETABLES
Apple with skin, 1 medium: **3 g**	Whole wheat, rye, or pumpernickel, 1 slice: **1 to 2 g**	Brown rice, ½ cup: **2 g**	Cooked dried beans (kidney, pinto, black, northern, navy), ½ cup: **6 g**	Canned corn, ½ cup: **3 g**
Banana, 1 medium: **2 g**	Muffin (bran, oat, corn), 1: **1 to 2 g**	Wild rice, ½ cup: **4 g**	Cooked dried peas, ½ cup: **4 g**	Broccoli, brussels sprouts, carrots, parsnips, spinach, ½ cup: **2 g**
Strawberries, 1 cup: **3 g**	Triscuits or Rye Krisp, 3: **3 g**	Barley, whole grain, ½ cup: **2 g**	Cooked lentils, ½ cup: **4 g**	Potato with skin, 1 medium: **2 g**
Pear with skin, ½ large: **3 g**	Whole wheat English muffin, 1: **2 to 4 g**	Whole wheat pasta, ½ cup: **2 g**	Cooked lima beans, ½ cup: **4 g**	
Prunes, 3: **3 g**	Corn tortilla, 1 small: **1 to 2 g**	Bulgur, ½ cup: **3 g**		
Raisins, ¼ cup: **3 g**	Whole wheat bagel, 1 small: **1 to 2 g**			
Raspberries, ½ cup: **3 g**				
Blueberries, ½ cup: **2 g**				
Orange, 1 medium: **2 g**				

Source: Adapted from American Cancer Society, *Eating Smart* (No. 87-250M-Rev 3/89-No. 2042).

Note: Dietary fiber is found only in foods of plant origin. Since the outer layer of fruits, vegetables, and grains is highest in fiber, leave the skin on your fruits and vegetables. Also, look for breakfast cereals that are high in fiber, such as all-bran cereals.

Sugars

We use table **sugar**, or *sucrose*, to prepare and sweeten foods and beverages. Other sugars occur naturally in a wide variety of foods, including fruits, vegetables, and milk. *Lactose* is the form of sugar found in milk and milk products; *maltose* is found in legumes and cereals; and *glucose* and *fructose* are found in honey and fruits, respectively.

Sugars provide energy but are of little other nutritional value. Consuming large amounts of sugar may satisfy your hunger and keep you from eating other foods that are richer in the nutrients your body requires, such as vitamins and minerals. Sugar also adds excess calories that can be converted into body fat and lead to overweight. Sugar contributes to tooth decay as well. It's not just the amount of sugar you consume that causes tooth decay, but also the form of sugar. Sugary foods that are chewy or sticky tend to stay on the teeth longer, thereby increasing the potential for decay. Sugary foods eaten between meals are also more likely to lead to decay than those consumed at mealtime.

Most of us are aware of table sugar, the most obvious form of sugar. Other forms of sugar, such as syrup, honey, and molasses, may be less obvious. Still less obvious are the sugars found in fruits and in many processed foods and baked goods.

On the whole, Americans consume too much sugar. You can cut back by making the following changes in your diet:

- Use table sugar, syrup, honey, and molasses sparingly if at all.
- Avoid drinking sugared soft drinks. The average 12-ounce can of cola contains a whopping nine teaspoons of sugar.
- If you buy canned fruit, buy fruit packed in water or juice, not in heavy syrup.
- Limit consumption of baked goods, candies, and sweet desserts.
- Use seasonings and spices when cooking and preparing food, rather than sugar. Experiment with cinnamon, ginger, nutmeg, and other spices.
- Select fruit juice rather than fruit drinks, which typically have added sugar besides the natural sugar found in the juice. Better yet, eat fresh fruits; fruit juices are higher in natural sugars.

Table 9-3 on the next page lists the amounts of added sugar in some commonly eaten foods.

sugar
A sweet-tasting simple carbohydrate, present in different forms in many of the foods we eat.

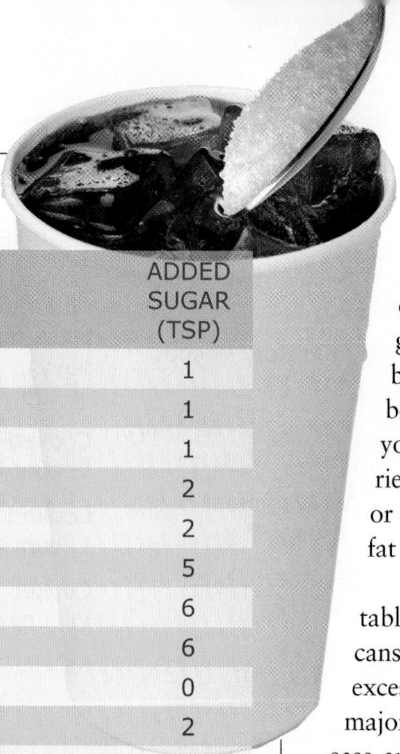

Table 9-3 Added Sugar in Common Foods

FOOD	ADDED SUGAR (TSP)
Muffin, 1 medium	1
Cookies, 2 medium	1
Danish pastry, 1 medium	1
Doughnut, 1 medium	2
Pound cake, no-fat, 1 oz	2
Angel food cake, 1/12 of cake	5
Cake, frosted, 1/16 of cake	6
Pie, fruit, 2-crust, 1/6 of pie	6
Fruit, canned in juice, 4 oz	0
Fruit, canned in light syrup, 4 oz	2
Fruit, canned in heavy syrup, 4 oz	4
Chocolate milk, 2%, 8 oz	3
Low-fat yogurt, plain, 8 oz	0
Low-fat yogurt, fruit, 8 oz	5
Ice cream, ice milk, or frozen yogurt, 4 oz	7
Chocolate shake, 10 oz	3
Syrup or honey, 1 tbsp	3
Chocolate bar, 1 oz	3
Fruit sorbet, 4 oz	3
Gelatin dessert, 4 oz	4
Sherbet, 4 oz	5
Cola, 12 oz	9
Fruit drink, 12 oz	12

Source: United States Department of Agriculture

Note: Four grams of sugar = one teaspoon (tsp).

Fats

Although the word *fat* is usually connected with all things negative, moderate amounts of **fats** are not bad for you. They play essential roles in the body: They nourish the skin, aid in the absorption of certain vitamins, help form cell membranes and hormones, help provide stamina, and insulate the body from extremes of temperature.

fat
Organic compound that forms the basis of fatty tissue of animals, including humans ("body fat"), and is also found in some plant materials.

LEARNING OUTCOME 4

Describe the functions of fats and health implications of excess fat intake

Fats are the most concentrated sources of food energy, or *calories*, in our diet. Each gram of fat packs more than twice the number of calories as each gram of protein or carbohydrate (see Table 9-4). Ounce for ounce, you consume more than twice as many calories by eating fats as you do by eating proteins or carbohydrates. People who consume a high-fat diet often become overweight.

All the fat you need amounts to about one tablespoon of vegetable oil daily. Most Americans face the opposite concern—consuming excessive amounts of fat. A high-fat diet is a major culprit in the two leading killers, heart disease and cancer. Eating less fat can lower the risk of heart disease and certain types of cancer, such as colorectal cancer and prostate cancer.

The list of high-fat foods includes cakes and cookies; fatty cuts of beef; poultry skin; lamb and pork products; dairy foods such as whole milk, sour cream, mayonnaise, cheese, yogurt, butter, and ice cream; nuts and seeds; lard and shortening used in cooking; vegetable oils used in cooking; margarine; and salad dressings. High-fat foods are tempting because fats absorb and retain the natural tastes of foods, enhancing their flavor.

Some sources of fat are highly visible, such as the "marbling" in steak, but most fat is not so obvious. For example, the blueberry muffin you pick up on the way to class or work contains a whopping 34 grams of fat, almost as much as a dish of ice cream or two Twinkies. People who are watching their weight may make the mistake of ordering a Caesar salad for lunch, thinking it is a healthier alternative. However, the dressing and cheese load their blood with 38 grams of fat—more fat than in an average burger and fries.

Confused about the fat values of the foods you eat? Check the fat content on the nutritional labels that appear on the side panels of containers of packaged

Table 9-4 Calories per Gram of Basic Nutrients

NUTRIENT	CALORIES PER GRAM
Proteins	4
Carbohydrates	4
Fats	9

Note: Calorie values are approximate.

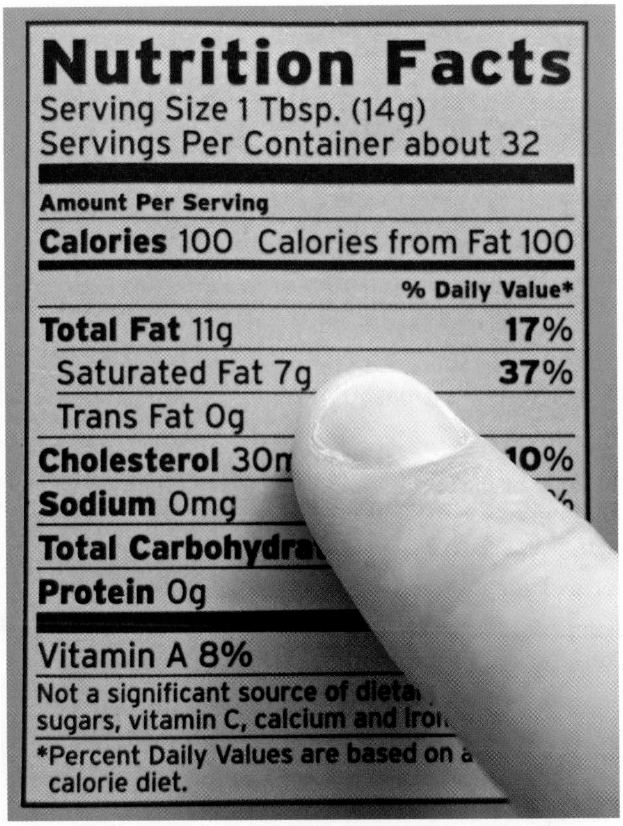

Nutrition Facts

Serving Size 1 Tbsp. (14g)
Servings Per Container about 32

Amount Per Serving

Calories 100 Calories from Fat 100

	% Daily Value*
Total Fat 11g	17%
Saturated Fat 7g	37%
Trans Fat 0g	
Cholesterol 30m...	10%
Sodium 0mg	%
Total Carbohydra...	
Protein 0g	

Vitamin A 8%

Not a significant source of dieta...
sugars, vitamin C, calcium and iron.

*Percent Daily Values are based on a ...
calorie diet.

and prepared foods. Substitute low-fat alternatives. A bagel, for instance, has but a fraction of the fat of a blueberry or raisin bran muffin. Preparing a salad without egg and cheese and skimping on the dressing brings the fat content way down. Don't mistake low fat for low calories. Some low-fat or even no-fat snack foods are loaded with calories, largely because of added sugar. For foods without food labels, use a diet guide that lists the fat content (along with the calories).

How Much Fat Should You Consume?

Health officials recommend that adults limit their total fat intake to between 20% and 35% of daily calorie consumption, and their saturated fat intake to less than 10% of calories consumed. To figure out your total fat limit, take the number of calories you consume daily and multiply that figure for total fat intake by 0.20 (20%) or 0.35 (35%) (depending on whether you choose the lower or higher end of the range) or 0.10 (10%) for saturated fat intake. Then divide by nine (one gram of fat contains nine calories). The result equals the recommended maximum number of grams of fat you should consume daily. Table 9-5 provides a quick conversion table for selected calorie levels. "Health Check 9-1" on page 192 will help you further evaluate the fat content of your diet.

Types of Fat

Fat consists of chemicals called *fatty acids*. Different kinds of dietary fat contain various amounts and kinds of fatty acids. There are three types of fatty acids: *saturated*, *monounsaturated*, and *polyunsaturated*. Each type differs in the amount of hydrogen it contains. Saturated fatty acids contain the most hydrogen, and polyunsaturated fats contain the least. Monounsaturated and polyunsaturated fats are also referred to as *unsaturated fats*. The greater the proportion of saturated fat, the harder the food product is at room temperature. Most saturated fats are solid at room temperature; these include butter, meat fat, cheese, and tropical oils such as coconut and palm oil.

The kinds of fatty acids have important health implications. The body converts dietary sources of fat into blood **cholesterol**, the fatlike substance that can clog arteries and lead to heart disease and strokes. The greater the proportion of saturated fat in a food, the greater the risk that fat will raise blood cholesterol levels. Consumption of high levels of saturated fat, typically from red meat and dairy products, increases risks of cardiovascular disease and certain types of cancer, such as colon and rectal cancer.[4] How much is too much? Investigators link higher colorectal

cholesterol
A natural, fat-like substance found in humans and animals.

Table 9-5 *Amount of Fat that Provides 30% of Calories at Indicated Calorie Levels*

CALORIES PER DAY IN THE DIET	SATURATED FAT DAILY LIMIT < 10% OF CALORIES CONSUMED	TOTAL FAT DAILY LIMIT: 20%/35% OF CALORIES CONSUMED
	Grams of fat	*Grams of fat*
1,500	16	33/58
2,000	22	44/77
2,500	27	55/97
3,000	33	66/116

Note: Grams of fat are rounded down.

PREVENTION 9-1

Vegetarianism: Does It Prevent Disease?

Vegetarianism is increasingly popular. Vegetarians exclude all or some types of meat and animal products from their diets. Some people adopt a vegetarian diet for moral reasons; they believe killing animals is wrong. Others view vegetarianism as a healthy alternative to the typical high-fat, meat-based American diet.

Following are types of vegetarians:

- A *vegan* follows a total vegetarian diet consisting only of plant foods and avoids all animal products, including dairy foods and eggs, as well as honey.
- A *lacto-ovo-vegetarian* eats dairy products and eggs as well as plant foods such as grains, fruits, vegetables, legumes, nuts, and seeds, but excludes meat, fish, and poultry.
- A *partial vegetarian* follows a diet composed of plant foods, dairy products, eggs, and some animal products, such as fish and perhaps chicken, but no red meat or pork.

Since protein is generally less plentiful in vegetables than in animals, vegetarians must be especially careful to obtain enough protein and other essential nutrients from vegetable sources.

Fruits and vegetables contain plant chemicals that may lower the risk of certain cancers, such as colorectal cancer. The question remains whether vegetarianism is healthier than alternative low-fat diets in which meat consumption is pared down but not eliminated. Vegetarians tend to be thinner and to have lower blood pressures than nonvegetarians, and excess body weight and hypertension does figure prominently in major health concerns such as cardiovascular disease.[5] Yet vegetarianism alone may not explain these differences, because vegetarians may differ from other people with respect to other healthy habits or even genetic factors that play a role in food preferences. Even so, people who don't adopt a vegetarian diet can benefit by eating ample portions of fruits and vegetables and reducing the level of fat in their diet.

cancer risk to daily consumption of at least three ounces or more for men (about one large fast-food hamburger) and two ounces or more for women over a period of 10 years. Regular consumption of processed meat, such as bologna and bacon, also increases the risk of colorectal cancer. The U.S. government recommends limiting saturated fat in the diet to less than 10% of total daily calorie intake.[6]

Health concerns about the risks posed by saturated fat have led millions of Americans to reduce their fat intake and switch from foods high in saturated fat to those containing mostly monounsaturated or polyunsaturated fats. Many Americans also follow vegetarian diets as an alternative to high-fat meat-laden diets (see "Prevention 9-1").

Table 9-6 offers suggestions for selecting leaner cuts of meat. Trim visible fat from meat before cooking or eating it. Many people have switched from butter to low-fat margarine and from whole milk to low-fat (1%) or skim milk. Butter consumption dropped dramatically as Americans came to understand that the unsaturated fats in margarine are a healthier choice than the saturated fats contained in butter. That being said, margarines may contain another unhealthy substance, as we discuss next.

Table 9-6 The Really Choice Cut: Leaner Is Better

FOOD	LEAN CUTS
Beef	Roasts/steaks: round, loin, sirloin, chuck, arm
Pork	Roasts/chops: tenderloin, center loin, ham
Veal	All cuts except ground
Lamb	Roasts/chops: leg, loin, foreshanks
Chicken and turkey	Light and dark meat, without the skin
Venison	Venison is very lean meat, and includes deer meat, elk meat, and moose meat
Fish and shellfish	Most are low in fat; those marinated or canned in oil are higher

Is Margarine Always the Healthier Choice?

Some forms of margarine and many processed foods contain an unhealthy type of fatty acid called **trans-fatty acids**. Trans-fatty acids (called *trans fat* for short) raise blood cholesterol levels at least as much as the saturated fatty acids found in butter. Trans fat is produced during the process of *hydrogenation*, which transforms liquid vegetable oils into the familiar hardened form of margarine that is shaped into sticks, as well as into Crisco-type vegetable shortening. Trans fat is also found in many processed foods, such as cookies.

It makes sense to limit your use of hydrogenated margarines in stick or tub forms, or to use squeezable liquid margarine instead. Also, limit consumption of processed foods that contain partially hydrogenated vegetable oil (check the list of ingredients on the food label). Store shelves are now stocked with snack foods that are free of trans fat, but the french fries, fried chicken, and many other dishes served at restaurants are still loaded with it.

Vegetable Oils

The vegetable oils used in salad dressings and cooking contain various proportions of saturated, monounsaturated, and polyunsaturated fats. Some vegetable oils, such as coconut and palm oil, are high in saturated fat, whereas others consist of predominantly monounsaturated fats (olive, canola, peanut, walnut, and avocado oils) or polyunsaturated fats (soybean, corn, safflower, sunflower, and cottonseed oils).

The oil that has long given Italian cooking its distinctive flavor—olive oil—has gained in popularity as more people have become aware of the need to reduce their consumption of saturated fat. Canola oil contains the least saturated fat of any oil. Its light flavor makes it a good choice in baked goods (olive or peanut oil may overpower the taste of bakery items) as well as in salad dressings and sauces.

Nevertheless, we shouldn't think of vegetable oils as health foods. All vegetable oils are 100% fat. Polyunsaturated and monounsaturated fats may be less unhealthy than saturated fats, but you should limit fats in general.[7]

How much fat is in your diet? "Health Check 9-1" on the next page will help you examine your own eating patterns. If you find that you have a high fat intake, the online feature "Health Skills 9-2" offers suggestions for cutting fat from your diet. While online, check out "Diversity 9-1" for suggestions on making healthy choices when enjoying food from other countries and cultures.

health skills

Access CourseMate for HLTH at www.cengagebrain.com.

diversity

Access CourseMate for HLTH at www.cengagebrain.com.

Cholesterol

Few words have become as strongly linked to the public's perception of health risks as *cholesterol*. Just what is cholesterol? Is it bad for us?

Cholesterol is a natural, fatlike substance in the body cells of humans and animals. The body uses cholesterol to produce hormones and cell membranes. Cholesterol is found in the lean and the fat of meat and in animal by-products, such as eggs, cheese, and milk. Organ meats such as liver and kidneys contain the highest concentrations of dietary cholesterol (see Figure 9-2 on the next page). One egg yolk contains about 10 times the amount of cholesterol found in one ounce of meat, poultry, or fish. (But research is mixed concerning the harmfulness of egg yolks.[8]) Cholesterol is not found in foods derived from plants, such as fruits and vegetables, grains, seeds, nuts, peas, and beans.

Our bodies make all the cholesterol they need. We do not need to consume additional cholesterol, but since there is cholesterol in all animal tissue, including meat, poultry, dairy products, shellfish, and in lesser amounts, fish, we may take in far more cholesterol than we can possibly use, increasing the level of cholesterol in our blood. The body also converts dietary fat into blood cholesterol. Excess blood cholesterol can result in the formation of fatty deposits on artery walls, impeding the flow of blood and increasing the risk of heart attacks and strokes. Blood cholesterol is usually considered high when it exceeds 200 to 240 milligrams per deciliter of blood.

Did you know that there are two types of cholesterol and that one of them is actually good for you? The culprit in clogging arteries is the so-called "bad" form of cholesterol, **low-density lipoprotein (LDL)**. A **lipoprotein** is a cluster of fat

trans-fatty acid
A type of fatty acid produced in the hardening process of margarine that can raise blood cholesterol levels.

low-density lipoprotein (LDL)
The so-called bad cholesterol because it can stick to artery walls, forming fatty deposits that restrict the flow of blood to vital body organs, setting the stage for heart attacks and strokes.

lipoprotein
A compound or complex of fat and protein by which fats are transported through the bloodstream.

HEALTH CHECK 9-1

How Much Fat Is in Your Diet?

Do the foods you eat provide more fat than is good for you? Answer the following questions, and then see how your diet stacks up.

HOW OFTEN DO YOU EAT:	SELDOM OR NEVER	1 OR 2 TIMES A WEEK	3 OR 4 TIMES A WEEK	ALMOST DAILY
Fried, deep-fat-fried, or breaded foods?				
Fatty meats such as bacon, sausage, luncheon meats, and heavily marbled steaks and roasts?				
Whole milk, high-fat cheeses, and ice cream?				
High-fat desserts such as pies, pastries, and rich cakes?				
Rich sauces and gravies?				
Oily salad dressings or mayonnaise?				
Whipped cream, table cream, sour cream, and cream cheese?				
Butter or margarine on vegetables, dinner rolls, and toast?				

Consider your answers. If several of your answers appear in the last two columns of this table, you may have a high fat intake. Is it time to cut back on foods high in fat?

Source: United States Department of Agriculture, Human Nutrition Information Service.

and protein that serves as a vehicle for transporting fats through the bloodstream. The other type of cholesterol, **high-density lipoprotein (HDL)**, is dubbed "good" cholesterol because it clears away cholesterol deposits from artery walls, bringing them to the liver, where they are processed and then excreted from the body. HDL helps lower the risk of cardiovascular disease.

Consuming saturated fat, trans fat, and dietary cholesterol raises the levels of "bad" (LDL) cholesterol, which in turn increases the risk of coronary heart disease (CHD). We can control how much fat and cholesterol we consume. Reducing dietary fat and cholesterol can reduce our risk of developing CHD.

Dietary cholesterol and saturated fat are often confused because both substances can increase blood cholesterol, especially harmful LDL. Some foods, such as red meat, are rich in both fat and

high-density lipoprotein (HDL) *The so-called good cholesterol because it sweeps away cholesterol deposits from artery walls for elimination from the body, thereby lowering the risk of cardiovascular disease.*

Figure 9-2 Cholesterol Content of Some Common Foods

Some of the highest amounts of cholesterol are found in organ meats, such as liver, and in egg yolks. Meat and dairy products contain significant but lesser amounts.

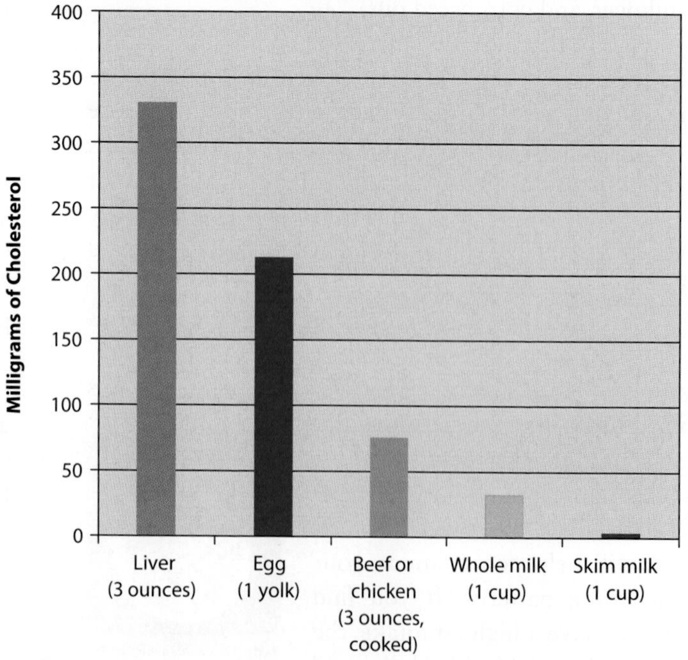

cholesterol. Eggs and organ meats are high in cholesterol but contain only moderate amounts of fat. Certain foods derived from plant materials, such as palm or coconut oil and peanut butter, have high levels of saturated fat but no cholesterol. Health officials recommend limiting intake of foods rich in cholesterol, total fat, and saturated fat. The U.S. government recommends limiting dietary cholesterol to less than 300 milligrams per day. To reduce cholesterol in your diet, you might start by becoming aware of the cholesterol content of foods in your diet and reducing your intake of cholesterol-rich foods (see Table 9-7).

Limiting the amount of meat and egg yolks you consume reduces your cholesterol intake. The yolk of a large egg contains about 214 milligrams of cholesterol. Also, reduce the size of your meat portions and substitute vegetable sources of protein several times a week. Switch to low-cholesterol products (the cholesterol contents are clearly labeled on packaging). Limit the number of egg yolks you use when preparing scrambled eggs or other dishes, or substitute egg whites whenever possible. Or skip egg dishes altogether. Be aware of hidden sources of cholesterol, such as cakes and muffins that are prepared with egg yolks or lard. Substitute grain products or popcorn when snacking.

Table 9-7 lists common foods high in cholesterol and saturated fats, along with some healthful alternatives. (For more tips, turn the page and read "Health Skills 9-3.")

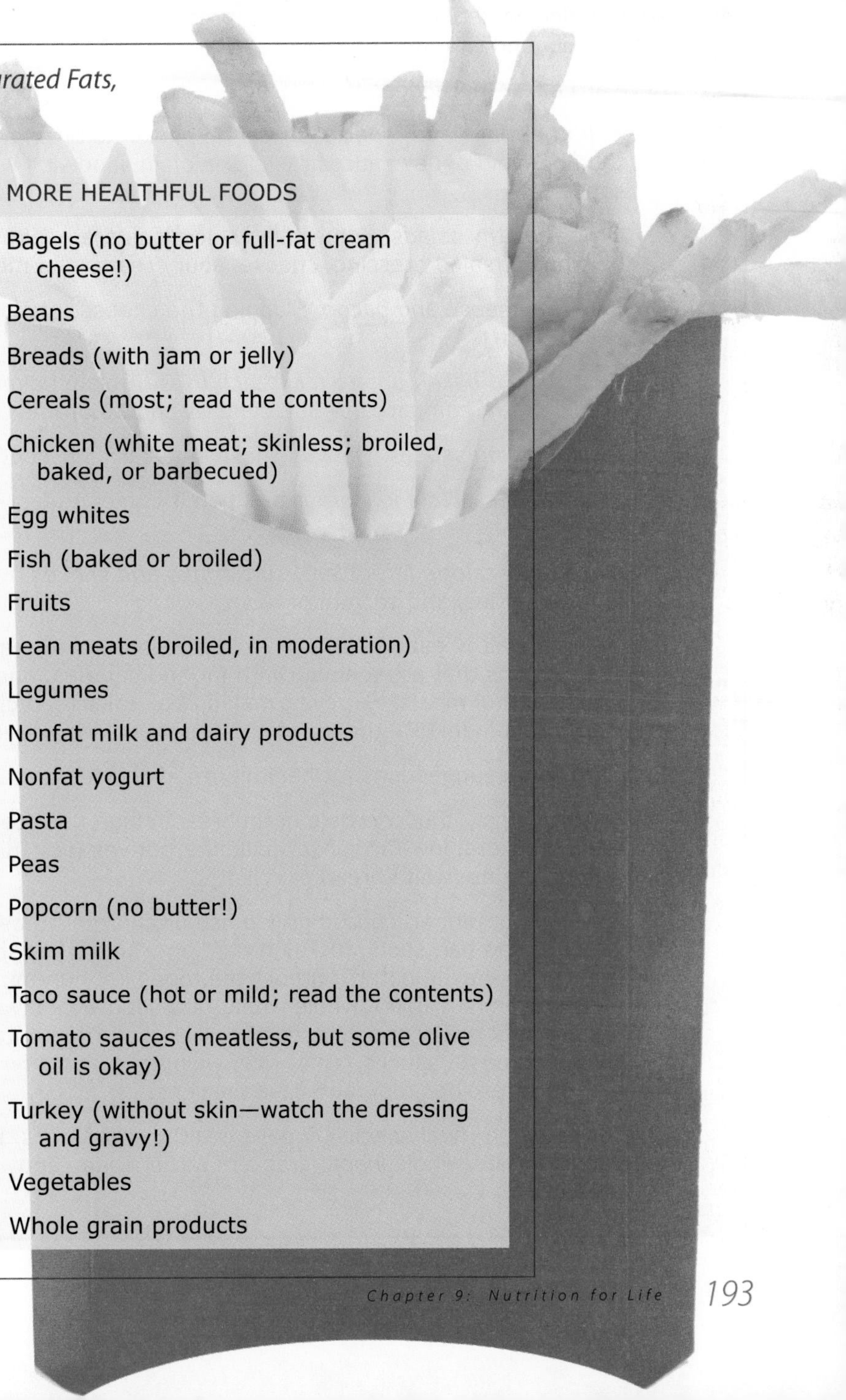

Table 9-7 Foods High in Cholesterol and Saturated Fats, and More Healthful Food Alternativies

FOODS HIGH IN CHOLESTEROL AND/OR SATURATED FATS	MORE HEALTHFUL FOODS
Bacon, sausage	Bagels (no butter or full-fat cream cheese!)
Beef	Beans
Butter, lard	Breads (with jam or jelly)
Cake	Cereals (most; read the contents)
Cheese (look for fat-free or low-fat cheeses)	Chicken (white meat; skinless; broiled, baked, or barbecued)
Crab	Egg whites
Cream	Fish (baked or broiled)
Croissants	Fruits
Eggs (yolks)	Lean meats (broiled, in moderation)
Frankfurters and luncheon meats	Legumes
French fries	Nonfat milk and dairy products
Fried foods	Nonfat yogurt
Ice cream (look for no-fat ice cream)	Pasta
Lobster	Peas
Organ meats (liver, kidneys, etc.)	Popcorn (no butter!)
Palm oil	Skim milk
Pie	Taco sauce (hot or mild; read the contents)
Potato chips	Tomato sauces (meatless, but some olive oil is okay)
Salad dressing (most; some olive oil is okay)	Turkey (without skin—watch the dressing and gravy!)
Whole milk	Vegetables
	Whole grain products

HEALTH SKILLS 9-3

Eating Fast Foods and Campus Foods the Healthy Way

You probably live or work no more than a few miles from a fast-food restaurant, and where there's one, there are usually others. We all know the arguments against fast food: It's high in calories, high in fat, and low in nutrition. But is it possible for fast food to be good for you, not just good tasting? The answer is a surprising yes—but only if you watch what you order.

Among the choices that are lowest in calories and fat are the basic hamburgers from any of the large chains. Although the meat isn't lean, the average hamburger contains only about 2 ounces of beef, which keeps down the fat and calorie content. Some people order fish or chicken in the belief that they are lower in fat and calories than the hamburger. It is true that grilled chicken sandwiches are among the healthiest choices, but breaded or fried chicken or fish, and chicken with skin, are typically loaded with fat and calories.

Here are a few more ideas for making healthier food choices:

- *Hold the mayo and "special sauce."* "Special" is often a euphemism for "high fat." As a rule of thumb, avoid gooey sauces. Ask for a plain sandwich with no sauce. Or use ketchup or a low-fat sauce.
- *Order healthy salads.* Some salad selections are healthy choices, but others contain heaping helpings of salad dressing, cheese, sour cream, and meat that add calories, fat, and sodium.
- *Skip the cheese and bacon.* Skipping the cheese, mayo, and bacon will save you calories, fat, and sodium.
- *Substitute a baked potato for french fries.* A plain baked potato has about 200 calories and 0 grams of fat, compared to 500 calories and 20 grams of fat for a large order of french fries.
- *Avoid dipping sauces.* Many of those finger-licking-good sauces are loaded with fat and calories.
- *Skip the desserts and fruit pies.* When it comes to fast-food restaurants, dessert is just another word for fat.
- *Avoid high-calorie ("regular") soft drinks and shakes*, and make sensible choices that are lower in fat, calories, and sodium.

Developing healthy eating habits at college can be challenging. Most food places on campus offer menu selections that are teeming with fat and calories, and most students feel too rushed to prepare healthful meals. However, making healthier food choices on campus can help you avoid the dreaded "Freshman 15"—the unwanted weight some first-year students put on.

Here are some suggestions for healthier food choices on campus:

1. For breakfast, *choose* whole grain breads, high fiber cereal, granola bars, fresh fruit, whole grain crackers, low-fat milk or milk alternatives (soy milk) *rather than* muffins, donuts, and refined grains (white bread or rolls).
2. For lunch or dinner, *choose* grilled fish or chicken breast or lean beef, veggie burgers, vegetable wraps, salad bar, sushi, turkey breast on whole wheat bread, fish, beans (but not refried beans) brown rice, baked potato without the toppings, hummus, low-fat yogurt, low-fat milk or milk alternatives (soy milk), whole wheat pita sandwiches with veggies or lean meat and salsa topping (not mayo or sour cream) *rather than* fried entrees, high-fat foods such as burgers and fries, rich pasta sauces, white rice, whipped cream, syrups, added sugar and salt, cheesy foods, high-fat dressings, or giant-sized portions.
3. For between-meal snacks, *choose* healthy snack bars, peanut butter crackers, trail mix, fruits, veggies, nuts, whole wheat crackers *rather than* candy bars, potato chips, cookies, or salted pretzels.

Vitamins

Vitamins are organic compounds that are needed, usually in minute amounts, to maintain normal physiological functioning. Vitamins serve a variety of vital functions, including helping to regulate the chemical reactions in the body that are involved in **metabolism**, the process by which food is converted into energy and assimilated into body tissue. Vitamins are found in small amounts in many of the foods we eat.

LEARNING OUTCOME 5

Describe the functions of vitamins and how to obtain them

There are 13 known vitamins, and they are divided into *fat-soluble vitamins* and *water-soluble vitamins*. The fat-soluble vitamins—A, D, E, and K—are carried in the fats we eat and stored in the liver and in fatty tissues of the body where they can accumulate until they are needed. Water-soluble vitamins, such as the B vitamins and vitamin C, travel freely in the bloodstream, and excess amounts are excreted in the urine rather than stored in body tissues.

The body synthesizes some vitamins, while others must be obtained from external sources, such as foods or supplements. For example, the body itself manufactures vitamin D in response to ultraviolet light, such as sunlight. Cloud cover, season of the year, latitude, and clothing limit direct sunlight. Thus, most of us must obtain additional vitamin D from dietary sources or supplements, such as vitamin D–fortified milk. Unfortunately, more than three-quarters of Americans have low levels of Vitamin D—a deficiency which can have damaging effects on bone health and general physical health.[9] The typical American diet is also deficient in *omega-3 fatty acids*, a type of saturated fat in fish oil found in fish such as salmon, tuna, and herring. Some evidence links higher levels of omega-3 fatty acids to reduced risks of heart-related problems.[10]

Most people can get the vitamins they need from a balanced diet. Vitamin A, for example, is found in orange produce, such as sweet potatoes and carrots, and in dark-green vegetables. Citrus fruits and juices are abundant sources of vitamin C. We can obtain the vitamin A we need by consuming fortified dairy products. Vitamin D is derived from sunlight. Ten minutes a day of exposure of arms and legs to the mid-day sun is sufficient for most people.

Vitamin B is plentiful in vegetables, legumes, nuts, and whole grain foods. Some substances, called *pro-vitamins*, are converted by the body into vitamins. *Beta-carotene*, for example, is classified as a pro-vitamin because it is converted into vitamin A during metabolism.

vitamins
Organic substances required in minute amounts to serve a variety of vital roles in metabolism, growth, and maintenance of bodily processes.

metabolism
The organic process by which food is changed into energy and assimilated into bodily tissue to sustain life and promote growth.

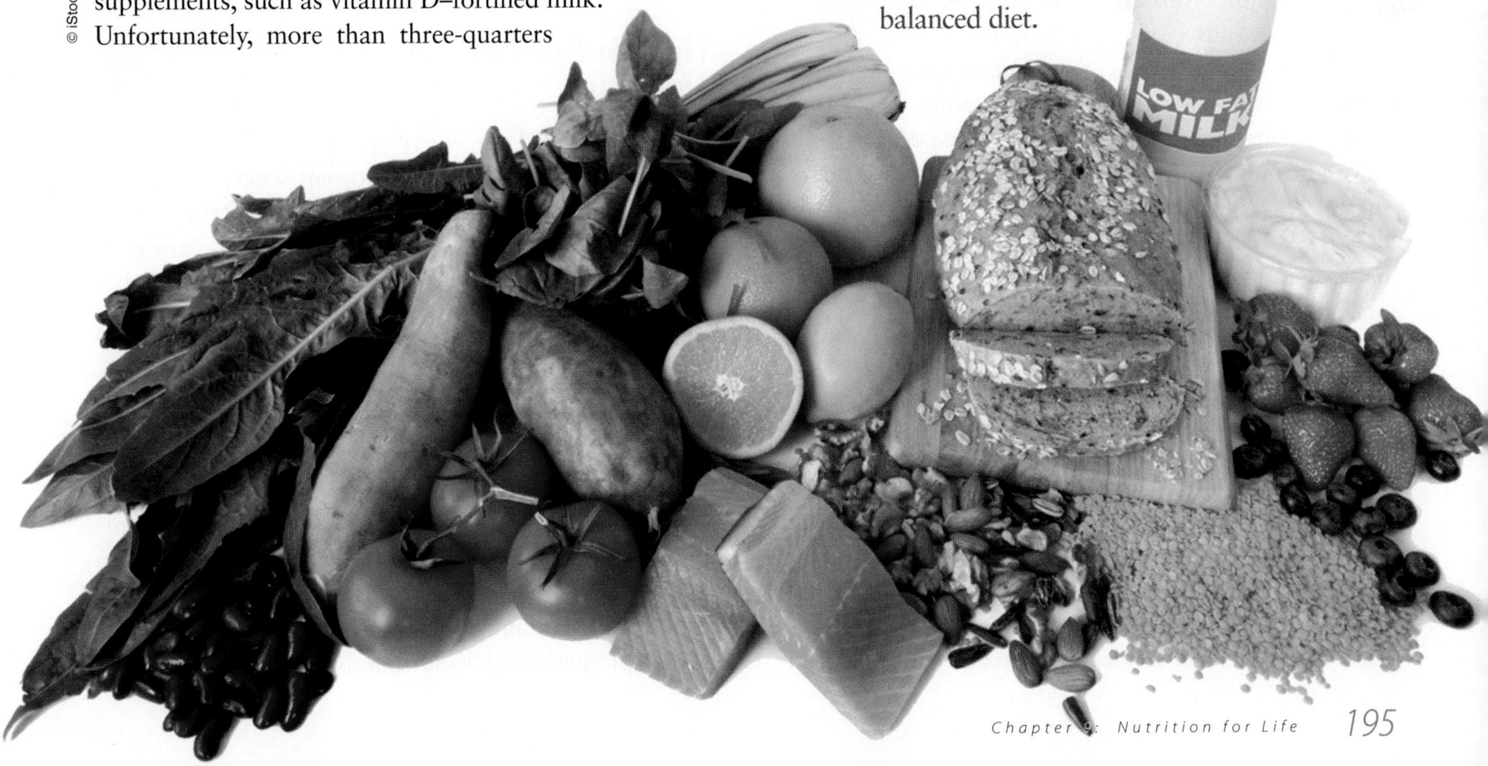

Most people can get the vitamins they need from a balanced diet.

© iStockphoto.com/Robyn Mackenzie

Table 9-8 Vitamins: Myths versus Facts

MYTH	FACT
Popping a vitamin pill can correct a poor diet.	Vitamin pills will not compensate for a poor diet. A multivitamin pill can ensure that you receive essential vitamins, but will not provide the other nutrients you need for your health.
The more vitamins you take, the better off you'll be.	Excess doses of vitamins can be harmful. For example, regularly taking high doses of niacin (vitamin B_3) and vitamin D can damage the liver.
Taking vitamin supplements will boost your athletic performance.	Vitamins will not improve your game or enhance your performance in sports.
Taking stress vitamins helps you cope with emotional problems.	So-called stress vitamins help the body counter the effects of physical stress, such as changes in temperature. There is no evidence that vitamins help people cope with emotional stress.
"Natural" vitamins are better than synthetic vitamins.	There is no evidence that your body can tell the difference between natural and synthetic vitamins.

Vitamin Deficiency Syndromes

Deficiency or underutilization of particular vitamins can lead to vitamin deficiency syndromes. *Scurvy*, a disease caused by vitamin C deficiency, is characterized by sore gums, painful joints, and hemorrhaging. Today in our society, scurvy is generally limited to two population groups: infants sustained exclusively on cow's milk and older people on limited diets. But that was not the case for the European explorers who ventured around the world in the 15th and 16th centuries. The Spanish explorer Vasco de Gama reported losing more than 60% of his crew of 160 sailors to the disease during his voyage around the Cape of Good Hope in 1498. Scurvy was quite common among seamen on long voyages because their diets lacked citrus fruits or other sources of vitamin C, although it wasn't until the early 1600s that lack of citrus fruits was actually linked to scurvy. By the early 1800s, the British Navy had begun issuing daily rations of citrus juice to sailors, a practice that led to the slang term "limey" to describe British seamen.

Another vitamin deficiency syndrome is *rickets*, a bone disease caused by the lack of vitamin D. The good news about rickets is that it has been virtually eliminated in the United States and Canada since milk supplies began to be fortified with vitamin D. Fortification of other dietary staples, such as bread and infant formula, have greatly reduced or virtually eliminated other deficiency syndromes in technological societies such as the United States and Canada. You can read "Prevention 9-2" online to learn about other vitamin deficiency syndromes and how to avoid them.

The online feature "Prevention 9-3" gives you information you need to know about the functions of various vitamins, their recommended daily levels, dietary sources, deficiency syndromes, and risks associated with excesses.

Health Benefits of Vitamins

Few of us need to worry about getting enough vitamin C to prevent scurvy or enough vitamin D to prevent rickets. But might vitamins have health benefits beyond preventing vitamin deficiency syndromes? Many people believe that the right mixture of vitamins can help them achieve optimum health, prevent cancer and other diseases, or thwart aging.

Let's separate the reality from the hype, first by focusing on outright distorted beliefs and myths that many people hold about the health value of vitamins (see Table 9-8).

Some health benefits of vitamins go beyond preventing vitamin deficiency syndromes. For example, vitamin D can help reduce the risk of osteoporosis. Supplementation with vitamin B_6 may help relieve symptoms of PMS (premenstrual syndrome) and asthma in some cases. Vitamin B_6 may also enhance the functioning of the immune system. Yet, the vitamin and pro-vitamin substances receiving the most attention from health researchers are those that function in the body as **antioxidants**, nutrients that counteract the damaging effects of oxidation that occur during metabolism.

Antioxidants: A Role in Prevention?

You have seen the corrosive effects of *oxidation* in the environment in the form of rust that is produced when oxygen and moisture come in contact with iron surfaces. Scientists believe that oxidation may also "corrode" the body. Oxidation occurs normally during metabolism and leads to the formation of metabolic waste products called **free radicals**. Free radicals are unstable molecules that can wreak havoc on cells by eating away their membranes and damaging their genetic material (DNA).

Damage caused by free radicals may hasten aging and contribute to the development of cancer and age-related diseases such as cataracts, immunological disorders, heart disease, strokes, and rheumatoid arthritis. Antioxidants protect cells from the damaging by-products of metabolism by scavenging free radicals and rendering them harmless. The best-known antioxidants are vitamins C and E and beta-carotene. Many fruits and vegetables are good sources of these antioxidants. Vitamin C is plentiful in citrus fruits, strawberries, and cantaloupe. Various grains and vegetables, including vegetable oils, contain vitamin E. Beta-carotene is found in dark yellowish and orange fruits, dark-green leafy vegetables, apricots, pumpkin, carrots, squash, spinach, broccoli, and cantaloupe. Table 9-9 lists food sources of the major types of antioxidant nutrients.

Table 9-9 Dietary Sources of Antioxidants

NUTRIENT	SOURCES
Vitamin C	Citrus fruits, broccoli, tomatoes, green peppers, potatoes
Vitamin E	Wheat germ, whole grains, oatmeal, peanuts, brown rice, vegetable oils
Beta-carotene	Carrots, broccoli, sweet potatoes, spinach, squash, peaches, cantaloupe

Do antioxidants help ward off diseases by protecting cells from the cumulative damage of free radicals? The short answer is that we don't know. Antioxidants may help prevent the clogging of blood vessels that can lead to heart attacks and strokes. However, hopes that supplements of vitamin E, which has antioxidant properties, might reduce the risks of heart disease or cancer have not panned out, based on the results of tightly controlled randomized experiments.[11]

Nor does use of vitamin C supplements prevent the common cold or reduce the frequency of colds.[12] Perhaps the mix of chemical substances naturally found in fruits and vegetables, and not antioxidants themselves, is responsible for lowering the

antioxidants
Agents that prevent or inhibit oxidation; they are believed to have healthful benefits by reducing the build-up of free radicals in the body.

free radical
Metabolic waste product produced during normal oxidation, which may damage cell membranes and genetic material.

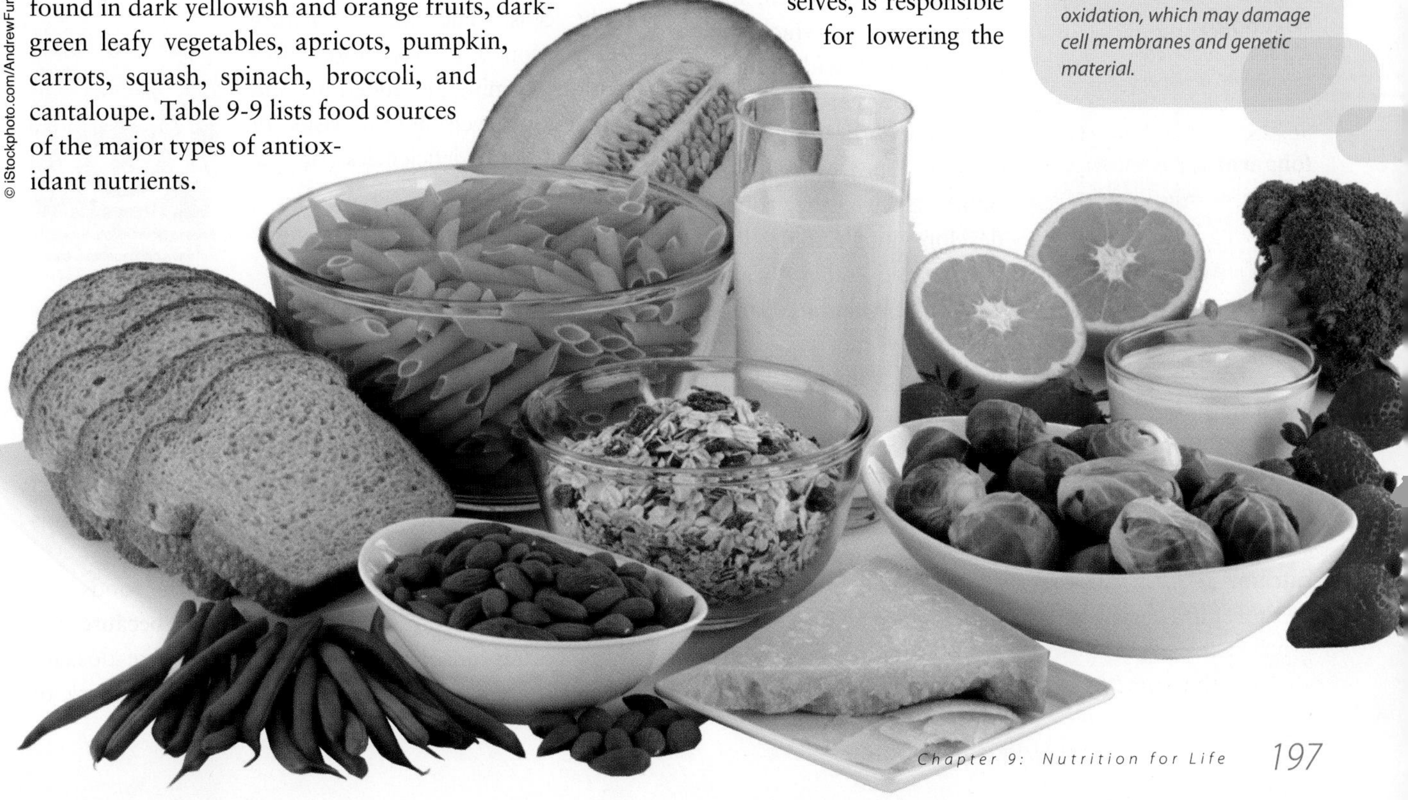

risks of disease. Plants contain more than 1,000 natural chemical substances called **phytochemicals**, many of which may help protect us from many types of diseases. The U.S. Department of Agriculture recommends that Americans consume a variety of fruits and vegetables daily, selecting from all five vegetable subgroups (dark green, orange, legumes, starchy vegetables, and other vegetables) several times a week.

Another set of antioxidants, called **flavonoids**, is found in various plant foods, including red grapes and chocolate. Flavonoids may have healthful benefits, such as reducing blood pressure and possibly decreasing the risks of heart disease and some cancers.[13] The greater the concentration of cocoa in chocolate, the higher the levels of antioxidant flavonoids. Dark chocolate is richer in cocoa content, so its flavonoid content is greater than that of milk chocolate. But chocolate is high in calories and saturated fat, so its potential antioxidant benefits might be offset by other health risks.

Folic Acid and Birth Defects: Did You Take Your Folic Acid Today?

The U.S. Public Health Service is calling for diet supplementation with **folic acid**, a B vitamin also known as *folate*. Daily consumption of folic acid during early pregnancy reduces the risk of neural tube defects (NTDs).[14] NTDs include *anencephaly*, in which the child is born without a brain and dies shortly after birth, and *spina bifida*, in which the child is born with a hole in the tube that surrounds the spinal cord. While most children born with spina bifida survive, they often develop intellectual deficiency and other health problems, including paralysis below the waist and difficulties with bladder or bowel control.

NTDs kill or disable nearly 2,500 newborns each year in the United States. NTDs develop early in pregnancy, often before the woman knows she is pregnant. Consequently, the U.S. Public Health Service recommends that all women of reproductive age who could possibly become pregnant consume 400 micrograms (0.4 milligrams) of folic acid daily. Most multivitamin pills contain 400 micrograms of folic acid, but health officials warn against taking higher doses because of potential adverse effects. Folic acid is found in such foods as leafy green vegetables, orange juice, and beans. The government also requires that certain foods, including enriched breads and cereals, be fortified with folic acid. The rate of spina bifida has declined significantly due to government requirements. But hopes that folic acid might have other important health benefits, such as reducing risks of heart disease or cancer, were dampened by results of a large-scale study that failed to show such benefits.[15]

phytochemical
Naturally occurring plant chemical.

flavonoids
A group of antioxidant compounds found in plants that may have healthful benefits.

folic acid
A B vitamin, known as folate, *which helps prevent neural-tube defects and may play a role in preventing heart disease.*

minerals
Inorganic elements obtained from the food we eat that are essential to survival.

hemoglobin
A protein in red blood cells, which gives blood its reddish color and transports oxygen to body cells.

calcium
A mineral essential to the growth and maintenance of bones.

Minerals

LEARNING OUTCOME 6

Describe the functions of minerals and how to obtain them

Minerals such as calcium, potassium, sodium, and magnesium are essential to health and are obtained from food. Minerals assist in the formation of bones and teeth, the transmission of nerve signals, and the manufacture of **hemoglobin** in red blood cells. Hemoglobin is the protein that gives blood its reddish color and transports oxygen to body cells. The online feature "Prevention 9-4" has more information on minerals' functions and sources, as well as the risks of excesses and deficiencies of the essential minerals.

prevention

Access CourseMate for HLTH at www.cengagebrain.com.

Calcium

Calcium is the most plentiful mineral in the body. Virtually all of the body's calcium—99%—is found in teeth and bones. Adequate calcium intake is important for bone health in adults as well as children. It is especially important in preventing osteoporosis, a bone disease that primarily affects older persons, especially postmenopausal women. Bone matter is continuously renewed, which is why we need calcium throughout our lives.

Calcium should be consumed from the foods you eat rather than from supplements, in part because it is more readily absorbed from food. Excessive dosages of calcium can lead to constipation, increased risk of kidney stone formation, and other kidney problems. Excess doses can also reduce the absorption of other necessary minerals, such as iron and zinc.

Because of the increased need for calcium during the growth years, the recommended daily intakes of calcium are 1,300 milligrams daily from age 9 through age 18, 1,000 milligrams from age 19 through age 50, and 1,200 milligrams afterward.[16]

Calcium is mainly obtained via dairy products. An eight-ounce cup of low-fat milk contains about 300 milligrams of calcium, or nearly a third of the adult recommended daily allowance of 1,000 mg/day. Other sources of calcium include kale, broccoli, and spinach (see Figure 9-3). Many processed foods are fortified with calcium, and bone material in our diets, such as the soft bones found in sardines and salmon, is also a rich source of calcium.

Figure 9-3 Sources of Calcium in the Diet

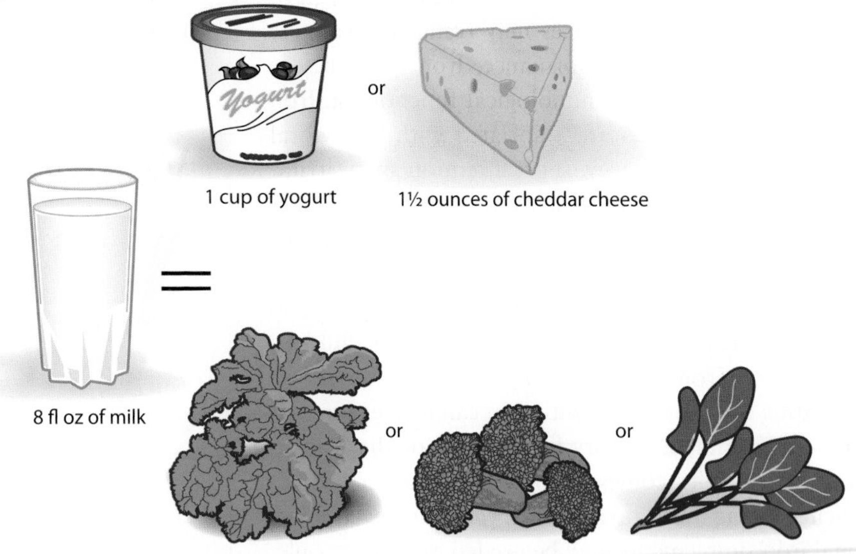

Source: *Dietary supplement fact sheet: Calcium.* (2004, August 1). Office of Dietary Supplements, National Institutes of Health.

Although milk and other dairy products are among the richest sources of calcium, some people need to avoid these foods because they cannot digest lactose, the sugar found in dairy products. They must satisfy their calcium needs in other ways or switch to milk products formulated for people who are lactose intolerant. Some lactose-intolerant people may need to take calcium supplements in order to obtain sufficient calcium from dietary sources.

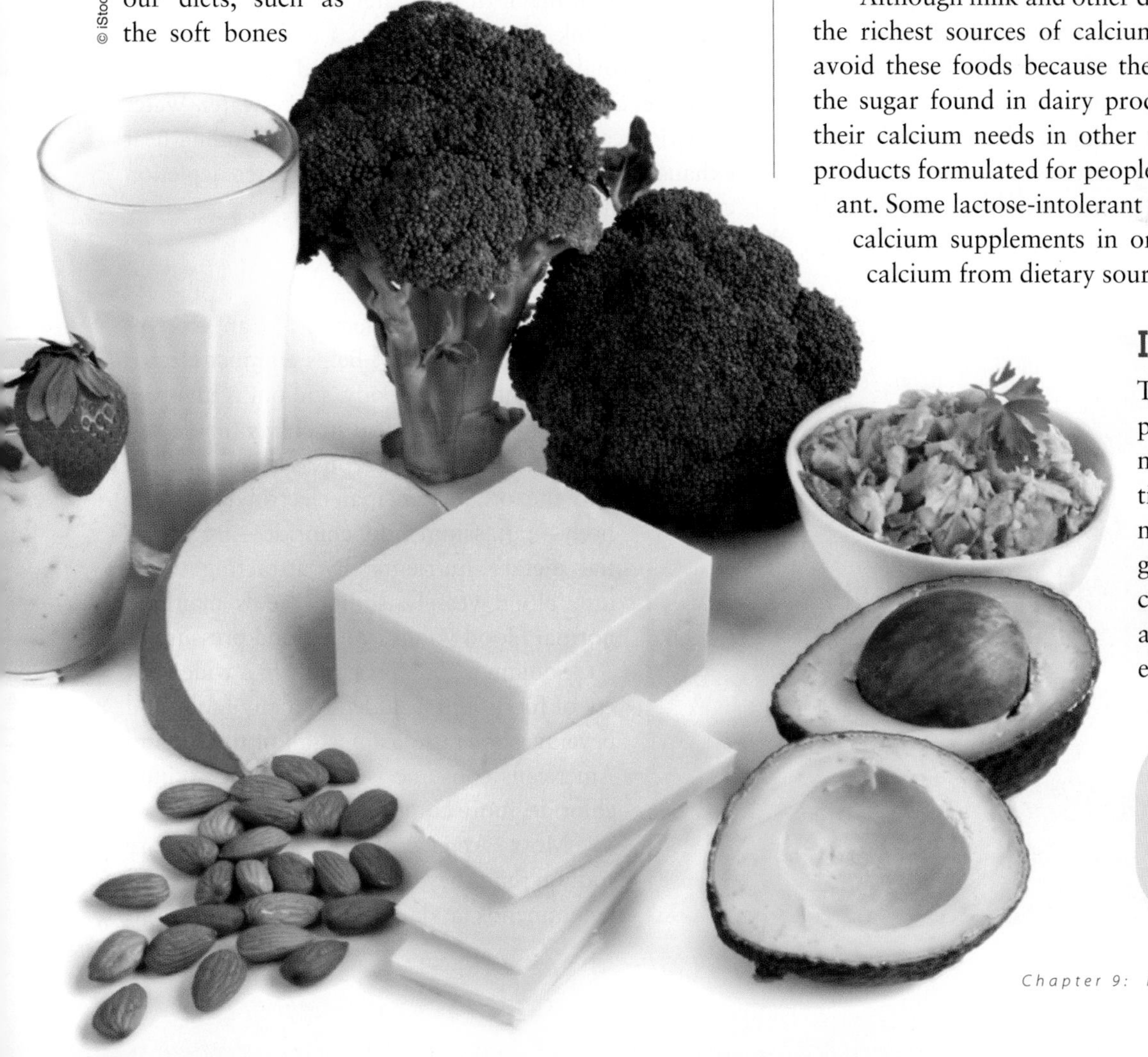

Iron

The metal iron forms part of the hemoglobin molecule. **Iron**, an essential nutrient, is found in meats, eggs, cereals, and grains (especially fortified cereal products), legumes, and green leafy vegetables. Iron deficiencies

iron
An essential mineral, it is a metallic element that forms part of the makeup of hemoglobin.

can lead to a condition called **anemia**, in which there is too little hemoglobin in the blood to carry oxygen to body tissues. Iron deficiencies may result in weakness and reduced physical performance. Iron deficiency is also linked to poorer immunological functioning. Iron deficiencies in children are associated with behavioral problems such as lethargy, short attention span, irritability, and learning disorders. Women need to be especially aware of their iron needs, because they tend to lose iron during menstruation, pregnancy, and breastfeeding. Yet, about 2,000 Americans experience iron poisoning each year, the majority involving children who swallow iron supplements.

Eating foods enriched with iron can help ensure adequate iron intake. Twenty-five percent of the iron in the American diet comes from fortified foods, such as enriched breads and breakfast cereals. However, additional iron supplements may be needed by some people, including pregnant women; menstruating women, especially those who bleed heavily; infants, children, and adolescents whose rapid growth requires high iron intake; long-distance runners and other endurance athletes; dieters whose bodies may eliminate iron during intense, prolonged exercise; and dieters who may skimp on foods rich in iron. Before taking any iron supplement, however, consult with your physician. Also, avoid taking doses exceeding 100 milligrams. High doses can hinder absorption of zinc, an essential mineral involved in metabolic and immune functioning.

anemia
A condition involving a lack of hemoglobin in the blood, causing such symptoms as weakness, paleness, heart palpitations, shortness of breath, and lack of vigor.

sodium
A metallic element that functions as an electrolyte in the body.

electrolyte
A substance that conducts electricity.

Water and Electrolytes

Water is often called "the forgotten nutrient," but without water, life would cease. Water serves a number of vital roles in the body, including transporting nutrients and removing wastes through the blood and regulating body temperature. One-half to perhaps four-fifths of our body weight is composed of water. Each day we need to replenish the 4% or so of our body weight in water that we lose through sweating and excretion of urine.

LEARNING OUTCOME 7

Describe the nutritional roles of water and electrolytes and the risks of excess sodium intake

We obtain much of the water we need in the beverages we drink. Yet water is also a major constituent of many solid foods. Many fruits and vegetables, for example, contain between 85% and 95% water. Water depletion can lead to various problems, including heat exhaustion and heatstroke. Prolonged water depletion can be lethal.

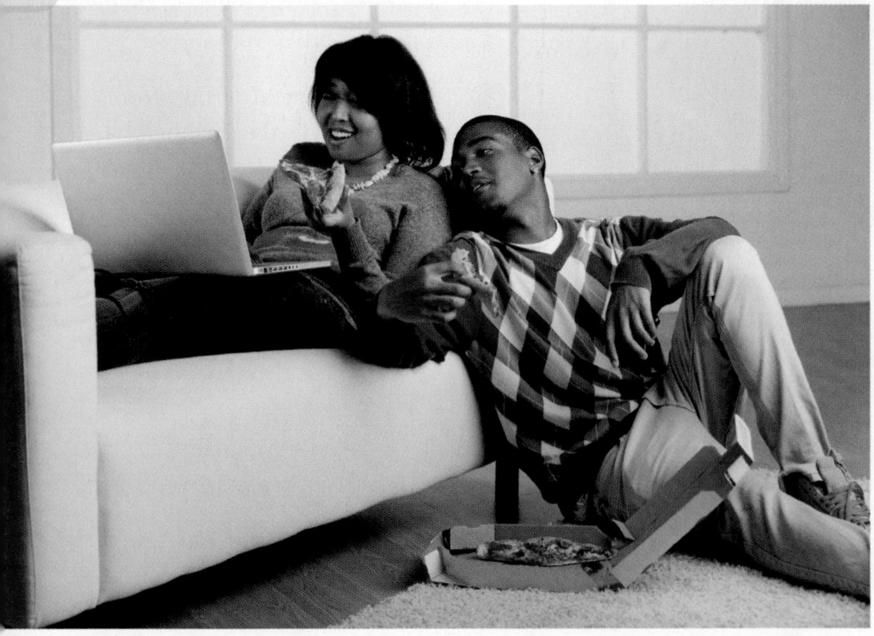

© iStockphoto.com/Blend_Images

Sodium

Sodium, a metallic element, is an **electrolyte**, a substance that helps conduct electrical currents. In the body, sodium is involved in conducting electrical impulses (nerve signals) through the nervous system. Sodium and the other principal electrolytes in the body—potassium and chloride—are essential dietary nutrients. By attracting water into blood vessels, sodium helps maintain normal blood volume and blood pressure.

Sodium is found naturally in a wide variety of foods and is added to many foods and beverages for taste. Almost all of the sodium Americans consume is derived from sodium chloride, more commonly called *table salt*.

Most Americans take in far more sodium than they need. The U.S. government recommends a daily sodium intake of no more than 1,500 milligrams for people aged 51 and older, children, African Americans, and people with hypertension, diabetes, or chronic kidney disease—and no more than 2,300 milligrams for other people.[17] Just how much (really, how little) is 2,300 mg? It is the amount of sodium found in a teaspoon of table salt. The average American consumes about 3,400 milligrams of sodium daily, mostly from salt in prepared and packaged foods as well as salt added at the dinner table.[18] Excess sodium intake increases the blood pressure, which can increase the risk of serious cardiovascular diseases, stroke, and kidney disease. Learn how to cut your sodium intake by reading the online feature "Health Skills 9-4."

health skills

Access CourseMate for HLTH at www.cengagebrain.com.

Salt is added to so many foods that it is difficult to know how much sodium we normally consume. Salt is second only to sugar among the ingredients food manufacturers add to processed foods as a preservative and flavor enhancer. Bread and bakery products, cured and processed meats, canned soup and vegetables, soy sauce, and cheese and other dairy products are especially high in salt.

> Food is needed to *sustain* life, but if food becomes contaminated by disease-causing bacteria it can also *endanger* life. The online feature "Prevention 9-5" will help you learn how to ensure food's safety.
>
> prevention
>
> Access CourseMate for HLTH at www.cengagebrain.com.

HEALTH APPS: YOUR LINK TO ONLINE HEALTH APPLICATIONS

health skills — **How to Cut Fat from Your Diet** Making healthy food choices does not require that you eliminate all sources of fat from your diet. Pick up tips on how to limit the overall amount of fat in your diet, especially saturated fat, in "Health Skills 9-2."

diversity — **Ethnic Food—Eating Out, Eating Smart** Tacos? Dim sum? Fettuccini Alfredo? Many of us enjoy food from other countries and cultures, but how can we know if what we are eating is really healthy for us? Read "Diversity 9-1" and find out.

prevention — **Preventing Vitamin Deficiency Syndromes** Can a lack of Vitamin A lead to blindness? Can a lack of Vitamin D lead to bone loss and rickets? Read "Prevention 9-2" to learn about vitamin deficiency syndromes and how to avoid them.

prevention — **Should You Take Vitamin Supplements?** A daily multivitamin may be advisable for those of us who don't eat what we should. But what about taking nutritional supplements beyond the daily recommended levels of vitamins and minerals? Is taking more of a good thing necessarily better? Go to "Prevention 9-3" to find out.

prevention — **Minerals** "Prevention 9-4" guides you through the functions, sources, recommended daily allowances, deficiency syndromes, and risks of excesses of the essential minerals.

health skills — **Cutting Back on Sodium** Most of us take in far more sodium than we need. "Health Skills 9-4" has six helpful suggestions for reducing your sodium intake.

prevention — **Ensuring Food Safety** Food can become contaminated by disease-causing bacteria and other microorganisms, or by poisonous substances that can enter our bodies and lead to serious illnesses, including cancer. Go to "Prevention 9-5" to learn how you can avoid falling victim to these health problems.

Go to the CourseMate for HLTH at www.cengagebrain.com for additional resources including flashcards, games, self-quizzes, review exercises, web exercises, learning checks, and more.

HLTH
Chapter 10

Managing Your Weight

"Unlike people with a drug habit, overweight people cannot just say no—they can't go evermore without food. Instead, they must say less."

We have some good news and some not-so-good news. First, the good news: The United States has such an agricultural abundance that Americans take in 200 billion calories a day more than their bodies need. How much is 200 billion calories? Enough to feed the nation of Germany—80 million people. Now, the not-so-good news: These excess calories are expanding our waistlines. Americans are heavier than ever (see Figure 10-1 on page 204).[1] About two out of three adults in the United States are overweight. More than half of those who are overweight are obese, and about one in seven is severely obese. Obesity is now on everyone's plate.[2]

Does it matter that we eat too much and weigh too much? Yes. The health problems connected with overweight are more than skin deep. Obesity is a major risk factor in many serious and life-threatening health problems, including cardiovascular disease, diabetes, respiratory illnesses, gallbladder disease, gout, and some forms of cancer.[3] Obesity accounts for more than 100,000 excess deaths in the United States every year and shaves six or seven years off the average person's life expectancy.[4] Life expectancy in the future may decline by another two to five years because of obesity.[5]

Losing weight has health benefits for overweight people. Even a modest loss of 10% to 15% of body weight can reduce health risks. But at least two-thirds of us can benefit from learning the skills needed to maintain a healthy weight.

We aim to help readers attain and maintain a *healthy weight*, not to conform to an idealized image of thinness. The contemporary social ideal has to

Learning Outcomes

1 Describe the relationship between calories and weight

2 Explain theories and evidence as to why people become overweight

3 Discuss the eating disorders, their origins, and their treatment

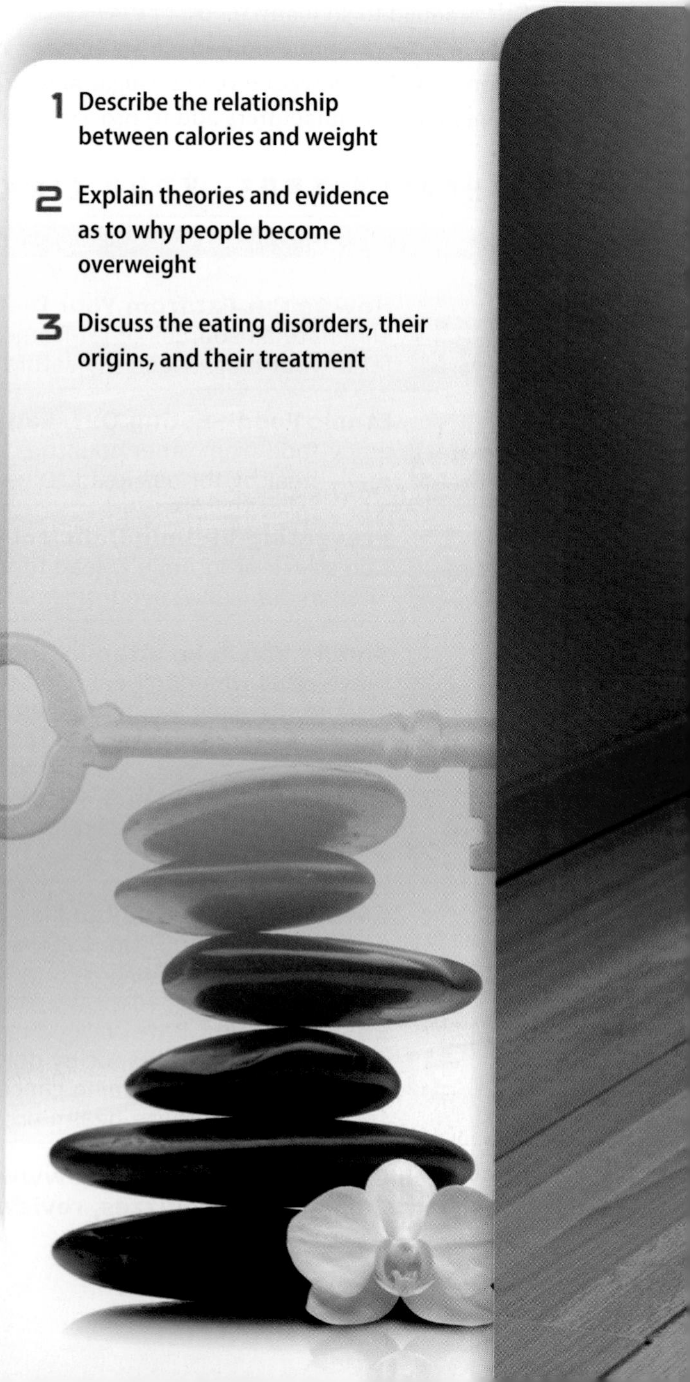

do with achieving a cosmetic goal of leanness, not a healthy weight. Social pressure to achieve an unrealistic standard of slenderness leads many people to become obsessed with their weight and dissatisfied with their bodies. A preoccupation with slenderness contributes to eating disorders such as anorexia and bulimia.

We are a nation of dieters. The pressure to be thin is so prevalent that dieting has become the normal eating pattern for many American women. Four out of five young women in the United States have gone on a weight-loss diet by the time they reach their 18th birthdays.

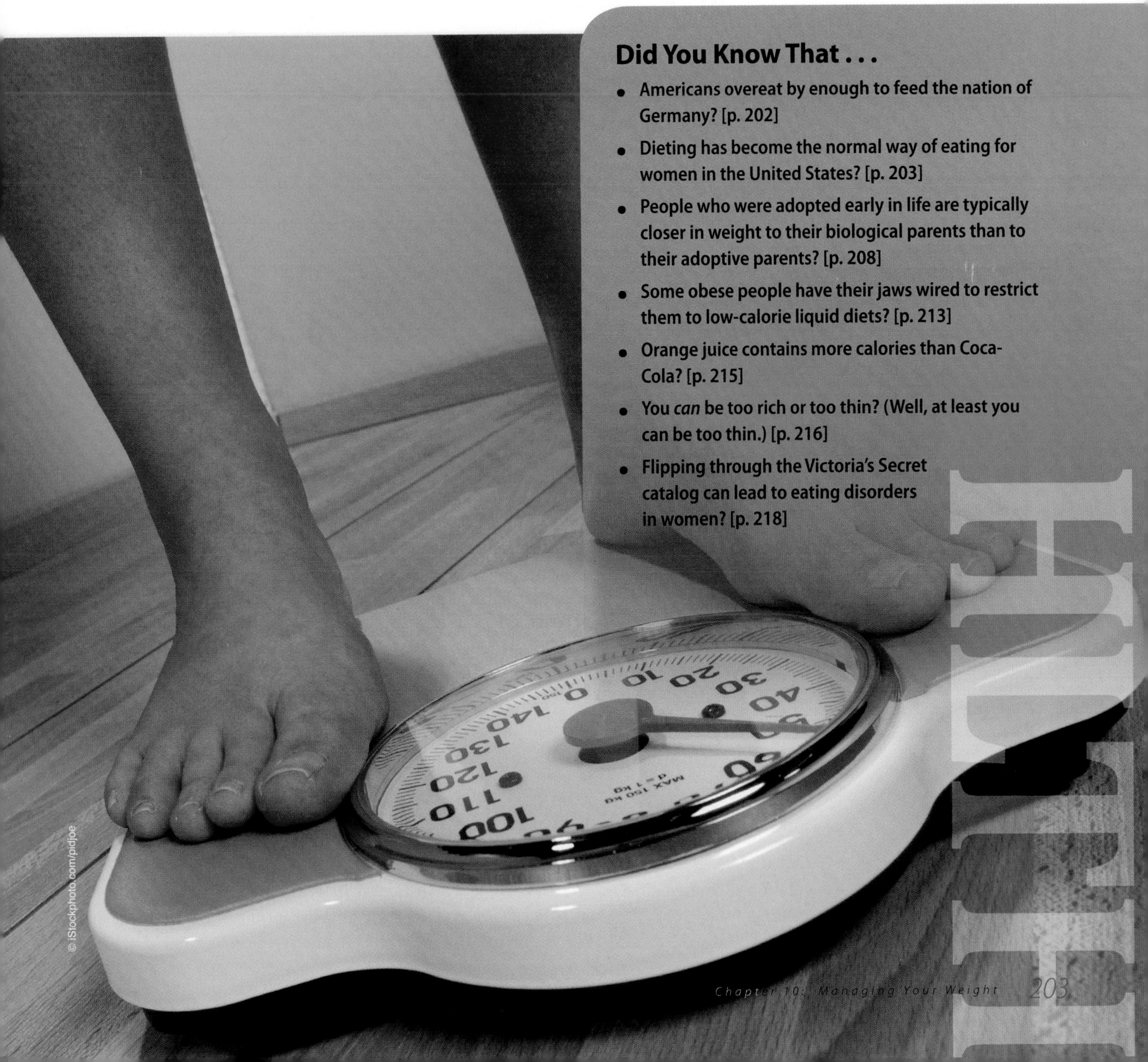

Did You Know That . . .

- Americans overeat by enough to feed the nation of Germany? [p. 202]
- Dieting has become the normal way of eating for women in the United States? [p. 203]
- People who were adopted early in life are typically closer in weight to their biological parents than to their adoptive parents? [p. 208]
- Some obese people have their jaws wired to restrict them to low-calorie liquid diets? [p. 213]
- Orange juice contains more calories than Coca-Cola? [p. 215]
- You *can* be too rich or too thin? (Well, at least you can be too thin.) [p. 216]
- Flipping through the Victoria's Secret catalog can lead to eating disorders in women? [p. 218]

Figure 10-1 Heavier than Ever

Americans have eaten themselves into a situation in which two-thirds of all adults are overweight, and more than half of the overweight are obese.

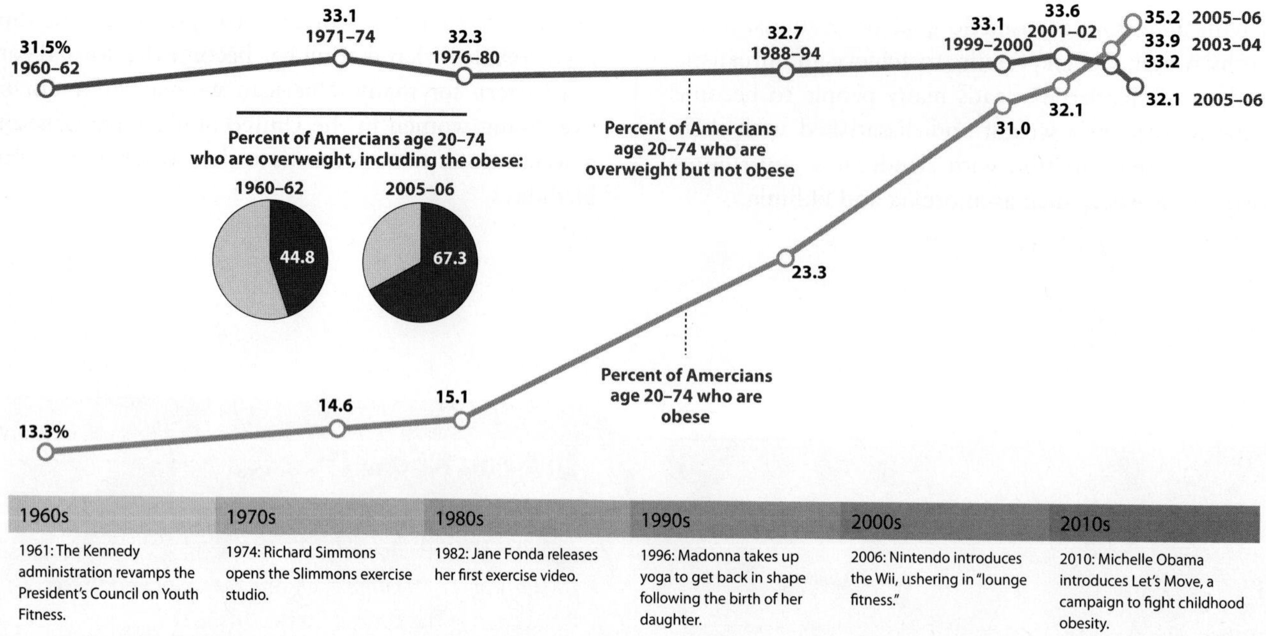

Source: Adapted from graphic in *The New York Times*, accessed online at http://www.nytimes.com/interactive/2011/01/30/weekinreview/30marsh.html?ref=weekinreview

Calories and Weight: A Balancing Act

Marathon runners can eat heaping portions of food day after day and never gain an ounce. Other people gain weight if they have an extra helping at Sunday dinner. Gaining weight is not simply a matter of what we eat. It also depends on the energy we expend in keeping the machinery of our bodies running. Our bodies burn calories—literally, food energy—to maintain normal body functions, such as breathing, circulation, and digestion. We also burn calories (expend energy) through physical activity and exercise. We gain weight when we consume more food energy in the form of calories than we expend (see Figure 10-2). Excess food energy becomes stored as fat. On the other hand, we lose weight when we expend more calories than we consume.

basal metabolic rate (BMR)
The minimum amount of energy needed to maintain bodily functions, apart from digestion.

resting metabolic rate (RMR)
The minimum energy that the body requires to maintain bodily functions including digestion.

LEARNING OUTCOME 1

Describe the relationship between calories and weight

Metabolic Rates

The **basal metabolic rate (BMR)** is the minimum amount of energy needed to maintain body functions apart from digestion. The **resting metabolic rate (RMR)** is the minimum energy the body requires to maintain body functions including digestion.

How many calories a day does your body need? The answer depends on many factors, including your gender, age, weight, and level of activity. Younger adults need more calories than older adults. Active people need more than sedentary people.

Men generally require more calories than women, even if they are of the same weight and are equally active. Why? Muscle tissue burns more calories than fat does, and a higher percentage of women's body weight is composed of fat. Men therefore tend to have a higher metabolic rate than women.

Consider the average woman 25 to 50 years of age. She's 5'4" tall and weighs 138 pounds. She engages in light to moderate physical activity during her day. She will need about 2,200 calories a day to maintain her weight. The average man of the same age is 5'10" tall and weighs 174 pounds. If he also engages in light to moderate physical activity, he will need about 2,900 calories daily to maintain his weight.

What happens if this average woman consumes more than 2,200 calories a day—or if the average man consumes more than 2,900? Excess calories are converted into fat. They add inches to our waists and other parts of the body where fat is stored. Our weight increases.

Nutrients—proteins, fats, and carbohydrates—supply various amounts of calories. Proteins and carbohydrates supply four calories per gram. Fats supply nine calories per gram. Ounce for ounce, fats provide more than twice as many calories as proteins or carbohydrates. That is why fat-laden desserts are so, well, fattening.

All fats have the same potential for increasing our weight. Switching from saturated to unsaturated fats makes good health sense because of its impact on cholesterol levels, but it won't change your weight.

People who regularly exercise, such as marathon runners, burn more energy than less active people. Thus, they can consume more calories without gaining weight. Physical activity not only burns calories but also increases the basal metabolic rate by building muscle. Muscular body tissue burns more calories than fatty body tissue.

Although excess calories are converted into body fat, taking in fewer calories than your body needs causes your body to convert stored fat into energy. Thus, you lose body fat and weight. Maintaining weight is a matter of balance between energy-in (calories consumed) and energy-out (calories expended through maintaining body processes and physical activity).

Figure 10-2 Weight Management: A Balance between Energy Input and Energy Output

When food is metabolized in the body, it releases energy. The amount of energy is measured in units called calories. A *calorie* is the amount of energy required to raise the temperature of one gram of water one degree Celsius.

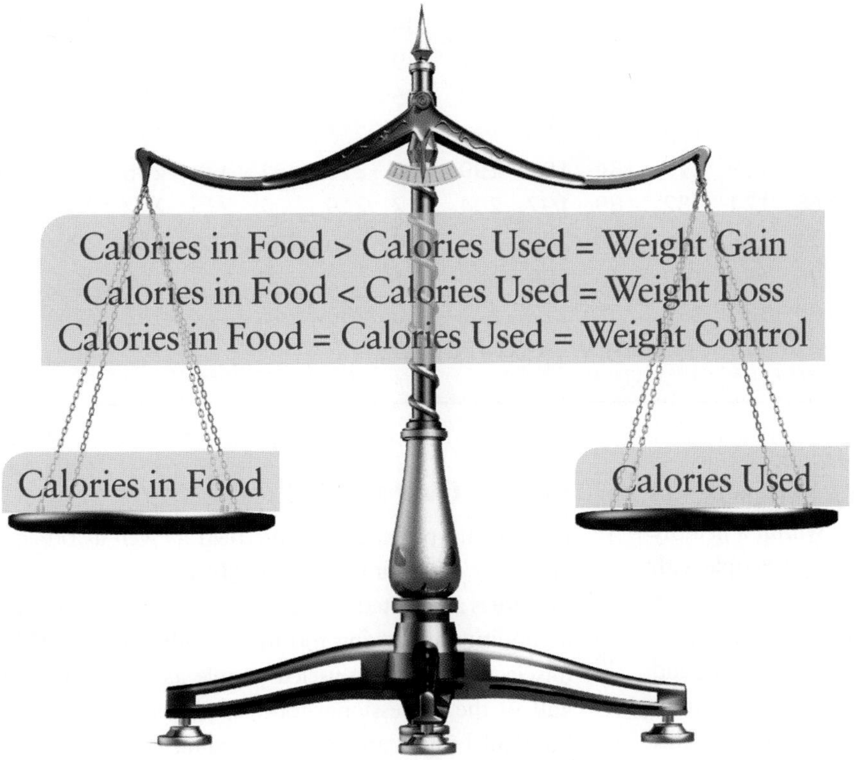

Source: *Physical activity and weight control.* (2006, November). National Institute of Diabetes and Digestive and Kidney Diseases (NIDDK). Retrieved from http://win.niddk.nih.gov/publications/physical.htm

How Much Should You Weigh?

The most widely used measure for determining whether you weigh more or less than you should is the **body mass index (BMI)**.

Body Mass Index

The BMI is a yardstick that takes height into account in determining whether a person's body weight falls in a healthy range. You can determine whether your own weight falls in the healthy range in "Health Check 10-1." According to the standard set by the National Institutes of Health, people with BMIs of 30 or greater are obese. Those with BMIs between 25

body mass index (BMI) *A measure of obesity that takes into account both weight and height. It is calculated by dividing body weight (in kilograms) by the square of the person's height (in meters).*

HEALTH CHECK 10-1

How Much Should You Weigh?

Are you in a healthy weight range? Overweight? Obese? To find out, use the body mass index (BMI) chart. Start by finding your height (no shoes!) at the left of the chart. Move to the right until you hit your weight. Go up from that point to the top of the chart, where you'll find your body mass index (BMI). Then use these standards to determine your weight group:

Healthy weight. A BMI from 18.5 to 24.9 is considered a healthy weight.

Overweight. A BMI from 25 to 29.9 is the overweight range.

Obese. People with a BMI of 30 or above are considered obese.

HEIGHT	BODY MASS INDEX (BMI)															
	19	20	21	22	23	24	25	26	27	28	29	30	31	32	33	34
58″	91	96	100	105	110	115	119	124	129	134	138	143	148	153	158	162
59″	94	99	104	109	114	119	124	128	133	138	143	148	153	158	163	168
60″	97	102	107	112	118	123	128	133	138	143	148	153	158	163	168	174
61″	100	106	111	116	122	127	132	137	143	148	153	158	164	169	174	160
62″	104	109	115	120	126	131	136	142	147	153	158	164	169	175	180	186
63″	107	113	118	124	130	135	141	146	152	158	163	169	175	180	186	191
64″	110	116	122	128	134	140	145	151	157	163	169	174	180	186	192	197
65″	114	120	126	132	138	144	150	156	162	168	174	180	186	192	198	204
66″	118	124	130	136	142	148	155	161	167	173	179	186	192	198	204	210
67″	121	127	134	140	146	153	159	166	172	178	185	191	198	204	211	217
68″	125	131	138	144	151	158	164	171	177	184	190	197	203	210	216	223
69″	128	135	142	149	155	162	169	176	182	189	196	203	209	216	223	230
70″	132	139	146	153	160	167	174	181	188	195	202	209	216	222	229	236
71″	136	143	150	157	165	172	179	186	193	200	208	215	222	229	236	243
72″	140	147	154	162	169	177	184	191	199	206	213	221	228	235	242	250
73″	144	151	159	166	174	182	189	197	204	212	219	227	235	242	250	257
74″	148	155	163	171	179	186	194	202	210	218	225	233	241	249	256	264
75″	152	160	168	176	184	192	200	208	216	224	232	240	248	256	264	272
76″	156	164	172	180	189	197	205	213	221	230	238	246	254	263	271	279
	BODY WEIGHT (POUNDS)															

and 29.9 are overweight. Those with a BMI of 18.5 to 24.9 are within a healthy weight range. People with a BMI of less than 18.5 are underweight.

People on either end of the continuum (either obese or underweight) stand an increased risk of premature death compared to people in the healthy weight range.[6]

overweight
A body weight exceeding desirable weight for an individual of a given age, height, and body frame, usually based on a criteria of a weight exceeding 20% above the desirable weight.

obesity
A condition of excess body fat.

Are You Overweight?

Health care providers use the BMI as well as other standards for determining **overweight** and obesity. Although **obesity** is associated with excess body weight, it is actually a condition of having too much body fat. The BMI can misclassify heavily muscled people as obese. More than half of the professional football players in the National Football League are obese according to the BMI index.[7] But BMIs don't consider differences in body composition, such as the ratio of *lean body mass* (*lbm*; muscle and bone) to body fat. Professional football players tend to be heavily muscled, so their BMIs may not indicate their body fat composition. On the other hand, some NFL players—especially linemen—are obese by any standard.

Assessing Your Body Composition

A measure of body composition provides a more precise indicator of whether or not a person has a healthy weight. One common standard is to consider men whose body fat percentage exceeds 24% to be obese; for women, a body fat content exceeding 33% would be considered obese. Women normally carry a higher percentage of body fat because they have more fat deposits than men in their breasts and hips.

There are several methods for assessing body fat, which should be conducted by health professionals, including skinfold measurement, hydrostatic weighing, and bioelectrical impedance analysis.

Skinfold Measurement: How Many Inches Can You Pinch? One widely used index of body fat is the thickness of skinfolds. **Skinfold thickness** is measured in such places as the waist, underarms, and back. Skinfold calipers (painlessly) pinch the skin to measure skinfold thickness. The measurements are used to estimate the percentage of body fat.

A convenient but crude measure of skinfold thickness is the *pinch test*. Want to pinch yourself? Hold one arm out to the side. Pinch the skin with your other hand at various points along the underside of the outstretched arm. (Pinch only the fat lying under the skin, not the adjoining muscle tissue.) Can you pinch more than an inch? If so, you have more body fat than is desirable.

Hydrostatic Weighing A more precise measure of body fat is provided by **hydrostatic weighing**, in which a person is weighed twice, once on land and again submerged in water. Body fat is lighter than water, while muscle and bone are heavier. Therefore, the body's weight when submerged largely reflects the density of body mass. The more people weigh submerged, relative to dry weight, the less body fat they carry.

Bioelectrical Impedance Analysis Water conducts electricity. Fat does not. **Bioelectrical impedance analysis** uses these facts to measure body fat. A harmless electrical current is passed through the body. A technician analyzes the shifts in electrical conductance (impedance) that occur to calculate the total amount of body water. The amount of body water is then used to compute percentages of lean and fat body weights.

Waist Circumference, Waist-to-Hip Ratio, and Apples and Pears

Two people may have the same BMI. They may even have the same amount of body fat. But they may have different health risks based on the distribution of fat on their bodies.

Men whose waists measure more than 40 inches and women whose waists exceed 35 inches may have

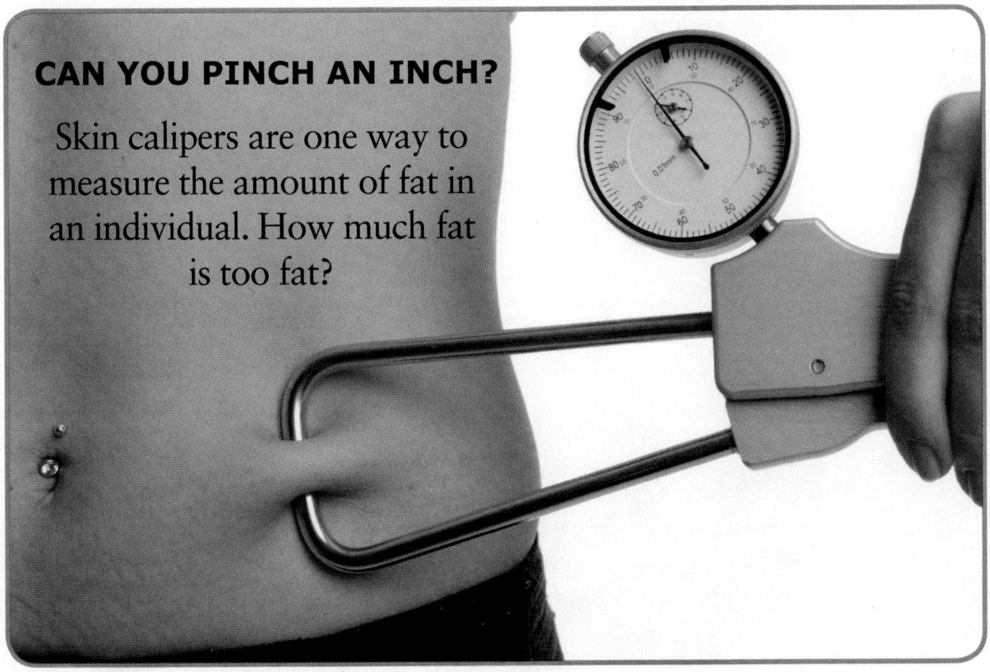

CAN YOU PINCH AN INCH?

Skin calipers are one way to measure the amount of fat in an individual. How much fat is too fat?

skinfold thickness *The thickness of the folds of skin, usually of the underarms, waist, or back, which is used to estimate the percentage of body fat.*

hydrostatic weighing *A method of measuring body weight by weighing a person both underwater and on dry land and comparing the results.*

bioelectrical impedance analysis *A method of measuring body fat composition by analyzing the changes in electrical conductance (impedance) as a mild electric current is passed through the body.*

greater health risks than men and women with smaller waists.[8] Also, men with a waist-to-hip ratio larger than 1 and women with a ratio larger than 0.8 stand greater health risks.[9]

What is your waist size? To measure the circumference of your waist, take a tape measure and run it around your bare abdomen just above your hip bone. Make the tape measure snug and keep it parallel the ground, but don't make it so tight that it pinches your skin. Take your waist measurement when you are relaxed and after you exhale.

We can classify people who carry excess fat around their midsections (waists) as "apples," whereas those carrying excess fat in their hips, buttocks, and thighs are "pears" (see Figure 10-3). Both patterns of excess weight are linked to health risks, but "apples" face even greater risks than "pears" of developing heart disease and diabetes.[10]

"Apples" may be at greater risk of health problems than "pears" because fat that accumulates around the pelvis (rather than the waist) is linked to higher blood levels of "good cholesterol," or high-density lipoprotein (HDL). HDL helps remove fatty deposits that accumulate in arteries. Artery-clogging deposits are an important risk factor in coronary heart disease and heart attacks. By contrast, carrying body fat around the waist is linked to lower levels of HDL. Men are more likely to be apples than women, so it is not surprising that they stand a greater risk of coronary heart disease at least until about age 65, when the rates between men and women even out.

Figure 10-3 Apples versus Pears

Apple-shaped people carry much of their excess weight around their waists, whereas pear-shaped people carry excess weight on their buttocks, thighs, and hips. Although both patterns of obesity are unhealthy, carrying excess fat around the waist is a greater risk factor for serious, potentially life-threatening diseases such as coronary heart disease, hypertension, and diabetes.

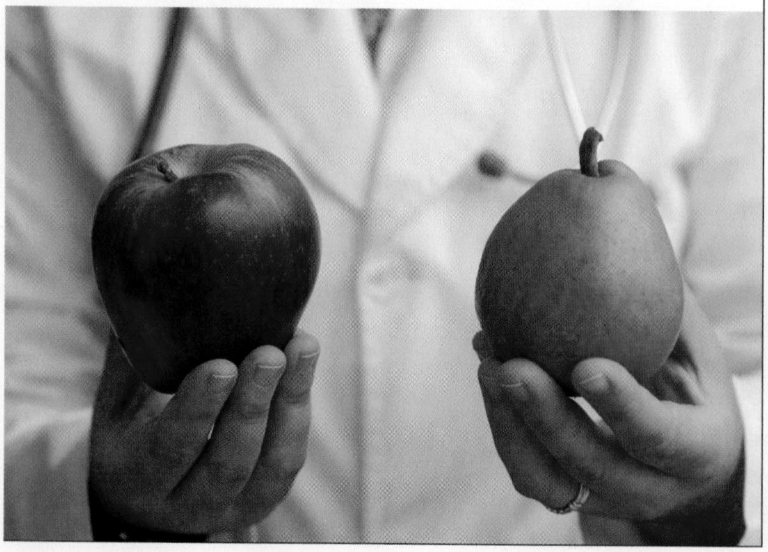

© iStockphoto.com/esolla

Why Do People Become Overweight?

People do not become overweight because they lack willpower. Overweight is a complex problem that involves many factors, including heredity, body metabolism, and activity level.

LEARNING OUTCOME 2

Explain theories and evidence as to why people become overweight

Heredity: All in the Family?

Overweight runs in families. People whose parents are overweight have a greater chance of becoming overweight themselves. Why does being overweight run in families? Some overweight parents may set poor examples for their children by consuming large portions of fattening foods. Early exposure to fattening diets may set the stage for obesity, but we have also learned that genetics plays an important role in body weight.[11]

A genetic contribution to body shape is supported by evidence that adults who were adopted in early life tend to have body weights closer to those of their biological parents than to those of their adoptive parents who reared them. Moreover, identical twins (who have the same genetic makeup) are closer in weight in adulthood than fraternal twins (who share only 50% of their genetic makeup). Whether reared apart or together, identical twins in one study weighed virtually the same in adulthood.

A gene regulates the production of *leptin* (derived from the Greek *leptos*, meaning "thin"), a hormone that helps put the brakes on eating by signaling the brain that the body has had enough. Scientists believe that this gene is but one of many involved in regulating body weight in humans.

Our genes may limit our ability to sculpt our bodies to match the cultural ideal. Still, even people whose genes are in the opposition's corner can achieve and maintain a healthy body weight by eating sensibly and exercising regularly.

Metabolic Factors: How Fast Do You Take It Off?

Heredity may also influence body weight through genes that regulate body *metabolism*—the rate at which the body burns calories to maintain itself at rest. Some people have a faster metabolic rate than others.

The human body is an efficient machine that allows us to store reserves of energy in fatty tissue until they are needed during times of famine. According to **set point theory**, the brain regulates body weight around a genetically predetermined level or "set point." When we either gain or lose weight, the brain adjusts the body's metabolic rate to keep weight around its set point.[12]

When people follow quickie diets to lose weight, their bodies react as if they were starving. Shifting into starvation mode, the brain slows down the body's metabolic rate in order to conserve remaining stores of fat. This phenomenon—called *adaptive thermogenesis*—would be helpful in times of famine but doesn't do dieters living among an abundance of tasty foods much good.[13] As fewer calories are burned, it becomes harder to continue to lose weight, even if people adhere to their diets. On the other hand, when people gain weight, their metabolism tends to speed up.[14] However, this boost does not compensate well for weight gains.

As you lose weight, your body requires fewer calories. Heavier bodies burn more calories than lighter bodies just to maintain their weights. Generally speaking, a loss of 10% of body weight in a healthy person translates into 10% fewer calories the body needs. Consider a 200-pound man who eats less and sheds 20 pounds, or 10%, of his body weight. At 180 pounds, his body requires about 10% fewer calories to maintain his new weight. Since the man needs 10% fewer calories than when he was heavier, he will regain weight if he returns to his pre-diet calorie intake.

You may be able to prevent adaptive thermogenesis by reducing food intake gradually and exercising regularly. Exercise may help offset reductions in metabolism. Muscle strengthening can also help because muscle tissue is more metabolically active than fat tissue—it burns more calories.

Fat Cells: Billions Served Daily

Fat cells? Despite their name, **fat cells** are not obese cells. Rather, they are cells that store fat. Fat cells are composed of **adipose tissue** (fatty tissue). Feelings of hunger are related to the number of fat cells in our bodies. As time passes since we have eaten, our blood sugar level drops. Low blood sugar leads to a release of fat from fat cells to fuel and nourish us. Depletion of fat in these cells is detected by the **hypothalamus**, a small structure in the midbrain. The hypothalamus triggers feelings of hunger that motivate us to eat. Eating, of course, replenishes fat cells and restores the blood sugar level.

Obese people have many billions more fat cells than do people of average weight. People with more fatty tissue in their bodies, and hence more fat cells, feel hungry sooner than people with less fatty tissue, even when they weigh the same amount. As a result, they may eat more often or feel food-deprived more often than people with fewer fat cells.

Heredity affects the number of fat cells in our bodies, but early dietary habits, such as excessive childhood eating, can also add fatty tissue. Unfortunately, we do not shed fat cells when we lose weight. Although fat cells sort of shrivel up, they continue to send signals to the hypothalamus that they need to be replenished. Thus, people who follow a calorie-reduction diet may experience nagging hunger, making it difficult to keep those extra pounds off.

Fatty tissue metabolizes, or "burns," food more slowly than muscle tissue. Two people may weigh the same amount and consume the same amount of food, yet they will metabolize food at different rates according to the proportions of fat and muscle in their bodies. People with higher fat-to-muscle ratios are thus more likely to put on extra pounds.

There is a gender difference in the fat-to-muscle ratio. Men's bodies average 40% muscle and 15% fat, while women's bodies average 23% muscle and 25% fat (see Figure 10-4 on the next page). Because of these differences, men typically burn off excess calories more quickly than do women of the same weight and activity level. Unfair as it may be, it is typically easier for men to keep off excess pounds.

set point theory
The theory that the brain regulates body weight around a genetically predetermined level or "set point."

fat cell
Body cell that stores fat.

adipose tissue
The body tissue in which fat is stored.

hypothalamus
A structure in the mid-brain that is involved in regulating body temperature, emotional states, and motivational states such as hunger and thirst.

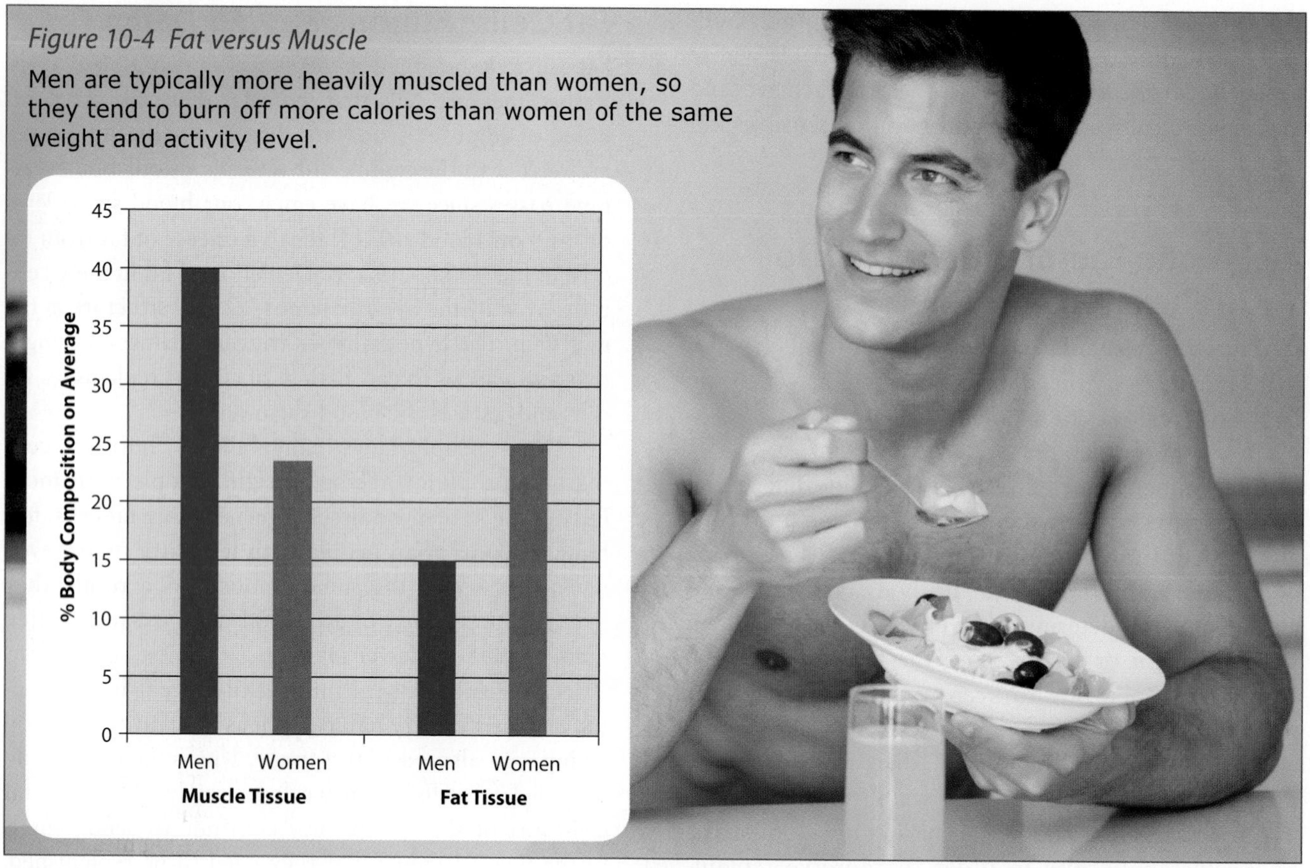

Figure 10-4 Fat versus Muscle

Men are typically more heavily muscled than women, so they tend to burn off more calories than women of the same weight and activity level.

Inactivity: Get a Move On!

Not enough people are exercising regularly, which is a major reason the nation's collective middles are expanding. Overweight people tend to be less active than other people. But which comes first, inactivity or weight gains? Actually, inactivity and weight gains *interact*. Inactivity contributes to weight gain, and people tend to become less active as they gain weight.

Metabolic rates also fluctuate according to our activity levels. Time spent in front of the "tube" is also time *not* spent walking, running, swimming, or doing other calorie-burning activities. Yet, even couch potatoes can increase their activity levels. While watching TV, they can walk around during commercial breaks or exercise in place. Using body sensors, researchers found that leaner people tend to move around more than obese people.[15] They stand, pace about, and fidget, all of which burn calories, while obese people tend to sit still for longer periods of time. This difference in activity levels translates to about 350 calories a day, which would amount to about 30 or 40 pounds of weight loss per year for an overweight person. Regardless of your weight class, here's one additional suggestion to consider while sitting (or standing) in front of the TV: Avoid mindless snacking.

Problem Eating Habits: Out of Sight, Out of Mouth?

Problem eating habits are another contributor to unwanted weight. Wolfing down your food does not give your brain the time it needs to register the sensation of satiety—the feeling of fullness. It takes about 15 minutes for your brain to catch up with your stomach, and you can consume a great deal of excess food in that amount of time! People seeking to lose weight should control not only what they eat and how much they eat, but also how quickly they eat.

Imagine a world in which there were no neon signs advertising fried chicken or pizza; no TV commercials filling your brain with images of melted cheese, drippy sauce, and scrumptious dessert fillings; and no magazines filled with pictures of cakes and pies that can be whipped up in a snap. In such a world, people might eat only in response to their internal hunger cues, or so we surmise. Modern civilization, however, bombards us with external food cues—ads and TV commercials displaying tempting foods, aromas that permeate the air as we walk by the local bakery, and so on. These environmental cues can trigger cravings for food even when our bodies are not registering hunger. Ads for fast-food restaurants typically feature burgers, shakes, and other high-calorie, high-fat items; more nutritious items, such as salads, are notably missing. We live in a fast-food–dominated culture, so much so that Ronald McDonald has become the most widely recognized figure among children today (after Santa Claus).[16]

Some of us may be better able to resist food-related cues than others, but we are all affected to one degree or another. That is why most weight-loss programs teach participants to limit their exposure to external cues. They recommend avoiding food-oriented magazines and keeping tempting treats or snacks out of sight (and preferably out of the house). To adapt a familiar expression, "Out of sight, out of mouth."

Emotional Eating: Using Food to Fill Emotional Needs

We need to eat to survive, but food means more than survival. There are connections between eating and emotional states such as love, anger, fear, and depression. The giving and receiving of food is among the first interchanges between parent and child. It is intimately connected with the emotional warmth of the parent-child relationship. Parents express love for children by feeding them, so food becomes a symbol of parental love. In fact, parents may feel hurt or unloved if Junior fails to clean his plate or does not appreciate the nutritious meals they have prepared.

We celebrate achievements, family reunions, and holidays with food. Offering food to guests is a sign of hospitality. Refusing an offer (or a second or third helping) can be perceived as a rejection of hospitality.

Some people also turn to food when their emotional needs are not being met. Food may become a substitute for love. Food can become a natural tranquilizer, mood elevator, or sedative. When we eat, the parasympathetic nervous system kicks into gear, activating digestive processes, lowering anxiety and tension, or inducing sleep. Some of us eat in anger, as though we were biting the enemy. Of course, eating because of negative emotions can compound emotional problems. It can lead to feelings of guilt for overeating and a negative body image when one gains weight.

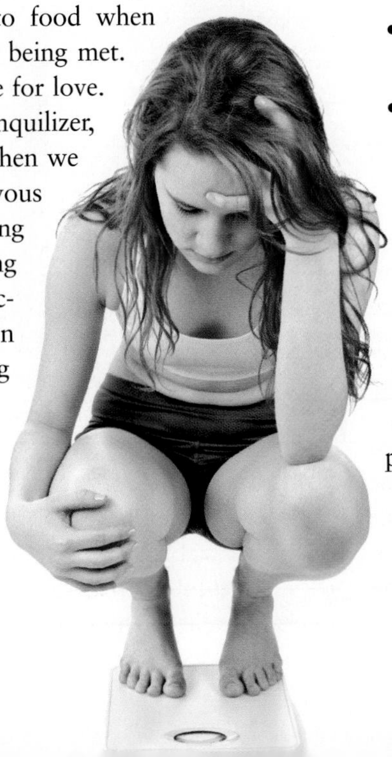

Negative emotions can also prompt *binge-eating*, the consumption of huge amounts of food within a short period of time. Have you ever dreaded an approaching test and downed a carton of ice cream to quell your anxiety? We may try to drown disturbing emotions like anxiety, fear, and depression in chocolate cake.

Many factors contribute to overweight: biological factors, inactivity, eating habits, and psychological factors. In "Diversity 10-1" on the next page, we explore the sociocultural aspects of obesity in America. "Prevention 10-1" on pages 214–215 can help you turn the tables and achieve or maintain a healthy body weight by developing sensible eating and exercise habits.

Eating Disorders

Is the saying true that you can never be too rich or too thin? Consider some facts about eating and eating disorders in the United States:[17]

- More than half of teenage girls and nearly one third of teenage boys use unhealthful methods to try to control their weight, including fasting, skipping meals, smoking, vomiting, and using laxatives.
- About two of five first- through third-grade girls would like to be thinner.
- More than four of five 10-year-old girls report fear of being fat.
- Nearly half of 9- to 11-year-old girls are "sometimes" or "very often" dieting.
- More than 90% of college women have dieted at some time.
- The average American woman is about 5'4" tall and weighs about 140 pounds. The typical American model is 5'11" and weighs 117 pounds.

☒ LEARNING OUTCOME 3

Discuss the eating disorders, their origins, and their treatment

Eating disorders are characterized by persistent, gross disturbances in eating patterns. In this section, we focus on an eating disorder in which individuals are too thin, *anorexia nervosa*, and one in which the person may be normal in weight but not in the methods used to maintain that weight, *bulimia nervosa*.

eating disorder
Disturbance of eating behavior, including anorexia nervosa and bulimia nervosa.

DIVERSITY 10-1

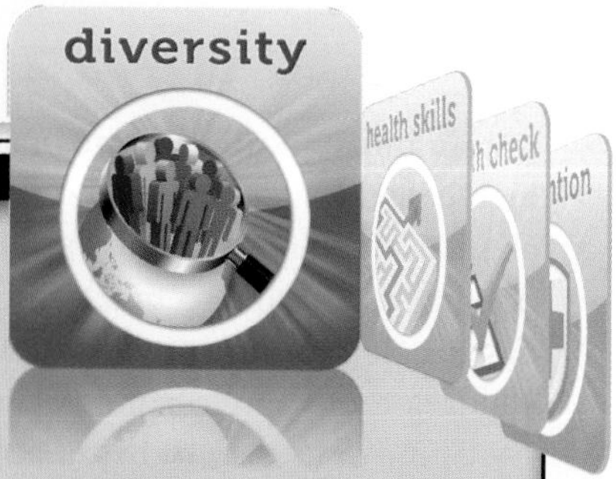

Socioeconomic, Sociocultural, and Ethnic Factors in Obesity

Rates of obesity vary across racial and ethnic groups. Obesity is more prevalent among people of color, especially African Americans and Native Americans, than among European Americans. Racial and ethnic differences are most pronounced among women. Figure 10-5 compares obesity among European American, African American, and Mexican American men and women.

Socioeconomic Factors

Obesity is more prevalent among poorer people. People of color are typically of lower socioeconomic status than European Americans, so it is not surprising that rates of obesity tend to be higher among African Americans and Mexican Americans, at least among women.

Why are people on the lower rungs of the socioeconomic ladder at greater risk of obesity? One reason is that more affluent people have greater access to information about nutrition and health and to health care providers. Furthermore, the fitness boom has been largely limited to more affluent people. Many poor people also turn to food as a way of coping with the stresses of poverty, discrimination, crowding, and crime.

Dietary Patterns

Cultural dietary customs may also contribute to obesity. African Americans, for example, are more likely than European Americans to consume high-fat, high-cholesterol foods.

Acculturation

Acculturation, the process by which immigrant or native groups adopt the cultural values, attitudes, and behaviors of the host or dominant society, helps immigrants adapt to a new culture. But it can become a double-edged sword when immigrants adopt unhealthy diets, such as the high-fat diet of many Americans. For example, Japanese Americans also stand a higher risk of developing diabetes and heart disease than do Japanese living in Japan.[18]

Figure 10-5 Prevalence of Obesity among Adult European Americans, Africans Americans, and Mexican Americans, by Gender[19]

Obesity varies with both gender and ethnicity. What factors might account for ethnic group and gender differences in obesity?

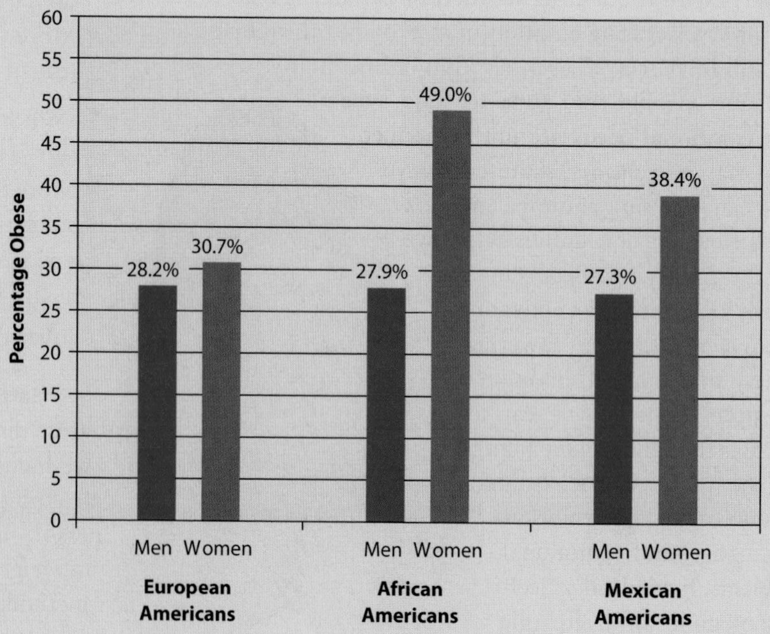

Rx

Are Weight-Loss Drugs or Surgery for You?

Medicine has done so much to cure or contain so many ills. There are medicines for weight control as well, but we're still awaiting the "magic pill" that will be safe and effective. Meanwhile, some people—especially extremely obese people—undergo surgery to help them control their weight. If you have tried various ways of losing excess weight and they have all failed, might one of these options be for you? Discuss them with your health care provider.

Weight-Loss Drugs

Over-the-counter (OTC) appetite suppressants work on the appetite control centers in the brain to temporarily stave off feelings of hunger or induce feelings of fullness. However, their effects are at best modest and temporary. Appetite suppressants can also have unpleasant side effects and possibly serious medical consequences. For example, the chemical *phenylpropanolamine hydrochloride* (PPA), an ingredient in many OTC appetite suppressants and some cold remedies, is associated with an increased risk of *hemorrhagic stroke* (bleeding in the brain). In the wake of a Food and Drug Administration (FDA) warning on the safety of PPA, many manufacturers of OTC drugs removed the ingredient from their formulations. You can take action yourself by reading OTC product labels and avoiding any product that still contains PPA.

Drug companies are spending millions (billions perhaps) to find medicines to combat obesity that will be both safe and effective over the long run. Even if an effective and safe anti-obesity pill were found, pills alone do not teach people more adaptive eating habits. Drugs are not a substitute for developing sensible eating and exercise habits.

Surgery

Surgery has revolutionized the treatment of *morbidly* obese people—that is, people whose weight exceeds *twice* the recommended level. Surgery may be indicated because of the serious health risks posed by morbid obesity. Other forms of treatment, such as dietary regimens, often prove ineffective for people struggling with extreme obesity.

One surgical technique is *gastric stomach bypass*. A section of the small intestine is surgically connected to a small pouch in the stomach. Not only is the stomach pouch too small to hold large amounts of food, but food now bypasses part of the stomach and small intestines so that fewer calories are absorbed. Bypass surgery has helped many morbidly obese people who could not lose weight through more conservative means, including the popular television weatherman Al Roker, who lost nearly 100 pounds following gastric bypass surgery. Although typical gastric bypass patients lose about 100 pounds within a two-year period after the surgery, many then start to slowly regain weight.

Another surgical method is *vertical-banded gastroplasty (VGB)*, in which much of the stomach is stapled off, leaving but a small pouch for food. As the person eats, the pouch quickly fills, leading to a feeling of fullness. This technique does not interfere with normal digestion.

Other surgical treatments include *jaw wiring*, which restricts eating to low-calorie liquids, *intestinal bypass* (shortening of the intestine to allow food to pass more quickly through), and insertion of a *stomach balloon* (to create a greater sense of fullness after eating). The outcomes of these techniques remain uncertain. A more common operation, which is not restricted to the morbidly obese, is a type of cosmetic surgery called *liposuction.* The surgeon removes excess fatty tissue from areas such as the hips or buttocks.

Serious risks and complications are associated with weight reduction surgery, so patients considering such procedures should carefully evaluate their options in consultation with their physicians.[20]

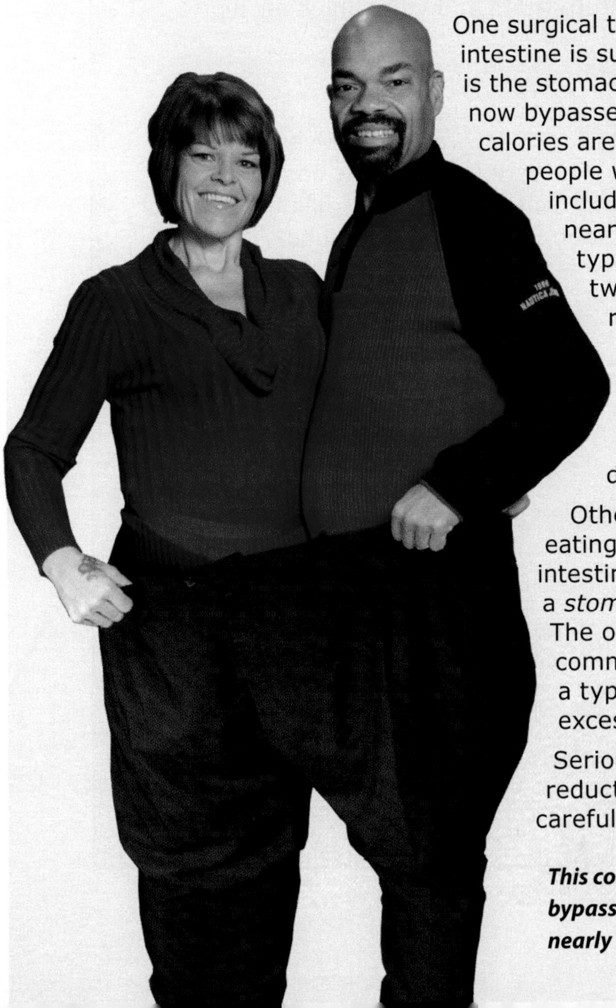

This couple had gastric bypass surgery and lost nearly 500 pounds together.

prevention diversity health check skills

Preventing Overweight

It is fortunate that body weight is not solely determined by genetics because there is little we can do to alter our genes. We *can*, however, adopt more healthful eating habits and a more active lifestyle to prevent ourselves from becoming overweight. Unlike people with a drug habit, overweight people cannot just say no—they can't go evermore without food. Instead, they must say less. And those who can, need to exercise.

Even a person with a genetic tendency toward becoming overweight may be able to maintain a healthful body weight. Effective weight management means balancing food energy consumed (calorie intake) with energy expended. Following are some tips to help you achieve this goal.

Follow a Nutritionally Balanced Diet. You needn't become a calorie counter, but you should become more aware of what you eat and how much you eat.

- *Follow the nutritionally balanced diet outlined in the MyPlate food plan (see Chapter 9).* You will eat several more servings of fruits and vegetables a day and take in ample minerals and vitamins.
- *Don't skip breakfast.* Skipping breakfast deprives your body of the nutrition it needs to get started for the day. It may also lead to overeating later in the day as your body seeks to make up for the missed meal. Avoid unplanned snacks.
- *Keep low-calorie, low-fat snacks handy for times when you may be tempted to binge.* You needn't give up snacking, but you do need to make smart choices. Choose fat-free popcorn over potato chips. Choose fat-free pretzels (read the labels). Switch from high-fat ice cream to low-fat or no-fat ice cream or frozen yogurt. Substitute fruits and vegetables for high-calorie snack foods.
- *Reach for an extra helping of vegetables or bread, not an extra entree.*
- *Cut fat from your diet.* Since fat is high in calories, switching to low-fat alternatives can help you control your weight. Substitute leaner cuts of beef. Alternate fish, poultry, and meat. Remove the skin from chicken before cooking or eating it. Switch from whole milk to low-fat or skim milk and from butter to diet margarine. Use low-fat or no-fat salad dressings.

Become Food Smart. You've heard of "book smarts" and "street smarts." Let us introduce you to "food smarts."

- *Use a guide that lists the caloric and nutritional values of common foods.*
- *Note that nuts may be more fattening than candy* (one ounce of roasted peanuts contains 165 calories).
- *Check out menu descriptions of meals.* Foods that are broiled, steamed, or cooked in their own juices are usually lower in fat and calories than foods that are pan-fried, sautéed, or described as "rich" or "crispy."
- *Beware of hidden calories.* Food add-ons, such as sauces, butter, syrups, gravies, and dressings, are major sources of hidden calories. A cup of fresh unsweetened peaches contains about 72 calories, but when the peaches are packed in heavy syrup, the calorie content jumps to 190. A baked potato contains about 220 calories and a trace of fat. One tablespoon of butter adds 11 grams of fat and 100 calories. Table 10-1 lists common foods that we don't usually think of as packing calories, but they do.

continued

Get Regular Exercise. Exercise helps you maintain a healthful weight in two important ways: It burns calories and increases your body's metabolic rate. Table 10-2 shows how many calories you can burn through various activities. Which of them can you include in your regular routine?

A half-hour swim at a typical pace burns about 200 calories for a 125-pound person. This compares to fewer than 40 calories expended by sitting quietly for the same amount of time. Over time, calories burned add up to weight lost.

Table 10-1 Sources of Hidden Calories

FOOD	CALORIES
Plain yogurt (8 oz)	145
Fruit-flavored yogurt (8 oz)	230
Cola (regular, 12 oz)	160
Orange juice (unsweetened, 12 oz)	180
Beer (regular, 12 oz)	150
Beer (light, 12 oz)	95
Wine, red (12 oz)	264
Wine, white (12 oz)	276
Liquor (90 proof, 1 oz)	75
Liquor (80 proof, 1 oz)	65

Focus on What You Eat, Not What You Weigh. Attend to what you eat, not what you weigh. Body weight fluctuates day to day due to water retention and other factors, which can make the daily ritual of weighing yourself a frustrating experience and discourage weight control efforts. Weigh yourself no more than once a week, without clothes and at the same time of day. Measure your waistline once a month or so. Or try our "closet test." See if you fit into those clothes hanging in the back of your closet—the ones you promised yourself you would wear again someday.

Take Corrective Action Early. Adjust your diet and activity level whenever your weight begins creeping upward or your clothes begin to feel tight. Think about making changes when you encounter a weight gain of, say, five pounds.

Don't go on a crash diet. Cut back gradually. Or switch from high-calorie foods to low-calorie substitutes. Increase your exercise level gradually. Don't risk injury. Take corrective action early, so that your weight remains within a stable range.

Table 10-2 Calories Expended in One Hour According to Activity and Body Weight

	BODY WEIGHT (IN POUNDS)				
ACTIVITY	100	125	150	175	200
Sleeping	40	50	60	70	80
Sitting quietly	60	75	90	105	120
Standing quietly	70	88	105	123	140
Eating	80	100	120	140	160
Driving, housework	95	119	143	166	190
Desk work	100	125	150	175	200
Walking slowly	133	167	200	233	267
Walking rapidly	200	250	300	350	400
Swimming	320	400	480	560	640
Running	400	500	600	700	800

Anorexia Nervosa

Consider the case of Rachel:[21]

> I wanted to be a runner. As a high school freshman, I trained hard, really hard and ate less. Lunch was lettuce sandwiches, carrots, and an apple. By my senior year, I was number three on the team and lunch was a bagel and an orange.
>
> I maintained a rigid schedule—running cross country and track, having a seat on student council, volunteering, and maintaining a 3.9 GPA throughout high school—while starving myself (1,000 calories per day). Several teammates were concerned, but I shrugged them off saying family members were tall and slender; I was a health nut, I didn't like fatty foods; I was a vegetarian; I didn't like sweets; I wasn't hungry; I wasn't starving.
>
> I dropped 10 pounds my freshman year—from 125 to 115 lbs. I was 5'8" tall and wore a size five. I was already taking birth control to regain my menstrual cycle; my weight was 15% below what was recommended for my height; I was always cold; I had chest pains and an irregular heartbeat; my hair was limp and broke off; my skin was colorless.
>
> It wasn't until I came to the University of Iowa and joined the varsity women's cross-country team that I began to see what I was doing to myself. A teammate had an eating problem. Every time I saw her, I felt sick to my stomach. She had sunken cheeks, eyes so big they swallowed her face. For one sick instant, I wondered if I would be happier if I were that thin. That is when I started to realize I was slowly killing myself.
>
> It's taken me three years to get where I am now. At 5'8¾" (I even grew as I got healthier) and 145 lbs, I look and feel healthier, have better eating and exercise habits, and I don't obsess about food as much as I used to. My eating disorder will haunt me for the rest of my life. If I'm not careful, it could creep back.

anorexia nervosa
An eating disorder characterized by the maintenance of an unusually low and unhealthy body weight and accompanied by an intense fear of gaining weight, a distorted body image, and, in females, an absence of menstruation (amenorrhea).

It was Wallis Simpson, the Duchess of Windsor who once said, "You can never be too rich or too thin." Most people make no objection to having a fat bank account, but as with Rachel, one can most certainly be too skinny. Rachel was diagnosed with **anorexia nervosa**, a life-threatening eating disorder characterized by extreme fear of being too heavy, dramatic weight loss, a distorted body image, and resistance to eating enough to reach or maintain a healthful weight.

Anorexia nervosa afflicts mainly women during adolescence and young adulthood.[22] The typical person with anorexia is a young European American female of higher socioeconomic status. Affluent females have greater access to fitness centers and are more likely to read the magazines that idealize slender bodies and shop in the boutiques that cater to females with svelte figures. All in all, they are regularly confronted with unrealistically high standards of slimness that make them unhappy with their own physiques.

The incidences of anorexia nervosa and bulimia nervosa have increased markedly in recent years. We also find eating disorders among some males, particularly among males who are compelled by their chosen activities—for example, wrestling or dancing—to keep their weight within a certain range or to remain very slender.[23] However, women with these disorders greatly outnumber the men who have them by more than six to one, although we lack precise data on their prevalence because so many people deny their disorders. A study of 985 European American women and 1,061 African American women found that 1.5% of the European Americans and none of the African Americans had met the diagnostic standards for anorexia nervosa at some time during their lives[24] (see Table 10-3).

Females with anorexia nervosa can drop 25% or more of their weight within a year. Severe weight loss triggers abnormalities in the endocrine system (that is, with hormones) that prevent ovulation.[25] General health deteriorates. Nearly every system in the body is affected. There are problems with the respiratory[26] and cardiovascular systems.[27] Females with anorexia are also at risk for premature development of osteoporosis, a condition characterized by loss of bone density that usually afflicts people in late adulthood.[28] Given all these problems, it is not surprising that the mortality rate for females with anorexia nervosa is approximately 5%.

In one common pattern, the girl sees that she has gained weight after reaching puberty, and she resolves she must lose it. But even after the weight is gone, she maintains her pattern of dieting and, in many cases, exercises at a fever pitch. This pattern continues as she plunges below her "desirable" weight—according to

Table 10-3 Incidence of Anorexia Nervosa and Bulimia Nervosa among African American Women and European American Women

	ANOREXIA NERVOSA	BULIMIA NERVOSA
African Americans	0%	0.4%
European Americans	1.5%	2.3%

standardized weight charts—and even after others tell her she is becoming all skin and bones.

Denial is a huge part of anorexia nervosa. Girls with the disorder tend to deny that they are losing too much weight. They are in denial about any health problems, pointing to their feverish exercise routines as evidence of their strength. Distortion of the body image—seeing oneself as heavier than one is—is a major feature of the disorder.[29]

Ironically, individuals with anorexia do not literally distance themselves from food. They may become as preoccupied with food as they are with their own body shape. They may develop a fascination with cookbooks, shop for their families, and prepare gourmet feasts—for other people, that is.

Bulimia Nervosa

Now consider the case of another young woman, who, like Rachel, was obsessed with remaining thin, but her strategy for keeping her weight down differed markedly:

> Every night that I throw up I can't help but be afraid that my heart might stop or something else happen. I just pray and hope I can stop this throwing up before it kills me. I hate this bulimia and I won't stop. It's hard for me to binge and throw up now (refrigerator is locked) and I just can't do it anymore. I just can't race through so much food so fast and then throw it up. I don't really want to. There are times that I do but not often. My new pattern is sure leaving me with an awful feeling in the morning. I eat dinner and kind of keep eating (snacking) afterwards to the point where I either feel too full or think (know) I've eaten too much, then I fall asleep (one hour or so) wake up and think I have to throw up. Half of me doesn't want to, the other half does and I always find myself throwing up. I try falling back asleep but it always seems like eventually sometime during the night I always throw up.[30]

Bulimia nervosa is sort of a companion disorder to anorexia nervosa. Bulimia nervosa also tends to afflict women during adolescence and young adulthood.[31] It entails repeated cycles of binge eating and purging. Binge eating often follows on the heels of food restriction—as in dieting.[32] There are various methods of purging. Some people vomit. Other avenues include strict dieting or fasting, the use of laxatives, and engaging in demanding, prolonged exercise regimens. Individuals with eating disorders tend to be perfectionists about their bodies. They will not settle for less than their idealized body shape and weight.[33] Bulimia, like anorexia, triggers hormonal imbalances: Studies find that many females with bulimia nervosa have irregular menstrual cycles.[34]

Eating disorders are upsetting and dangerous in themselves, of course, but they are also often connected with deep depression.[35] However, it seems that depression is more likely to occur *with* eating disorders than to be caused by them.[36]

Do you have an eating disorder, or are you at risk of developing one? "Health Check 10-2" on page 219 might provide some insight.

Origins of Eating Disorders

Health professionals have done a great deal of research into the origins of eating disorders. Yet they will be the first to admit that many questions about these disorders remain unanswered.

According to some psychoanalysts, anorexia nervosa may symbolize a young woman's efforts to cope with sexual fears, especially fear of pregnancy. Anorexia is connected with **amenorrhea** (lack of menstruation); therefore, some psychoanalysts interpret anorexia as a female's attempt to regress to her lifestyle prior to puberty. Anorexia nervosa prevents some adolescents from separating from their families and assuming adult responsibilities. Their breasts and hips flatten

bulimia nervosa
An eating disorder characterized by repeated episodes of binge eating followed by purging, and accompanied by persistent fears of gaining weight.

amenorrhea
Absence of menstruation.

again due to the loss of fatty tissue. In the adolescent's fantasies, perhaps, she remains a sexually undifferentiated child.

Many parents are obsessed with getting their children—especially their infants—to eat. Thus, some psychoanalysts suggest that children now and then refuse to eat as a way of engaging in warfare with their parents. ("You have to eat something!" "I'm not hungry!") It often seems that warfare does occur in the families of adolescents with eating disorders. Parents in such families are often unhappy with the family's functioning. They frequently have eating and dieting issues themselves. They may act out against their daughters—informing them that they consider them unattractive and that they should lose weight.[37]

A particularly disturbing risk factor for eating disorders in adolescent females is a history of child abuse, particularly sexual abuse.[38] One study compared 45 pairs of sisters, one of whom was diagnosed with anorexia.[39] Those with anorexia were significantly more likely to be exposed to high parental expectations *and* to sexual abuse.

We must also consider sociocultural factors that may contribute to eating disorders. Slimness is idealized in the United States, but when you check out *Cosmopolitan* or the Victoria's Secret catalog, you are looking at models who, on average, are 9% taller and 16% thinner than the typical female—and who still manage to have ample bust lines. Miss America, the annually renewed American role model, has also been slenderizing herself over the years. Over the past 80 years, the winner has added only 2% in height but has lost 12 pounds in weight. In the early days of the 1920s, Miss America's weight relative to her height yielded a body mass index (BMI) of 20 to 25, which is considered normal by the World Health Organization (WHO). The WHO labels people as malnourished when their BMIs are lower than 18.5. However, recent Miss Americas come in at a BMI near 17,[40] which is clearly underweight.

Yes, flipping through the Victoria's Secret catalog can contribute to eating disorders among women. As the cultural ideal slenderizes, women with desirable body weights according to the health charts feel overweight, and overweight women feel gargantuan.

©Kristian Dowling/Getty Images

Slimness is idealized in the United States. On average, models are 9% taller and 16% thinner than the typical female.

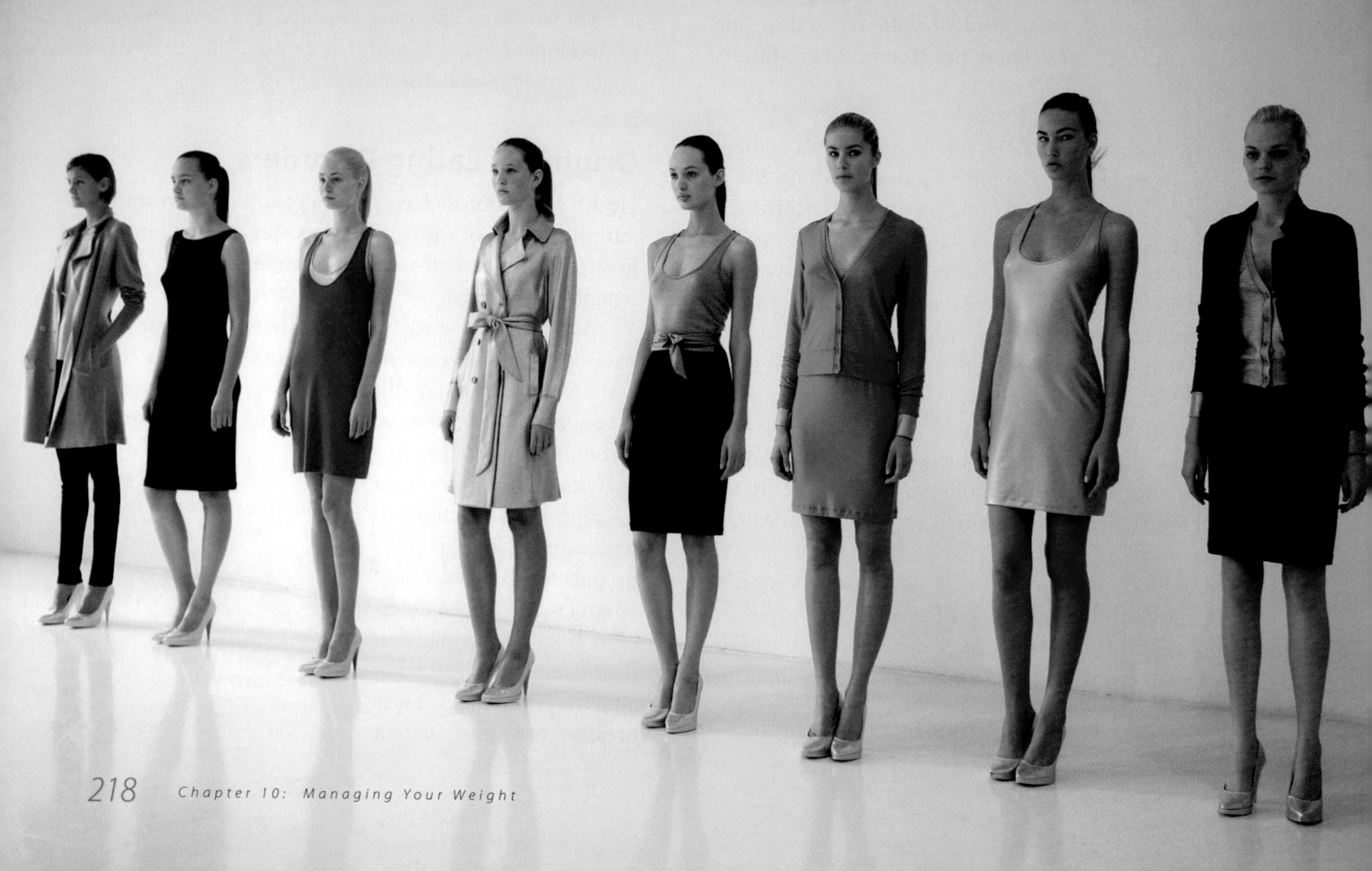

HEALTH CHECK 10-2

Eating Disorders Quiz[41]

The following are some questions that may help identify the presence or potential for an eating disorder. These are not a substitute for evaluation by a professional in the field.

1. Are you preoccupied about your weight or shape? (Note: Some concern is normal in our society.)
2. If you are dieting, have you lost a significant amount of weight or have you lost weight rapidly?
3. (If you answered yes to question 2) Are your family, friends, or your doctor concerned about your weight loss?
4. (If you answered yes to question 2) Is your weight more than 10% under a healthy weight for your age and height?
5. (If you answered yes to question 2) Do you feel colder than your friends or family?
6. (If you answered yes to question 2) Has your energy level decreased significantly?
7. (If you answered yes to question 2) Females: have your periods stopped or become irregular?
8. (If you answered yes to question 2) If you are still growing, have you failed to increase weight as you have become taller and older?
9. Do you experience binge eating or "grazing" with a sense of loss of control that causes physical or psychological distress?
10. Do you purge after eating by inducing vomiting, using laxatives, taking water pills, using diet pills, skipping meals, or do you compensate in other ways for eating more than you thought you should?
11. Do you compulsively exercise—to the point where your friends or family are concerned, your coach is concerned, or you have medical symptoms from excessive exercise?
12. Are you using any bodybuilding steroids to increase your muscle mass?
13. Do you experience yo-yo (up and down) weights on a regular basis?
14. Do you have a significant increase in carbohydrate craving or binge eating or grazing in the fall and winter months?
15. Do you have a continuing negative attitude toward your body weight or shape to the extent that it interferes with the quality of daily life or preoccupies you much of the time?

The above questions address only some of the signs and symptoms of an eating disorder. If you answered "yes" to any of the above questions, there is a possibility that you have an eating disorder, and you may want to seek assistance. If you answered "yes" to five or more items, you should seriously consider seeking professional advice.

Many individuals with eating disorders are involved in activities that demand weight limits, such as dancing, acting, and modeling. As noted earlier, male wrestlers and other athletes also feel the pressure to stay within an "acceptable" weight range.[42] Men, like women, experience pressure to create an ideal body, one with power in the upper torso and a trim abdomen.

Eating disorders tend to run in families, which raises the possibility of the involvement of genetic factors.[43] Genetic factors might be involved in the obsessionist and perfectionist personality traits that often accompany the need to be super thin.[44] Genetically inspired perfectionism, cultural emphasis on slimness, self-absorption, and family conflict may create a perfect recipe for the development of eating disorders.

Treatment of Eating Disorders

People with anorexia who become dangerously thin or malnourished are often hospitalized and force-fed, if necessary. The immediate goals of treatment are regaining weight and stabilizing body chemistry through normalizing eating behavior.

Since the neurotransmitter serotonin induces feelings of satiation, drugs that stimulate appetite by curbing the actions of serotonin can lead to weight gains in patients with anorexia.

Antidepressant drugs have the opposite effect. They increase the serotonin available in the brain, which suppresses appetite. Thus, antidepressant drugs that target serotonin activity in the brain can help reduce cravings for food and tendencies to binge in people with bulimia and **binge-eating disorder**.[45] Since people with both bulimia and binge-eating disorder are often depressed, antidepressants may have a secondary benefit of helping alleviate underlying depression.

binge-eating disorder
A type of eating disorder characterized by recurrent binges that are not accompanied by purging.

behavior modification
A set of psychological interventions that apply the principles of learning to help people change their behavior.

Psychological approaches also play important roles. When patients need to be hospitalized because of anorexia, a program of behavior therapy (sometimes called **behavior modification**) may offer them reinforcements or rewards, such as increased ward privileges, contingent on eating or gaining weight. With bulimics, behavior therapists may use the technique of *exposure* (to forbidden foods) together with *response prevention* (preventing the purging ritual). For example, a patient with bulimia might be instructed to eat modest amounts of "forbidden" foods, with a therapist standing by to help prevent vomiting until the urge to purge passes. In this way, people with bulimia learn to tolerate deviations from their rigid dieting rules without resorting to purging.

Psychodynamic treatment explores the psychological roots of the problem. Family therapy helps resolve family conflicts that contribute to or worsen eating disorders. Cognitive-behavioral psychologists help people with eating disorders replace distorted beliefs about their bodies, food, and dieting with more rational beliefs. (For advice on losing extra weight in healthful ways, read the online feature "Health Skills 10-1.")

health skills

Access CourseMate for HLTH at www.cengagebrain.com.

Patients are encouraged not to define their self-worth in terms of their body weight. Although promising results of psychological and drug therapies are reported, many adolescents with eating disorders experience recurrent episodes into adulthood.

HEALTH APPS: YOUR LINK TO ONLINE HEALTH APPLICATIONS

health skills

Skills of Effective Weight Management *Super Diet!! Diet Power!! So easy, they call it a miracle diet! Lose weight fast, effortlessly! The Atkins Diet!! (The New Atkins Diet!!) The Ornish Diet!! Take off excess weight permanently . . . in your sleep! Hollywood stars reveal their diet secrets!*

These are but a few of the magazine headlines promising quick, easy, permanent weight loss. There are literally thousands of approaches to helping people lose weight, everything from low-carb, high-protein diets to diets named after trendy locales, such as the South Beach diet. Read "Health Skills 10-1" to learn how to separate the diet wheat from the diet chaff and for advice on losing extra weight in healthful ways.

Go to the CourseMate for HLTH at www.cengagebrain.com for additional resources including flashcards, games, self-quizzes, review exercises, web exercises, learning checks, and more.

HLTH
Chapter 11

Combating Cardiovascular Disease, Cancer, and Other Major Diseases

"This chapter is about major health problems and killer diseases that we can ignore at our own peril or take steps to protect ourselves against."

Learning Outcomes

1. Describe the cardiovascular system
2. Discuss the major forms of cardiovascular disease
3. Describe methods of diagnosing and treating cardiovascular disease
4. List and discuss the risk factors for cardiovascular disease
5. Discuss the nature of cancer and how it develops
6. List and discuss the causes of cancer
7. Discuss the similarities and differences among various types of cancer
8. Discuss the nature, incidence, and control of diabetes
9. Discuss the major forms of chronic obstructive pulmonary disease

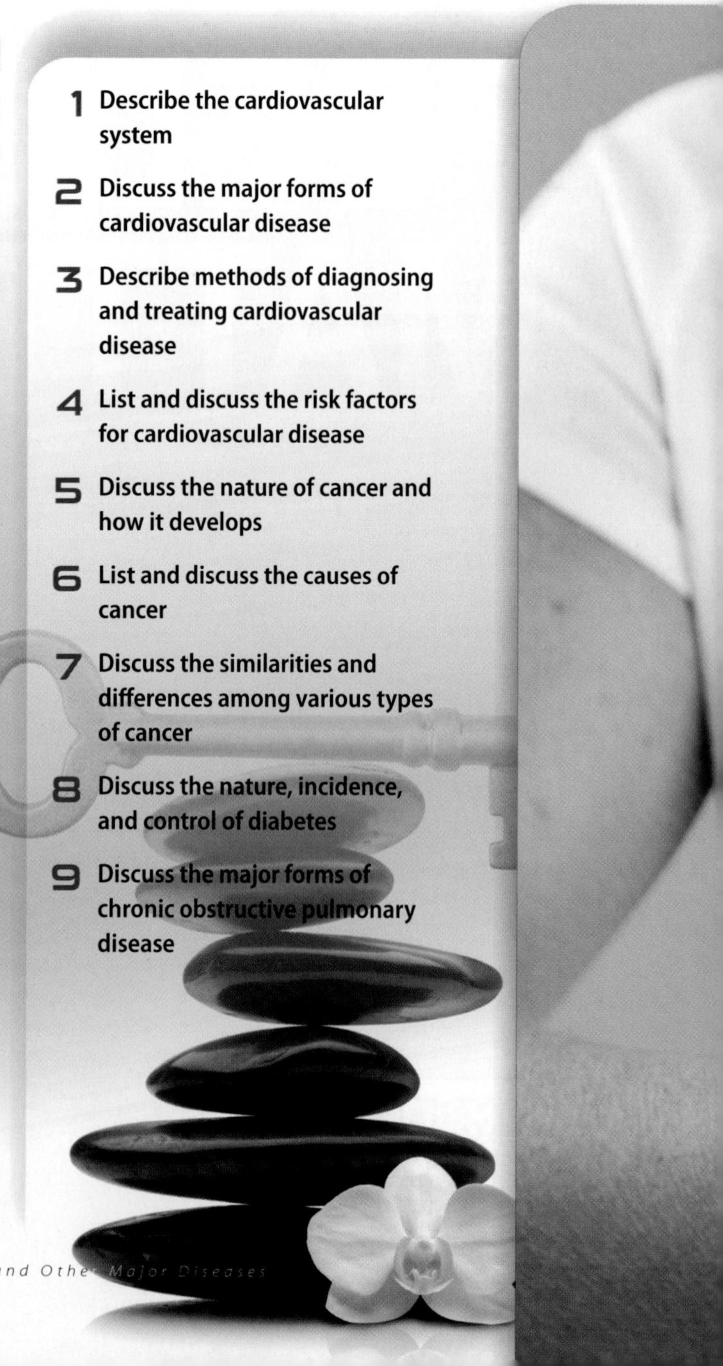

© iStockphoto.com/ mykeyruna

This chapter is about major health problems and killer diseases that we can ignore at our own peril or take steps to protect ourselves against. Most young people have healthy hearts and assume that those hearts will beat for many years to come. What can you do to increase the odds that you are correct? You probably know someone who had cancer or died from it. If you are cancer-free, what can you do to try to remain that way? Twenty-six million Americans have diabetes and another 79 million Americans have *pre-diabetes*. What can you do to avoid becoming one of them? Then there are those who have chronic breathing problems. What can you do so that you will not someday be gasping for breath?

This chapter is not about pleasant topics, but it does give you the knowledge you need to lower your risk factors for these problems and, if they occur, to deal with them early and effectively. We begin with cardiovascular disease.

CARDIOVASCULAR DISEASE

This section is about your highway of life—your cardiovascular system. Your cardiovascular system is the network that connects your heart and blood vessels. It furnishes the cells in your body with oxygen and nutrients, and trucks away their wastes.

But there are accidents along this highway. Many of them are in the form of cardiovascular disease. **Cardiovascular disease** (disease of the heart and blood vessels), or **CVD**, is the leading killer in the United States and around the world.[1] It claims about 1 million lives annually and accounts for more than 35% of all deaths in the United States, most often from heart attacks or strokes.[2] It leaves millions more disabled or impaired.

cardiovascular disease (CVD)
A disease of the heart or blood vessels.

But road signs alert us to dangers to our cardiovascular system. In this section we emphasize prevention of cardiovascular disease through a heart-smart lifestyle. How much do you already know about heart disease? The online feature "Health Check 11-1" will help you evaluate your "heart smarts."

health check

Access CourseMate for HLTH at www.cengagebrain.com.

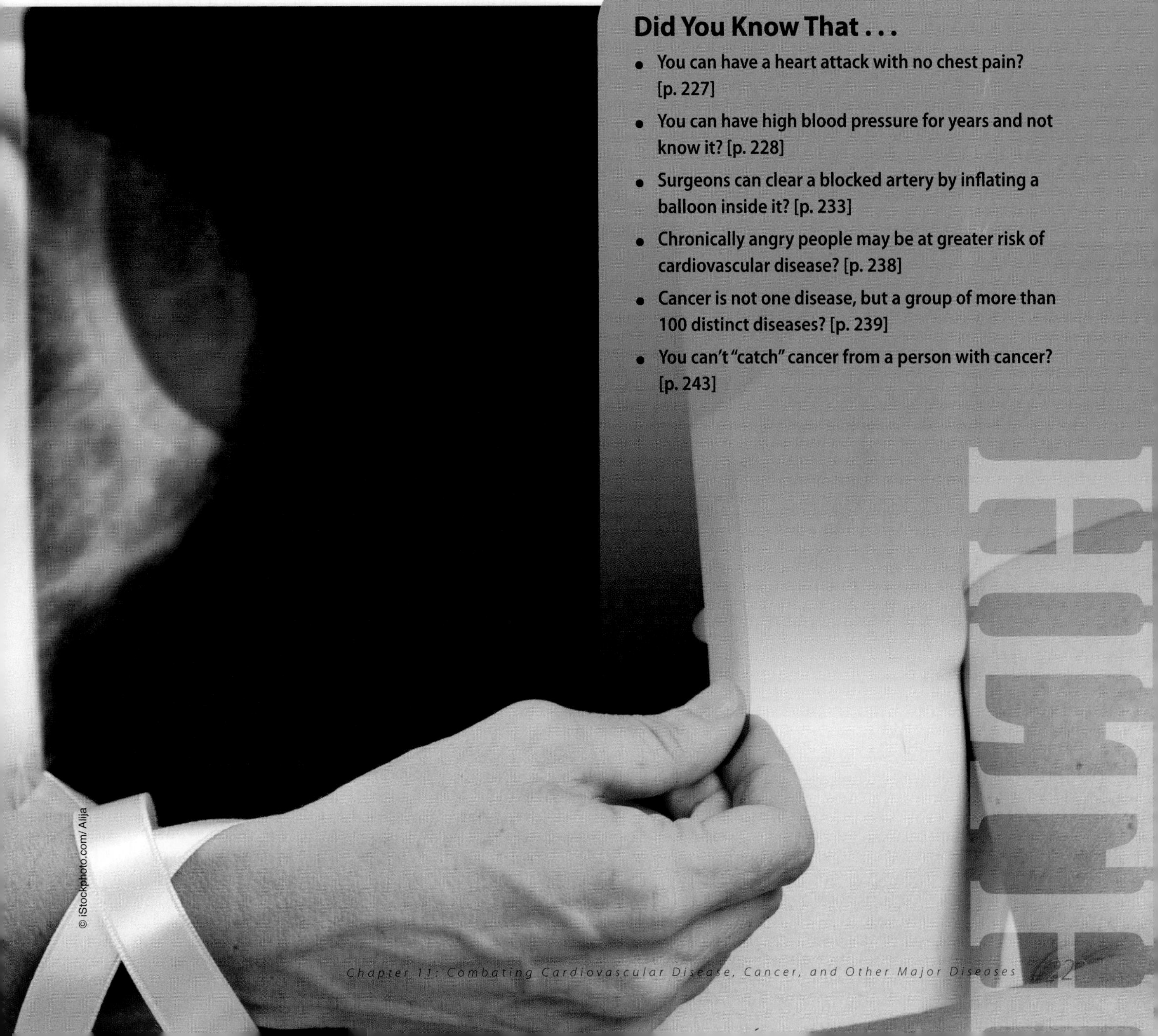

© iStockphoto.com/ Alija

Did You Know That . . .

- You can have a heart attack with no chest pain? [p. 227]
- You can have high blood pressure for years and not know it? [p. 228]
- Surgeons can clear a blocked artery by inflating a balloon inside it? [p. 233]
- Chronically angry people may be at greater risk of cardiovascular disease? [p. 238]
- Cancer is not one disease, but a group of more than 100 distinct diseases? [p. 239]
- You can't "catch" cancer from a person with cancer? [p. 243]

The Cardiovascular System

The cardiovascular system consists of the heart, the circulatory system, and blood.

The Heart

The heart is a strong, muscular pump. It is about the size of a clenched fist, and weighs a mere 11 ounces. Yet this powerhouse pumps five or more quarts of blood through your circulatory system every minute, some 2,000 gallons a day.

LEARNING OUTCOME 1

Describe the cardiovascular system

Over the course of an average lifetime, the human heart will beat (contract and expand) more than 2.5 billion times. It beats about 72 times a minute while your body is resting and faster when you exert yourself. That works out to about 100,000 beats per day. Once it stops beating for more than a few minutes, life ends.

Places in the Heart

You may think your heart is shaped like a valentine, but it looks more like an upside-down pear (see Figure 11-1). The heart is situated between your lungs in the middle of your chest. It lies in a moistened sac that is located behind the breastbone and is protected by the rib cage.

The interior of the heart contains open spaces called *chambers*. On each side of the heart there is an upper chamber called an **atrium** (plural *atria*) and a lower chamber called a **ventricle** (see Figure 11-1).

atrium
The upper chamber in each half of the heart.

ventricle
The lower chamber in each half of the heart.

circulatory system
The system or network of blood vessels that carries blood throughout the body.

The Circulatory System

The **circulatory system** is the network of blood vessels that bring oxygen and nutrients to the organs and tissues of the body and cart away cellular waste products. The circulatory system is so complex that if you laid all the blood vessels in an adult's body in a straight line, it would be nearly 100,000 miles long!

When blood leaves the heart through the aorta, it is funneled from larger to smaller blood vessels. Along the way, it delivers oxygen to cells, and cells deposit their waste products into the bloodstream. Some wastes are filtered through the liver and kidneys before being eliminated from the body as urine. Oxygen enables cells to metabolize sugars and fats into energy, and *carbon dioxide* is a resultant waste product that is carried by the circulatory system to the lungs, which expel it from the body.

The circulatory system also carries hormones that assist organs in carrying out their functions. It transports armies of disease-fighting white blood cells and

Figure 11-1 Places in the Heart

The heart has four chambers. The upper chambers are called *atria* and the lower chambers are *ventricles*. Unoxygenated blood enters the right atrium. It then passes into the right ventricle, from where it is pumped through the *pulmonary artery* into the lungs. In the lungs, the blood releases carbon dioxide and picks up oxygen. The oxygenated blood then enters the left atrium and from there is pumped into the left ventricle, which drives the blood into the *aorta*, the body's main artery. Blood vessels branch off from the aorta, eventually reaching every cell in the body.

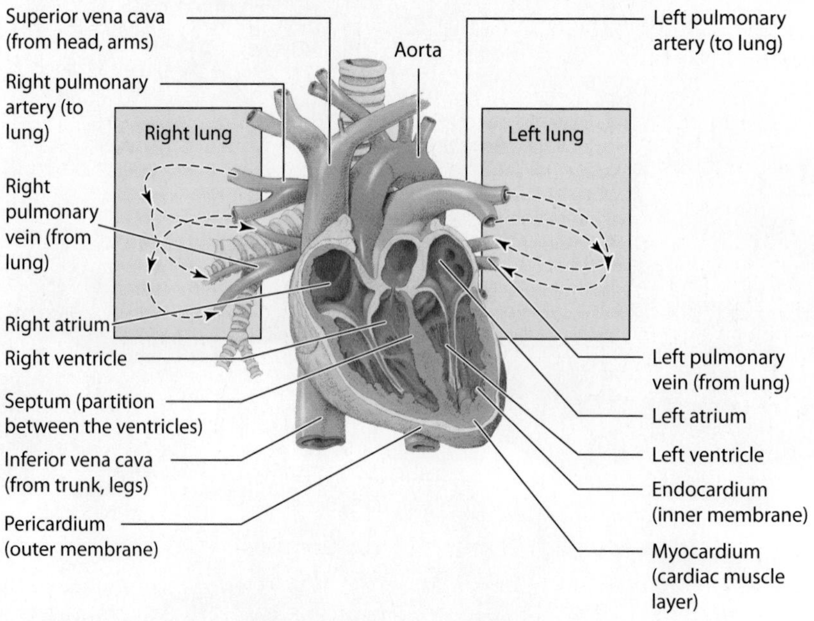

antibodies that enable the body to defend itself against invading microorganisms and rid itself of diseased, cancerous, and worn-out cells.

Types of Blood Vessels

There are three types of blood vessels. **Arteries** funnel oxygen-rich blood from the heart into increasingly narrower arterial vessels that eventually connect to the smallest blood vessels—**capillaries**—which bring blood directly to cells. Carbon dioxide and other waste products are deposited by cells into other capillaries, which are connected to **veins**. Veins transport blood back to the heart, widening as they near it.

The largest veins, the **vena cava**, carry the oxygen-poor blood into the right atrium of the heart, from where it repeats its journey (see Figure 11-1). The *superior vena cava* carries blood from the upper body. The *inferior vena cava* carries blood from the lower body. On the way to the heart, the blood passes through the liver and kidneys, where cellular waste products are removed for excretion in urine.

Blood

Blood is the fluid that travels through the heart and circulatory system. Blood carries oxygen, nutrients, hormones, and antibodies cells and carts away cellular waste products and carbon dioxide. The straw-colored or yellowish liquid part of blood is called *blood plasma.*

Erythrocytes, or red blood cells, carry oxygen to cells. Red blood cells contain *hemoglobin*, the red, iron-rich substance that gives blood its reddish color. In the lungs, hemoglobin binds to oxygen, which carries it in the bloodstream for transport to body tissues. In the capillaries, hemoglobin releases oxygen so that it can pass into body cells.

Leukocytes, or white blood cells, comprise part of the immune system. They protect the body by destroying invading microbes.

Platelets are small, colorless bodies that accumulate when the wall of a blood vessel is damaged or punctured. They form clots that plug holes in the walls of the injured blood vessels. The process of clot formation (or *coagulation*) is completed by specialized proteins called *clotting factors*, which are also carried in the plasma. Without platelets we would bleed to death from the slightest wound.

New blood is continuously manufactured by the body to replace old or defective blood cells and blood lost through injury. Most blood cells are manufactured in the bone marrow, the soft material that fills the inner cavities of bones. Some white blood cells, called *lymphocytes*, are produced in lymph glands and other organs in the lymphatic system.

Major Forms of Cardiovascular Disease

Cardiovascular diseases affect the functioning of the heart and circulatory system. The major forms of cardiovascular disorder include coronary heart disease (CHD), hypertension, rheumatic fever, congenital heart disease, arrhythmias, and stroke.

LEARNING OUTCOME 2

Discuss the major forms of cardiovascular disease

Coronary Heart Disease (CHD)

The heart is made of muscle tissue, which like other body tissue requires oxygen and nutrients carried by the blood. The harder the heart works, the more oxygen it needs. In **coronary heart disease** (**CHD**; also called *coronary artery disease*), the flow of blood to the heart is insufficient to meet its needs. The word *coronary* derives from the Latin *corona* ("crown") and suggests the way in which the arteries encircle the heart in a crown-like manner. CHD is the most common type of heart disease and accounts for most deaths resulting from cardiovascular disease, making it the leading cause of death in the United States. CHD results in about 600,000 deaths annually, or about one death in five.

Approximately one in eight adults (12%) in the United States has been

arteries
Blood vessels that carry blood from the heart and connect to capillaries that deliver oxygen-rich blood to body tissues.

capillaries
Tiny blood vessels that carry blood from the smallest arteries directly to the cells and connect to the tiniest veins for transport of deoxygenated blood and cellular waste products.

veins
Blood vessels that carry blood back to the heart.

vena cava
The largest veins, which carry blood directly into the heart.

erythrocytes
Red blood cells; they carry oxygen to cells.

leukocytes
White blood cells; they combat infection.

platelets
Round or oval disks in the blood that help blood clot when there is a wound or injury.

coronary heart disease (CHD)
A disease usually caused by damage to coronary arteries in which the blood supply to the heart is reduced to a level that is insufficient to meet the heart's needs.

diagnosed with some form of heart disease, and about 6% has been diagnosed with CHD.[3] One of every two men, and one of every three women, will eventually develop CHD.[4]

CHD most commonly results from **arteriosclerosis** or hardening of the arteries, a condition in which the walls of the arteries become thicker and harder. Arteriosclerosis can impair circulation and increase the risk of a blood clot becoming lodged in an artery. If the blood clot chokes off the blood flow, a heart attack or stroke can result.

Figure 11-2 Atherosclerosis

Atherosclerosis, the major form of arteriosclerosis, is a condition in which fatty deposits or plaque build up along artery walls. As a result, arteries become narrower, setting the stage for blockage by blood clots that can result in heart attacks or strokes. This figure shows (a) a normal artery cross-section; (b) moderate buildup along the artery wall; and (c) severe buildup along the artery wall.

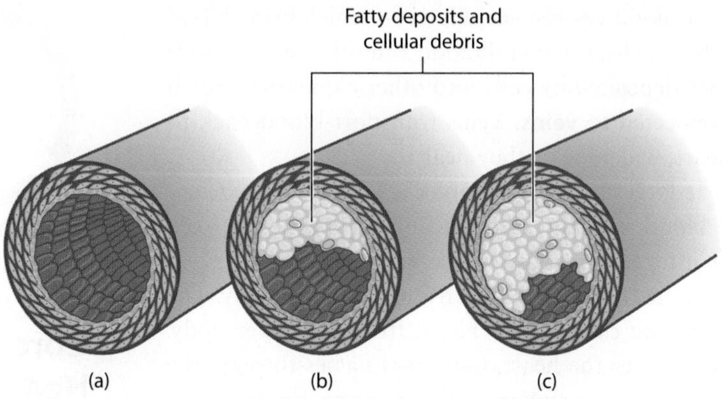

Atherosclerosis

The most common form of arteriosclerosis is atherosclerosis—the buildup of fatty deposits called *plaque* on the inner wall or lining of arteries (see Figure 11-2). The word *atherosclerosis* is derived from the Greek *athero* (meaning "paste") and *sclerosis* (meaning "hardness"), which is an apt description of the "hardening" of this artery-clogging "paste" (plaque).

In CHD, plaque builds up in *coronary arteries*, the small blood vessels that provide life-sustaining oxygen and nutrients to the heart. The arteries may no longer be able to supply the heart with enough blood, especially during physical exertion, leading to chest pain or *angina*. Blood clots may become lodged in arteries narrowed by atherosclerosis. If a blood clot (*thrombus*) forms in a coronary artery narrowed by atherosclerosis, it may nearly or even completely block the flow of blood to a part of the heart, resulting in a *heart attack*. If the blood vessel is one that services the brain, the result can be a **stroke**.

The medical term for heart attack is **myocardial infarction (MI)**. The word *myocardial* derives from the Greek roots *myo* ("muscle") and *kardia* ("heart"). An *infarct* is an area of dead or dying tissue. A myocardial infarction is the death of heart tissue arising from an insufficiency of blood supply (called *ischemia*). Within minutes of a disruption of its blood supply, the heart tissue served by the blocked artery begins to die. As the area of the infarct expands, the heart may no longer be able to pump enough blood to sustain life. Brain death can occur within minutes if the heart fails to pump enough blood. Though CHD typically develops slowly over a period of years, the first sign may be a heart attack. About every 30 seconds in the United States, someone suffers a heart attack.[5]

arteriosclerosis
A condition in which the walls of arteries become thicker and harder and lose elasticity. Commonly called hardening of the arteries.

stroke
The sudden loss of consciousness and resulting paralysis, loss of sensation, and other disability or death resulting from blockage of blood to a part of the brain or bleeding in the brain. Also called a cerebrovascular accident *or* CVA.

myocardial infarction (MI)
A condition involving damage or death of heart tissue due to insufficient blood flow to the heart, usually as the result of a blockage in one or more coronary arteries.

Inflammation

Inflammation in blood vessels can cause fatty deposits (plaque) along artery walls to burst, which then can form blood clots that block the flow of blood to the heart. The result can be a heart attack.

Heart specialists are zeroing in on a specific marker of inflammation, a type of protein produced by the liver called *C-reactive protein* (CRP).[6] The liver produces C-reactive protein whenever there is inflammation in the body. The inflammation may arise in the arteries but also from other sources such as the body's response to infection. Elevated levels of CRP in the blood are associated with increased risk of cardiovascular disease. Medical researchers are investigating the health benefits of screening people for CRP and also how to treat people with high levels of the protein.

Signs of a Heart Attack

Heart attacks are medical emergencies that require immediate attention. The first minutes and hours are critical to survival, as most people who die of heart attacks succumb within two hours. Yet about half of the people who suffer a heart attack wait two hours or more before getting help. Many people minimize their symptoms or attribute them to more benign causes, like indigestion or heartburn.

Whether or not one survives a heart attack depends on the extent of damage to heart tissue and to the electrical system that controls the heart rhythm. Death rates from heart disease have declined steadily during the past 50 years, in part because fewer people are smoking (smoking is a major risk factor) and because of improvements in treatment.

Becoming aware of the signs of a heart attack can save a life, perhaps your own. Though not all of the following symptoms need be present, the signs of a heart attack may include:

- Intense, prolonged chest pain, described as crushing not sharp, which may be experienced as a feeling of heavy pressure or tightness in the chest. Some describe a squeezing sensation in the chest, or a sensation like a giant fist enclosing the heart. Yet some people have heart attacks without chest pain.
- Pain extending beyond the chest to the left shoulder and arm, the back, even into the jaws and gums.
- Prolonged pain in the upper abdomen.
- Shortness of breath.
- Fainting or weakness.
- Heavy perspiration, nausea, or vomiting.
- Anxiety and fear.

What to Do in Case of a Heart Attack

If you experience the signs of a heart attack or are with someone who does, seek medical attention immediately. Call 911 or your local emergency operator and follow their instructions. If the person stops breathing, administer CPR if you have been trained in the procedure. If not, an emergency technician may be able to explain CPR over the phone until help arrives.

Angina Pectoris

Although the first signs of CHD may be a sudden heart attack, many heart attacks are preceded by a series of attacks of chest pain called **angina** (technical term: *angina pectoris*). Angina is similar to but less severe and prolonged than the pain of a heart attack. Angina is experienced below the breastbone and may extend to the left jaw and shoulder and down the left arm. It may feel like an ache or pressure. There may be feelings of heaviness or tightness in the chest or a burning sensation. Sometimes the pain is mistaken for heartburn or indigestion.

Angina is a symptom, not a disease, that is caused by insufficient blood reaching the heart—the same process that can result in a heart attack. In angina, however, the restriction of blood is not as complete or as prolonged as in a heart attack. Sometimes the obstruction of blood flow is caused by a spasm in an artery serving the heart, but most cases are caused by a buildup of plaque.

Angina attacks usually, but not always, occur during periods of exertion, as during exercise, when more oxygenated blood is needed by the heart. (If you should experience chest pain during exercise or when walking up the stairs, stop the activity immediately and call your doctor.) Angina may be relieved by the drug *nitrogylerine*, which dilates (opens) coronary arteries, allowing blood to flow more freely to the heart. It is usually taken in tablet form and dissolved under the tongue.

Angina attacks usually subside in a few minutes without lasting damage to the heart. Many people with angina never experience a heart attack, but many heart attacks are preceded by angina. Thus, angina should be treated seriously.

angina
Heart pain arising from insufficient blood flow to the heart.

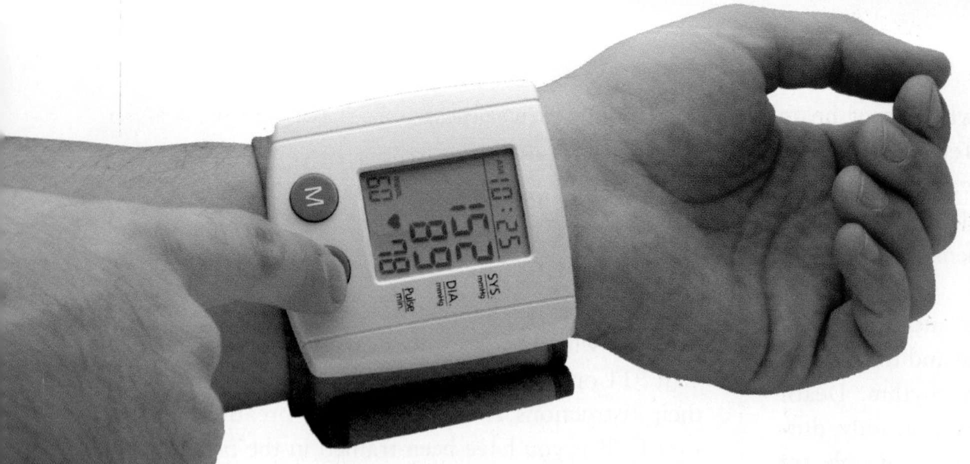

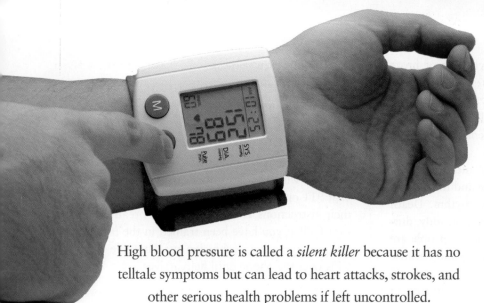

High blood pressure is called a *silent killer* because it has no telltale symptoms but can lead to heart attacks, strokes, and other serious health problems if left uncontrolled.

Hypertension

Hypertension, or high blood pressure, is a leading risk factor for cardiovascular disease. It can lead to heart attacks, congestive heart failure, kidney damage, stroke, even blindness. About one in three Americans has hypertension.[7]

Blood pressure is the force or pressure applied by the blood against the walls of a blood vessel. Blood pressure is defined by two numbers:

- The first number is the **systolic blood pressure (SBP)**. This is a measure of the maximum pressure in the arteries when the heart contracts or beats and pushes blood into the body.
- The second number is the **diastolic blood pressure (DBP)**, which is the minimum pressure remaining in the arteries when the heart relaxes between beats.

Based on the latest medical guidelines, an SBP of about 110–120 mm Hg and a DBP of about 75–80 mm Hg is considered desirable. A blood pressure of 120 SBP and 80 DBP is written in the form 120/80 mm Hg (read that 120 *over* 80 millimeters of mercury).

SBP at a level of 120 to 139 mm Hg, or DBP at a level of 80 to 89 mm Hg, falls within a category of *prehypertension* (see Table 11-1). People with blood pressures in this prehypertensive range may be encouraged to make changes in their diet and exercise patterns (such as losing weight, reducing salt intake, exercising more regularly, and curbing alcohol intake) to prevent their blood pressure from rising into the hypertensive range. The risks of cardiovascular and other diseases (such as kidney disease) begin to climb when blood pressure levels rise above 115/75 mm Hg. Taking both systolic and diastolic BPs into account helps doctors better appraise cardiovascular risk than either type alone.[8]

People with an SBP consistently equal to or greater than 140 mm Hg systolic and/or a DBP consistently equal to or greater than 90 mm Hg have hypertension. Even people with normal blood pressure at age 55 have a high risk of eventually developing hypertension.[9] In some cases, hypertension can be traced to identifiable physical problems or defects, such as kidney malfunction. But in *essential hypertension* (also called *primary hypertension*), which accounts for about 90% of cases, the cause remains unclear.

The risk of developing hypertension increases with age. Until age 55, men stand a higher risk than women, but gender differences then level off until age 75, at which point women begin to incur greater risks.[10] About 20% of people with hypertension don't know it because hypertension rarely produces noticeable symptoms.[11] Only about half of people with hypertension have it under control.[12] People usually become aware of hypertension when it's detected during a routine physical exam. No wonder hypertension is called a silent killer.

hypertension
High blood pressure, generally determined by a blood pressure reading of 140 (systolic)/90 (diastolic) or higher.

systolic blood pressure (SBP)
The maximum pressure in the arteries that occurs when the heart contacts with each heartbeat.

diastolic blood pressure (DBP)
The minimum pressure that remains in the arteries when the heart relaxes between beats.

Table 11-1 Blood Pressure Categories: Are You Hypertensive?

	SYSTOLIC BLOOD PRESSURE (MM HG)	DIASTOLIC BLOOD PRESSURE (MM HG)
Desirable	100–120	75–80
Prehypertension	120–139	80–89
Hypertension	140 or higher	90 or higher

Deaths resulting from underlying high blood pressure are often attributed to other causes, such as heart attacks and strokes. Yet hypertension is a killer disease and should be treated as such. Hypertension accelerates the process of atherosclerosis, which increases the risk of heart attacks and strokes. There are steps you can take to lower your risk of developing hypertension (see Table 11-2). A range of effective treatments is also available to help people who suffer from hypertension. As you'll read in the online feature "Diversity 11-1," African Americans are more likely than European Americans to develop.

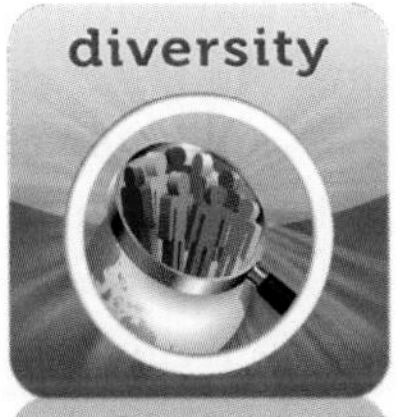

Access CourseMate for HLTH at www.cengagebrain.com.

Congestive Heart Failure

In **congestive heart failure**, damage to the heart prevents it from pumping out all the blood it receives from the veins. Blood thus backs up or pools (congests) in the veins and elsewhere, such as the lungs and lower extremities. Congestive heart failure claims some 50,000 lives per year in the United States. It may result from such causes as congenital heart defect, loss of muscular tissue in the heart due to a heart attack or disease, rheumatic fever, or high blood pressure.

The signs of congestive heart failure include edema (swelling), especially in the ankles and legs, and shortness of breath, which results from congestion in the lungs. If the kidneys fail to get an adequate supply of blood, excess fluid can build up in the body, contributing to edema and weight gain. Inadequate blood flow to the muscles may lead to a loss of muscular endurance, causing early fatigue during physical exertion.

Though congestive heart failure is a serious and life-threatening condition, it is treatable in most cases. Treatment may involve rest and modified daily activities to conserve energy, a carefully monitored exercise program to strengthen the heart, proper diet, avoidance of alcoholic beverages, and weight control.

Drugs may bring down swelling (edema) and improve the heart's pumping efficiency. *Diuretics* (sometimes called "water pills") reduce edema by increasing the secretion of urine. *Digitalis* preparations, such as *digoxin*, are drugs derived from the digitalis plant. They improve the heart's pumping ability by increasing the force of contractions. *Vasodilators* make it easier for the heart to pump blood by expanding the arteries. They also reduce blood pressure. Surgery may be required to repair or replace a damaged or diseased heart valve that may be allowing blood to back up. In extreme cases, when the heart is damaged beyond repair, a heart transplant may be needed.

Congenital Heart Defects

The word *congenital* (from the Latin *congenitus*, meaning "with birth") means inborn or innate. **Congenital heart defects** are thus present at birth and comprise defects in which the heart or the connections between the heart, lungs, and blood vessels fail to develop normally.

A congenital heart defect is the most common type of birth defect, occurring in about one in every 100 live births.[14] The cause in most cases remains unknown, but some cases can be traced to a viral infection experienced by the mother during pregnancy, such as *rubella* (German measles). Other common causes include maternal use of alcohol or other drugs, such as cocaine, during pregnancy, and Down syndrome, a chromosomal disorder that produces mental retardation and characteristic features such as a rounded face and a wide, flattened nose.

Table 11-2 Steps You Can Take to Reduce Your Risk of Hypertension[13]

☑ Adopt a diet rich in fruits, vegetables, whole grains, and low-fat dairy foods and sparing in saturated fat, total fat, and cholesterol.
☑ Reduce salt and sodium in your diet.
☑ Maintain a healthy weight (a body mass index [BMI] between 18 and 24.99).
☑ Be physically active for 30 minutes a day.
☑ Limit alcohol intake to one drink a day for women or two drinks a day for men.
☑ Quit smoking, or don't start smoking.

congestive heart failure
A condition in which the heart is unable to pump out as much blood as it receives, leading to a backing-up or pooling of blood in the veins, lungs, and extremities.

congenital heart defect
A heart defect that is present at birth.

Most heart defects require open-heart surgery. Such surgery is riskier with newborn babies, so surgeons prefer to wait until early childhood to operate. In many cases, the defect can be repaired and the person can lead a normal life.

Arrhythmias

The heart normally beats about 72 times per minute when a person is at rest. An **arrhythmia** is an abnormal heartbeat or rhythm. An abnormally fast heartbeat is called *tachycardia*. An abnormally slow beat is termed *bradycardia*. Sometimes the heart beats irregularly or the chambers of the heart contract in an uncoordinated fashion, reducing the heart's efficiency.

Some arrhythmias are common and hardly noticed. Most people occasionally skip a heartbeat, which is not usually a problem unless it becomes recurrent or persistent. Nor is it unusual for people to experience occasional episodes of tachycardia, in which the heart suddenly speeds up to about 160 beats per minute. Tachycardia may be experienced as "palpitations" or a fluttering sensation.

Arrhythmias can be dangerous, even life threatening. Most dangerous arrhythmias result from heart disease, although some are due to congenital defects. Loss of consciousness or death may result if the heart beats too slowly. Heart attacks can damage the heart muscle and lead to a disruption in the electrical impulses that regulate the heartbeat, causing potentially fatal arrhythmias such as *ventricular fibrillation*. Most deaths resulting from heart attacks are actually caused by ventricular fibrillation, in which the two ventricles, or lower chambers of the heart, contract irregularly and are unable to pump effectively. Ventricular fibrillation may be stopped by an electrical device called a *defibrillator*, which shocks the heart through electrodes placed on the chest and restores the normal heartbeat (a technique no doubt familiar to viewers of medical dramas on TV). Ventricular fibrillation can trigger *cardiac arrest*, in which the heart suddenly stops beating, resulting in loss of consciousness and cessation of breathing and other bodily functions. Death occurs shortly as the brain and other vital body organs fail to receive blood. The defibrillator can help jolt the stopped heart back to a normal rhythm.

Cardiopulmonary resuscitation (CPR) techniques, including cardiac massage, may be able to restart the heartbeat of someone in cardiac arrest. (CPR is a lifesaving technique that everyone should learn *before* a life-threatening emergency occurs. Classes that train lay people in CPR techniques are offered in most communities. Contact your local health department or hospital center.)

Stroke

The brain, like other body tissue, needs a constant flow of blood to supply it with oxygen and nutrients (glucose) and cart away metabolic waste products. A stroke (also called a *cerebrovascular accident* or *CVA*) occurs when the flow of blood to an area of the brain is blocked by an obstruction in an artery serving that part of the brain. Deprived of its blood supply, even for a few minutes, the affected parts of the brain may be damaged or destroyed. In some strokes, brain tissue is destroyed by blood seeping out of a ruptured blood vessel. Because brain tissue does not regenerate, the functions controlled by affected parts of the brain may be lost or severely impaired.

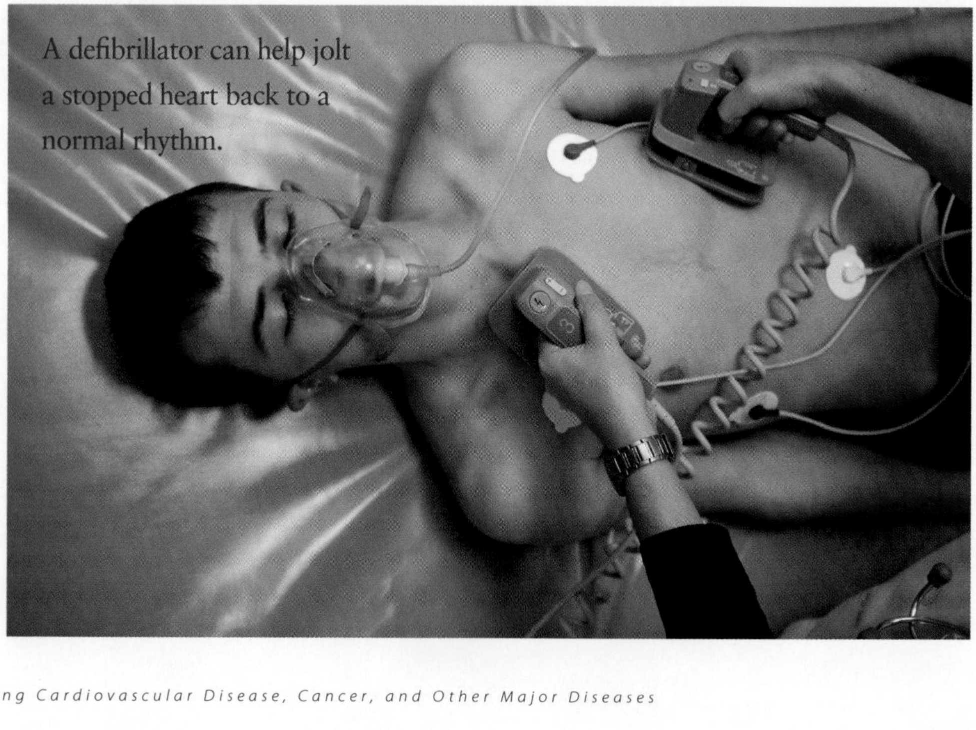
A defibrillator can help jolt a stopped heart back to a normal rhythm.

© iStockphoto.com/muratseyit

arrhythmia
An irregular heart rhythm.
cardiopulmonary resuscitation (CPR)
An emergency medical treatment used to restore coronary and pulmonary functioning following cardiac arrest.

Strokes are among the leading killers of Americans, striking about 800,000 people annually and causing about one in 18 deaths annually in the U.S., which amounts to about 150,000 lives each year.[15] African Americans have nearly double the risk of suffering strokes than do European Americans, in large part because of an increased frequency of risk factors such as high blood pressure and cigarette smoking. Hypertension is the leading risk factor for stroke.

Types of Strokes

There are three major types of strokes (see Figure 11-3):

1. *Cerebral thrombosis.* This type of stroke accounts for about three strokes in four. It occurs when a blood clot (a *thrombus*) blocks an artery that supplies blood to the brain. The clot usually becomes lodged in a blood vessel narrowed by atherosclerosis.
2. *Cerebral embolism.* An *embolism* is an obstruction of a blood vessel. In a cerebral embolism, a blood clot or some other particle that forms in another part of the body travels through the circulatory system and lodges in an artery that serves the brain, blocking the flow of blood.
3. *Hemorrhagic stroke.* A hemorrhagic stroke, or *cerebral hemorrhage*, is the least common but most severe type of stroke. It results in death about half the time. A blood vessel in the brain ruptures so that blood leaks into brain cavities, damaging brain tissue. Hemorrhagic strokes are often linked to high blood pressure. Bleeding in the brain can also result from a head injury or a burst *aneurysm*. An aneurysm is a blood-filled sac or pouch that balloons out from a weak artery wall.

Effects of Stroke

The symptoms of stroke may include loss of speech or difficulty understanding speech; loss of feeling, numbness, weakness, or paralysis of a limb or the face; or sudden loss of consciousness. There may also be unexplained severe headaches, blurred or double vision, and dizziness or loss of balance or coordination. Stroke usually affects one side of the brain. The resultant loss of sensation or movement is limited to the other side of the body, because each side of the body is controlled by the opposite side of the brain.

Depending upon the site and extent of damage, the effects of a stroke can be relatively minor or result in serious disabilities, coma, and death. If the sensory or motor areas of the brain are affected, survivors may lose sensation or develop paralysis. Damage to the speech centers can lead to a general loss of speech or to problems with articulation. There may be declines in cognitive abilities involving memory, reasoning, and judgment.

Transient Ischemic Attacks (TIAs)

Transient ischemic attacks (TIAs) are brief stroke-like episodes resulting from an insufficient blood supply, or *ischemia*, to the brain. Symptoms may be similar to those of stroke and may include numbness, weakness, tingling, dizziness, headache, blurred or double vision, and temporary blindness. There may be momentary loss of motor function on one side of the body or difficulty speaking.

Unlike stroke, TIAs resolve quickly, usually within five minutes, and do not cause permanent disability, such as paralysis. However, TIAs need to be taken seriously. They are often early warning signs of stroke. About one in 10 strokes is preceded by TIAs. Among people who have had one or more TIAs, more than a third will eventually have a stroke.[16] Timely medical treatment following a TIA may help prevent a stroke. Anticoagulants may be used to thin the blood and prevent the formation of clots. Surgery may remove fatty deposits that clog arteries.

Figure 11-3 Types of Strokes

There are three types of strokes: thrombosis, embolism, and cerebral hemorrhage. Though any stroke is a potential killer, the cerebral hemorrhage is the most lethal.

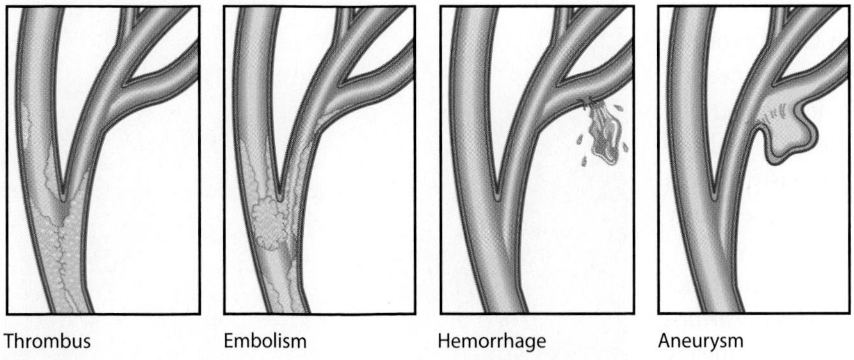

Diagnosis and Treatment of Cardiovascular Disorders

Several techniques are used to diagnose and treat cardiovascular disorders.

Diagnostic Tests

> **LEARNING OUTCOME 3**
>
> **Describe methods of diagnosing and treating cardiovascular disease**

Doctors use various techniques to probe the cardiovascular system for abnormalities. The doctor may push against the patient's chest to feel for an enlarged heart. A stethoscope is used to listen for irregular heart rhythms or other unusual sounds in the chest, such as a *heart murmur*. A heart murmur occurs when blood passes through a heart valve that is normally closed. Blood tests provide information about the blood levels of fats such as cholesterol and triglycerides that are associated with coronary artery disease. Blood is also analyzed for the level of thyroid hormone because overactivity of the thyroid gland is implicated in some arrhythmias.

A chest X-ray may reveal abnormalities in the heart or the blood vessels that serve the heart. The *electrocardiogram* (*ECG* or *EKG*) prints out a record of the heart's electrical activity. In an EKG, electrodes are attached to the skin on various sites of the body to measure the electrical discharges emanating from the heart when it beats. The EKG reveals abnormal heart rhythms that may be caused by congenital birth defects, CHD, or heart attacks. Sometimes abnormal heart rhythms may not be detected unless the heart is stressed. Therefore, an *exercise electrocardiogram* (*stress test*) may be used to chart the heart's activity while the person exercises on a treadmill or stationary bicycle.

The stress test helps to uncover heart problems, but as many as one in four people with CHD produce normal stress test results. Some arrhythmias are fleeting and don't show up during the EKG. To detect intermittent arrhythmias, people may wear a portable 24-hour EKG, called a *Holter monitor*, that continuously records the heart's electrical activity as they go about their daily activities.

Scanning techniques reveal the structure and functioning of the heart and the arteries. The *echocardiogram* uses the reflection or "echo" of high-frequency sound waves bounced against the chest to create an image of the heart on a monitor. The echocardiogram can reveal damage to the heart muscle, the presence of tumors or blood clots, valve disorders, and aneurysms.

Radionuclide imaging can detect blockages in the blood flow in and around the heart. Small amounts of radioactive substances called *radionuclides* are injected into a vein in the arm, usually as the person is exercising on a treadmill. A specialized scanning device creates images from their movement through the heart to detect any blockages.

Magnetic resonance imaging (*MRI*) uses a strong magnetic field to generate a computerized image of the structure of the heart or of other parts of the body. It can detect congenital heart defects, heart damage from previous heart attacks, and abnormalities in the blood vessels around the heart.

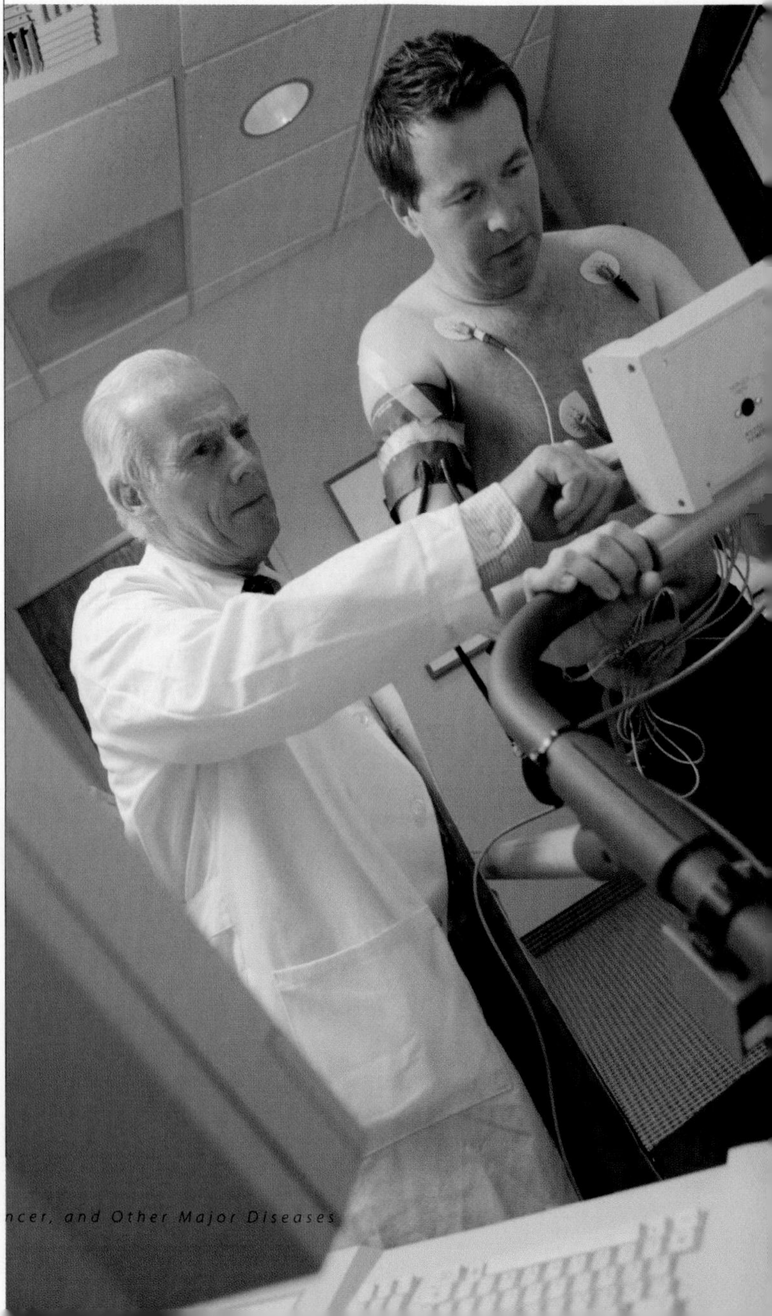

A more invasive procedure called a *coronary angiography* (also called an *angiogram*) involves a specialized X-ray technique that reveals blockages in coronary arteries, the blood vessels that bring blood to the heart. Because of the costs and potential risks of the procedure, its widespread use is debated among health professionals.

Specialized diagnostic tests are used to determine the causes of strokes, the extent of damage, and the most appropriate treatment. An *electroencephalogram (EEG)* measures brain waves and can reveal abnormal brain wave activity that results from damage to the brain.

Imaging techniques such as MRI and *computed tomography (CT) scan* (also called *computerized axial tomography scan* or *CAT scan*) may reveal areas of the brain damaged by a stroke. The CT scan is a specialized X-ray machine that takes pictures from different angles to display a three-dimensional image of the brain. These imaging techniques can help doctors determine whether a stroke was caused by a blood clot (thrombus) or a hemorrhage.

Treatment of Heart Disease

Major advances have been made in the treatment of heart disease in recent years. In most cases, people with heart disease can be successfully treated with medication or with such techniques as balloon angioplasty, coronary bypass surgery, and heart transplantation. The general goals of treatment are to reduce pain, improve circulation, and regulate the heart rhythm.

Heart Medications

Statins are a class of cholesterol-lowering drugs that can help prevent the buildup of fatty deposits (plaque) along artery walls that can lead to heart disease. *Anticoagulants* help prevent the formation of blood clots in people with narrowed arteries. Clot-dissolving drugs, called *thrombolytic agents* (*streptokinase* is one), can dissolve blood clots following a heart attack. *Beta blockers* reduce the pumping demands placed on the heart, which is useful in treating angina. *Vasodilators*, such as *angiotensin converting enzyme (ACE) inhibitors*, expand blood vessels narrowed by fatty deposits. ACE inhibitors may also be used after a heart attack to help the heart pump blood better. *Calcium channel blockers* interfere with the normal flow of calcium through the channels in the heart muscle. This can have several beneficial effects with cardiac patients by helping to expand the coronary arteries, which allows more blood to flow to the heart, and reducing blood pressure and pumping demands on the heart. *Nitroglycerine* dilates coronary arteries, increasing blood flow to the heart and relieving angina attacks. Even the common household aspirin may be used in the both the treatment and prevention of heart attacks (see the online feature "Prevention 11-1").

prevention

Access CourseMate for HLTH at www.cengagebrain.com.

Coronary Artery Bypass Graft Surgery

In *coronary artery bypass graft surgery* (*CABG*; sometimes pronounced *cabbage*), surgeons take a piece of a vein from elsewhere in the body, usually a leg, and construct grafts that direct the flow of blood around a blocked or narrowed coronary artery. One end of the graft is attached to the artery just above the blockage. The other end is connected to the artery just below the blockage. Typically, four or five bypasses are needed. The bypass allows blood to circumvent the blockages and flow more freely to the heart. Bypass surgery is typically recommended when blockages are severe or when the symptoms of coronary artery disease do not respond to other forms of treatment. CABG carries some risk, but the risk of dying is less than 1% for patients who are otherwise healthy. CABG does not correct the underlying disease process: atherosclerosis. Thus, the person must still follow a strict regimen consisting of proper diet, regular exercise, and avoidance of smoking.

Percutaneous Transluminal Coronary Angioplasty

Percutaneous transluminal coronary angioplasty (*PTCA*, also called *balloon angioplasty*) is used to clear coronary arteries of fatty deposits that obstruct the flow of blood to the heart (see Figure 11-4 on the next page). Under local anesthesia, a catheter is inserted into a leg artery and threaded into a blocked coronary artery. Once it reaches its destination, a tiny balloon is inflated. The balloon widens the blocked artery by flattening the blockage against the artery wall. Widening improves circulation to the heart.

Through a procedure called an *atherectomy*, blockages are surgically removed rather than just compressed as in traditional angioplasty. A laser may also be used to clear away blockages.

About three times as many angioplasty procedures are performed than bypass surgeries. Angioplasty is less costly, avoids the trauma of open-heart surgery, and shortens recovery. However, angioplasty is not problem-free. Angioplasty is generally more successful in clearing some blockages than others, depending

Figure 11-4 Tools for Unclogging Arteries[17]

(a) Balloon angioplasty. A balloon catheter is used to flatten plaque and stretch artery walls. (b) Atherectomy. Special devices remove plaque from artery walls. (c) Coronary stenting. A device called a *stent* is placed inside the artery and props it open.

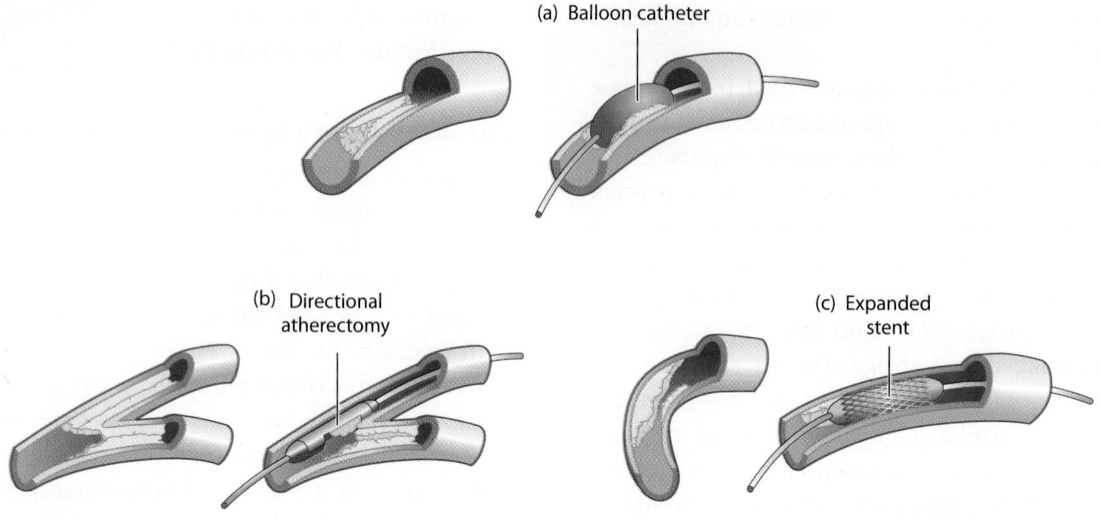

on the location and shape of the blockage. It generally succeeds in widening arteries, but blockages often return, requiring bypass surgery or repeat angioplasty. A variation on the procedure involves the use of a *stent* to open a clogged artery and keep it open (a stent typically remains in place permanently). Stents can also be used to prevent aneurysms from bursting.

Heart Transplants

Heart transplant operations are the most dramatic and risky of the procedures used to treat heart disease. The defective or diseased heart is replaced with a healthy heart from a donor whose death did not damage the heart. The donor's heart is preserved for transport in a special solution and is inserted in the recipient's chest cavity once the recipient's heart is removed.

People who are not expected to live more than two or three years with their current heart may be candidates for a heart transplant. These include people whose hearts have been severely damaged by previous heart attacks or by **cardiomyopathy**, a weakening of the heart muscle due to disease, and those with severe congestive heart failure. Though never routine, heart transplantation has become accepted medical practice as a treatment of last resort for people who otherwise have little or no hope for survival. About four of five recipients live for at least a year following the procedure. Many have survived for a decade or more with their new heart. The major problem with heart transplants is the risk that the body will reject it. Drugs suppress organ rejection and increase the chances of survival of heart transplant patients.

cardiomyopathy
A disease of the heart muscle or myocardium.

Treating a Heart Attack

Delays in health care following a heart attack cost lives. Many people who have a heart attack die before receiving medical attention. Emergency medical system (EMS) teams in most cities can reach people with heart attacks in minutes, apply life-saving techniques such as CPR, and stabilize them en route to the hospital. Most people who die before receiving medical help either ignore their symptoms or delay seeking help. But of those who reach the hospital alive, the great majority survive.

In the Hospital . . .

Various tests are used to diagnose a heart attack and determine the extent of the damage. An EKG reveals patterns of electrical impulses that indicate whether a heart attack has occurred and irregular heart rhythms that may have resulted. Blood tests detect enzymes that are released by damaged heart tissue. An angiogram may be performed to diagnose blocked arteries.

Blood clots that lodge in arteries already choked off by fatty deposits cause heart attacks. Doctors race against the clock to dissolve the clot before the blockage leads to permanent damage or death. They may use a drug like *streptokinase*. Or they may use *balloon angioplasty* or a related procedure to clear a blocked coronary artery. Angioplasty may also be used to clear fatty deposits in coronary arteries.

Nitroglycerine may be administered through a vein during or following a heart attack to increase the blood flow to the heart and decrease the heart's needs for oxygen. *Beta-blockers* may be used to reduce the oxygen requirements placed on the heart by slowing down the heart rate and reducing the force of heart contractions. *Aspirin* also eases the flow of blood through the circulatory system.

People who are alive two hours after a heart attack are likely to survive. Nevertheless, there may be complications. Damage to the heart muscle may affect the electrical system that controls the heartbeat, leading to life-threatening arrhythmias (irregular heart rhythms). In some cases the heart beats abnormally slowly, which may require the implantation of a pacemaker, a small electrical device that helps maintain a normal heartbeat. The extent of damage to the heart muscle in some patients is so severe that congestive heart failure develops.

After the Hospital . . .

Most people who recover from a heart attack are able to resume their normal lives within a few weeks. However, they will need to make lifestyle adjustments if they want to improve their chances of avoiding another attack—quitting smoking, decreasing intake of dietary cholesterol and fat, losing excess weight, exercising regularly, and keeping blood pressure under control.[18]

Treating a Stroke

As with a heart attack, delays in seeking medical attention following a stroke can be fatal. There is perhaps a three- to six-hour window of opportunity during which treatment has its greatest benefits. Knowing the signs may be critical in getting help soon enough to save a life.

Common Warning Signs of Stroke

Anyone who experiences these symptoms should treat them as a medical emergency and dial 911. Immediate treatment can spell the difference between life and death or between rapid recovery and permanent disability.[19]

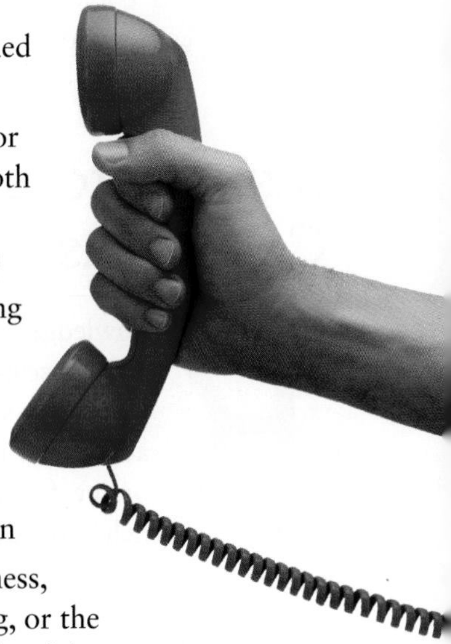

- Sudden, severe, unexplained headache
- Sudden blurring of sight or loss of vision in one or both eyes
- Sudden confusion, loss of speech, or trouble speaking
- Sudden difficulty understanding simple statements
- Sudden dizziness or loss of balance or coordination
- Sudden weakness, numbness, or paralysis of an arm, leg, or the face, especially on one side of the body

In the Hospital . . .

Diagnostic tests can help pinpoint the cause of the stroke. If the stroke was due to a thrombus, clot-dissolving drugs such as *tissue-plasminogen activator* (*t-PA*) may be used to disperse the clot or prevent it from growing. Clot-dissolving drugs may be used to restore the flow of blood to the brain, saving brain tissue or minimizing damage. However, clot-dissolving drugs may cause more bleeding and further brain damage if the stroke was due to a cerebral hemorrhage. Therefore, health professionals need to diagnose the *type* of stroke. If an embolism is suspected, doctors may attempt to track down its source and remove it surgically. Surgery may also be used to widen narrowed arteries in order to improve the blood supply to the brain.

After the Hospital . . .

Changes in diet and lifestyle may help reduce the risk of recurrent strokes: avoiding smoking, restricting intake of saturated fat and dietary cholesterol, and controlling blood pressure. In some cases, blood thinners (*anticoagulants*) may be needed indefinitely to prevent clotting.

Rehabilitation after a stroke depends on the nature of the disability. Physical therapy can improve muscle strength and coordination and help the person use mechanical aids, such as crutches or walkers, to compensate for loss of motor function. Occupational therapy can help improve eye–hand coordination and improve skills needed for daily living, such as bathing, dressing, and cooking. Speech and language therapy can help people whose speech has been affected.

Risk Factors for Cardiovascular Disease

Knowledge of the risk factors for cardiovascular disease will inform you of whether you are at special risk and would be well-advised to take preventive measures. The online feature "Health Check 11-2" will help you evaluate your personal risk of having a heart attack. You have no control over some risk factors, namely your age, gender, family history, and ethnic background. You do have control over others, by making changes in your lifestyle or obtaining appropriate treatment. Even if you are healthy and have no current risk factors, taking preventive measures now may help avert the later development of cardiovascular disease.

☒ LEARNING OUTCOME 4

List and discuss the risk factors for cardiovascular disease

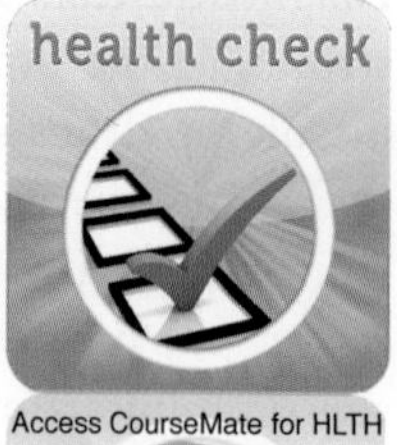

Access CourseMate for HLTH at www.cengagebrain.com.

Risk Factors You Can't Control

Age With men, the risk of CHD rises sharply with age after about age 40. Among women, CHD is uncommon until menopause and then rises sharply with increasing age. Stroke most often affects people over the age of 65.

Gender Men face a greater risk of heart disease (CHD), the major form of CVD, than women do, at least until about age 65. The relative risks for men and women begin to even out after age 65 (see "Diversity 11-2").

Heredity CVD tends to run in families, so people with a family history of cardiovascular disease are at greater risk than other people. This is especially so for people with a close male relative who had a heart attack or died suddenly before the age of 55, or a close female relative who suffered these consequences before the age of 65.

Race/Ethnicity African Americans are much more likely than European Americans to die from coronary heart disease and stroke (see Figure 11-5). Greater prevalence of hypertension, obesity, and diabetes among African Americans is largely responsible for elevated risks of cardiovascular disease.[20] Economic differences also enter the picture. Poorer people typically have more risk factors for cardiovascular disease, including smoking, obesity, high-fat diets, inactivity, and stress. African Americans as a group face greater economic hardships than European Americans do.

African Americans are also less likely than European Americans to receive aggressive treatments for heart conditions, such as coronary artery bypass surgery and angioplasty. The lack of aggressive treatments results in many needless deaths. This dual standard of care may reflect discrimination and possible cultural factors, such as mistrust of black patients toward the medical establishment. Investigators suspect that the stresses associated with racism contribute to the increased risk of cardiovascular disease faced by African Americans.[22]

Figure 11-5 Racial/Ethnic Differences in Death Rates Due to Cardiovascular Disease in the United States[21]

These data compare death rates from heart disease of ethnic/racial minorities to those of European Americans. African Americans have the highest mortality rate from heart disease, a rate that is 1.3 times higher than that of European Americans. Native Americans, Latin Americans, and Asian Americans all have lower death rates from heart disease than European Americans. The death rate for Asian Americans is half that of European Americans. What factors might account for these differences?

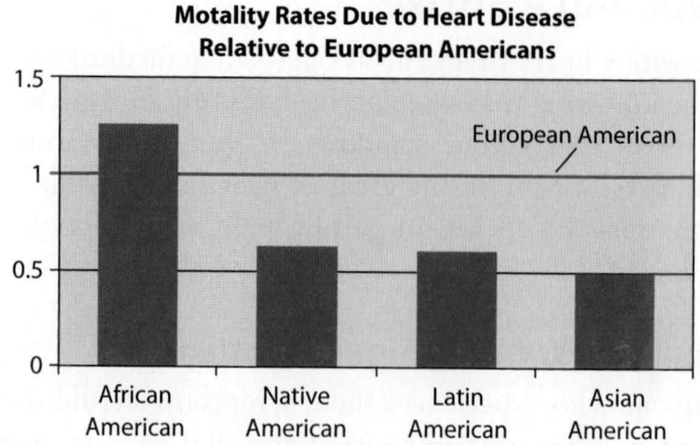

Risk Factors that May Be Controlled

Hypertension Hypertension is a major risk factor for CHD and stroke. Control of hypertension is largely credited with a reduction of about 60% in the incidence of strokes in recent years.

Blood Cholesterol Another prominent risk factor for cardiovascular disease is cholesterol. High blood levels of *low-density lipoproteins* (*LDL*, or "bad" cholesterol) form plaque that clings to artery walls. The buildup of plaque (*atherosclerosis*) can eventually choke off blood flow, leading to heart attacks or strokes. "Good" cholesterol, or *high-density lipoproteins* (*HDL*), lowers your risk of heart disease by carrying excess LDL to the liver for elimination from the body.

Having high total blood cholesterol or low HDL increases your risk of heart disease. Generally speaking, desirable blood cholesterol levels are less than 200 mg/dL for total cholesterol, LDL under 100 mg/dL, and HDL of 40 mg/dL or higher for men and 50 mg/dL or higher for women.

When evaluating heart risks, consider the ratio between total cholesterol and HDL; divide the total cholesterol level by the level of HDL. The optimal ratio is 3.5:1.[23] Therefore, if your HDL cholesterol is 36 mg/dL and your total cholesterol is 200, your risk ratio is 200/36, or 5.55. A ratio of 5:1 or higher puts you at risk.

Dietary sources of cholesterol and saturated fats increase LDL levels, but your genes also play a role. Heredity influences how quickly LDL is produced in the body and how fast it is removed from the blood. Blood cholesterol levels also tend to rise with age.[24]

Diet modification and exercise are generally recommended as the first steps in reducing high blood levels of cholesterol (see the online feature "Health Skills 11-1"). If diet and exercise are insufficient, drugs called *statins* have proven effective in lowering LDL and often raising HDL. Statins slow the body's production of cholesterol and increase the liver's ability to remove LDL.[25] However, some patients develop abnormal liver function or muscle problems. Therefore, patients treated with statins are regularly monitored to detect possible side effects.

health skills

Access CourseMate for HLTH at www.cengagebrain.com.

triglycerides
The main type of fat carried through the bloodstream and stored in the body's fatty tissue.

Triglycerides **Triglycerides** are the most common type of fat in the bloodstream and in the body's

diversity

DIVERSITY 11-2

Women and Heart Disease

Heart disease affects one in two or three American women, and one woman in four dies from it.[28] Heart disease is the leading cause of death in women.

CHD typically develops more gradually in women than in men. Before age 65, a woman's risk of dying from a heart attack lags that of a man's by about 10 years. That is, a 60-year-old woman has about the same chance of dying of a heart attack as a 50-year-old man. Though a woman's risk of dying from heart disease increases as she ages, it still lags the risk faced by men of the same age.

Prior to menopause, women may have a lower risk of CHD and heart attacks than men because of the protective effect of high estrogen levels. Estrogen boosts HDL. After menopause, however, estrogen production is cut and the risk of CHD rises. LDL also tends to increase following menopause and with advancing age.

Women are twice as likely as men to die from a heart attack, more likely to have a second heart attack, and less likely to survive after CABG and balloon angioplasty. Several factors appear to account for the poorer outcomes in women. For one thing, women with heart disease tend to be older than their male counterparts. Heart disease tends to be recognized sooner and treated more aggressively in men than in women.[29] Treatment differences may reflect the misperception that heart disease is essentially a male problem. Women are also more likely than men to experience a "silent" heart attack—one without chest pain.

fatty tissue. They store energy and are derived from fats and carbohydrates in foods we eat. High triglyceride levels are a risk factor in heart disease and stroke, perhaps because they are often associated with obesity and high levels of cholesterol.[26] The normal level of triglycerides in blood serum is less than 150 mg/dL. People with high triglyceride levels should ask their health care providers whether they would benefit from drugs to lower triglycerides.

Diabetes Diabetes is an endocrine disorder that stems from an insufficient production or utilization of the hormone insulin. People with diabetes have a higher risk of CHD, hypertension, and stroke. Diabetes damages blood vessels, hastening the process of atherosclerosis that can lead to heart attacks and strokes, and contributing to hypertension.

Obesity Obesity increases the risk of cardiovascular disorders such as CHD, stroke, and hypertension, in part because obesity is associated with high blood cholesterol. People with excess fat around their midsections ("apples") have a greater risk of CHD and higher mortality rates than those with excess weight around the hips ("pears").

Overweight and obesity is part of a complex of health problems commonly referred to as *metabolic syndrome*. People with metabolic syndrome are at increased risk of Type 2 (adult-onset) diabetes. Other risk factors in metabolic syndrome include high blood pressure, increased sugar in the bloodstream (indicative of *insulin resistance*, a condition in which the body fails to use insulin properly), high levels of triglycerides, high levels of LDL, and low levels of HDL. Fifty million Americans are estimated to have metabolic syndrome.[27]

Smoking Smoking more than doubles the chances of having a heart attack and is linked to more than one of five deaths due to CHD. Smokers also have twice the risk of stroke. Smokers are less likely to survive a heart attack, and smoking doubles the risk of sudden cardiac death. Tobacco smoke damages artery walls, making them more receptive to the formation of plaque. The nicotine in tobacco smoke accelerates the heart rate and blood pressure. Smoking increases total blood cholesterol while reducing levels of HDL. The carbon monoxide in tobacco smoke reduces the supply of oxygen reaching vital body organs, including the heart. Smoking also increases the risk of blood clots by making platelets "stickier." Exposure to secondhand smoke in the home increases the risk of CHD for nonsmokers.

cancer
Any of more than 100 diseases characterized by the development of malignant tumors, which may invade surrounding tissues and spread to other sites in the body through the lymphatic system and bloodstream.

Inactivity A sedentary life increases the risk of heart disease and strokes.

Negative Emotions Occasional feelings of anger may not do any damage, but chronic hostility and proneness to anger may be as dangerous to the heart as obesity, smoking, heredity, and a high-fat diet.[30] Anxiety and depression also raise the risk of CHD.[31] Holding in anger may also stress the heart and circulatory system. (Cool down, but when you get upset, don't explode—discuss your feelings as rationally as possible.)

Negative emotions may damage the cardiovascular system because they are associated with release of the stress hormones epinephrine and norepinephrine, which speed up the heart rate and raise blood pressure. Stress hormones may also increase the stickiness of blood platelets.

CANCER

Nearly every reader knows people who have had **cancer** or have died from it. Nearly 1.5 million Americans are diagnosed with cancer each year, and more than half a million die from it. Cancer accounts for about one in five deaths in the United States and is the nation's second leading cause of death, after heart disease (see Figure 11-6).[32]

Yet this section is not about doom and gloom. Although cancer remains a life-threatening disease, it can be cured or controlled in many cases. By following the advice in this section, you will achieve two health goals:

1. You will place yourself in lower risk categories for developing cancer.
2. By learning about the warning signs of cancer and screening methods for early detection, you will be better able to detect cancer at its earliest and most treatable stage.

Cancer is a chronic, *noncommunicable* (noninfectious) disease. Despite the threat of infectious diseases like influenza, pneumonia, and STDs, people in the United States, Canada, and other industrialized nations are more likely to die from chronic, noncommunicable diseases such as heart disease, cancer, and diabetes. Even stroke, another leading killer, typically follows years of buildup of artery-clogging plaque in arteries that service the brain.

What Is Cancer?

Cancer is not one disease but a group of more than 100 distinct diseases characterized by uncontrolled growth of body cells. Normally, new cells are formed by cell division only when the body needs them. Genes cause them to replicate themselves in an orderly way. But cells sometimes lose the ability to regulate their growth. They multiply when new cells are not needed, forming masses of excess body tissue called **tumors**.

LEARNING OUTCOME 5

Discuss the nature of cancer, its diagnosis, and its incidence

Tumors can be *benign* (noncancerous) or *malignant* (cancerous). Benign tumors do not spread to surrounding tissues and only rarely threaten life. They can generally be removed surgically and don't recur. Malignant tumors invade and destroy surrounding tissue. Cancerous cells in malignant tumors may also break away from the primary tumor and travel through the bloodstream or lymphatic system to form new tumors, called **metastases** or *secondary tumors*, in other parts of the body. They damage body organs and systems and often lead to death.

How Does Cancer Develop?

Cancer begins when a cell's DNA, its genetic material, changes such that the cell grows abnormally. The change is triggered by *mutations* in the DNA. Mutations are caused by internal or external factors. Internal factors include heredity, immune conditions, and hormonal influences. External cancer-causing agents are called **carcinogens** and include some viruses, chemical compounds in tobacco, and ultraviolet radiation from the sun.

tumor
A mass of excess body tissue or growth that may or may not be cancerous.

metastases
Secondary tumors that arise from the primary growth in a new location in the body. Cancers that metastasize are those that spread from one body part to another.

Two types of genes play roles in the development of

Figure 11-6 Chronic Diseases: America's Leading Killers

Chronic diseases are America's leading killers, with heart disease and cancer topping the list of the "top ten." Other killer chronic diseases include respiratory diseases and diabetes.

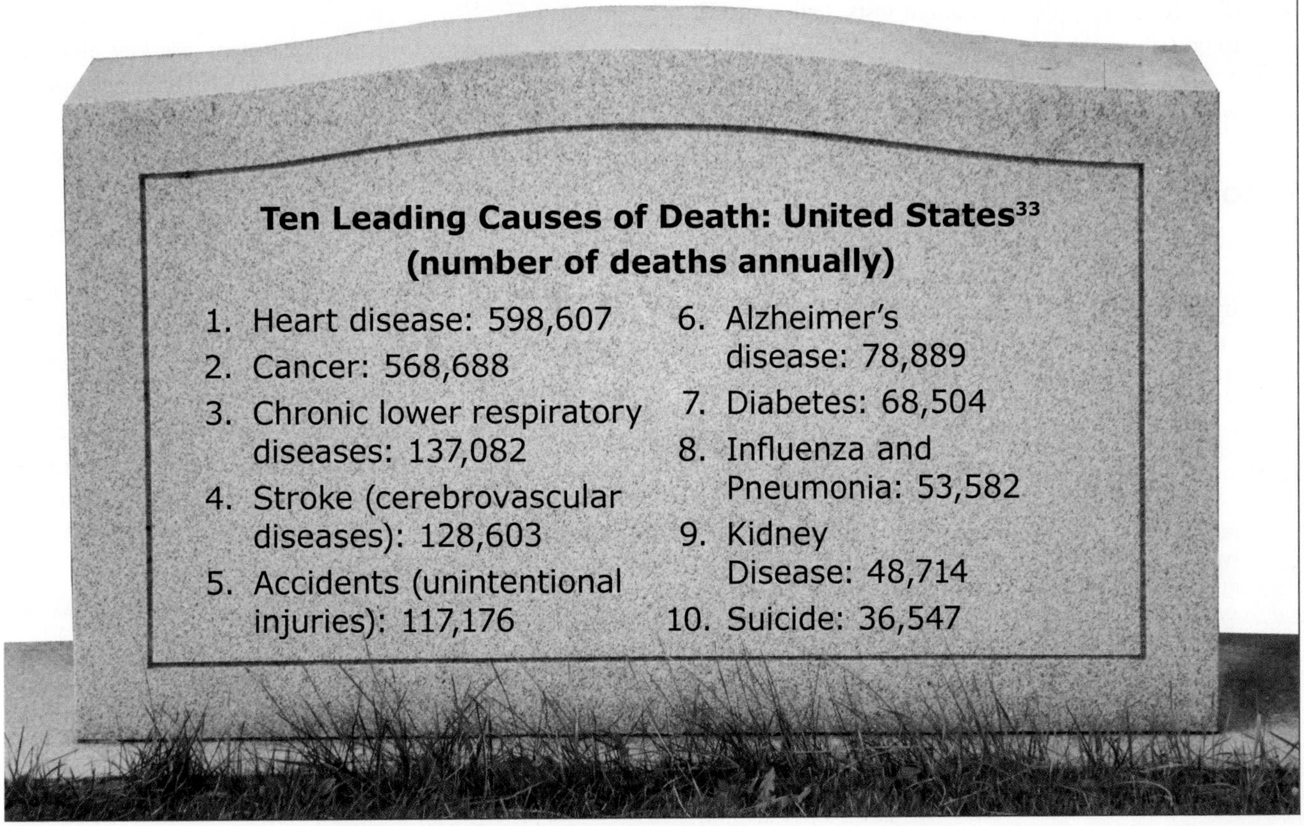

cancer. **Oncogenes** play a direct causal role. They cause uncontrolled proliferation of body cells, leading to tumors. (Physicians who specialize in the treatment of cancer are called *oncologists*.) Oncogenes are mutated forms of *proto-oncogenes*—the normal genes that control replication and differentiation (specialization) of cells. We can liken proto-oncogenes to the accelerator pedal on a car.[34] A gas pedal controls the speed of a car; similarly, proto-oncogenes control the rate at which cells divide. Like a car with a stuck gas pedal and no brakes, oncogenes foster runaway cell replication, leading to uncontrolled growths or tumors. More than 100 oncogenes have been identified, and scientists are attempting to develop drugs to stop or inhibit them.

Other genes—**suppressor genes**—normally curb cell division and suppress the development of tumors. They also prevent cancers from developing or growing. One particular suppressor gene stands guard against the most frequent type of skin cancer, basal cell carcinoma, suppressing its development. If the gene is defective, basal cell cancers may develop unchecked.

Diagnosing Cancer

Physicians conduct physical examinations to feel for any suspicious lumps on the patient's body and to look closely at growths on the skin. They may order a *biopsy* in which a sample of tissue is removed and analyzed for cancerous cells. They may order specialized tests, such as a CT scan, to determine the size of a tumor and whether it has spread. They are alert to symptoms that may represent early warning signs of cancer (see "Prevention 11-2").

Who Gets Cancer?

The odds of eventually developing some form of cancer are high. About half of Americans develop cancer.[35] Although cancer may develop at any age, most cases, about three-fourths, occur in people age 55 and older. Only 10% of cases are diagnosed in people under the age of 45.[36]

carcinogen
A cancer-causing substance.

oncogenes
Genes involved in regulating cell growth that in mutated form can promote the development of cancerous growths.

suppressor genes
Genes that curb cell division and suppress development of tumors.

On the other hand, the American Cancer Society estimates that more than half of all cancer deaths could be prevented if people made healthful changes in their lifestyle by exercising, avoiding tobacco use, eating healthier foods, and undergoing regular screening. Moreover, the incidence of cancer and cancer death rates are declining, with deaths dropping by about 2% per year.[37] Health experts largely credit reductions in smoking and improved early detection and treatment. Smoking is the leading cause of cancer-related deaths in the United States.[38] Yet there remain significant differences in the relative risks of developing and dying of cancer among different racial and ethnic groups in our society (see the online feature "Diversity 11-3").

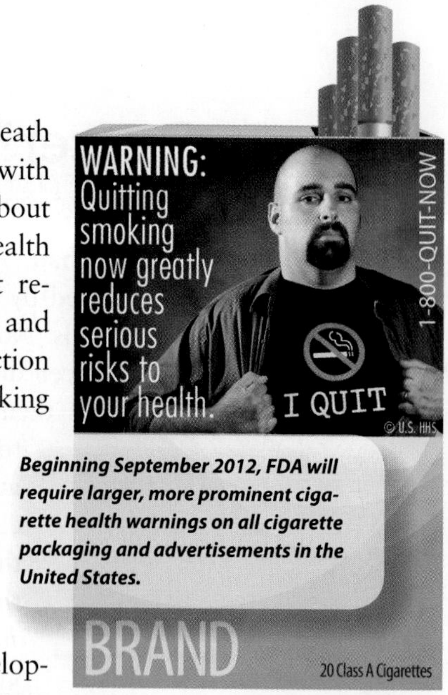

Beginning September 2012, FDA will require larger, more prominent cigarette health warnings on all cigarette packaging and advertisements in the United States.

© REN HAIJUN/Xinhua/Landov

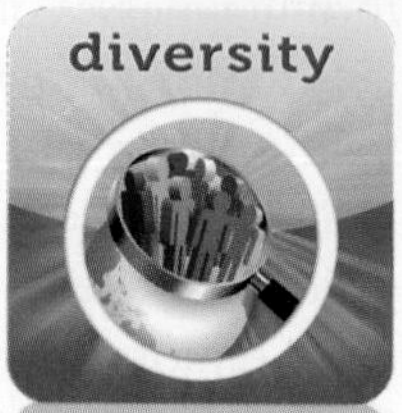

Access CourseMate for HLTH at www.cengagebrain.com.

Surviving Cancer

At the turn of the 20th century, few people diagnosed with cancer survived longer than a few years. By the 1940s, the five-year survival rate had jumped to one in four. By the mid-1970s, about half survived. Today, the odds of surviving cancer five years after diagnosis have risen to about 66%.[39]

Early detection and treatment are key elements in long-term survival. The American Cancer Society estimates that if all Americans followed their recommendations for early detection of breast, colon, rectal, cervical, prostate, testicular, oral cavity, and skin cancers, the five-year survival rate for people with cancer would be about 95%.

Surviving five or more years is a widely used measure of success in the war against cancer, but reaching this threshold doesn't necessarily mean that cancer is cured. Some cancers return 10 years later or more. The American Cancer Society considers a person to be cured of cancer if he or she shows no further evidence of the disease and has the same life expectancy as a person who has never had cancer. Some cancers that had a bleak outlook decades ago can often be cured today, including Hodgkin's disease, testicular cancer, most skin cancers, some forms of lymphoma, bone cancer, and leukemia and kidney cancer in children (see the online feature "Health Skills 11-2" for a tour of cancer treatments under

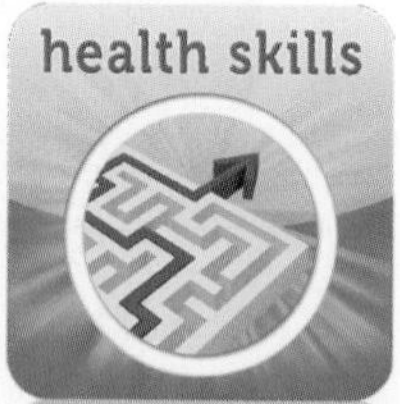

Access CourseMate for HLTH at www.cengagebrain.com.

prevention diversity health check skills

Early Signs and Symptoms of Cancer[40]

The chances of surviving cancer are greater if it is detected and treated early. The American Cancer Society identifies general and cancer-specific warning signs. But because these symptoms may result from other causes, they should be brought to the attention of a health care provider to arrive at a diagnosis.

GENERAL SIGNS AND SYMPTOMS

- **Unexplained weight loss:** The first sign of cancer may be an unexplained weight loss. Be alert to any weight loss of about 10 pounds that cannot be explained by dieting or another obvious cause.
- **Fever:** Fever is a common symptom of cancer. Although it usually occurs at later stages of disease, it may be an early sign of some cancers, such as Hodgkin's disease.
- **Fatigue:** Fatigue can occur in the early stages of some cancers. However, it usually becomes a more prominent symptom in more advanced cases.
- **Pain:** Be alert to any symptoms of pain. Pain is the body's early warning sign of injury or disease. Though pain can stem from many causes, it can be an early symptom of some cancers, including bone cancers and testicular cancer. Typically, pain is a symptom of more advanced cancers.
- **Skin changes:** Be aware of any changes in the skin, such as growths, yellowing, itching, darkening, or excessive hair growth, or changes in the size or color of a mole. Skin changes can be a symptom not only of skin cancers but also of some internal cancers.

CANCER-SPECIFIC SIGNS AND SYMPTOMS

- **Changes in bowel habits or bladder function:** Be aware of any changes such as pain during urination, blood in the urine, diarrhea, chronic constipation, changes in the size of the stool, or changes in frequency of urination.
- **Sores that do not heal:** Persistent sores that don't heal may be signs of cancers, such as oral cancer and skin cancer. Also be aware of any sores on the penis or vagina, which could be signs of infection or an early cancer.
- **Unusual bleeding or discharge:** Any unexplained bodily discharge or bleeding should be investigated immediately. Blood in the stool may be a sign of colon or rectal cancer, whereas blood in the urine might indicate bladder or kidney cancer. Bleeding from a nipple may be a sign of breast cancer.
- **Thickening or lump in the breasts or other parts of the body:** Lumps or thickening under the skin can be a sign of either early or late cancer, especially when it involves the breast, testicles, glands (lymph nodes), and soft tissues of the body.
- **Indigestion or difficulty swallowing:** Cancers of the esophagus, stomach, or pharynx (throat) may be accompanied by symptoms of indigestion or difficulty swallowing.
- **Recent changes in warts or moles:** Check your skin at regular intervals. Note changes in the size, color, or shape of any warts or moles. Bring them to the attention of a physician. They may be signs of melanoma, a lethal type of skin cancer, which can be treated successfully if it is detected early.
- **Nagging cough or hoarseness:** A nagging cough that won't go away may be a sign of lung cancer. Persistent hoarseness may indicate a cancer of the larynx (voice box) or thyroid.

development). In addition to the millions who have been cured of cancer are millions more who are surviving day to day and year to year. No one has to go it alone: the online feature "Health Skills 11-3" lists organizations that help people who are living with cancer.

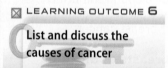

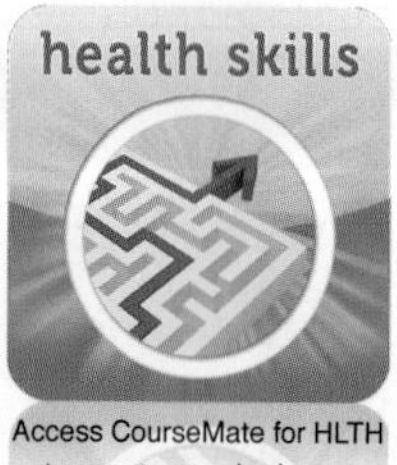

Access CourseMate for HLTH at www.cengagebrain.com.

Important challenges remain, however. Only limited progress has been made in survivability of some forms of cancer in adults, such as cancers of the lung, pancreas, and liver (see Table 11-3). These cancers have poor survival rates even when they are diagnosed at a localized stage before the cancer has spread to other parts of the body.

Causes of Cancer

There are many causes of cancer, including genetic factors, exposure to cancer-causing chemicals, and exposure to certain viruses. But two out of three cancer deaths in the United States are the result of two factors you can control: smoking and diet.[41]

LEARNING OUTCOME 6

List and discuss the causes of cancer

Smoking

Cigarette smoking is responsible for approximately 80–90% of lung cancer deaths in the United States and one-third of all cancers and cancer deaths overall. It is also responsible for most cancers of the mouth, larynx, pharynx, esophagus, and bladder. Cigarette smoking can also cause kidney, pancreatic, cervical, and stomach cancers, and leukemia.[43] Smoking may also be connected to breast cancer and cervical cancer. Secondhand smoke contributes to several thousand cancer deaths per year, and other forms of tobacco use, including pipe and cigar smoking, and smokeless tobacco, also cause cancer.

Diet

Dietary factors may account for as many as 30% of all cancers in the United States and other Western nations.[44] The prime culprit is saturated fat, especially animal fat. But does switching to a low-fat diet actually reduce the risks of cancer and other chronic diseases, such as CHD? One study tracked the health of nearly 49,000 women aged 50 to 79 for eight years and found that those assigned at random to a low-fat diet did not significantly differ in rates of breast cancer, colorectal cancer, heart attacks, and strokes from those who followed their own diets.[45] One limitation of the study is that it targeted total dietary fat rather than focusing on saturated fat. Perhaps direct targeting of saturated fat is needed to reduce these health risks. Another limitation is the problem of compliance; that is, we cannot be certain that participants assigned to low-fat diets actually adhered to them.

Obesity

Obesity is a risk factor for many forms of cancer, including cancers of the colon, breast (in postmenopausal women), prostate, endometrium (the lining of the uterus), kidney, esophagus, and possibly pancreas.[46] The connection between fat intake and the risk of breast cancer remains unclear.[47]

Alcohol

Heavy alcohol consumption raises the risk of several cancers, including cancers of the mouth, pharynx, esophagus, larynx, breast, and liver.[48] But even moderate drinking may increase the risks of some forms of cancer, such as breast cancer in women.[49] The more

Table 11-3 Five-Year Survival Rates for Selected Cancer Sites[42]

CHANCE OF 5-YEAR SURVIVAL	SELECTED CANCER SITES
Less than 10%	Pancreas
10% to 29%	Liver, esophagus, gallbladder, lung and bronchus, stomach
30% to 59%	Brain and nervous system, ovary
60% to 89%	Bones and joints, colon and rectum, kidney and renal pelvis, cervix, Hodgkin's disease, larynx, non-Hodgkin's lymphoma, oral cavity and pharynx, urinary bladder, corpus and uterus
90% or better	Breast (females), prostate, testes, thyroid, melanoma of the skin

alcohol women consume, the greater their risk of breast cancer. The American Cancer Society recommends that for people who consume alcohol, intake should be limited to two drinks a day for men and one drink a day for women.

Environmental Factors

Many chemicals can cause cancer in humans—benzene, asbestos, vinyl chloride, coal tars, and arsenic. Still other chemicals are probable carcinogens. **Ionizing radiation**, a form of radiation found in X-rays and radon gas, can cause cancer. Links also exist between heavy use of organic solvents in the home (used in some hobbies or home projects) and childhood leukemia.

Most environmental causes of cancer can be prevented by protecting the quality of our air and water. The federal government sets safety standards for chemical or radiation exposure in the environment and the workplace.

Sun Exposure

Ultraviolet (*UV*) *radiation* in the form of sunlight is the main cause of a worldwide increase in all forms of skin cancer among Caucasians. Prolonged exposure can lead to the development of *basal cell* and *squamous cell carcinomas* (discussed in detail on page 253). These are the most common forms of skin cancers that tend to occur later in life. They are relatively benign and can be removed surgically. Sunburns are believed to play a major role in the development of *melanoma*, the most deadly form of skin cancer.

Infectious Agents

Cancer is not contagious (you can't "catch" it from someone) but some forms of cancer are caused by infectious agents such as viruses and bacteria. Viruses—especially those transmitted sexually—are the major microbial offenders. For example, *human papillomavirus* (HPV), the virus that causes genital warts and that is rampant on college campuses, is also responsible for the great majority of cases of cervical cancer.

HIV, the virus that causes AIDS, is a cause of Kaposi's sarcoma, a rare soft-tissue cancer that is characterized by the development of purplish spots on the body. HIV is also a risk factor in non-Hodgkin's lymphoma.[50] Other sexually transmissible organisms, such as the hepatitis B and hepatitis C viruses, can cause liver cancer. The Epstein-Barr virus, which causes mononucleosis, may contribute to some cases of cancer of the pharynx and stomach, and several forms of lymphoma. *Human T-cell leukemia virus-I* (HTLV-1), a virus belonging to the same family of viruses as HIV, is implicated in some forms of leukemia and lymphoma.[51]

How do viruses cause cancer? Some viruses inject themselves into the cell's DNA and activate genes that lead to tumor growth or *de*activate genes that suppress tumors. Viruses like HIV also weaken the immune system, making it less capable of ridding the body of cancerous cells.

The bacterium *H. pylori* is associated with stomach cancer. It can lead to stomach ulcers, which in some cases may contribute to the development of cancer.

ionizing radiation
Powerful, high-energy radiation capable of causing atoms to become electrically charged or ionized.

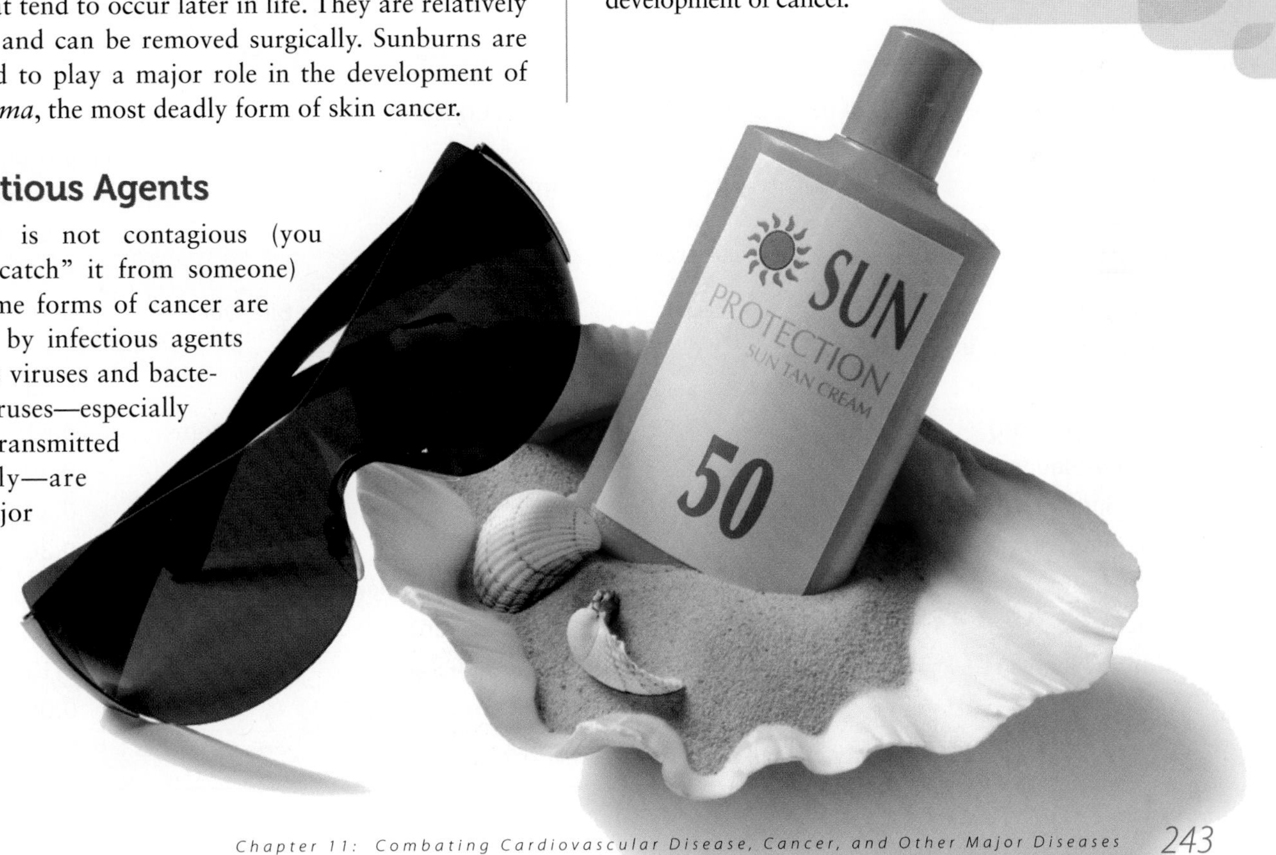

Genetic Factors

Some cancers, perhaps 5% to 10%, are inherited. Cancer is a disease in which genes function abnormally. People may inherit defective or mutant genes that lead to the development of cancer, including some forms of colorectal cancer, skin cancer, prostate cancer, leukemia, ovarian cancer, and breast cancer.[52]

carcinoma
Cancer that originates in the epithelial tissues of the body.

sarcoma
Cancer that originates in connective tissues of the body.

lymphoma
Cancer that forms in the cells of the lymphatic system.

leukemia
Cancer that forms in the blood and blood-forming tissues of the body.

melanoma
A potentially deadly form of cancer involving the formation of cancerous growths in melanin-forming cells, most commonly in the skin but sometimes in other parts of the body containing such cells, such as the eye.

Inactivity

Physical inactivity may also contribute to the risk of cancer, especially colorectal cancer.[53] Sedentary workers have higher rates of colorectal cancer than physically active workers.

Will you get cancer? Your risk depends on many factors, especially diet, smoking, exposure to the sun, and family history. Table 11-4 shows the risks faced by American women and men for selected cancers. "HealthCheck 11-3" can help you assess your personal risk potential.

Types of Cancer

Cancer can develop in any organ or tissue of the body. There are several major types of cancer including the following:

LEARNING OUTCOME 7

Discuss the similarities and differences among various types of cancer

- **Carcinoma** is the most common type of cancer. It refers to malignant tumors that form in *epithelial tissue*, the tissue that covers body surfaces and lines body cavities. The most common sites for such cancers include the epithelial layers of the skin, the large intestine, the lungs, the prostate gland in men, and the breasts in women.
- **Sarcoma** is a malignancy of the connective tissue in the body, such as the muscles or bones.
- **Lymphoma** forms in the lymph system.
- **Leukemia** arises in the blood and blood-forming tissues of the body.
- **Melanoma** begins in melanin-containing cells, most commonly found in the skin.

Most cancers are named after the organ or type of cell in which the cancer originally forms. The original

Table 11-4 Lifetime Risk (%) of Being Diagnosed with Various Cancers[54]

SITE	ALL RACES/ ETHNICITIES (%)	SITE	ALL RACES/ ETHNICITIES (%)
All Sites Combined	40.77	Thyroid	0.90
Prostate (Men)	16.22	Stomach	0.88
Breast (Women)	12.15	Liver and Intrahepatic Bile Duct	0.76
Lung and Bronchus	6.95	Cervix (Women)	0.68
Colon and Rectum	5.12	Myeloma	0.64
Uterus (Women)	2.58	Brain and Other Nervous System	0.61
Urinary Bladder	2.39	Esophagus	0.50
Non-Hodgkin Lymphoma	2.10	Testes (Men)	0.37
Melanoma of the Skin	1.93	Larynx	0.36
Kidney and Renal Pelvis	1.49	Hodgkin Lymphoma	0.23
Pancreas	1.41	Breast (Men)	0.13
Ovary (Women)	1.39	Mesothelioma	0.12
Leukemia	1.30	Kaposi's Sarcoma	0.05
Oral Cavity and Pharynx	1.02		

HEALTH CHECK 11-3

Assessing Your Personal Risk of Cancer

Cancer can strike anyone, but some of us are at greater risk than others. Your relative risk depends on many factors, especially your family history and lifestyle. Examining your risk profile can help you identify those risk factors that you can change.

"Yes" Answers to the Following Questions Are Associated with an Increased Cancer Risk:

_____ 1. Do you have a member of your immediate family who suffers or has suffered from cancer, excluding basal and squamous skin cancers?

_____ 2. Do you or any member of your immediate family have a history of precancerous growths?

_____ 3. Are you 45 years of age or older?

_____ 4. Do you currently smoke or use other tobacco products, such as smokeless tobacco or snuff? Or are you a former smoker, having smoked regularly for at least a year or more?

_____ 5. Are you overweight?

_____ 6. Do you drink two or more drinks of alcohol daily?

_____ 7. Have you had a history of severe sunburns, even back in childhood? Do you enjoy sunbathing and fail to adequately protect your skin with sunscreen lotion?

"Yes" Answers to the Following Questions Are Associated with a Lower Cancer Risk:

_____ 1. Do you watch your fat intake, making sure not to consume more than 30% of your total caloric intake in the form of dietary fat?

_____ 2. Do you follow a diet rich in fruits, vegetables, and dietary fiber?

_____ 3. Do you generally avoid foods that are smoke-, nitrite- or salt-cured?

_____ 4. Do you limit your alcohol intake to fewer than two drinks per day?

_____ 5. Do you use sunscreen protection (SPF value of 15 or higher) when you go out in the direct sun for longer than a few minutes?

_____ 6. Do you protect your skin from overexposure to the sun by wearing protective clothing?

_____ 7. Do you avoid use of all tobacco products?

_____ 8. Do you exercise regularly and take generally good care of your health?

_____ 9. Do you get regular health checkups and follow recommended cancer screening guidelines given your age and family history, such as Pap smears, prostate cancer screening tests, clinical breast exams and mammography, and digital rectal exams?

_____ 10. If you are a woman, do you regularly examine your breasts for lumps? If you are a man, do you regularly examine your testicles for lumps?

_____ 11. Do you limit your exposure to environmental hazards such as asbestos, radiation, and toxic chemicals?

_____ 12. Do you avoid tanning salons and home sunlamps?

_____ 13. Is your diet rich in sources of essential vitamins and minerals?

No particular score translates into a precise risk estimate. The more "Yes" answers to the first set of questions and the fewer "Yes" answers to the second set, the greater your overall cancer risk. Examine these risk factors carefully. Ask yourself which risk factors you can change to help improve your chances of remaining healthy and cancer-free.

site of a cancer is called the *primary cancer* or *primary tumor*. If cancer spreads to other sites, they are called *secondary tumors*. For example, breast cancer begins with the formation of small tumors in the breast but can spread to other parts of the body, such as the liver. If it does, the disease is called *metastatic* breast cancer, not liver cancer. Because cancer may spread, it is important to detect it early, while it remains *in situ* (localized where it developed). Let's now look more closely at several major forms of cancer, beginning with breast cancer.

Breast Cancer

One in eight women develops breast cancer, the second most common form of cancer among women (after skin cancer) and the second leading cancer killer of women (after lung cancer).

Breast cancer usually strikes in middle to late adulthood (see Figure 11-7). The average age of women at diagnosis is 61. Most women who die of breast cancer are over the age of 65. Nonetheless, breast cancer is also the leading cause of death of women between the ages of 35 and 54. About 200,000 women are diagnosed with breast cancer each year in the United States, and more than 40,000 die of the disease. Breast cancer in men is rare, with 1,400 new cases reported annually.

The incidence of breast cancer is declining at the same time that the odds of survival are increasing.[55] The five-year survival rate for women in the early 1950s who had breast cancer was 60%. Today, the five-year survival rate has risen to nearly 90%.

Figure 11-7 Age at Diagnosis with Breast Cancer (%)[56]

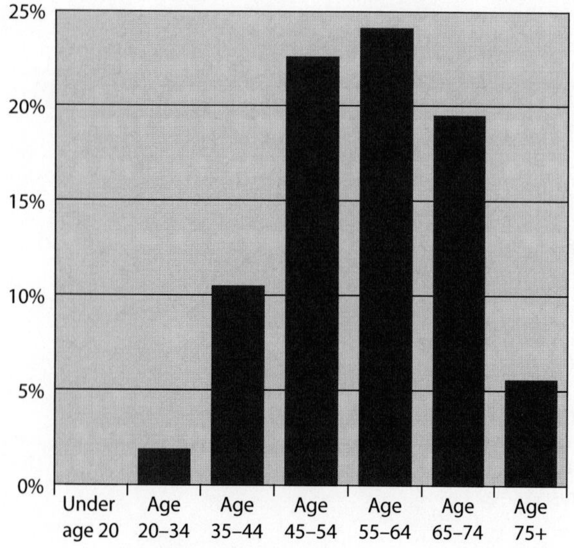

The chances of survival depend largely on when the disease is detected. Early detection of breast cancer is discussed further in "Prevention 11-3." Women with localized breast cancer have better than a 95% chance of surviving five years, as compared with about 20% of those whose cancers have metastasized.

Women whose mothers, sisters, or daughters have breast cancer have twice the risk of developing breast cancer themselves. Some 5% to 10% of breast cancer cases can be traced to two mutated forms of genes labeled BRCA1 and BRCA2.[57] These are mutated suppressor genes that fail to keep cellular growth in check. However, as many as 70% of women with breast cancer have no family history of the disease.

Other risk factors include a history of an abnormal breast biopsy, being overweight or obese, radiation therapy to the chest, hormone-replacement therapy (HRT) in postmenopausal women, and hormonal factors such as early age at first menstruation (before age 12), late completion of menopause (after age 55), no childbearing, or bearing a first child after age 30. These hormonal factors are related to greater exposure to estrogen at a time in life when the breasts may be most susceptible to the possible cancer-causing properties of the hormone.

Women who have used oral contraceptives ("the pill") have a slightly greater risk of breast cancer. Women with a family history of breast cancer or other risk factors should carefully consider their choice of contraception in consultation with their doctors.

Treatment

The four standard ways of treating breast cancer include surgery, chemotherapy, radiation, and hormone treatment. A combination is usually used. Depending on the size and location of the tumor, treatment may involve either *breast-conserving surgery* in which all or part of the breast is spared or one of several forms of *mastectomy* in which the entire breast is removed. In breast-conserving surgery, the surgeon either performs a *lumpectomy*, in which the tumor and some surrounding tissue are removed, or a *partial mastectomy*, which removes the part of the breast that contains the cancerous growth and some surrounding tissue. If the tumor has spread to the adjoining lymph nodes in the armpits, these too would be surgically removed.

Radiation therapy uses high-energy X-rays or other types of radiation to destroy cancer cells in the breast. *Chemotherapy* involves the use of anticancer drugs to kill cancer cells or stop their growth. In *hormone therapy*, drugs such as *tamoxifen* are used to block the effects of the female hormone estrogen in the breast.

PREVENTION 11-3

Early Detection of Breast Cancer

Three primary screening techniques are used to detect early signs of breast cancer: the breast self-exam, the mammogram, and the clinical breast exam (CBE). The American Cancer Society recommends the following three-pronged strategy for early detection.[58]

1. *Breast self-examination.* Women can conduct a breast self-examination (BSE) to check for any lumps or other changes in the breasts.

   A women may perform an initial breast self-examination with her physician in order to determine the degree of "lumpiness" that seems normal for her. She can then perform a breast self-examination on a regular schedule arranged in consultation with her health care provider and then report any changes promptly to her physician or nurse. Here are some general suggestions for performing a BSE, but women should first consult with their health care provider to ensure they are doing it correctly.

   a. *In the shower.* Examine your breasts during bath or shower; hands glide more easily over wet skin. Keep your fingers flat and move gently over every part of each breast. Use the right hand to examine the left breast and the left hand for the right breast. Check for any lump, hard knot, or thickening.

   b. *Before a mirror.* Inspect your breasts with your arms at your sides. Next, raise your arms high overhead. Look for any changes in the contour of each breast, a swelling, dimpling of skin, or changes in the nipple. Then rest your palms on your hips and press down firmly to flex your chest muscles. Your left and right breasts will not exactly match—few women's breasts do. Regular inspection shows what is normal for you and will give you confidence in your examination.

   c. *Lying down.* To examine your right breast, put a pillow or folded towel under your right shoulder. Place your right arm behind your head—this distributes breast tissue more evenly on the chest. With your left hand, fingers flat, press gently with the finger pads (the top thirds of the fingers) of the three middle fingers in small circular motions around an imaginary clock face. Begin at the outermost top of your right breast for 12 o'clock, then move to 1 o'clock, and so on around the circle back to 12. A ridge of firm tissue in the lower curve of each breast is normal. Then move in an inch, toward the nipple. Keep circling to examine every part of your breast, including the nipple. This requires at least three more circles. Now slowly repeat the procedure on your left breast. Place the pillow beneath your left shoulder, your left arm behind your head, and use the finger pads on your right hand.

   After you examine your left breast fully, squeeze the nipple of each breast gently between your thumb and index finger. Any discharge, clear or bloody, should be reported to your doctor immediately. In addition to lumps, women should also be sensitive to other changes and report them to their physicians. These include changes such as thickening, swelling, dimpling, skin irritation, pain, discomfort, discharge, or any change in tenderness of the nipple.

2. *Clinical breast examination.* Once every three years, women in their 20s and 30s should receive a *clinical breast examination* (CBE) in which a physician or other health professional carefully examines the breast and under the arms for any lumps or abnormalities. After age 40, the American Cancer Society recommends that women have an annual clinical breast exam. In a small percentage of cases, tumors not revealed on a mammogram can be detected by a woman or physician.

3. *Mammograms.* A *mammogram* is a specialized X-ray that can find tumors that are too small to be felt. The American Cancer Society advises women over age 40 to have an annual mammogram.[59] Early detection from mammography is associated with reductions in the number of breast cancer deaths.[60] However, mammography sometimes produces false alarms that lead to unnecessary treatment.

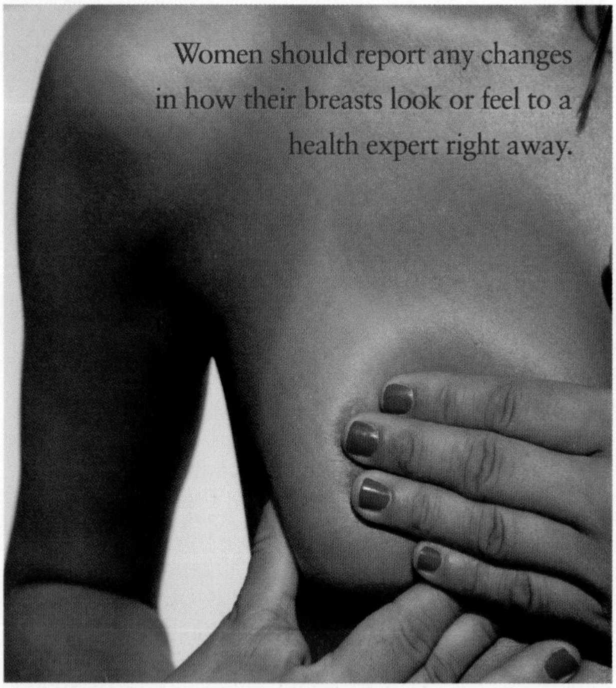

Women should report any changes in how their breasts look or feel to a health expert right away.

©iStockphoto.com/Hüseyin Tuncer

The decision to have a lumpectomy or mastectomy can be agonizing. As with other important medical decisions, women need to make informed decisions based on consultation with their physicians.

Prevention

The National Cancer Institute suggests that lifestyle changes such as exercise and avoiding gaining weight may lower the risk of breast cancer.[61] Regular exercise reduces secretion of female hormones, which may in turn lower the risk of breast cancer, especially in younger women.

The American Cancer society recommends a diet rich in fruits and vegetables and low in saturated fat.[62] Women should avoid regular heavy drinking and ask their gynecologists about the risks of light drinking.

Women at increased risk of developing breast cancer may also ask their gynecologists about *tamoxifen*, a breast-cancer treatment drug that interferes with the activity of estrogen in the breast.[63]

Pap test
The scraping of a "smear" of cells from the vagina and cervix for microscopic examination to reveal the presence of cancer. Also called a Pap smear; named after its developer, George Papanicolaou (1883–1962).

Ovarian Cancer

The lives of more women are lost to ovarian cancer (cancer of the ovaries) than to any other gynecological cancer, including uterine and cervical cancer. About 22,000 new cases of ovarian cancer are diagnosed and about 14,000 women die of it each year.

Ovarian cancer is difficult to detect at an early stage because of a lack of noticeable symptoms. Only about two of three women with ovarian cancer survive five or more years when the cancer has spread beyond the ovaries. But survival rates jump to better than 90% when the cancer is detected before it has metastasized.[64] Unfortunately, ovarian cancers are diagnosed early in only about *one in five* cases.

We lack an effective screening test for ovarian cancer. Women over the age of 40 are advised to have an annual cancer-screening examination, including a pelvic examination. But even a pelvic examination may fail to pick up early signs of ovarian cancer.

Risk Factors

Most cases of ovarian cancer occur after menopause, but ovarian cancer can also occur in younger women. Other risk factors include a family history of the disease; not having borne children; a history of breast, endometrial, or colon cancer; early age at first menstruation; and going through menopause after the age of 50. Conversely, having had several pregnancies and having used oral contraceptives appear to afford protection against the disease.

Treatment

Treatment of ovarian cancer may involve surgery, radiation, chemotherapy, or a combination of treatments. The extent of surgery depends on the state of the disease. It may include removal of one or both ovaries (*oophorectomy*), the uterus (*hysterectomy*), and the fallopian tubes (*salpingectomy*).

Cervical Cancer

About 12,000 cases of cervical cancer are diagnosed in the United States annually, and about 4,000 women die of it. The number of cervical cancer deaths has declined as use of the screening method called the *Pap test* has become widespread. Cervical cancer tends to strike women between the ages of 30 and 55, although it may occur in younger and older women. The disease is highly curable if it is detected and treated before it metastasizes. Overall, the five-year survival rate is about 70%. But the rate rises to nearly 100% when the cancer is detected at its earliest stage.

Detection

Because of the importance of early detection, a woman's best defense against cervical cancer is an annual **Pap test.** In this test, a sample (called a *smear*) of cervical tissue is examined for the presence of abnormal cell changes. The American Cancer Society recommends that all women start having regular Pap tests about three years after first engaging in sexual intercourse but no later than age 21.[65] Women should also report early signs of cervical cancer, including abnormal uterine bleeding or spotting and an abnormal vaginal discharge.

Risk Factors and Treatment

Virtually all cases of cervical cancer are linked to HPV infection.[66] A vaccine is now available that protects against several strains of HPV that cause cervical cancer, but it is less effective with women who are already infected. Although HPV infection is the most common sexually transmitted infection in the United States, only a small percentage of women with untreated HPV eventually develop cervical cancer.[67]

Risk factors for cervical cancer include those that increase the risk of HPV infection, such as having sex at an early age and with many partners, unprotected sex, as well as sex with uncircumcised men. Other risk factors include lack of Pap tests, HIV infection, family history, overweight, long-term oral contraceptive use, and smoking. Surgery or radiation, or a combination of these approaches, are used to treat cervical cancer.

Uterine (Endometrial) Cancer

About 40,000 women develop uterine cancer each year in the United States, and 8,000 die of the disease. Uterine cancer is cancer of the uterus, the hollow, pear-shaped organ in which the fetus develops. The cancer usually develops in the endometrium, the inner layer of the uterine wall, and is called *endometrial cancer*. Endometrial cancer is the most common cancer of the female reproductive organs.

The risk of endometrial cancer increases with age. Most cases are diagnosed in women aged 50 or above.[68] Other risk factors include early age at first menstruation, late menopause, family history, infertility, a high-fat diet, failure to ovulate, diabetes, use of the drug *tamoxifen* (a breast cancer drug), hormone-replacement therapy, and obesity.

Detecting endometrial cancer early is difficult. Pelvic exams tend to pick up only advanced cases, and the Pap test, effective in detecting early cervical cancer, often fails to detect uterine cancer. As women age, they need to be alert to bodily changes that might suggest early signs of the disease, such as unusual bleeding, spotting, or other discharge.

Treatment

Treatments for uterine cancer include surgery to remove cancerous tissue, radiation, hormone therapy, and chemotherapy. Surgery often involves removal of the uterus (hysterectomy) and nearby structures. In advanced cases, a *radical hysterectomy* may be performed, in which the surgeon removes the cervix, uterus, fallopian tubes, ovaries, part of the vagina, and, possibly, nearby lymph nodes. Like other forms of cancer, the chances of recovery depend upon whether the cancer has metastasized. The five-year survival rate is about 95% if it is detected and treated at the early stage of the disease. However, survival rates decline precipitously, to about 25%, if the cancer has spread distantly within the body.

Lung Cancer

Each year nearly 225,000 Americans are diagnosed with lung cancer, and more than 150,000 die from the disease. Lung cancer typically develops in middle and later life, but the damage to lung tissue from smoking is years in the making. Lung cancer is the leading cancer killer of both men and women in the United States.

Prevention of lung cancer is straightforward: If you haven't started smoking, don't. If you do smoke, quit. Avoid exposure to secondhand smoke. Exposure to high levels of radon, a gaseous radioactive element, causes about 21,000 lung cancer deaths each year. Radon detectors installed in the home can inform you of unsafe levels.

Commonly reported symptoms of lung cancer include shortness of breath, a persistent cough, wheezing, coughing up blood, chest pain, fever, and weight loss. But some people have no symptoms.

Lung cancer is especially deadly. The type of treatment depends on the stage of the disease and the extent to which it has spread, but it usually involves a combination of surgery (removal of all or part of the diseased lung) and radiation, chemotherapy, or both. Five-year survival rates are low, about 15%. Still, there is a reasonable chance of survival if the cancer is detected and removed while it is confined to the lungs. However, since the disease produces few symptoms in the early stages, relatively few cases are detected before they have spread.

Testicular Cancer

Testicular cancer is relatively uncommon, affecting only about 8,500 men annually in the United States and accounting for about 350 deaths. It generally affects men in the 15 to 40 age range, although it can occur at any age, even in infancy. It is also among the most

PREVENTION 11-4

Testicular Self-Examination

Self-examination of the testicles is best performed shortly after a warm shower or bath, when the skin of the scrotum is most relaxed. The man should examine the scrotum for evidence of pea-sized lumps. Each testicle can be rolled gently between the thumb and the fingers. Lumps are generally found on the side or front of the testicle. The presence of a lump is not necessarily a sign of cancer, but it should be promptly reported to a physician for further evaluation. The American Cancer Society lists these warning signals:

- A slight enlargement of one of the testicles.
- A change in the consistency of a testicle.
- A dull ache in the lower abdomen or groin. (Pain may be absent in cancer of the testes, however).
- Sensation of dragging and heaviness in a testicle.

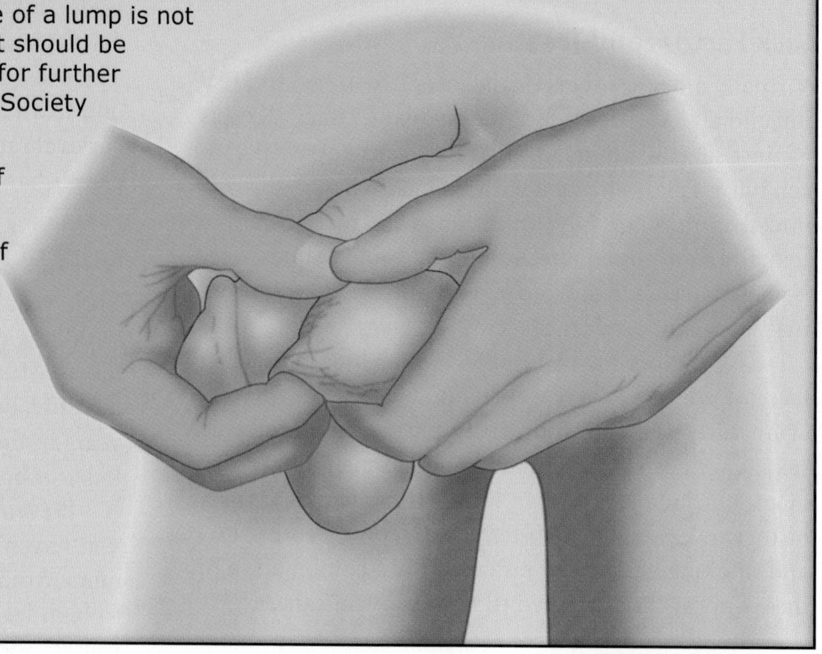

curable kinds of cancer if detected early. In 90% of cases, the cancer can be recognized by a lump in the testicle or swelling of the testicles. Any swelling, lump, or aching in the testicles should be reported to a health professional. Five-year survival rates are 95% overall and 99% when the cancer is detected and treated while it remains localized. Doctors will remove the affected testicle and may recommend chemotherapy to kill remaining cancer cells. About one-third of testicular cancer patients have an inherited predisposition to the disease. Regular self-examination of the testicles is one way to help assure that abnormalities in the testicles will be detected early (see "Prevention 11-4").

Colorectal Cancer

Colorectal cancer is cancer of the colon or rectum. It is the second leading cancer killer in the United States, after lung cancer, and the third most commonly diagnosed form of cancer. About 143,000 new cases of cancer of the colon and rectum are diagnosed each year in the United States and more than 50,000 Americans die of the disease each year.[69] Colon cancer alone kills more women than cervical and ovarian cancers combined. One in twenty Americans eventually develops colorectal cancer, making it the third most frequently occurring non-skin cancer in both men (after prostate cancer and lung cancer) and women (after breast cancer and lung cancer).

polyps
Bulging masses of tissue in the colon, which may become cancerous.

Colorectal cancer tends to grow slowly. Though it can occur at any age, more than 90% of cases occur in people over the age of 50. If colorectal cancer is detected at an early stage, it can be cured in more than 90% of cases.

Risk factors for colorectal cancer include family history of the disease, advanced age, ulcerative colitis, Crohn's disease, and a history of colorectal **polyps.** Lifestyle factors in colorectal cancer include inactivity; a diet rich in saturated fat but poor in fruits, vegetables, and fiber; obesity; alcohol consumption; and tobacco use. High fat intake may cause the body to secrete more acid for digestion, which may irritate the lining of the bowel. Fiber intake helps speed waste products through the colon and rectum, reducing the length of exposure to possible carcinogenic substances. Cutting back on saturated fat in the diet, combined with other healthful changes in diet and regular exercise, may reduce the risk of colorectal cancer. Exercise helps speed the stool through the colon, which may have a preventive effect.

The key to preventing colorectal cancer is identifying and removing precancerous polyps or growths.[70] Colorectal cancer usually begins as benign polyps that turn cancerous in 5 to 10 years. Overall, the five-year survival rate for cancers of the colon and rectum is now 65%, which is up substantially from the 50% survival rate 30 years ago. Physicians now recommend one or a combination of the following screening methods for most adults aged 50 and above:

1. An annual *fecal occult blood test* (*FOBT*). This is a home test for hidden blood in the stool. Fecal blood may indicate bleeding from a precancerous or cancerous polyp.
2. Every five years: *Flexible sigmoidoscopy*. In a flexible sigmoidoscopy, the physician inserts a hollow, flexible lighted tube to detect polyps in the rectum and lower third of the colon.
3. Every 5 to 10 years: *Colonoscopy.* A colonoscopy allows the physician to view the entire colon and to remove any small polyps. Larger polyps may be removed in follow-up surgery. The physician uses an elongated scope to see the inner surfaces of the colon. The procedure is typically performed as an outpatient procedure while the patient is sedated.
4. Every five years: *Double-contrast barium enema*. The double-contrast barium enema test uses a series of X-rays of the colon and rectum. The patient is first given an enema containing barium dye, which is followed by injection of air in the lower bowel.

Other screening tests include the *stool DNA test* and the *CT colonography* (also called a "virtual colonoscopy"), a type of CT scan that can detect polyps and cancerous growths. Ask your health care provider which of these tests you should use and the age at which you should begin.

Colorectal cancer can usually be cured if it is detected in its early, localized stage, but it is often "silent" in the early stages. If people wait until symptoms such as rectal bleeding, diarrhea, and constipation appear, colorectal cancer may have metastasized, reducing the chances of recovery. Five-year survival rates plummet from about 90% for cases detected at the localized stage to about 10% for those in which it has metastasized.

Treatment for colorectal cancer involves surgical removal of precancerous and cancerous growths. Chemotherapy and/or radiation is usually given when cancer has spread into the bowel wall or lymph nodes. Improvements in cancer treatment have greatly minimized the need for a *colostomy bag*, an external bag worn to collect fecal wastes from an artificially constructed abdominal opening after surgery for colon cancer.

Prostate Cancer

Prostate cancer is the second most common cancer in American men, after skin cancer. It is also the second leading cancer killer of men, after lung cancer. Each year nearly 200,000 men are diagnosed with prostate cancer and about 30,000 die of the disease.

The prostate is a male reproductive gland that secretes most of the seminal fluid that carries sperm. Many men with prostate cancer don't know they have the disease, since it typically does not produce any symptoms in its early stages. Since prostate cancer usually affects older men and grows slowly, most men with the disease eventually die of other causes. For some, especially younger men, the disease is more aggressive. Five-year survival rates have improved steadily during the past 50 years to the point at which virtually all American men diagnosed with prostate cancer (99%) survive for at least five years, as compared to a 50% survival rate 30 years ago.

Though the incidence of prostate cancer has been rising in recent years, medical researchers believe that the increase reflects improved screening and early detection and not changes in underlying disease patterns. Early detection received a significant boost with the introduction of a blood test that measures the levels in the blood of a protein, *prostate-specific antigen* (*PSA*), which is produced by the prostate gland and is often elevated in men with prostate cancer.[71] However, it is uncertain whether PSA reduces death rates from prostate cancer.[72] Heightened PSA levels may also occur because of an enlarged prostate, underlying infection, or other causes. The diagnosis of prostate cancer is confirmed by a biopsy in which a sample of prostate tissue is removed and examined for cancerous growths.

Early, localized prostate cancer does not usually produce pain or other symptoms. Men may notice some difficulty in urination, but such symptoms are more often associated with other causes, such as an enlarged prostate or *prostatitis*. The American Cancer Society recommends that men over age 50 should discuss prostate cancer screening with their health care providers.[73] Men with a family history of prostate cancer are advised to consult their health care providers by the age of 40. The health care provider may use the following screening tests: (1) a *digital rectal exam* (*DRE*), in which the doctor feels for the presence of bumps or hard spots in the prostate (Figure 11-8); (2) a *PSA test*, which measures the level of a naturally-occurring substance made by cells in the prostate and is used to detect localized prostate cancers that might not be felt by examination; and (3) a *transrectal ultrasound* (*TRUS*), in which sound waves reflected by the prostate form an image of the gland. Any abnormal results from these tests may be followed up with a biopsy.

Treatment

The choice of treatment depends on the stage of development of the cancer, the man's age, and general health. For men with localized cancers of the prostate, one treatment alternative is surgical removal of the prostate—*radical prostatectomy.* Removal minimizes the risk that the cancer will metastasize but may have side effects such as urinary incontinence (loss of control over urinating) and erectile disorder (problems obtaining and maintaining erection). Alternative treatments include radiation, which kills or shrinks cancer cells in the gland, and hormone therapy. Since the male sex hormone testosterone stimulates the growth of prostate cancer cells, hormone therapy is used to reduce testosterone levels.

Figure 11-8 Digital Rectal Examination

In a digital rectal examination, a physician presses against the prostate gland, searching for bumps or hard spots that may signify prostate cancer.

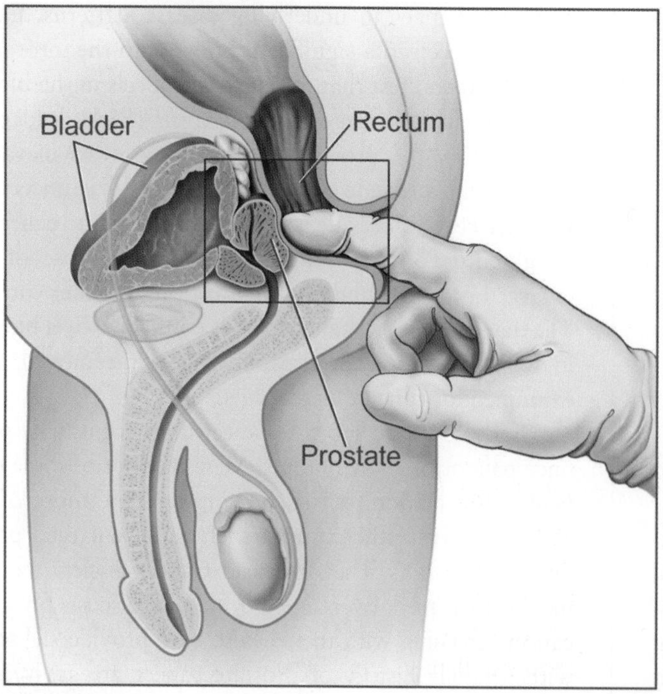

Source: National Cancer Institute

Some men with early prostate cancer may be advised by their doctors to "wait and watch" rather than have surgery and radiation. "Watchful waiting" is best suited to older men without symptoms and for whom this slow-growing cancer is unlikely to shorten their lives. Metastatic prostate cancer is usually treated with a combination of radiation therapy, chemotherapy, and hormone therapy.

Risk Factors

The primary risk factor for prostate cancer is age.[74] Other risk factors include race, family history, and dietary fat. Men in countries such as China and Japan, where low-fat, high-fiber diets are the norm, have lower rates of prostate cancer than men in Northwestern Europe and North America, where fat intake is higher.[75]

Prevention

Since prostate cancer may be linked to diet, it makes sense for men to curb their intake of high-fat foods and increase their consumption of vegetables, fruits, and grains. Reducing fat intake may also help prevent other health problems, including cardiovascular disease and adult-onset diabetes. Tomatoes may also help. Yes, tomatoes. Plant chemicals called *lycopenes*, the substances that give tomatoes their red color, may help prevent damage to DNA, which in turn might possibly reduce the risk of prostate cancer and some other cancers as well.[76] Pink grapefruit and watermelon are also good sources of lycopenes. Another possible preventative is antioxidant-rich green tea.[77]

Skin Cancer

Skin cancer is the most common and most rapidly increasing type of cancer in the United States. Skin cancer can occur anywhere in the skin, but is most common in areas commonly exposed to sunlight, such as the face, neck, hands, and arms. It affects one in six Americans. Two possible reasons for the increase are the popularity of sunbathing and the thinning of the ozone layer of the atmosphere. The ozone layer surrounding the Earth filters harmful ultraviolet (UV) radiation from the sun.

The two major types of skin cancer are *nonmelanoma skin cancer*, which consists of two highly curable forms, basal cell and squamous cell carcinomas, and *melanoma*, the most deadly form of the disease (see Figure 11-9). Nonmelanoma cancers are far more common, with more than 1 million new cases diagnosed annually in the United States, as compared to about 68,000 cases of melanoma,

Figure 11-9 Major Types of Skin Cancer

(a) The two forms of nonmelanoma skin cancer, basal carcinoma (shown here) and squamous cell carcinoma, are the most common forms of skin cancer and the most easily treatable when detected early. (b) A melanoma, like the one shown here on a lower leg, is the most deadly form of skin cancer, accounting for more than 8,000 deaths annually in the United States.

(a)

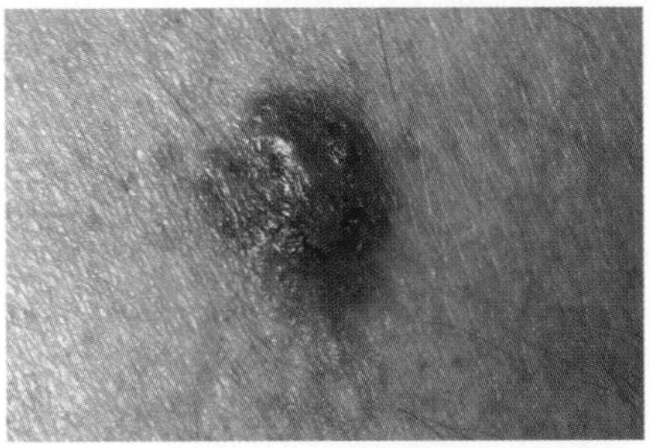

(b)

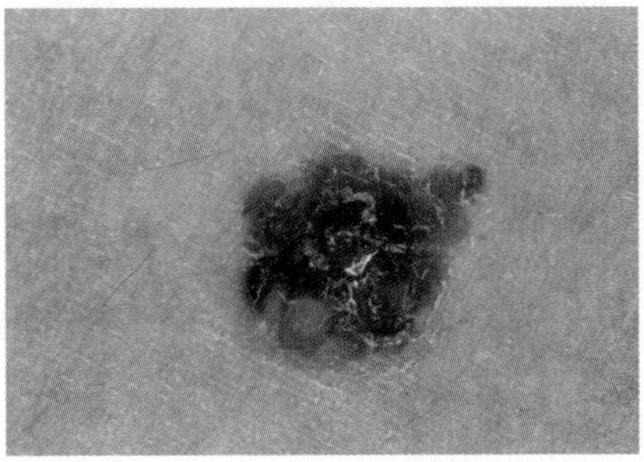

a cancerous (malignant) tumor that begins in melanin-forming cells, most commonly in the skin.[78] Melanin is the pigment that gives color to the skin, hair, eyes, and some other body parts. Non-melanoma skin cancers account for fewer than 1,000 deaths annually in the United States, as compared to 8,700 deaths due to melanoma.

Basal cell carcinoma (BCC) is a translucent, pearly raised tumor found mostly on the skin of the face, neck, hands, and trunk. The tumor may crust, ulcerate, and bleed. **Squamous cell carcinoma (SCC)** is a raised red or pink nodule that generally appears on the face, hands, or ears. It may grow and spread to other parts of the body. Early detection and treatment lead to a cure in 95% or more cases of nonmelanoma skin cancers. They primarily affect older people after a lifetime of exposure to the sun.

Risk Factors and Prevention

Sun, sun, sun. No, this is not a refrain from an old Beach Boys song. It is the principal risk factor for skin cancer. Lighter-skinned people and people with more sensitive skin who burn easily are at greater risk of skin cancers.

Two types of ultraviolet radiation found in sunlight, **ultraviolet A (UVA)** and **ultraviolet B (UVB)**, are largely responsible for skin damage and skin cancer. UVB rays quickly redden the skin, producing dangerous sunburns. They are responsible for more than 90% of skin cancers and are especially dangerous because they can damage cellular DNA. UVA rays, once thought to be harmless "tanning" rays, actually play a role in some skin cancers.[79]

Cumulative sun exposure over the years is thought to be responsible for most skin cancers other than melanoma. A history of sunburns, especially in childhood, increases the risk of melanoma. Nearly 80% of a person's lifetime exposure to the sun occurs before age 18.

Preventing skin cancer and minimizing its damage rest on adoption of sun-sensible behaviors (limiting exposure to the sun and using sunscreen with an SPF, or *sun protection factor*, of 15 or higher) and early detection by means of regular self-examinations and head-to-toe medical examinations. But many people remain in the dark about skin cancer.

Exposure to tanning lamps can lead to skin cancer, including both basal cell carcinoma and melanoma. Because their lamps rely mainly on ultraviolet A (UVA) radiation and are less likely to produce a sunburn, tanning salons would have you believe that they are safe. They do not say (or do not know) that both types of ultraviolet radiation (UVA and UVB) can damage the skin and promote skin cancer. Save your money and your skin. Stay out of tanning salons. Home sunlamps are no safer.

In addition to sun, a high-fat diet may also promote the growth of basal and squamous cell carcinomas. Practicing sun-sensible behaviors and following a low-fat diet are your best line of defense against skin cancer.

Warning Signs of Skin Cancer

Can you identify the moles and other spots, bumps, and growths on your body? Have you examined your skin from head to toe, front and back? Awareness of moles or areas of pigmentation on your skin establishes a benchmark for evaluating changes that might raise suspicions of cancer. The

basal cell carcinoma (BCC)
A form of nonmelanoma skin cancer; it is easily curable if detected and treated early. It appears as translucent, pearly raised tumors, usually found on the skin of the face, neck, hands, and trunk.

squamous cell carcinoma (SCC)
A form of nonmelanoma skin cancer, which like basal cell carcinoma, is easily curable if detected and treated early. It appears as a reddish or pinkish raised nodule, usually on the face, hands, or ears.

ultraviolet A (UVA)
A form of ultraviolet radiation from sunlight that can damage the skin and eyes.

ultraviolet B (UVB)
A more dangerous form of ultraviolet radiation from sunlight that is principally responsible for sunburns.

warning signs and symptoms of skin cancer include any unusual skin condition, particularly a change in the size, shape, or pigmentation of moles or other dark areas of skin. Take notice of any bleeding, ulceration, scaliness, or other changes in any nodule, growth, bump, or "beauty mark." Notice any changes in sensation (pain, tenderness, itchiness) of skin marks or a spreading of pigmentation. Notify your doctor of any changes or suspicious-looking moles or growths. Applying the "ABCDE" rule to moles on your body can help identify warning signals of melanoma (see Figure 11-9):[80]

- *A is for asymmetry*. One half of the mole does not match the other half.
- *B is for border irregularity*. The edges are ragged, notched, or blurred.
- *C is for color*. The pigmentation is not uniform. Shades of brown, tan, and black are visible.
- *D is for diameter greater than six millimeters*. Any sudden or progressive increase in size should be of special concern.
- *E is for evolving*. "E" is to alert people to be aware of any evolving changes in the shape, size, color, or symptoms (itching, hurting, bleeding, etc.) of the mole.

Examine your skin monthly. Report any suspicious findings to your family physician or dermatologist without delay. It may be "just a mole," but it is best to play it safe when it comes to melanoma.

Treatment

Early skin cancers are excised (removed surgically) in most cases, though other methods are sometimes used to destroy cancerous growths, such as the use of heat (*electrodessication*), freezing (*cryosurgery*), and radiation therapy. For melanoma, the primary growth and some surrounding healthy tissue are removed surgically, sometimes along with nearby lymph nodes that may harbor some migrating cancer cells. Though early melanomas can usually be cured, the chances of recovery are slim if they are detected after they have metastasized. The chances of surviving five years following diagnosis of melanoma are better than 90% if the cancer is small and is removed before it can spread to other parts of the body. The odds drop precipitously to about 15% to 20% if it has metastasized.[81] However, more than four of five melanomas are detected before they have done so.

Oral Cancer

Oral cancers include cancers of the mouth, lips, tongue, and throat. Some 37,000 new cases of oral cancers are diagnosed annually, and more than 8,000 deaths result from them. The disease is most common in men, especially men over 40. Early signs of oral cancer include a sore in the mouth or on the lips that bleeds easily and doesn't heal; a lump, thickening, or persistent red or white patch in the mouth, lips, tongue, or throat; and difficulty chewing, swallowing, or moving the tongue or jaw.

Most oral cancers result from tobacco use—smoking cigarettes, cigars, or pipes; using chewing tobacco; and dipping snuff. So too is excessive use of alcohol. Excessive sun exposure can also lead to cancer of the lip.

The principal methods of treatment are surgery and radiation therapy. Oral cancers can be disfiguring when cancerous parts of the oral cavity and jaw are removed. But with early treatment, cure rates are excellent.

The key to fighting oral cancer is prevention: avoidance of smoking, smokeless tobacco, and excessive use of alcohol. Limiting exposure to the sun, wearing a hat that shades the lips, and using lip balms or lotions containing sunscreen can reduce the risk of cancer of the lip.

Leukemia

Many people think of leukemia as a childhood disease since it accounts for one in three cancer cases in children. However, it affects about ten times more adults than children, some 43,000 cases in total, and causes about 22,000 deaths a year.[82]

Leukemia is cancer of the blood cells, which are made by the bone marrow—the soft spongy material in the center of bones. In most cases the abnormal cells are white blood cells, the body cells that fight infection. In leukemia, abnormal blood cells accumulate in the bloodstream and lymph nodes, interfering with vital body organs. Different types of leukemia are classified by how quickly the disease progresses and the type of blood cells that are affected.

If leukemia is suspected, a biopsy of the bone marrow and blood tests are used to confirm a diagnosis. Though the causes of leukemia remain a mystery in most cases, a rare form of the disease is caused by a type of virus, *human T-cell leukemia virus-I* (*HTLV*-1). Exposure to high levels of radiation, or to certain chemicals such as benzene, may also play a part. People with certain genetic abnormalities are also at higher risk.

Treatment typically involves chemotherapy with cancer-fighting drugs that interfere with the ability of cancerous cells to grow and spread. A bone marrow transplant from a compatible donor may be used to restore healthy blood cells. Some patients undergo stem cell transplantation in which they receive healthy stem cells that hopefully will develop into new, cancer-free blood cells. The five-year survival rate overall remains relatively low, 57% overall.

Lymphoma

Lymphomas develop in the lymph system, which is part of the body's immune system. In lymphoma, lymph cells grow abnormally and can metastasize. **Hodgkin's disease** (also called *Hodgkin lymphoma* or *Hodgkin's lymphoma*) is a rare form of lymphoma that primarily affects people age 15 to 34 or over 55. Estimates are that about 74,000 Americans are diagnosed with lymphoma each year, and about 21,000 people die of the disease.[83]

The majority of lymphomas, about nine of 10 cases, are **non-Hodgkin's lymphomas (NHL)**. The incidence of non-Hodgkin's lymphoma has increased sharply during the past two decades, while the rate of Hodgkin's disease has declined. A few decades ago, few people survived non-Hodgkin's lymphoma. Today, advances in treatment have increased the chances of surviving five or more years to 67%. Five-year survival rates from Hodgkin's disease are even higher: 85%.

Diagnosis is made from biopsy of a lymph node. Exposure to certain viruses, impaired immune system functioning, following a high-fat diet, being older, and having a history of organ transplantation (which can alter immune system functioning) increase the risk of certain lymphomas. In a few cases (fewer than 1% in the United States), lymphomas are caused by the HTLV-1 virus. Treatment depends upon the type of lymphoma and the stage of the disease and may involve chemotherapy, radiation therapy, and surgery.

Pancreatic Cancer

Pancreatic cancer is most deadly. It is newly diagnosed in some 43,000 people in the United States each year and kills about 37,000.[84] It is "silent" in the early stages; by the time it produces symptoms, cure is almost out of the question. The disease primarily strikes people between the ages of 65 and 79. Only about 6% of patients diagnosed with the disease live five years or longer. Though little is known about the causes of pancreatic cancer, people who smoke have double or triple the risk of developing the disease. Other risk factors include a high-fat diet, diabetes, male gender, and a history of chronic infection of the pancreas. Treatment involves surgery, radiation therapy, and chemotherapy.

DIABETES

An estimated 26 million people in the United States have **diabetes mellitus**, but more than one in four of them don't know it.[85] Ignorance of diabetes is anything but bliss, however. Failure to diagnose and control diabetes can lead to serious complications—for example, double the risk of CHD and strokes—and death.

What Is Diabetes?

Diabetes affects more than 11% of adults in the United States over the age of 20, claiming some 70,000 lives annually but also contributing to more than 200,000 deaths, mostly from heart disease. Diabetes it also a common chronic disorder of children and adolescents.

☒ LEARNING OUTCOME 8

Discuss the nature, incidence, and control of diabetes

The cells in our body use *glucose* (sugar) as the major source of fuel for

Hodgkin's disease
A rare type of lymphoma characterized by enlargement of the lymph nodes, named after Thomas Hodgkin (1798–1866), a London physician who described its symptoms.

non-Hodgkin's lymphomas
All forms of lymphoma (cancers of the lymphatic system) other than Hodgkin's disease.

diabetes mellitus
A metabolic disease involving insufficient production of insulin or a failure of cells to utilize the insulin that is produced, which leads to high glucose levels building up in the blood while cells remain starved for the glucose they need.

There is no guaranteed way to prevent diseases such as cancer, but you can lower your risk. While it's true that you can't control factors such as age and heredity, there are risk factors you *can* control. Read the online feature "Health Skills 11-4" to learn more.

health skills

Access CourseMate for HLTH at www.cengagebrain.com.

growth and energy. The liver converts most food into glucose and releases it into the bloodstream to circulate and be taken up by cells. **Insulin**, a hormone produced by the **pancreas**, allows cells to draw glucose from blood. Like a key fitting into a lock, insulin opens glucose receptors on cells. The pancreas regulates the amount of insulin the body needs. In diabetes, the pancreas produces too little insulin or none at all, or cells in the body fail to efficiently utilize the insulin that is available. Thus too much glucose circulates in the blood. It is eventually excreted in urine while cells remain starved for nourishment. Lacking glucose, the cells begin burning fat and even muscle as fuel. Unless diabetes is controlled, excess glucose in the blood can damage organs, cause nerve damage and circulatory problems, and lead to the types of health problems shown in Table 11-5.

An estimated 35% of American adults aged 20 and above—79 million people—have a condition called *pre-diabetes*, in which their blood sugar levels are higher than normal but not yet high enough to be diagnosed as diabetes. Half of them are aged 65 or older.[86] Development of Type 2 diabetes is not inevitable for pre-diabetics and may be delayed or prevented through weight loss, exercise, and medication.

Types of Diabetes

The two major types of diabetes are easy enough to remember—Type 1 and Type 2. A third type of diabetes, *gestational diabetes*, affects pregnant women.

Type 1 Diabetes

In **Type 1 diabetes** (previously called *insulin-dependent diabetes mellitus* [*IDDM*] or *juvenile-onset diabetes*), the body's own immune system destroys insulin-producing cells in the pancreas. Type 1 diabetes typically develops in children and young adults and accounts for 5% to 10% of diagnosed cases. People with Type 1 diabetes require daily injections of insulin. If insulin-dependent diabetes goes untreated, the person can lapse into a life-threatening coma.

Type 2 Diabetes

Type 2 diabetes (formerly called *non-insulin-dependent diabetes mellitus* [*NIDDM*] or *adult-onset diabetes*) is more common than Type 1 and accounts for 90% to 95% of cases, usually occurring in middle or late adulthood and among overweight people.[87] Type 2 diabetes typically begins with *insulin resistance*, a

insulin
A hormone produced by the pancreas that allows cells to take up glucose from the bloodstream.

pancreas
A gland located near the stomach that secretes a digestive fluid into the intestines and manufactures the hormone insulin.

Type 1 diabetes
A form of diabetes that usually develops in childhood or young adulthood in which the person requires daily doses of insulin to make up for the deficient production by the pancreas. Previously called juvenile diabetes *or* insulin-dependent diabetes mellitus (IDDM).

Type 2 diabetes
A type of diabetes that usually develops in middle or later life involving a breakdown in the body's use of insulin. Previously called adult-onset diabetes *or* noninsulin-dependent diabetes mellitus (NIDM).

Table 11-5 Complications of Diabetes[88]

COMPLICATION	EFFECTS
Heart disease and strokes	Diabetic adults have two to four times the death rates of normal people from heart disease and strokes.
High blood pressure	About two-thirds of diabetic people have blood pressure equal to or greater than 140/90 mm Hg or use prescription medications for hypertension.
Blindness	Diabetes is the leading cause of new cases of blindness among adults aged 20–74 years.
Kidney disease	Diabetes is the leading cause of kidney failure, accounting for 44% of new cases.
Nervous system disease	About 60% to 70% of people with diabetes have mild to severe nervous system damage, impairing sensation or causing pain in the feet or hands, slowing digestion of food, and causing carpal tunnel syndrome.
Amputations	More than 60% of lower-limb amputations occur in people with diabetes.
Dental disease	Almost one-third of people with diabetes have severe periodontal (gum) disease.
Complications of pregnancy	Poorly controlled diabetes before conception and during the first trimester can cause major birth defects in 5% to 10% of pregnancies and spontaneous abortions in 15% to 20% of pregnancies.

condition in which cells in the body fail to use insulin properly. Though the pancreas pumps out enough insulin, the body cannot use it effectively. Too little glucose gets through to the cells, and blood glucose rises to unhealthy levels. With increased demands, over time the pancreas eventually loses its ability to produce insulin. The symptoms of Type 2 diabetes typically occur gradually and may go unnoticed. They include fatigue; feeling ill; frequent urination, especially at night; increased thirst; weight loss; and blurred vision.

Gestational Diabetes

Gestational diabetes is a form of insulin resistance that affects some women during pregnancy. Women with the condition require medical treatment to ensure that their blood glucose levels remain normal during pregnancy. The disorder usually disappears after childbirth but increases the risk that women may later develop Type 2 diabetes.

Risk Factors for Diabetes

Key risk factors for developing diabetes include excess body weight and family history (heredity).[89] Although your family history is fixed, you can reduce your risk of diabetes by controlling your weight.[90]

Although the incidence of pre-diabetes is comparable for various racial/ethnic groups in the United States, African Americans and Mexican Americans have a 70% to 80% greater risk of developing Type 2 diabetes than European Americans do.[91] Native Americans have the highest rates of Type 2 diabetes. Genetic factors may contribute to these differences, but eating and exercise habits, especially overweight and obesity rates, play roles.

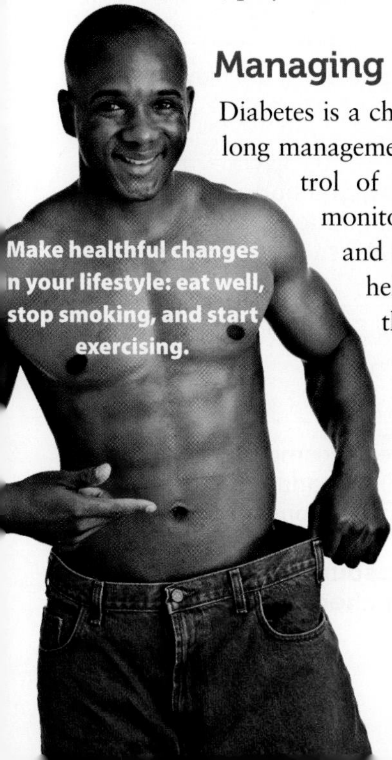

Make healthful changes in your lifestyle: eat well, stop smoking, and start exercising.

©iStockphoto.com/Stockphoto4u

Managing Diabetes

Diabetes is a chronic disease that requires lifelong management. Treatment emphasizes control of blood glucose levels through monitoring, sugar-restrictive diet, and regular physical activity, which helps clear excess glucose from the blood. People with Type 1 diabetes also need daily doses of insulin, which may be administered by injection or a pump. Many people with Type 2 diabetes also need daily insulin, but others control their blood glucose with diet, exercise, and oral medication.

CHRONIC OBSTRUCTIVE PULMONARY DISEASE (COPD)

Chronic obstructive pulmonary disease (COPD) (also called *chronic obstructive lung disease* or *COLD*) is a general term for chronic lung disease. In COPD, the breathing passageways (tubes carrying air into and out of the lungs) are partially obstructed, making breathing difficult. COPD is the fourth leading cause of death in the United States, and affects more than 12 million adults.[92]

Types of Chronic Obstructive Pulmonary Disease

The major forms of COPD are emphysema and chronic bronchitis. In most cases of COPD, both emphysema and chronic bronchitis are present. COPD can cause severe disability and death. COPD is the second leading cause of disability in the United States, after CHD. As the American Lung Association puts it, "When you can't breathe, nothing else matters."

LEARNING OUTCOME 9

Discuss the major forms of chronic obstructive pulmonary disease

Emphysema

Emphysema is a progressive disabling disease in which the walls of the air sacs (*alveoli*) in the lung are destroyed, reducing the lung's ability to exchange oxygen and carbon dioxide and causing shortness of breath, especially following exertion. People with emphysema may find it difficult to walk short distances or climb a flight of stairs. Smoking is the primary cause of emphysema, but exposure to air pollution and dust may contribute. There is also a rare inherited form of the disorder.

gestational diabetes
Diabetes developed during pregnancy.

emphysema
A lung disease involving destruction of the walls of the air sacs (alveoli) in the lungs. The most common symptom of emphysema is breathlessness upon exertion.

Chronic Bronchitis

Chronic bronchitis is an inflammation of the lining of the bronchial tubes, the airways that connect the windpipe to the lungs. Inflammation obstructs the flow of air and leads to the buildup of mucus or phlegm. As a result, people experience a hacking, persistent cough; shortness of breath; and wheezing. You may have had acute bronchitis on the heels of a cold or the flu. Usually it passes within several weeks. In chronic bronchitis, the symptoms persist for months or years and cannot be explained by an underlying infection. It is often called a "smoker's cough" because, like emphysema, cigarette smoking is the most common cause. Prolonged exposure to air pollution also irritates the lungs, leading in some cases to bronchitis.

Treatment of COPDs

Since smoking figures prominently in the development of these chronic respiratory diseases, quitting smoking is a critical element in treatment. Treatment may include regular exercise or conditioning to improve overall fitness and strengthen the respiratory muscles. Bronchodilators are medications administered by an inhaler that can help open clogged airways and reduce shortness of breath.

HEALTH APPS: YOUR LINK TO ONLINE HEALTH APPLICATIONS

health check
Heart Quiz How much do you know about that pumping station in your chest? "Health Check 11-1" can help you evaluate whether or not you are heart smart.

diversity
High Blood Pressure and Ethnicity Why do African Americans have higher blood pressure than any other ethnic group in the United States? How does it contribute to their risk of cardiovascular disease? For possible answers to these questions, go to "Diversity 11-1."

prevention
Aspirin: Not Just for Headaches Anymore The common aspirin in your medicine cabinet not only reduces headache and fever, but may be helpful in preventing and treating blood clots, including clots that can cause heart attacks when they become lodged in arteries narrowed by fatty deposits. Learn more in "Prevention 11-1."

health check
Estimating Your Risk of a Heart Attack What is your personal risk of suffering a heart attack within the next 10 years? "Health Check 11-2" can help you find the answer.

health skills
Dieting to Cut Your Cholesterol Level The guidelines in "Health Skills 11-1" may help you reduce your blood cholesterol level. They will also help you manage your weight and are consistent with dietary guidelines for minimizing the risks of cancer and other chronic diseases.

diversity
Racial/Ethnic Differences in Cancer Risk Cancer is not an equal-opportunity destroyer. African Americans and Native Americans have a greater risk of death than European Americans for many kinds of cancer. Go to "Diversity 11-3" to learn more.

health skills
New Methods of Combating Cancer Surgery, radiation, chemotherapy, and hormone therapy remain the mainstays of cancer treatment, but they have their limitations, such as killing healthy tissue along with cancerous tissue and unpleasant side effects. "Health Skills 11-2" will take you on a tour of methods under development.

health skills
Living with Cancer Living with cancer is a challenge, but patients need not go it alone. Go to "Health Skills 11-3" to learn about organizations that can be of help.

health skills
Protecting Yourself from Cancer and Other Chronic Diseases When it comes to protecting yourself from disease, you cannot control risk factors such as age and heredity, but "Health Skills 11-4" will help you get a handle on the risk factors you *can* control.

Go to the CourseMate for HLTH at www.cengagebrain.com for additional resources including flashcards, games, self-quizzes, review exercises, web exercises, learning checks, and more.

Infection and Immunity

"As you are reading this page, countless microscopic warriors within your body are carrying out search-and-destroy missions against foreign agents."

You may be reading this page at your desk, at the library, or in your bed. You may also be listening to music or have the TV murmuring in the background. But something else is happening, something vital to your health: countless microscopic warriors within your body are carrying out search-and-destroy missions against foreign agents. And the great majority of the time, you win.

In Europe in 1348, millions of people lost. Bodies littered the streets. The bubonic plague leapt from town to town and so ravaged the populace that it was said that the living were scarcely able to bury the dead before they too were claimed as victims. Their symptoms included high fever, vomiting of blood, aching limbs, and most noticeably, the swelling of the lymph nodes in the neck, armpits, and groin. Protruding lymph nodes turned blackish, from which the plague drew its name, "the black death."

The bubonic plague was caused by something too small to see with the naked eye: a *bacillus* that was transmitted to humans by fleas that fed off the blood of rats. Rats died, people died. The bacillus thrived until those who remained had developed immunity.

In 1918 the so-called Spanish influenza swept the world. The outbreak claimed 675,000 lives in the United States—more than in the Civil War, more than in all the wars of the twentieth century combined.

A far more prevalent and devastating condition, AIDS (acquired immune deficiency syndrome), has become one of history's worst **epidemics**. More than 40 million people worldwide are infected with HIV, the virus that causes AIDS, and about 25 million have died from it.[1] HIV infects some 55,000 Americans each year.

epidemic
The occurrence of disease above usual levels in a given group or community.

LEARNING OUTCOMES

1. Discuss the nature of infection, types of pathogens, and the course of infections
2. Describe the body's defenses against infection
3. Discuss immunity and immunization
4. Describe common infectious diseases
5. Discuss the causes, transmission, symptoms, diagnosis, and treatment of sexually transmitted infections

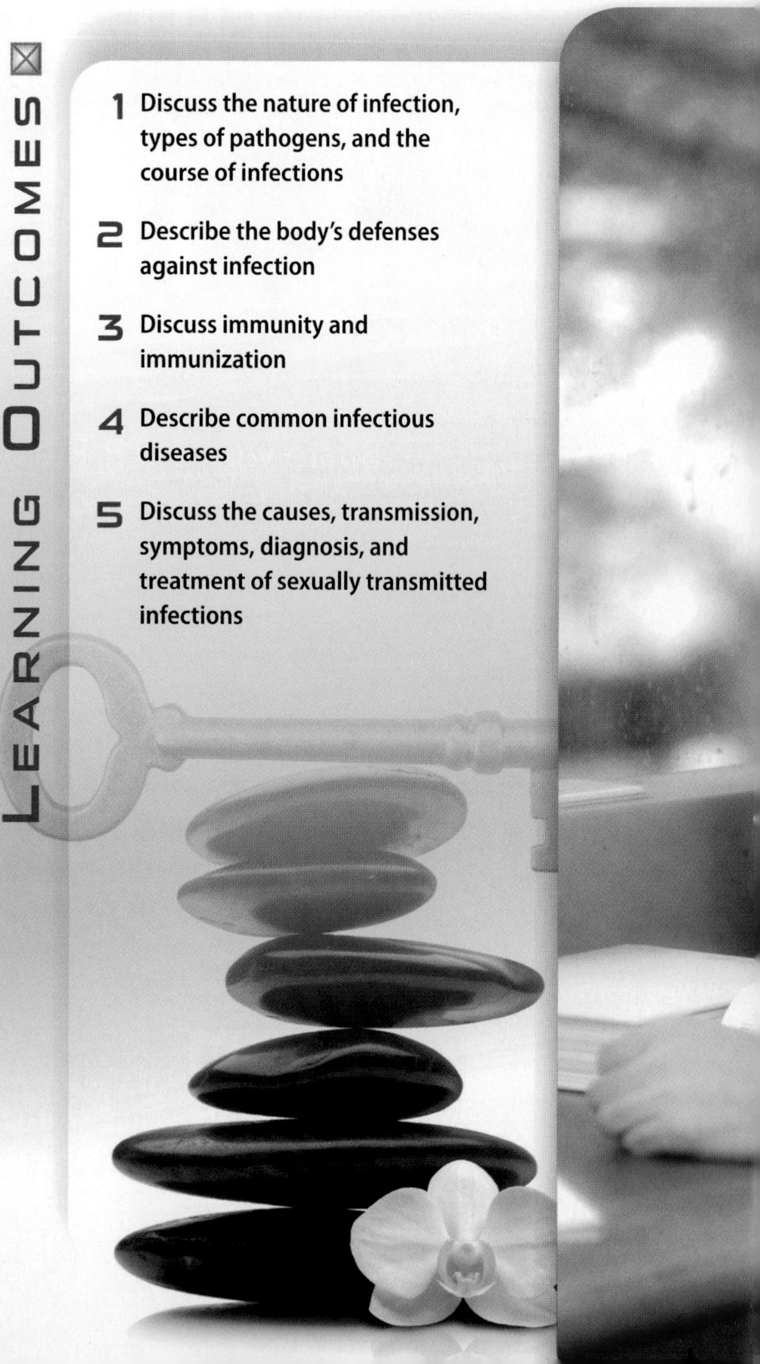

The Basics of Infection and Immunity

Bubonic plague, influenza, and HIV/AIDS are all forms of infectious disease—diseases caused by microorganisms. Because of globalization, someone who sneezes in Bangkok might infect a traveler who spreads the disease to any part of the world in a day.

The environment is a veritable soup of infectious organisms, so it is not surprising that infectious diseases such as colds, the flu, sinus infections, and sore throats are among the most commonly identified health impediments that affect the academic performance of college students today (see Table 12-1 on the next page).

LEARNING OUTCOME 1

Discuss the nature of infection, types of pathogens, and the course of infections

Infectious diseases are also called *communicable diseases*. They are caused by contact with **pathogens** that multiply within

pathogen
Disease-causing organism, including bacteria, viruses, fungi, and parasites.

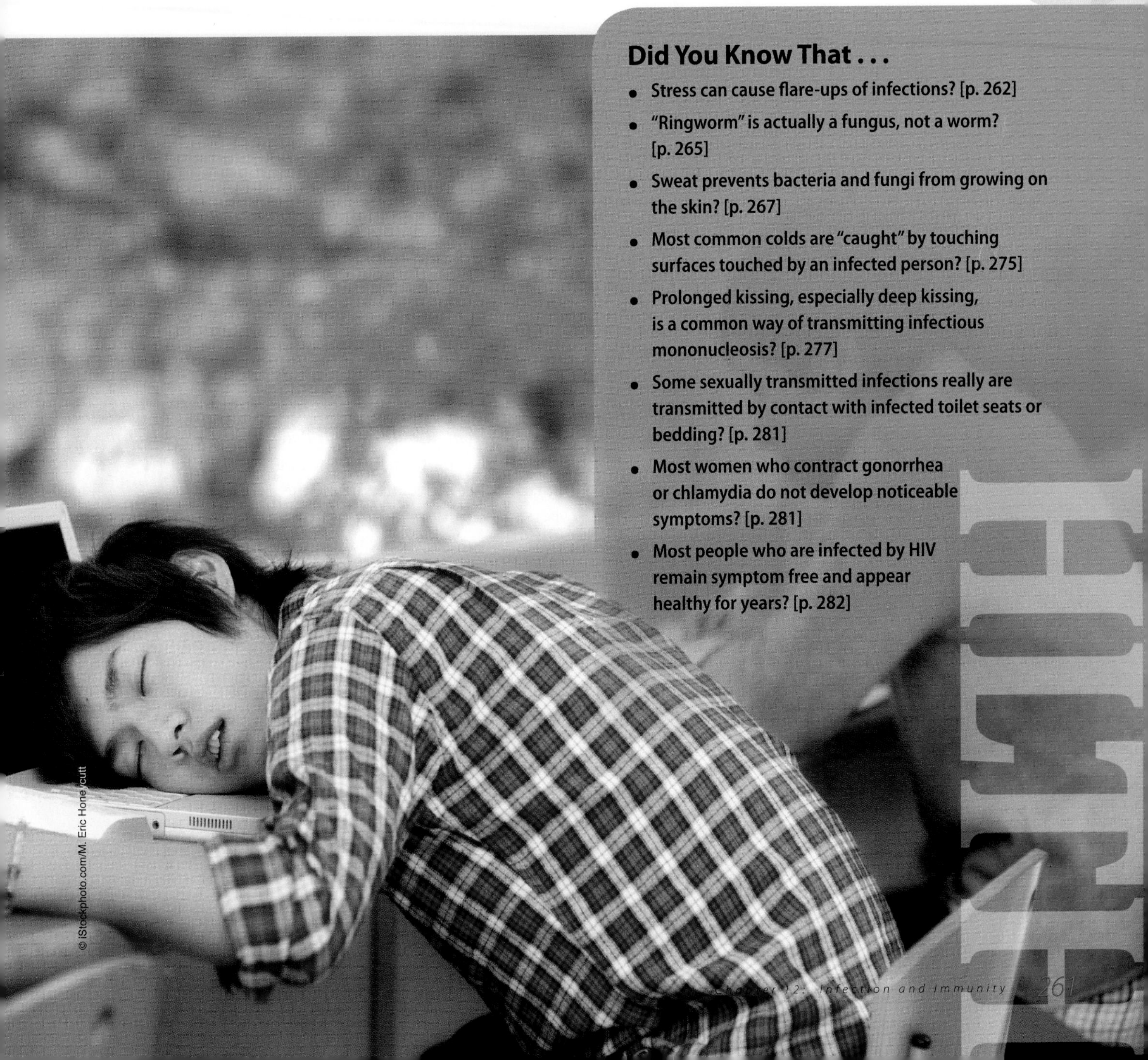

Did You Know That . . .

- Stress can cause flare-ups of infections? [p. 262]
- "Ringworm" is actually a fungus, not a worm? [p. 265]
- Sweat prevents bacteria and fungi from growing on the skin? [p. 267]
- Most common colds are "caught" by touching surfaces touched by an infected person? [p. 275]
- Prolonged kissing, especially deep kissing, is a common way of transmitting infectious mononucleosis? [p. 277]
- Some sexually transmitted infections really are transmitted by contact with infected toilet seats or bedding? [p. 281]
- Most women who contract gonorrhea or chlamydia do not develop noticeable symptoms? [p. 281]
- Most people who are infected by HIV remain symptom free and appear healthy for years? [p. 282]

Table 12-1 *Top 10 Reported Health-Related Impediments to Students' Academic Performance (%)*[2]

RANK	HEALTH IMPEDIMENT	TOTAL	FEMALE	MALE
1	Stress	33.9%	37.5%	27.2%
2	Cold/flu/sore throat	28.8	31.0	24.7
3	Sleep problems	25.6	26.6	23.8
4	Concern about troubled friend or family member	18.8	20.9	14.7
5	Internet use/computer games	16.9	18.1	12.5
6	Depression/anxiety disorder/seasonal affective disorder	16.1	18.1	12.5
7	Difficulty with relationships	15.9	17.0	14.0
8	Sinus infection/ear infection/bronchitis/strep throat	9.3	11.1	5.9
9	Death of a friend or family member	9.3	11.1	5.9
10	Alcohol use/abuse	7.8	6.9	9.5

the body. Pathogens include bacteria, viruses, fungi (yeasts and molds), and parasites such as insects and worms (see Figure 12-1). Most pathogens are microorganisms—too small to be seen by the naked eye. They reproduce in a *host*, a plant or animal that provides a breeding ground. Pathogens enter the body through ports such as tiny pores or sores in the skin, or through the oral or nasal cavities. Unchecked, they can establish beachheads in the body. They can use the body's own resources to multiply and produce illness. Infectious organisms are transmitted by contact with infected people or animals, insect bites, or via contaminated food, air, soil, or objects (see Figure 12-2). Some microorganisms are normally found in the body. They become a problem only when they overgrow or sprout colonies in parts of the body where they are not normally found.

meningitis
An inflammation of the membranes (meninges) of the spinal cord or brain.

Types of Infection

Infectious diseases may be *localized*, or restricted to a particular part of the body, as in some skin infections. They may instead be *generalized* or *systemic*, involving many organs and systems. Infections can also be *acute*, producing fever and other symptoms rapidly, or *chronic*, developing slowly and producing milder but more enduring symptoms. Most acute infections such as the common cold or flu run their course in days or weeks. But some acute infections, such as bacterial **meningitis**, can overcome the body's ability to defend itself, leading to death. Some chronic infections can enter acute phases, and some acute infections may progress to chronic infections.

It may take months or years from the time pathogens enter the body for symptoms to occur. These *latent* ("hidden") *infections* are symptom-free but can turn active, especially when the person's health is compromised by stress or other diseases. The virus causing genital sores (*herpes simplex II*) may lie dormant for lengthy periods after its initial outbreak.

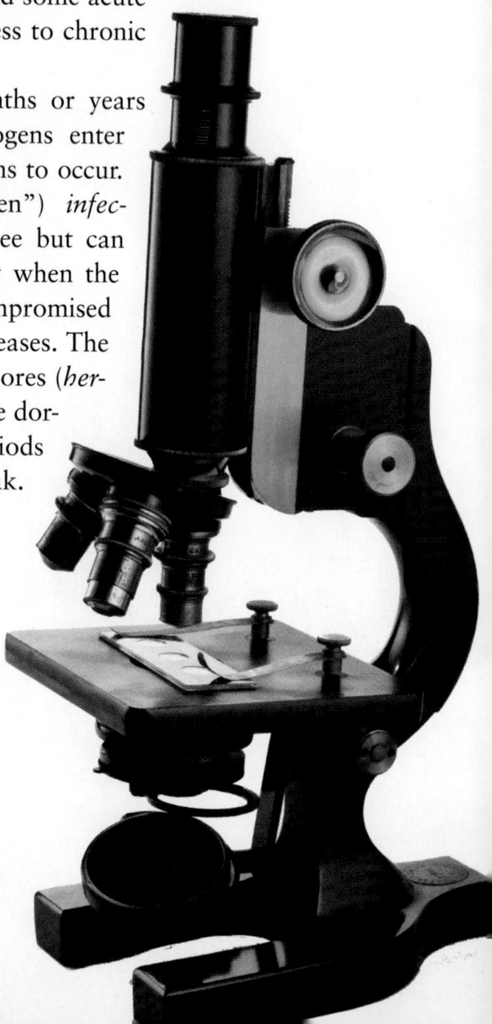

Figure 12-1 *Kinds of Pathogens*

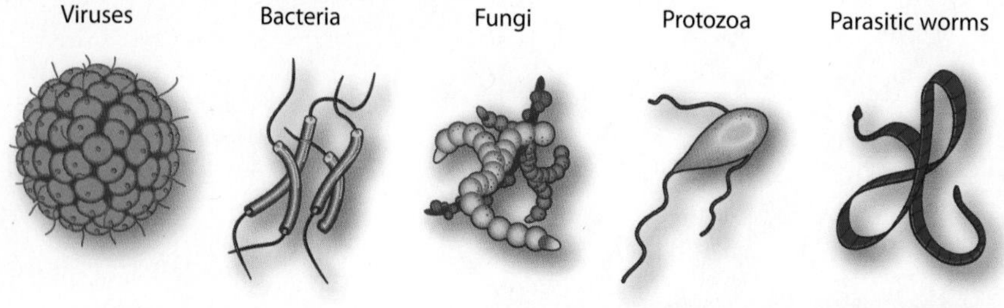

Figure 12-2 How Infectious Diseases Are Transmitted

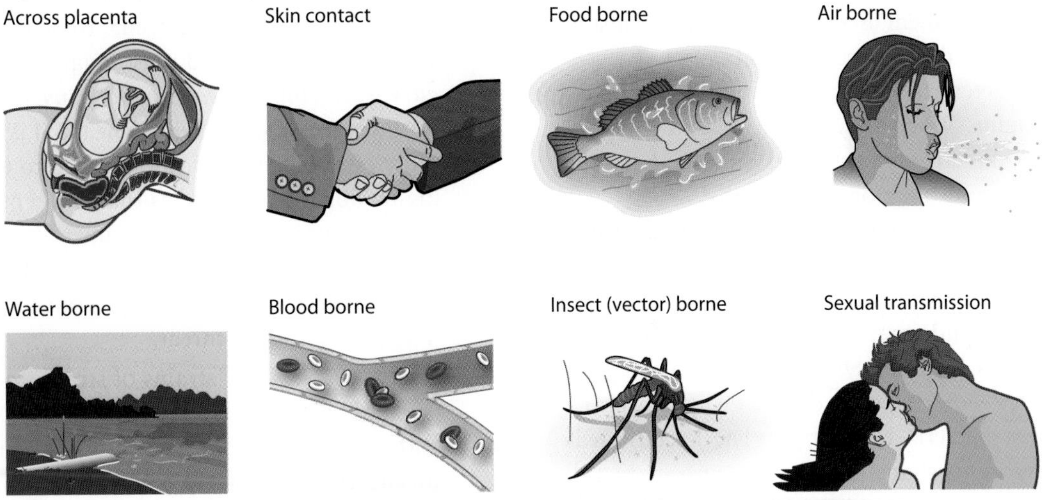

Pathogens

Countless microorganisms surround us each day. Most of them are not pathogenic, or disease causing. Some are essential to our survival. Some bacteria play key roles in digestion. Microorganisms also degrade waste material. Yet many microbes are dangerous to our health, and some are deadly.

Endogenous versus Exogenous Microbes

Microorganisms are *endogenous* or *exogenous*. **Endogenous microorganisms** originate within the body. **Exogenous microorganisms** originate outside the body. Endogenous microorganisms generally live peacefully, making up our body's natural flora and fauna (plant and animal life). *Candida albicans*, for instance, is a yeast-like fungus that is naturally present in the intestinal tract and elsewhere in healthy people. It helps prevent other potentially harmful fungi and bacteria (including *E. coli*) from overgrowing. The bacterium *Escherichia coli* (E. coli) normally dwells in the colon, where it helps digest food.

When imbalances occur in the body's flora and fauna, the body's **immune system** (the network of specialized cells, tissues, and organs that defends against pathogens) becomes weakened, allowing normally harmless endogenous organisms to overbreed and turn pathogenic or grow in parts of the body where we don't normally find them. Overgrowth of *candida* can cause vaginal infections. *E. coli* may start growing in the urethra, causing inflammation (*urethritis*) and spread to the bladder and kidneys.

Exogenous microorganisms, such as the bacteria that cause tuberculosis and flu viruses, pose greater risks. They cause acute, sometimes severe infections. Let's look at types of pathogens.

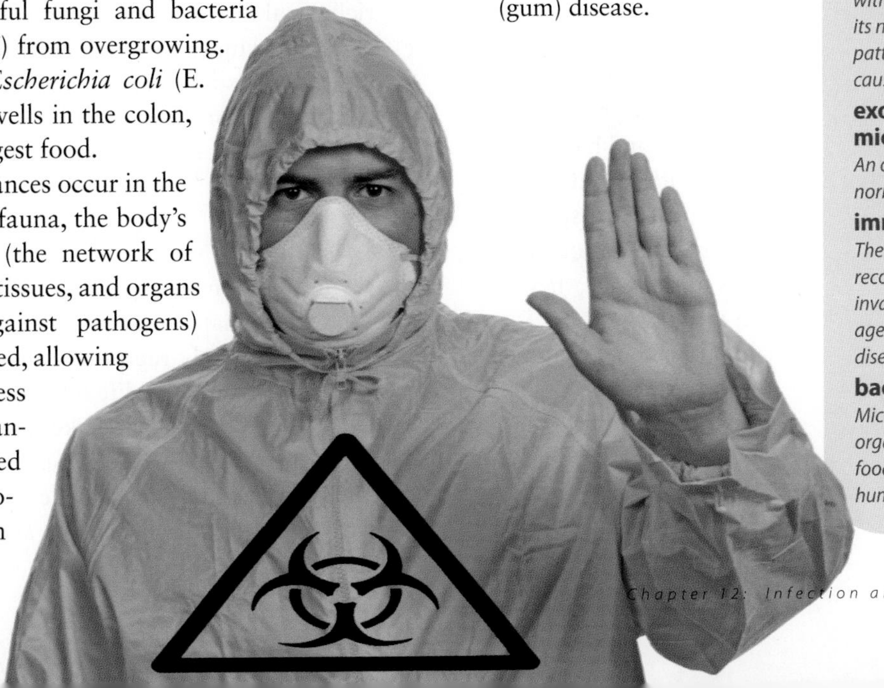

Bacteria

Bacteria (singular: bacterium) are microscopic, single-celled organisms that live in soil, air, plants, and animals, including humans. They cause tuberculosis, some kinds of pneumonia, urinary tract infections, Lyme disease, dysentery, botulism (food poisoning), and periodontal (gum) disease.

endogenous microorganisms
Organisms normally living within the body that constitute its natural flora; if growth patterns are disturbed, it can cause infection.

exogenous microorganism
An organism that does not normally inhabit the host.

immune system
The body system that recognizes and destroys invasive disease-causing agents and rids the body of diseased or worn-out cells.

bacteria
Microscopic, single-celled organisms that live in air, soil, food, plants, animals, and humans (singular: bacterium).

Some bacteria are sphere-shaped (*cocci*), others resemble a rod (*bacilli*), still others have a spiral shape (*spirochetes*). Each of them uses nutrients from the host to reproduce. They divide into two identical cells.

Harmful bacteria release poisonous chemical substances, or toxins. When they invade body cells, they destroy tissue directly or reproduce so fast that they prevent organs from functioning normally.

Though some bacterial infections can be identified by the person's symptoms, a definitive diagnosis is often made from laboratory tests. In some cases, a sample of blood is analyzed under a microscope to identify bacteria. In other cases, a throat swab or sample of a bodily fluid is *cultured*—that is, placed in a dish with nutrients that allow bacteria to multiply. The bacterium is then identified by its shape and growth pattern. In still other cases, stains made of colored dyes are mixed with bacteria-laden cells on a microscope slide. The stains bind to different bacteria in characteristic ways, allowing identification.

Bacterial infections are typically treated with antibiotics. Some antibiotics, such as *penicillin*, destroy bacteria outright; others, such as *tetracycline*, slow their rate of reproduction. Some bacterial infections, such as diphtheria, whooping cough, and tetanus, can be prevented by **vaccination**. Bacteria are grouped in families:

- *Staphylococci.* Staphylococci ("staph") are naturally present in the skin and harmless, but if they infect the bloodstream, spinal fluid, bladder, or other parts of the body, they can produce serious staph infections. Staph infections include urinary tract infections, acne, and blood infections. One type of staphylococcus, *staphylococcus aureus*, normally lives on the skin and hair. When it enters the body, it can cause wound infections, pneumonia, toxic shock syndrome (TSS), and food poisoning. *Staphylococcus aureus*, *E. coli*, and *salmonella* cause food-borne illnesses. **Toxic shock syndrome (TSS)** is a potentially fatal but rare infection linked to the use of highly absorbent tampons that are kept in place for six hours or more. Most super-absorbent tampons have been removed from the market. Leaving diaphragms in the body for prolonged periods may pose a similar threat.
- *Streptococci.* Many strains of streptococci ("strep") are found in the throat, tonsils, skin, and anal area. *Group A streptococci* cause **strep throat**, rheumatic fever, scarlet fever, and **impetigo**. *Group B Streptococci* cause urinary tract infections, wound infections, and endometritis. *Streptococcus pneumoniae* cause bacterial pneumonia.
- *Chlamydia.* Strains of chlamydia cause respiratory tract infections, eye disease, and genital tract infections. *Chlamydia pneumoniae* is linked to "walking pneumonia," a common form of pneumonia in the United States, especially among young adults. *Chlamydia trachomatis* can cause *trachoma*, a cause of blindness found among Native Americans in the southwest. *Chlamydia trachomatis* can also be transmitted sexually.
- *Rickettsiae.* **Rickettsiae** are bacteria-like organisms that inhabit insects and other parasites. Lice, fleas, ticks, and mites transmit them by biting humans. Most diseases caused by rickettsiae are rare in developed nations, except for Rocky Mountain spotted fever, which accounts for most cases of rickettsial disease in the United States. The most common symptoms—high persistent fever and a rash—may disappear in two weeks or so but sometimes worsen and can lead to complications, even death. Rickettsial diseases are treated with antibiotics.

Viruses

Viruses are the smallest pathogens. They consist of a core of genetic material surrounded by a coat of protein. Viruses can only reproduce; they cannot metabolize food or perform other life functions. Therefore, they "hijack" the machinery that makes the host's cells work. When a virus invades a cell, it injects its DNA or RNA into the cell, providing the genetic code for replication while the host provides the energy and materials.

vaccination
A means of introducing a weakened or partial form of an infectious agent into the body so as to produce immunity without incurring the full-blown illness caused by the infectious agent.

toxic shock syndrome (TSS)
A rare and sometimes fatal bacterial infection linked to tampon use.

strep throat
A bacterial infection caused by streptococcal bacteria; characterized by a painful and reddish sore throat, fever, ear pain, and enlarged lymph nodes.

impetigo
A contagious skin disease, primarily affecting the skin around the mouth and nose, caused by different types of bacteria including streptococci.

rickettsiae
Bacterial-like organisms that grow inside insects and other parasites; transmitted to humans via bites by lice, fleas, ticks, and mites.

viruses
Submicroscopic particles consisting of a core of nucleic acid containing DNA or RNA and a surrounding coat of protein; incapable of replicating outside of cells of living plants or animals.

Some viruses remain dormant within host cells for long periods. Others reproduce quickly and burst out from cells with a vengeance, producing acute infections such as influenza—the "flu." Some viruses have mild effects, such as cold sores or warts; others, such as HIV, produce lethal conditions. Table 12-2 lists virus families and the infections they cause.

Viruses can enter the body via the skin, eyes, nose, mouth, and genital tract. They can be inhaled from airborne droplets, ingested, or transmitted sexually. Some viruses are contracted by contact with infected blood or semen. Others, like **rabies**, are passed through skin punctures from bites by infected animals.

Health care providers diagnose viral infections on the basis of symptoms and laboratory examination of bodily specimens for the presence of **antibodies**. Health professionals usually test for HIV by examining a sample of blood, urine, or saliva for HIV antibodies.

Antibiotics are useless against infections and are not used for the common cold and flu. Some drugs have antiviral properties, including *acyclovir* (used in treating herpes) and *amantadine* (used with influenza). HIV/AIDS is typically treated with a "cocktail" of antiviral drugs that can contain the virus. This treatment—highly active antiretroviral therapy (HAART)—has helped many HIV/AIDS patients survive, but it does not eradicate the virus, and side effects may become problematic. The best weapon against viruses is prevention.

Fungi

Fungi are primitive plants such as yeasts and molds. Fungal infections typically occur on the skin.

- *Ringworm.* Dermatomycosis, or **ringworm**, is a fungal infection of the hair, skin, or nails. The pathogen is the fungus *dermatophyte*. About one in 10 Americans develops ringworm each year. Athlete's foot (*tinea pedis*), jock itch (*tinea cruris*), and scalp itch (*tinea capitis*) are ringworm infections, symptomized by itching, scaling, and occasionally by painful lesions. Treatment includes powders to dry the affected area and topical antifungal medications such as *miconazole* and *clotrimazole*.
- *Candida.* Candida is a yeast-like endogenous fungus. Overgrowth may result from a weakened immune system or the use of antibiotics, causing

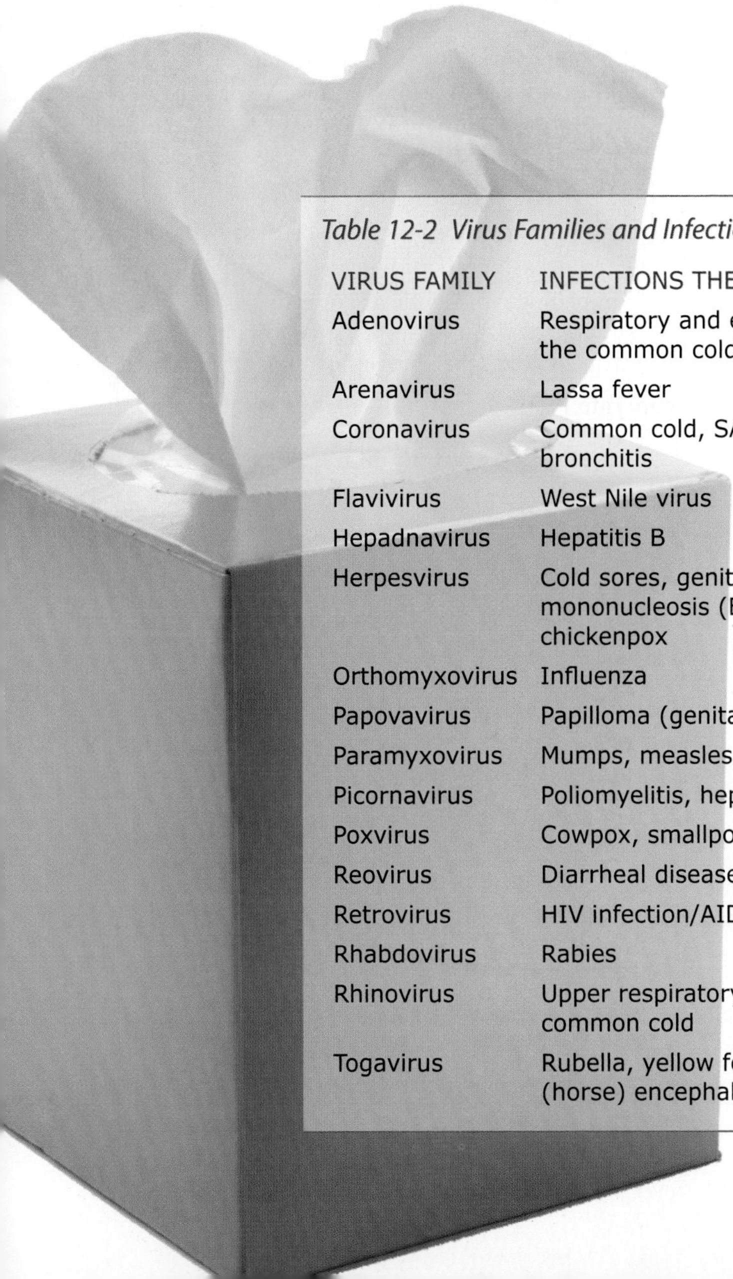

Table 12-2 Virus Families and Infections They Cause

VIRUS FAMILY	INFECTIONS THEY CAUSE
Adenovirus	Respiratory and eye infections, including the common cold
Arenavirus	Lassa fever
Coronavirus	Common cold, SARS, possibly infectious bronchitis
Flavivirus	West Nile virus
Hepadnavirus	Hepatitis B
Herpesvirus	Cold sores, genital herpes, infectious mononucleosis (Epstein-Barr virus), chickenpox
Orthomyxovirus	Influenza
Papovavirus	Papilloma (genital warts)
Paramyxovirus	Mumps, measles, parainfluenza
Picornavirus	Poliomyelitis, hepatitis A, common colds
Poxvirus	Cowpox, smallpox (eradicated)
Reovirus	Diarrheal disease
Retrovirus	HIV infection/AIDS, human T-cell leukemia
Rhabdovirus	Rabies
Rhinovirus	Upper respiratory infections, like the common cold
Togavirus	Rubella, yellow fever, dengue, equine (horse) encephalitis

rabies
A viral disease that primarily affects the central nervous system and can lead to paralysis and death if not treated immediately with the rabies vaccination.

antibodies
Protein molecules that mark antigens for destruction by other cells. Also called immunoglobulins.

fungi
Primitive vegetable organisms such as yeasts and molds.

ringworm
A fungal skin infection characterized by red patches, itching, and scaling, such as athlete's foot.

candidiasis (also known as *moniliasis*, *thrush*, or most commonly, a *yeast infection*). Yeast infections are treated with antifungal medications applied topically, in a suppository, or in a pill.

Protozoa

Protozoa—single-celled aquatic animals—are the largest microorganisms. Some are visible to the naked eye. Protozoal diseases such as malaria and diarrhea are a major health problem in tropical climates and developing nations.

- *Giardiasis.* *Giardiasis lamblia* is a highly contagious diarrheal disease found most commonly in the United States among children. Also called *traveler's diarrhea*, it affects children in day-care centers and people with impaired immune systems. In developing countries, it causes several million deaths a year among young children. Contaminated water and oral–fecal contact are common sources of transmission. Giardiasis is treated with the antiprotozoal drugs *quinacrine* or *metronidazole*.

- *Malaria.* Malaria is transmitted to humans by bites from the female mosquito of the *Anopheles* species. Symptoms include flu-like aches and fever; if left untreated, death can result. Travelers to high-risk areas are sometimes advised to take antimalarial drugs as a precaution and to use insect repellents. The development of antimalarial drugs such as *chloroquine* and insect control programs raised hopes that malaria was poised for elimination. Although developed countries are largely free of malaria, about 300 million people worldwide are infected each year, and some 700,000 to 1 million die of the disease, mostly children in sub-Saharan Africa.[3] Rates of malaria are especially high in countries in Africa, Southeast Asia, and Latin America (see Figure 12-3).[4]

helminths
Multicellular parasites, or worms (flat or round) ranging in size from tiny microscopic flukes to 20-foot-long tapeworms that flourish in the intestines.

Parasitic Worms

Parasitic worms (**helminths**) are flat or round and flourish in the intestines. They range in size from microscopic flukes to tapeworms, whose length can be measured in feet. Worms cause "pinworms" and schistosomiasis.

- *Pinworms.* Nearly 20% to 30% of American children and perhaps half as many adults are infected with pinworms. They hatch in the intestines and are transmitted by oral–anal contact, as by scratching or touching the anal cavity and then bringing the fingers to the mouth. The entire family, not just the apparently infected member, should be treated with an anthelmintic drug. But even without treatment, most cases disappear in about a month.

- *Schistosomiasis.* Schistosomiasis, a waterborne disease, is caused by a parasitic worm called a *fluke*. The worm lays its eggs in snails. When the eggs hatch, they burrow into the skin of bathers or of people working in infested water. Once the worm invades the body, it can survive for five years or more, taking refuge in the intestines or bladder, where it produces as many as 3,500 eggs a day. Over time, the eggs can clog the veins serving many of the body's organs, obstructing blood flow and occasionally proving lethal. Some 200 million people worldwide are infected, especially those living in tropical and subtropical climates. Drugs used to combat this disease have a high cure rate.

Figure 12-3 Geographic Distribution of Malaria

■ Malaria transmission occurs throughout ☐ Malaria transmission occurs in some parts ■ Malaria transmission is not known to occur

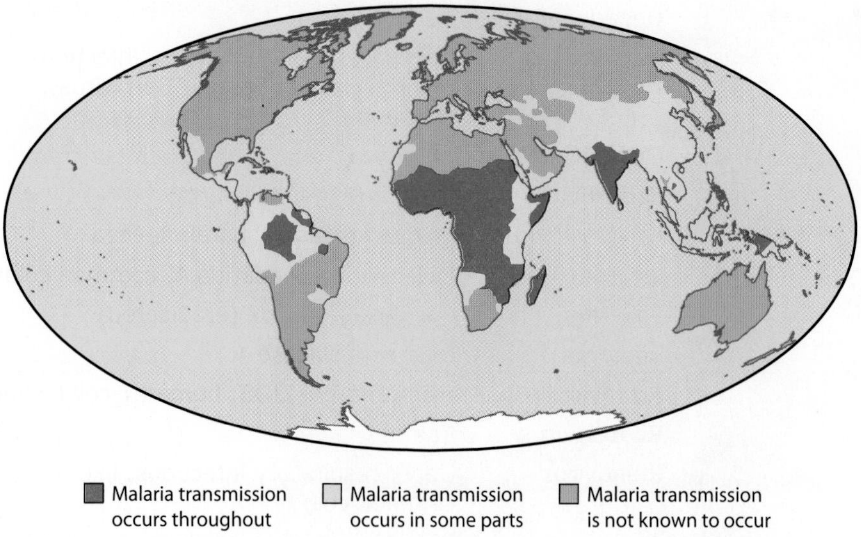

Source: Centers for Disease Control and Prevention. (2010, February). *Where malaria occurs.* Retrieved from http://www.cdc.gov /malaria/about/distribution.html

The Course of Infections

Whether you suffer a common cold or life-threatening infection, infections progress through a sequence of common stages leading, most often, to recovery. Pathogens multiply during the *incubation period*—the time between infection and the development of symptoms. Incubation periods can last from one to two days for the flu to 10 years or more for HIV/AIDS. Symptoms first appear in the *prodromal stage.* Initial symptoms are often nonspecific, such as low-grade fever, fatigue, and general aches and pains. We are typically most contagious during this stage. The *clinical stage* is characterized by development of full-blown symptoms specific to the infection. For rubella, for example, there is a characteristic red rash. In the *decline stage*, symptoms subside. *Convalescence* is the period between the end of the disease state and the return to normal. In some infections such as herpes, hepatitis, and syphilis, some of the pathogen may remain in the body, and "carriers" may be symptom-free but also be contagious.

The Body's Defenses against Infection

LEARNING OUTCOME 2

Describe the body's defenses against infection

Our best defense against infection is not a miracle drug. It is the body's own multilayered defense system. First-line defenses include physical and chemical barriers such as skin surfaces, saliva, and tears. Far more complex is the immune system.

Cells in the immune system recognize and destroy invasive disease-causing agents ("germs") such as bacteria and viruses. The immune system marshals the resources of an army of specialized cells that seek out, attack, and destroy infectious agents. It also rids the body of worn-out cells and cancerous cells that it recognizes as alien. You can help your body's immune system by regularly washing your hands to prevent the spread of infection (read the online feature "Prevention 12-1"), getting regular medical checkups, and getting enough sleep. People who get less than seven hours of sleep—hello, college students!—are nearly three times more likely than those getting eight or more hours of sleep to develop the common cold after exposure to cold viruses.[5]

prevention

Access CourseMate for HLTH at www.cengagebrain.com.

First-Line Defenses against Infection

Many pathogens never make it past the body's physical and chemical barriers. These include the *skin*, the moist body-lining tissue called *mucous membranes*, hairlike structures called *cilia* that line certain body passageways and sweep away pathogens, and *chemical secretions* produced by the body that wage chemical warfare against invading pathogens. Infections can occur when these lines of defense are breached, as when the skin is penetrated via lacerations, puncture wounds, burns, or insect bites; when organisms are inhaled and penetrate the mucous membranes of the respiratory system; when an organism is ingested (via food or water) and penetrates the mucous membranes of the gastrointestinal tract; or when an organism breaches the lining of the reproductive or urogenital systems.

- *The skin.* Skin is composed of layers of tightly-knit cells that provide a waterproof-like covering that prevents many pathogens from entering the body. The skin also secretes protective chemical substances such as sweat and sebum. *Sebum* is an oily substance secreted by sebaceous glands under the skin. Sebum and sweat help prevent bacteria and fungi from growing on the skin.
- *Mucous membranes.* Mucus is a slippery, "slimy" fluid that coats mucous membranes and keeps them from drying out. Mucous membranes line body openings—including the eyes, mouth, nose, and respiratory, gastrointestinal, reproductive, and urogenital tracts—and serve as barriers to pathogens. Mucus contains disease-fighting cells and traps and disposes of many contaminants.
- *Cilia.* Cilia are hairlike structures on the surface of cells. They sweep away invading organisms before they can invade tissue lining. Cilia line the respiratory tract, where they continually work to remove (via mucus that is coughed or blown away) invading pathogens from the lining of the lungs and windpipe.
- *Chemical defenders.* Chemical substances in your digestive tract, saliva, and tears also destroy pathogens. Acids kill many kinds of bacteria. The enzyme muramidase, found in tears and in the urogenital tract, kills many pathogens.

Figure 12-4 Like a Key in a Lock

A particular antibody fits a particular antigen like a key in a lock. Once locked in, the antibody marks the antigen for destruction by other cells of the immune system.

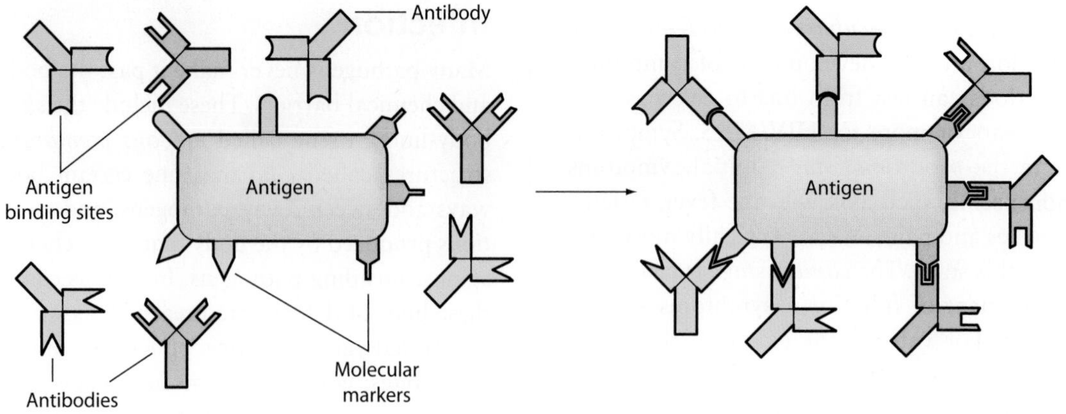

The Immune System: Search and Destroy

When invading pathogens breach the body's external barriers, the immune system springs into action. Sometimes it conquers the invaders so quickly that we are not aware we have been infected. In other cases, the infection takes root and we "get sick."

The immune system commands an army of billions of specialized **white blood cells** in the bloodstream and body tissue. These cells—**lymphocytes**—circulate continuously throughout the body, alert to foreign agents or **antigens** (literally *anti*body *gen*erators). An antigen is a substance that the immune cell recognizes as foreign to the body, such as a bacterium or virus—even a cancerous or worn-out body cell. Chemically, antigens are proteins on cell surfaces that stimulate an immune response.

The *immune response* is the sequence of events that takes place when lymphocytes detect antigens and destroy them. Some lymphocytes directly attack and destroy antigens. Others produce *antibodies*. Antibodies are molecules of protein called *immunoglobulins*. A particular antibody fits an invading antigen like a key fitting a lock (see Figure 12-4). By locking into an antigen, the antibody marks it for destruction by other immune cells. There are several kinds of immune responses:

- *Cell-mediated immunity.* When immune cells directly attack and kill antigens without the aid of antibodies, the response is called *cell-mediated immunity*.
- *Antibody-mediated immunity.* When antibodies join the fray, the response is called *antibody-mediated immunity*.
- *Nonspecific immune response.* When the body is invaded by a pathogen, a nonspecific immune response is initiated. This first line of defense is carried out by **phagocytes** (large white blood cells called "cell eaters") and **NK cells** ("natural killer" cells).

Phagocytes and NK cells are referred to as *scavenger cells* because they continuously roam the bloodstream and body tissues, hunting foreign microbes and cellular debris. When phagocytes encounter antigens, they swallow and digest them. NK cells also destroy antigens by filling them with a lethal burst of poisonous chemicals. The body defends itself by consuming its own diseased parts, and NK cells perform this function. Phagocytes also play a key role in inflammation—the body's nonspecific defense reaction to tissue damage (such as in cuts, burns, or splinters) caused by invading

white blood cells
Specialized blood cells that comprise part of the body's immune system by combating invading pathogens. Also called leukocytes.

lymphocytes
White blood cells of the immune system that attack antigens; may be T-lymphocytes ("T cells") or B-lymphocytes ("B cells").

antigen
Any substance that the immune system recognizes as foreign to the body and which induces it to produce antibodies.

phagocytes
A major class of white blood cells that seek out and destroy antigens in the bloodstream. Also called cell eaters.

natural killer (NK) cell
A type of white blood cell that destroys many kinds of antigens, especially viruses and tumor cells.

pathogens. When an area is infected, capillaries (small blood vessels) at the site enlarge to allow more white blood cells to flow to the injury. This activity causes the redness, swelling, warmth, and pain characteristic of inflammation. The pus that often accompanies inflammation contains the aftermath of the battle between immune cells and antigens. It contains dead cells and fluids that participated in the fight.

Tough as they are, some antigens are too powerful to be dealt the deathblow by immune cells comprising the nonspecific response team alone. In such cases, phagocytes signal other lymphocytes to move into action, initiating a specific immune response. These other lymphocytes act in concert with phagocytes to disarm and destroy antigens. Figure 12-5 shows the structure of the immune system.

Lymphocytes and the Lymphatic System

Lymphocytes are produced in the bone marrow and various organs of the **lymphatic system**, including the lymph nodes, spleen, and thymus. The lymphatic system is the body's other circulatory system. It carries the fluid **lymph**, which is collected from tissues throughout the body, through its network of vessels. Lymph passes through the **lymph nodes**, or glands, where lymphocytes cleanse it of infectious agents and debris. This is why your lymph nodes become swollen when you come down with an infection. Lymphocytes are also released into the bloodstream where they battle invaders.

There are two major types of lymphocytes: *T-lymphocytes* (simply, T cells) and *B-lymphocytes* (or B cells). Both T cells and B cells attack and disarm antigens but in different ways.

Helper T cells prowl the bloodstream for antigens, much like free-floating phagocytes. Once they find them, they secrete chemical messengers called *cytokines*. Cytokines alert *killer T cells* and phagocytes to swing into action. Killer T cells have a receptor that matches only one antigen. When it finds that antigen, it "locks" into the antigen and injects it with lethal chemicals. At birth, each of us is endowed with enough T cells to recognize at least 1 million different kinds of invading organisms, including viruses, bacteria, and even dust mites.

Helper T cells also trigger production of B-lymphocytes—immune cells that produce antibodies that attack antigens. Antibodies do not kill

lymphatic system
The system of vessels, nodes, ducts, organs, and cells that manufactures and stores lymphocytes and helps destroy infectious agents.

lymph
The fluid, usually clear or colorless, found in lymphatic vessels.

lymph nodes
Lymphatic glands located throughout the body, primarily under the arms and in the groin, neck, and elbow, that produce and store lymphocytes and serve an immune system function by filtering out infectious agents.

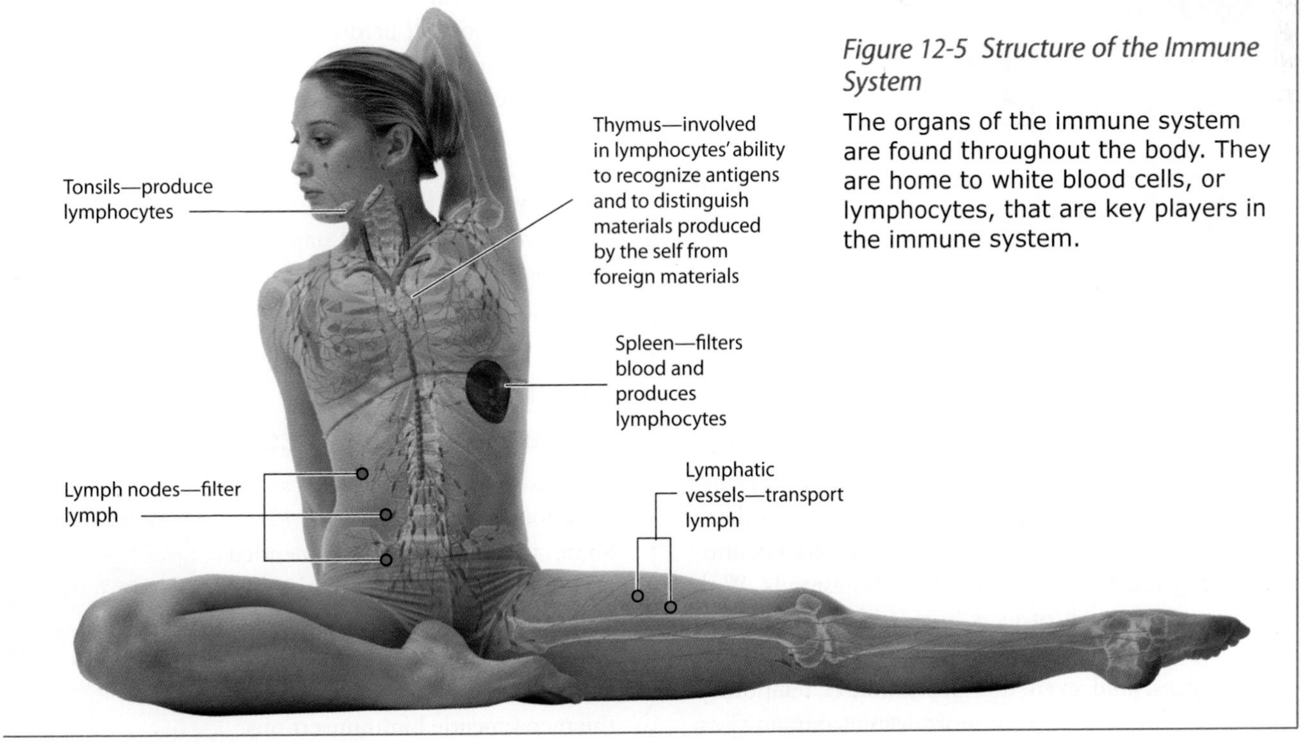

Figure 12-5 Structure of the Immune System

The organs of the immune system are found throughout the body. They are home to white blood cells, or lymphocytes, that are key players in the immune system.

memory cell
A type of B cell that recognizes and disposes of antigens that are reintroduced in the body, sometimes years after initial infection.

suppressor T cells
Immune cells that regulate the activities of T and B cells; suppressor T cells prevent lymphocytes from damaging healthy cells near the site of infection.

gamma globulin
Antibody-rich serum (blood fluid) from the blood of another person or animal used to induce passive immunity.

antigens themselves. They act as "vises" that hold antigens in place so that T cells and other immune cells can destroy them. Each B cell makes only one kind of antibody that targets a particular antigen. Surrounded by phagocytes, T cells, and antibodies, most antigens don't stand much of a chance.

Memory cells are specialized B-lymphocytes that remain after the battle against a specific antigen is over, even for a lifetime. They are called *memory cells* because they produce antibodies that have a "memory" for the antigens to which they were exposed. This allows them to react swiftly when the same antigen invades the body again. Because of them, you will not come down with chicken pox twice. Memory cells specific to the chicken pox virus remain poised in your body, ready to rapidly disarm it should it reappear.

Suppressor T cells regulate the activities of B cells and other T cells. They prevent the immune response from getting out of hand and damaging healthy cells in the vicinity of the infection. Suppressor T cells also signal the various T and B cells to cease activity when the infection has been eradicated.

Immunity and Immunization

The human body is capable of several kinds of immunity, or ways of protecting itself against disease. Let us begin as people begin, with innate immunity.

LEARNING OUTCOME 3

Discuss immunity and immunization

Innate Immunity

Inborn or *innate immunity* results from transmission of the mother's antibodies to the fetus. Following birth, additional antibodies are passed along to the baby in breast milk. With rare exceptions, each of us is born with innate immunities. Babies are protected for only a limited number of pathogens, and even this protection is temporary. As we develop, we acquire more lasting immunity to many kinds of pathogens. To survive the continuous onslaught, we need acquired immunity.

Acquired Immunity

Acquired immunity develops after birth. Acquired immunity can be active or passive. *Active immunity* can develop naturally, as when we are infected by a pathogen and the immune system produces antibodies against it. It can develop artificially, as by vaccination. In naturally acquired active immunity (NAAI), foreign agents cause an infection, which leads memory lymphocytes to develop antibodies that target the specific antigen. The antibodies protect us from reinfection. However, many viral and bacterial organisms mutate, or change their genetic structure. This is especially true of influenza, which is why a case of the flu during one flu season does not protect us when we are exposed to a different strain the following year.

Artificially acquired active immunity (AAAI) involves the use of an immunizing agent such as a vaccine. A vaccine—also called an "immunization"—contains a killed or weakened pathogen to stimulate production of antibodies. Many vaccines, such as those for diphtheria, measles, and mumps, are administered in early childhood and provide long-term immunity. Teenagers and adults may be given booster shots to enhance their effects. Some vaccines are injected. Others are taken orally.

Some infections—such as those produced by snakebite toxin—act so fast that they can prove lethal unless passive immunity is induced. *Passive immunity* is a short-lived form of protection against infections that can damage or kill before the immune system can produce antibodies. It is used in the treatment of snakebites, rabies (along with a vaccine), and other infections for which there are no vaccines.

Passive immunity can be transferred from one person to another through injecting antibody-rich blood serum (*antiserum*) called **gamma globulin** into the person needing protection. Once in the recipient's bloodstream, the antibodies attack antigens.

Immunization and Preventable Diseases

Vaccination is used to prevent many infectious diseases (see Table 12-3). Some vaccines are recommended for children through age six (see Figure 12-6). However, as discussed in the online feature "Diversity 12-1," not all children receive the recommended immunizations.

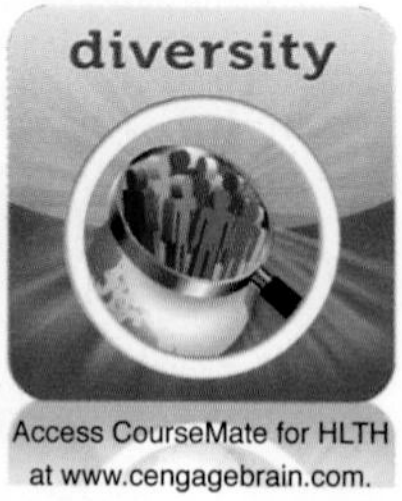
diversity
Access CourseMate for HLTH at www.cengagebrain.com.

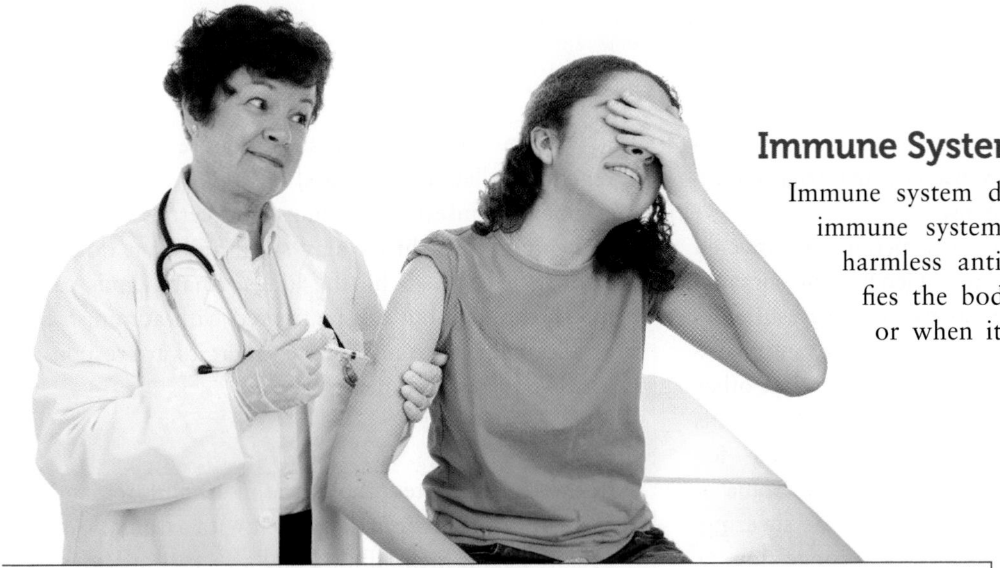

Immune System Disorders

Immune system disorders occur when the immune system overreacts to normally harmless antigens, when it misidentifies the body's own cells as foreign, or when it is unable to protect the body from common pathogens.

Allergies: An Overly Sensitive Alarm

One of every five Americans—about 60 million people—has allergies. An allergy is hypersensitivity to a normally harmless substance such as dust, foods, mold, pollen, animal dander, and insect bites. An allergic reaction occurs when the immune

Table 12-3 Some Vaccine-Preventable Infectious Diseases

Anthrax	Hepatitis A	Pneumococcal pneumonia
Bacterial meningitis	Hepatitis B	Polio
Chicken pox	Influenza (flu)	Rabies
Cholera	Measles	Rotavirus
Diphtheria	Mumps	Rubella
Haemophilus influenzae type B	Pertussis	Tetanus

Figure 12-6 Recommended Vaccinations for Children in the United States from Birth through Age Six[6]

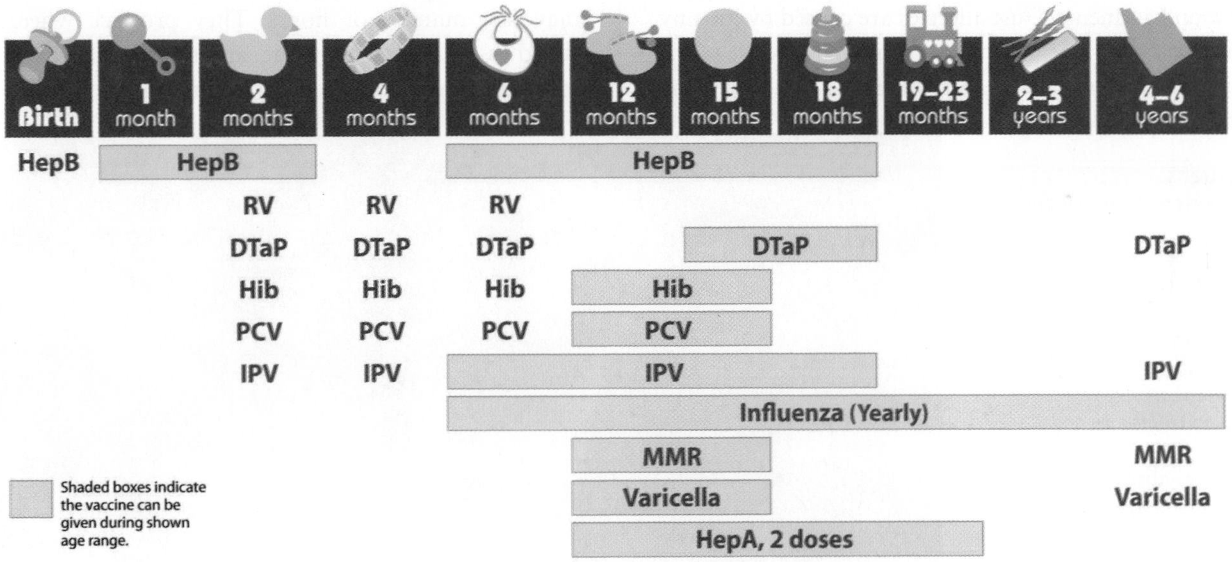

Key:

HepB: Vaccine that can prevent hepatitis B infection

HepA: Vaccine that can prevent hepatitis A infection

IPV: Vaccine that can prevent polio

RV: Vaccine that can prevent rotavirus, a common cause of severe diarrhea in children

HiB: Vaccine that can prevent haemophilus influenza type B

PCV: Vaccine to prevent pneumococcal disease, the most common type of bacterial pneumonia

Varicella: Vaccine that can prevent varicella (chickenpox)

DtaP: Combination vaccine that can prevent diptheria, tetanus, and pertussis

MMR: Combination vaccine that can prevent measles, mumps, and rubella

system mounts too vigorous a response to substances that actually pose no threat. Substances that trigger allergic reactions are called **allergens**.

It remains unclear why some people are affected by allergies and others are not. Genetics presumably plays a role. The immune systems of allergy sufferers respond to allergens by releasing **histamine**, an inflammatory chemical that causes a runny nose and other symptoms typical of allergies. The particular symptoms depend in part on where histamine is released—for instance, in the nose, chest, skin, or intestine. Some of the most common allergic responses include sneezing, itchy skin, hives, eczema, diarrhea, nasal congestion, or constriction of the lungs such that one finds it difficult to breathe.

Allergic rhinitis, commonly called *hay fever*, occurs when airborne allergens such as pollen, dust, mold, and particles of dried dog or cat saliva enter the nose and throat of an allergic person. Common symptoms include puffy and itchy eyes, a runny or stopped-up nose (or both), and sneezing. People who are sensitive to pollens and ragweed suffer most during the pollination seasons of spring and fall.

Mold allergies involve reactions to seeds or spores of plants in the fungus family. Molds can survive anywhere there is moisture, including piles of fallen leaves and walls of damp basements. Dust allergies are caused by the tiny droppings (feces) of microscopic bugs called *dust mites*, which dwell in mattresses, carpeting, and upholstery.

Some allergy sufferers experience severe allergic reaction called **anaphylaxis**, or *anaphylactic shock*, in response to insect bites, stings, and certain foods, such as peanuts. The throat may swell and shut down and fluid may begin to fill the lungs. Anaphylaxis can be life-threatening but can be treated with administration of adrenaline. Nut and peanut allergies are responsible for several hundred deaths a year.

Asthma

In the United States, about one in 10 children and one in 12 adults have been diagnosed with asthma.[7] Asthma usually begins in childhood and affects more boys than girls, but in adulthood, equal numbers of men and women are affected. Though some children outgrow it, it may persist.

Asthma is a chronic, noninfectious lung disease in which the bronchial airways, or bronchi—the tubes in the lungs—become temporarily obstructed or blocked. Muscles in the walls of the bronchial tubes tighten and go into spasm, making breathing difficult. The bronchial tubes also become inflamed, swollen, and blocked with mucus, further impairing the flow of air. Asthma can result from allergies, respiratory infections, and exposure to environmental pollutants such as soot and cigarette smoke. Stress can trigger or heighten attacks. Attacks may last minutes or hours. They produce wheezing, shortness of breath, coughing, and tightness in the chest. In severe cases, blockage of breathing can be lethal.

allergens
Commonly occurring antigens such as dust, food, pollen, and dander that trigger an allergic reaction in persons with allergies.

histamine
A powerful inflammatory chemical that causes symptoms of allergies and asthma.

allergic rhinitis
One of the most common kinds of allergies, caused when airborne allergen particles (pollen, dust, mold, animal dander, and so forth) enter the nose and throat of an allergic person. Also called hay fever.

anaphylaxis
A severe allergic reaction ranging from hives and wheezing to convulsions; treated with injections of adrenaline.

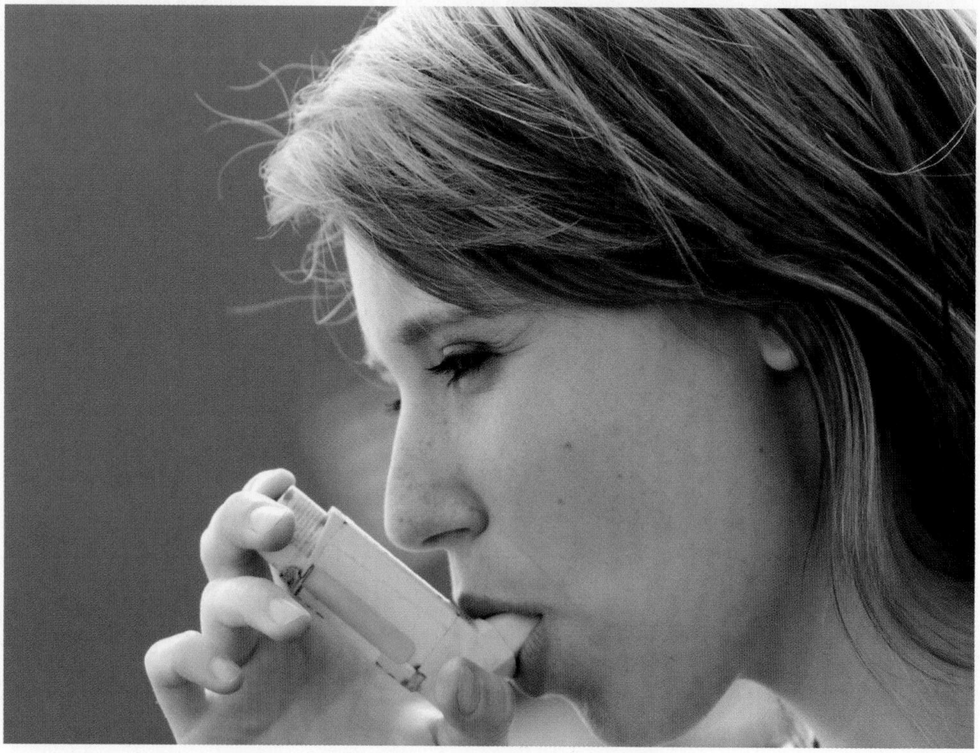

HEALTH CHECK 12-1

Is It a Cold or an Allergy?

This exercise is intended to raise your awareness about the similarities and differences in the symptoms of the common cold and airborne allergies. Match the symptom with what you think is the frequency of occurrence for the cold or allergy (circle your answers).

SYMPTOMS	COMMON COLD	AIRBORNE ALLERGIES
1. Cough	Never, Rare, Sometimes, Common, Usual	Never, Rare, Sometimes, Common, Usual
2. General aches and pains	Never, Rare, Sometimes, Common, Usual	Never, Rare, Sometimes, Common, Usual
3. Fatigue and weakness	Never, Rare, Sometimes, Common, Usual	Never, Rare, Sometimes, Common, Usual
4. Itchy eyes	Never, Rare, Sometimes, Common, Usual	Never, Rare, Sometimes, Common, Usual
5. Sneezing	Never, Rare, Sometimes, Common, Usual	Never, Rare, Sometimes, Common, Usual
6. Sore throat	Never, Rare, Sometimes, Common, Usual	Never, Rare, Sometimes, Common, Usual
7. Runny nose	Never, Rare, Sometimes, Common, Usual	Never, Rare, Sometimes, Common, Usual
8. Stuffy nose	Never, Rare, Sometimes, Common, Usual	Never, Rare, Sometimes, Common, Usual
9. Fever	Never, Rare, Sometimes, Common, Usual	Never, Rare, Sometimes, Common, Usual

Note the differences and similarities of duration, treatment, prevention, and complications for colds and allergies, too:

	COLD	AIRBORNE ALLERGIES
Duration	3–14 days	Many weeks
Treatment	Antihistamines Decongestants Nonsteroidal anti-inflammatory medicines	Antihistamines Decongestants Nasal steroids
Prevention	Wash your hands often with soap and water Avoid close contact with anyone with a cold	Avoid those things that you are allergic to such as pollen, house dust mites, mold, pet dander, cockroaches
Complications	Sinus infection Asthma Middle ear infection	Sinus infection Asthma

Answers:

Cold: 1. Common, 2. Sometimes, 3. Sometimes, 4. Rare or Never, 5. Usual, 6. Common, 7. Common, 8. Common, 9. Rare

Airborne Allergies: 1. Sometimes, 2. Never, 3. Sometimes, 4. Common, 5. Usual, 6. Sometimes, 7. Common, 8. Common, 9. Never

Did this exercise raise your awareness about the similarities and differences between colds and allergies? In what ways? (Bear in mind that a formal diagnosis should only be made by a qualified health care provider.)

Source: U.S. Department of Health and Human Services, National Institutes of Health, National Institute of Allergy and Infectious Diseases. (2011, April). Retrieved from http://www.niaid.nih.gov/topics/allergicdiseases/documents/coldallergy.pdf

As with allergies, reducing exposure to allergens helps prevent attacks (see "Health Skills 12-1"). Avoiding smoking or secondhand smoke is a must.

Two types of asthma medications are bronchodilators and anti-inflammatories. *Bronchodilators* open bronchial passages by relaxing the muscles surrounding the air tubes, making it easier to breathe. *Anti-inflammatories* help prevent attacks by keeping bronchial tubes open. With proper management, people with asthma can participate in virtually any activity. Several Olympic medalists have had asthma, but it did not deter them.

autoimmune disorder *Disease in which the immune system mistakenly identifies the body's own cells as foreign and attacks them.*

antihistamines *Medications designed to counter the effects of histamine, the chemical produced in an allergic reaction.*

Autoimmune Disorders

In **autoimmune disorders**, the immune system attacks healthy cells as though they were foreign. Two of the more prevalent autoimmune disorders are *rheumatoid arthritis*, a painful, potentially disabling condition involving chronic inflammation of the membranes that line the joints, and *lupus erythematosus*, a chronic inflammatory disorder of connective tissue. Both diseases strike women more often than men. These diseases are treated with varying degrees of success with drugs that suppress the immune response.

Multiple sclerosis (MS) is a chronic and often crippling nervous system disorder in which *myelin*, the coating that insulates nerve cells in the brain and spinal cord, is damaged or destroyed. When myelin is damaged, communication between the brain and spinal cord breaks down, leading to symptoms that can impair speech, walking, or writing. MS strikes women about twice as often as men. MS may be an autoimmune disease in which white blood cells attack the body's nerve cells, causing inflammation that depletes myelin. A viral infection may trigger the autoimmune response, but no specific causal agent has been found.

Immune Deficiencies

In rare instances, generally resulting from a genetic defect, children are born with immune systems that fail

HEALTH SKILLS 12-1

health skills

Protecting Yourself from Allergies

Allergies can be diagnosed by a skin test in which a drop of the suspected allergen is injected just below the skin. Depending on the type of allergy, you can take the following steps to control it or reduce discomfort.

- *Environmental engineering.* Avoiding allergens is the most direct way of preventing an allergic response. People who are sensitive to pollens might benefit from checking the daily pollen count in their local newspaper or on the Internet. On days when the pollen count is especially high, they might minimize outdoor activities. If you are sensitive to dust mites, keep your home and workplace as free of dust as possible. Venetian blinds, down-filled blankets, feather pillows, and wall-to-wall carpeting are natural dust collectors. Protect your bedding with allergen-proof covering and wash it regularly. You can dust furniture but vacuuming may raise more dust than it removes. (There are low-emission vacuum cleaners.) You might use cleaning products containing *acaricides*, which kill dust mites.
- *Allergy medications.* Allergy medications help control the symptoms of allergies. Your primary health care provider or allergist can help identify the nature of the allergen(s) causing your symptoms and the appropriate course of treatment. **Antihistamines** counteract histamines and are useful in treating sneezing, runny nose, and itchy eyes and throat. Decongestants help unclog stuffy noses. Follow the instructions on the label. Steroid nasal sprays offer greater relief of nasal congestion than nasal decongestants do. Another type of nasal spray contains the anti-inflammatory drug *cromolyn sodium*.
- *Allergy injections.* Allergy shots contain tiny amounts of an offending allergen and gradually desensitize the individual. Though effective in most cases, they must be taken regularly for months or years. People who cannot control their exposure to a particular allergen are especially good candidates for allergy shots.

to protect them from common pathogens. They must live in a sterile environment to prevent exposure to pathogens that children with healthier immune systems fight off. In the case of HIV/AIDS, a virus attacks the immune system, crippling it and leaving the person vulnerable to "opportunistic" infections. Immune system deficiencies have also been implicated in the development of cancer. Cancer cells that would normally be eradicated may grow out of control if the immune system is weakened by age or other factors.

Common Infectious Diseases

Now that we have considered the nature of pathogens and immunity, let's discuss a number of respiratory tract infections and other common infectious diseases. Then we turn to a number of infections that are already too familiar: sexually transmitted infections.

☒ LEARNING OUTCOME 4

Describe common infectious diseases

Respiratory Tract Infections

Respiratory tract infections range from the common cold and milder cases of flu to more serious conditions like pneumonia and tuberculosis. Though bacteria and viruses are most often the pathogens involved, smoking and exposure to pollutants increase susceptibility to these infections.

The Common Cold

The common cold is a contagious viral infection of the upper respiratory tract. Colds are the most common infectious illness. Most adults get two to four colds per year; children have about six to 10.[8] About 200 different viruses cause the common cold, with *rhinoviruses* (from the Greek *rhino*, meaning "nose") causing 30% to 35% of them. Symptoms include nasal congestion, sore throat, fatigue, headache, and perhaps a low-grade fever. Colds typically last one to two weeks.

Some colds are transmitted by airborne exposure to viruses expelled by an infected person through sneezing, coughing, or just talking. Most common colds, however, are contracted by touch, that is, by contact with a surface (for example, a tissue, door knob, or hand) that contains nasal secretions left by an infected person.

The best way to recover from a cold is to rest and drink plenty of fluids. No medications or vaccines prevent or cure the common cold, but many medications alleviate the symptoms.

Influenza

Influenza or "the flu" is a highly contagious viral disease that affects the lungs and other parts of the body. It is transmitted like the common cold and caused by three families of influenza viruses: type A, type B, and type C. Type A influenza is most common and associated with the most severe outbreaks. Now and then new strains of influenza virus emerge, which may lead to worldwide epidemics, or **pandemics**, because few people have antibodies against the strain.

After an incubation period of one to three days, infected people experience a fever between 102° and 104° Fahrenheit, chills, headache, general aches and pains, fatigue, weakness, and possibly a sore throat, dry cough, nausea, and burning eyes. The fever usually subsides after two or three days, but chest and nasal congestion may develop. In most healthy persons, flu symptoms disappear in about a week. In vulnerable groups, however, such as children, older people, and people with other health problems, the flu can lead to serious, possibly fatal complications (read about flu vaccinations in "Prevention 12-2" on the next page).

As with colds, the flu is best treated with rest, fluids, and pain and fever relievers. When taken one to two days after the onset of infection, antiviral drugs may reduce symptoms. (Not sure whether you have a cold or the flu? Learn how to tell the difference in "Health Check 12-2" on page 277.)

Pneumonia

Pneumonia is a serious lung infection in which invading pathogens cause the air sacs in the lungs—the alveoli—to fill with pus and other liquid, making it difficult for oxygen to reach the blood. Lack of oxygen may cause death. Pneumonia claims more than 50,000 lives annually in the United States.[9] Most cases involve viral or bacterial infection, but pneumonia may also result from irritation to the lungs due to pollutants or, in hospitalized patients, from lung

influenza
An acute lower-respiratory-tract infection caused by several viruses. Abbreviated form: flu.

pandemic
An epidemic affecting a whole country, continent, or the entire world.

pneumonia
An acute infectious disease of the respiratory tract that results from pathogens causing fluids to build up in tiny air sacs called alveoli, *making breathing difficult.*

PREVENTION 12-2

Flu Shots

Anyone can get the flu. The best protection against the flu is an annual flu shot or vaccination. Health professionals strongly recommend annual vaccinations for persons aged 65 and older, those with other diseases or in general poor health, children six months and older with respiratory disorders, and health care and other workers who come into contact with infected patients. If you are uncertain about whether you should obtain a flu shot, check with your primary health care provider or pharmacist—but don't wait until the flu season strikes.

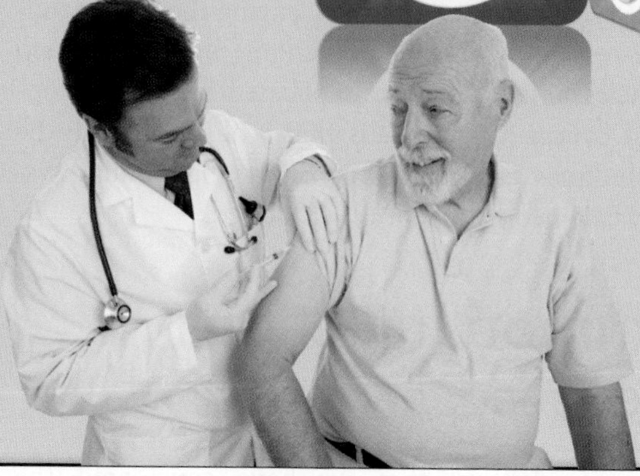

© iStockphoto.com/Lisa F. Young

irritation caused by anesthesia or intravenous foods and liquids. Symptoms usually include fever and chills; chest pain; a cough with rust-colored, yellow, or greenish sputum (mucus-laden material coughed up from deep inside the lungs); and difficulty breathing. Pneumonia is especially dangerous in older people and the very young.

Bacterial pneumonia is treated with antibiotics. Though there are no effective drugs for viral pneumonia, most cases resolve on their own. Rest, fluids, proper diet, and avoidance of smoking are all helpful. A vaccine is available for *pneumococcal pneumonia.*

Legionnaire's Disease

Legionnaire's disease is a deadly bacterial pneumonia so named because it attacked people attending an American Legion convention. A search for the cause led to the discovery of a bacterium now called *legionella* that dwelled in the water of the air-conditioning system of the hotel. Legionnaire's disease has also been found on cruise ships.

Legionnaire's disease is spread through exposure to airborne droplets of *legionella*. Person-to-person transmission is rare. Symptoms include headache, muscular and abdominal pain, diarrhea and vomiting, and a dry cough, followed by high fever, shaking chills, sputum, and drowsiness. Legionnaire's disease is treated with antibiotics.

tuberculosis (TB)
A bacterial infection that usually affects the lungs and sometimes other parts of the body, including the brain, kidneys, or spine.

Lyme disease
An infectious disease spread to people and animals by ticks; caused by the bacterium Borrelia burgdorferi.

Tuberculosis

Tuberculosis (TB) was one of our most dreaded diseases until the 1940s and 1950s, when antibiotics were discovered. TB is a chronic infection caused by the bacterium *mycobacterium tuberculosis*, which usually affects the lungs and sometimes other parts of the body, including the brain, kidneys, or spine. Symptoms include a racking cough, fever, night sweats, fatigue, hoarseness, chest pain, weight loss, and blood in the sputum.

The prevalence of TB is at a low ebb in the general population, but there is a high incidence of the disease among people who use intravenous drugs, people with HIV/AIDS, homeless people, and people in confined living conditions. TB is generally contracted through months of contact with infected people and is transmitted via sneezed or coughed airborne droplets. The bacteria multiply in the air sacs in the lungs, forming cheese-like clumps or lesions called *tubercles*. If left untreated, the entire lung can become scarred with these clumps, leading to respiratory failure and death.

The presence of the TB bacterium is detected by a tuberculin skin test (or *Mantoux* test), in which a small amount of fluid, called *tuberculin*, is injected under the skin of the forearm. If a red welt appears 48 to 72 hours later, TB may be present. Additional diagnostic tests determine whether an infected person has TB. Treatment for TB involves the prolonged use of antibiotics.

Lyme Disease

When summer comes around again, Americans head outdoors to the mountains and countryside or to stroll through wooded areas close to home. Today, many of us are filled with trepidation as we or our children—and even our house pets—venture into wooded areas, even our own backyards. The fear is that we will contract **Lyme disease**, named after a town on the Connecticut sea-

HEALTH CHECK 12-2

Is It a Cold or Is It the Flu?[10]

Though the symptoms of the common cold and flu may be similar, it is frequently possible to distinguish between them. The flu is more likely than the cold to be associated with headaches and feeling exhausted, and to linger for two to three weeks.

SYMPTOMS	COLD	FLU
Fever	Rare	High (100–102 degrees for three to four days)
Headache	Rare	Common
General aches and pains	Slight	Usual and often severe
Fatigue, weakness	Sometimes	Usual, can last up to three weeks
Exhaustion	Never	Usual in the beginning
Stuffy nose	Common	Sometimes
Sneezing	Usual	Sometimes
Sore throat	Common	Sometimes
Cough	Mild to moderate hacking cough	Common, can be severe
Complications	Sinus congestion Middle ear infection Asthma	Bronchitis Pneumonia Worsened chronic conditions

board. There are 25,000 to 30,000 new cases in the United States each year.[11] The online feature "Prevention 12-3" has suggestions for protecting yourself from the disease.

prevention

Access CourseMate for HLTH at www.cengagebrain.com.

Lyme disease is caused by a spiral-shaped bacterium (spirochete), *Borrelia burgdorferi*, which is spread to people and animals by ticks that inhabit the fur of deer and mice in wooded areas. When an infected tick bites, the bacterium can be injected into the host's blood.

Between 3 and 30 days after being bitten, a slowly expanding circular, triangular, or oval-shaped red-ringed rash begins to form around the bite in most infected people (see Figure 12-7 on the next page). Within the first few days or weeks after exposure, the person may suffer flu-like symptoms, such as fever, fatigue, chills, swelling of the lymph nodes, and painful or swollen joints. People should seek medical attention if they suspect they have been infected, because the disease, if left untreated, can progress to cause incurable heart or nerve damage or crippling arthritis.

Lyme disease is most often cured by antibiotics, especially when treatment is begun early. The disease is made evident by examination of the characteristic symptoms and the red bull's-eye rash. A blood test is also available.

Infectious Mononucleosis

Infectious mononucleosis is caused by the *Epstein-Barr virus* (*EBV*). "Mono" is often referred to as the "kissing disease" because the virus reproduces in salivary glands, making saliva especially contagious. Other means of transmission include sharing toothbrushes and eating utensils.

Mono typically affects young adults in the 16- to 30-year age range, but almost everyone catches "mono" at some point in their lives. Symptoms begin to develop after an incubation period of perhaps 30 to 50 days and may include fever, sore throat, swollen glands, and fatigue, followed by high fever (101° to 105°F), sore throat (caused by enlarged, often pus-covered tonsils), and swollen lymph glands in the neck, arm, and groin.

infectious mononucleosis
A viral disease caused by the Epstein-Barr virus and characterized in the acute stage by enlarged lymph nodes and spleen, fever, and sore throat.

Figure 12-7 Lyme Disease Rash

A rash in the form of a reddish bull's-eye or ring may spread outward from the bite in the early stages of Lyme disease.

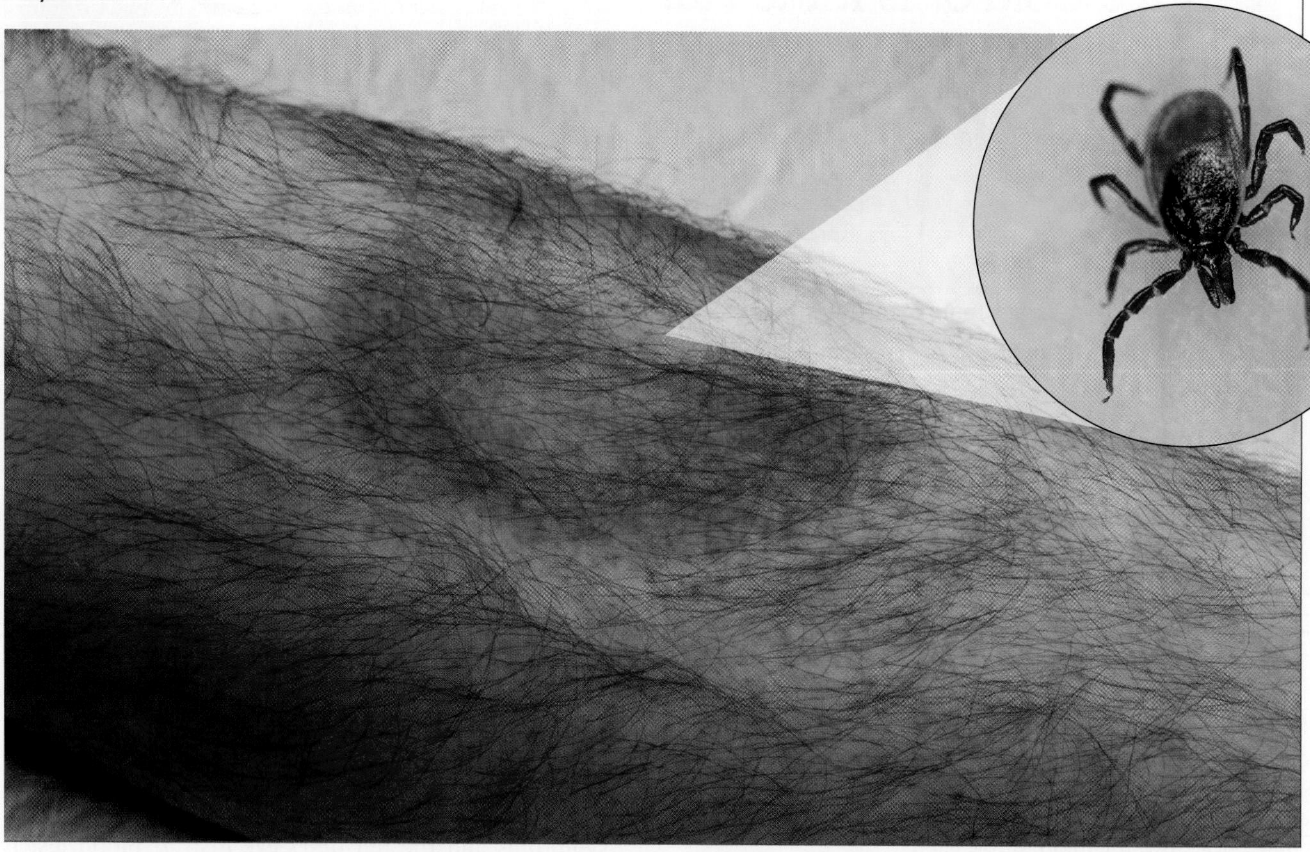

The clinical stage typically lasts two to three weeks, although some symptoms linger for months.

A blood test is used to detect EBV. No drugs or vaccines are available to cure or prevent mono. Rest, ample fluids, and a balanced diet are the best route to recovery. Pain relievers may be used for headaches and other discomfort. Sore throats may be treated with salt gargles.

Emerging Infectious Diseases

Strides have been made in combating infectious diseases, thanks largely to large-scale immunization programs, introduction of powerful antimicrobial drugs, and development of water purification systems. Scourges like polio, tetanus, smallpox, cholera, and diphtheria have been all but eliminated from the United States and other developed nations.

Yet victory in the war against infectious disease is nowhere in sight. Only one infectious disease—smallpox—has been eradicated. New threats have also emerged because of factors such as:

- *Increase in world travel.* More people than ever travel the globe, bringing pathogens with them.
- *Changing ecological conditions.* With the eradication of many wilderness areas in the world's developing nations, humans are coming into greater contact with animal carriers of infectious agents of diseases. For example, the construction of the Aswan High Dam in Egypt created a new lake that became a breeding ground for virus-bearing mosquitoes.
- *Rise of drug-resistant strains.* Many infectious organisms mutate into strains that are resistant to commonly used drugs, such as antibiotics. We face drug-resistant strains of microorganisms, including those causing malaria, tuberculosis, pneumonia, and staph infections.
- *Increasing urbanization.* Because of increasing urbanization, more than a third of the world's population now lives in cities, often under crowded and unsanitary conditions that promote transmission of pathogens.

Table 12-4 Emerging Infectious Diseases

DISEASE	INFECTIOUS AGENT	CONTRIBUTING FACTORS
Avian flu (bird flu)	Influenza A (H5N1) virus—also called *H5N1 virus*	During an outbreak among poultry, possible risk to people who have contact with infected birds or surfaces that have been contaminated with birds' excretions
Cholera	*Vibrio cholerae* 0139 (bacterium)	Evolution of new strain of bacteria combining increased virulence and long-term survival in the environment
Ebola hemorrhagic fever	*Filoviridae* family (virus)	Unknown natural reservoir; transmission in medical settings
Lassa fever	*Arenaviridae* family (virus)	Urbanization and other conditions that favor the rodent host; transmission in medical settings
Severe acute respiratory syndrome (SARS)	Coronavirus	Spread mainly by close human contact
West Nile virus	Flavivirus	Most common in Africa, West Asia, Europe, and the Middle East; first found in the United States in 1999; transmitted mainly by mosquitoes

Table 12-4 lists a number of emerging infectious diseases.

Sexually Transmitted Infections (STIs)

Sexual relationships can be sources of pleasure and personal fulfillment. They also carry some risks and responsibilities. One of the risks is that of contracting HIV/AIDS or other sexually transmitted infections (STIs). Although media attention usually focuses on HIV/AIDS, other STIs are more widespread. Nearly 3 million new chlamydia infections occur each year, with the incidence among college students especially high.[12] Chlamydia is a major cause of pelvic inflammatory disease, which often leads to infertility. (Sexually active people who are not in a monogamous relationship are advised to practice "safer sex." The online feature "Health Skills 12-2" explains what that means.)

LEARNING OUTCOME 5

Discuss the causes, transmission, symptoms, diagnosis, and treatment of sexually transmitted infections

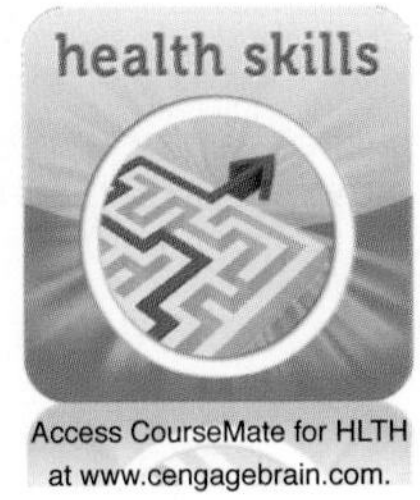
health skills
Access CourseMate for HLTH at www.cengagebrain.com.

Most college students are informed about HIV transmission and AIDS, yet many are unaware that chlamydia can go undetected for years. A survey of first-year college students also found a great deal of ignorance about human papilloma virus (HPV) and genital warts.[13] Although nearly all (96% of the males and 95% of the females) had heard of genital warts, only 4% of the males and 12% of the females knew that HPV caused them. Nationwide, only about 55% of women know that HPV infection is linked to cervical cancer.[14] Yet as many as 1 million new cases of HPV infection occur each year in the United States—more than syphilis, genital herpes, and AIDS combined.

Various bacteria, viruses, fungi, protozoans, and parasites are transmitted sexually. The modes of transmission, symptoms, diagnosis, and treatment of major STIs are described in Table 12-5 on the next page. We'll look at a few of them more closely.

Bacterial STIs

Bacteria also cause the STIs gonorrhea, syphilis, and chlamydia. They are all treated with antibiotics.

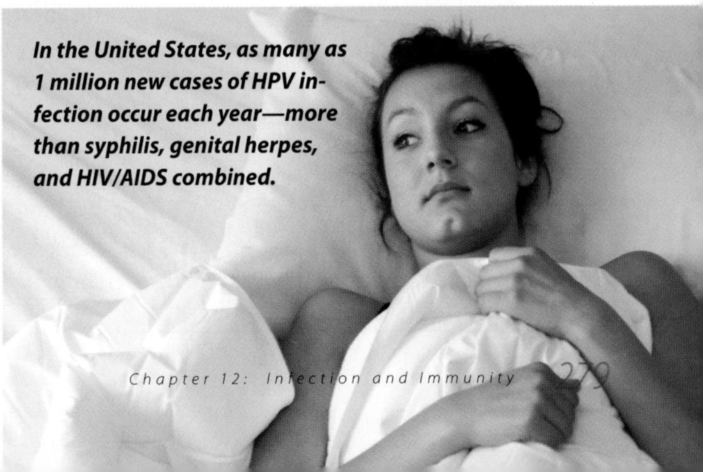

In the United States, as many as 1 million new cases of HPV infection occur each year—more than syphilis, genital herpes, and HIV/AIDS combined.

Table 12-5 Causes, Transmissions, Symptoms, Diagnosis, and Treatment of Sexually Transmitted Infections (STIs)

STI AND PATHOGEN	MODES OF TRANSMISSION	SYMPTOMS	DIAGNOSIS	TREATMENT
HIV/AIDS (*AIDS stands for acquired immune deficiency syndrome and HIV stands for Human immunodeficiency virus*)	• Sexual intercourse • Injection of contaminated blood • From mother to child during childbirth or breast-feeding	• Flu-like symptoms • May be asymptomatic for a decade or so • Chronically swollen lymph nodes and intermittent weight loss, fever, fatigue, and diarrhea • Opportunistic infections • Potentially lethal	• Blood, saliva, and urine tests can detect HIV antibodies in the bloodstream • Other tests detect the virus itself	• HAART (highly active antiretroviral therapy) reduces the amount of HIV in the blood and prolongs life
Bacterial vaginosis: *Gardnerella vaginalis* bacterium and others	• Sexual contact	• In women, a vaginal discharge, genital irritation, and mild pain during urination • In men, inflammation of the penis, urethritis, and cystitis • May be asymptomatic	• Culture and examination of bacterium	• Oral treatment with metronidazole
Candidiasis (moniliasis, thrush, "yeast infection"): *Candida albicans*—a yeast-like fungus	• Sexual contact • Sharing a washcloth or towel with an infected person	• In women, vulval itching, discharge, soreness, or swelling of genital tissues • In men, itching and burning on urination, or inflammation of the penis	• Diagnosis usually made on basis of symptoms	• Vaginal suppositories, creams, or tablets with miconazole, clotrimazole, or teraconazole
Chlamydia and nongonococcal urethritis (NGU): *Chlamydia trachomatis* bacterium in women, and several in men	• Vaginal, oral, or anal sexual activity	• In women, frequent and painful urination, abdominal pain and inflammation, and vaginal discharge • In men, burning or painful urination, slight discharge; may be asymptomatic	• Analysis of a cervical smear in women	• Antibiotics
Genital herpes: *Herpes simplex virus-type 2 (HSV-2)*	• Vaginal, oral, or anal sexual activity • Most contagious during flare-ups	• Painful, reddish bumps around the genitals • Bumps become blisters or sores that fill with pus and break, shedding viral particles • Burning urination, fever, aches and pains, swollen glands, and vaginal discharge possible	• Clinical inspection of sores • Culture and examination of fluid drawn from sore	• Antiviral drugs may provide relief and prompt healing but are not cures
Gonorrhea ("clap," "drip"): Gonococcus bacterium (*Neisseria gonorrhoeae*)	• Vaginal, oral, or anal sexual activity	• In men, thick discharge, burning urination • In women, may be symptom-free or there may be increased discharge, burning urination, irregular menstruation	• Clinical inspection • Culture of discharge	• Antibiotics

continued

Table 12-5 continued

STI AND PATHOGEN	MODES OF TRANSMISSION	SYMPTOMS	DIAGNOSIS	TREATMENT
HPV infection/ genital warts: *Human papilloma virus (HPV)*	• Sexual contact • Other forms of contact, as with infected towels or clothing	• HPV infection may be symptom-free • Painless warts resembling cauliflowers on the genitals or anus or in the rectum • Some HPV strains cause cervical cancer	• Clinical inspection • Pap tests	• Immune system often clears infection • Vaccine developed • Removal of warts
Pubic lice ("crabs"): *Pthirus pubis* (an insect, not a crab)	• Sexual contact • Contact with infested towel, sheet, or toilet seat	• Intense itching in pubic area and other hairy regions to which lice can attach	• Clinical examination	• Pyrethrins or piperonal
Syphilis: *Treponema pallidum* bacterium	• Vaginal, oral, or anal sexual activity	• Hard, round painless chancre (sore) appears at site of infection within two to four weeks • May progress through additional stages if not treated • Potentially lethal	• Clinical examination or examination of fluid from a chancre • Blood test	• Antibiotics
Trichomoniasis ("trich"): *Trichomonas vaginalis*—a protozoan	• Almost always transmitted sexually	• In women, a discharge, itching or burning in vulva • Mild urethritis in men • May be asymptomatic	• Microscopic examination of vaginal secretions • Culture of sample	• Metronidazole

Gonorrhea

There are some 500,000 to 600,000 new cases of gonorrhea in the United States each year.[15] Most of them are contracted by young adults—ages 20 to 24. Gonorrhea is caused by the bacterium *Neisseria gonorrhoeae*. Most men experience symptoms two to five days following infection, including a penile discharge and, because of an inflamed urethra, a burning sensation while urinating. Women may be asymptomatic. However, women should be tested for gonorrhea as a matter of course, since the bacterium can spread throughout the reproductive organs, leading to pelvic inflammatory disease (PID) and blocked fallopian tubes.

Syphilis

Syphilis is caused by the spirochete bacterium, *Treponema pallidum* (*T. pallidum*, for short). There are about 36,000 new cases reported in the United States each year.[16] Syphilis develops through several stages. In the first or *primary*

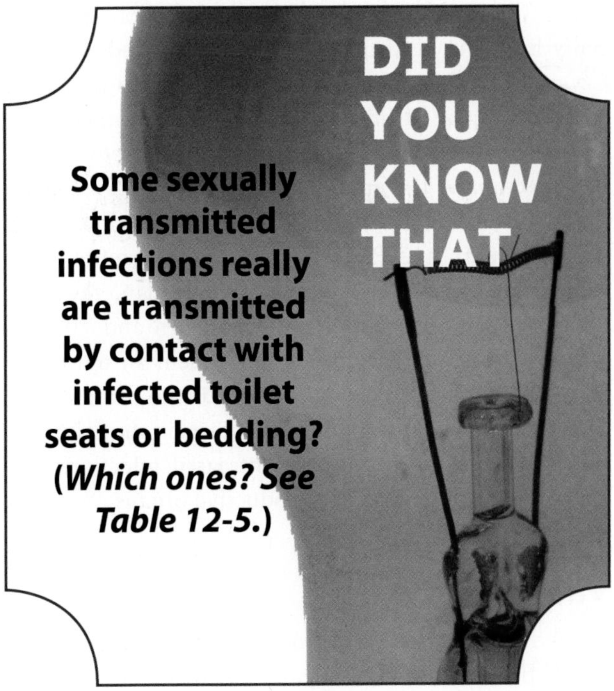

DID YOU KNOW THAT

Some sexually transmitted infections really are transmitted by contact with infected toilet seats or bedding? (*Which ones? See Table 12-5.*)

stage, a painless chancre (a hard, round, ulcer-like lesion with raised edges) appears at the site of infection two to four weeks after contact. When women are infected, the chancre may form on the vaginal walls or the cervix and not be visible. With men, the chancre usually forms on the penile glans, scrotum, or penile shaft. If the mode of transmission is oral or anal, the chancre may appear on the lips, tongue, or rectum. The chancre disappears in a few weeks, but if the infection remains untreated, syphilis develops into a *secondary stage* within a few weeks or months, characterized by a painless skin rash that bursts, oozing a discharge, and often by sores in the mouth, painful swelling of joints, a sore throat, headaches, and fever. These symptoms also disappear. Syphilis then enters the *latent stage* and may lie dormant for one year to a lifetime. In many cases, the disease eventually progresses to a *tertiary stage*, in which a large ulcer may form on the skin, muscle tissue, digestive organs, lungs, liver, or other organs. More serious damage can occur to the central nervous system or the cardiovascular system. Either outcome can be fatal. *Neurosyphilis* can cause brain damage, resulting in paralysis or mental illness.

Chlamydia

Chlamydia is the most common bacterial STI, with as many as 3 million new cases in the United States each year.[17] The incidence of chlamydia infections is especially high among teenagers and college students. The *Chlamydia trachomatis* bacterium can cause several different types of infection, including *nongonococcal urethritis* (*NGU*) in men and women, *epididymitis* (infection of the epididymis) in men, and *cervicitis* (infection of the cervix), *endometritis* (infection of the endometrium), and PID in women. The symptoms of chlamydia are similar to, but milder than, those of gonorrhea, but as many as 25% of men and 70% of women notice no symptoms. In women, an untreated chlamydial infection can spread throughout the reproductive system, causing PID and scarring the fallopian tubes, resulting in infertility. Untreated infections can also damage the internal reproductive organs of men.

Viral STIs

Many viral infections are transmitted sexually, including HIV/AIDS, herpes, viral hepatitis, and genital warts.

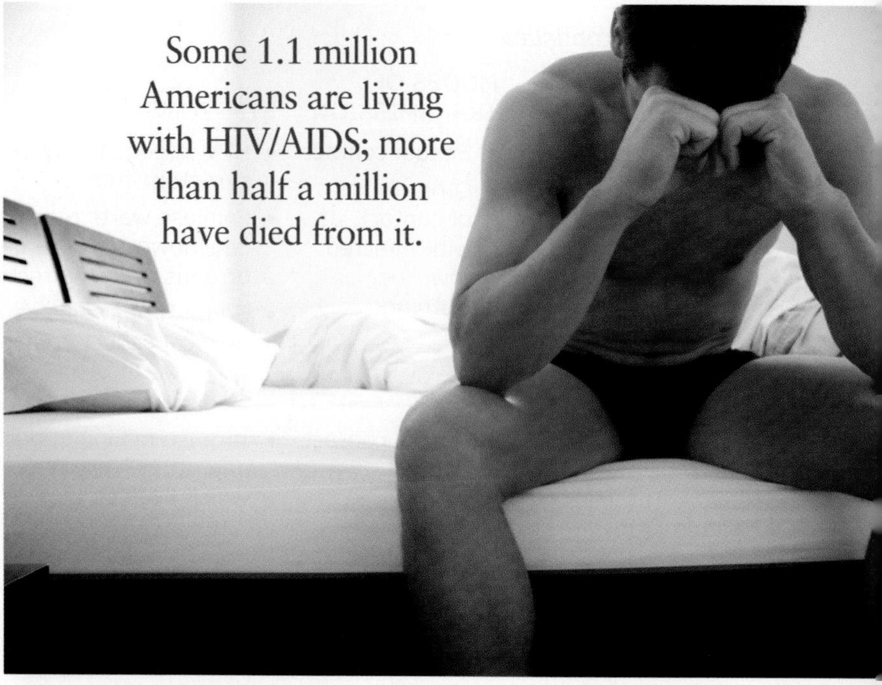
Some 1.1 million Americans are living with HIV/AIDS; more than half a million have died from it.

© iStockphoto.com/becon

HIV/AIDS

AIDS is considered a fatal condition, despite the fact many people are living with HIV/AIDS due to the development of highly active antiretroviral therapy (HAART). HIV attacks and disables the immune system such that the individual develops infections that would not otherwise take hold. Cancerous cells might also proliferate.

Some 1.1 million Americans are living with HIV/AIDS, and more than half a million have died from it.[18] Many people with HIV are unaware of being infected and so are not receiving antiviral treatment.

Worldwide, more than 40 million people are infected with HIV, with the majority involving transmission of the virus through male–female sex. Worldwide, nearly 3 million people are infected with HIV each year. Yet progress is being made in combating the epidemic in many hard-hit countries, as the number of new HIV infections and the number of AIDS-related deaths have declined worldwide by almost 20% during the past 10 years.[19] In the United States, HIV/AIDS is predominantly found among men who engage in sexual activity with other men, male–female sex partners, or those who share needles when injecting drugs (see Table 12-6).

Most people who are infected with HIV remain symptom free for years. About half develop AIDS within 10 years of infection. AIDS is termed a *syndrome* because it is typified by a variety of symptoms such as swollen lymph nodes, fatigue, fever, night sweats, diarrhea, and weight loss that cannot be attributed to dieting or exercise. HIV/AIDS is connected with the appearance of diseases such as pneumocystis carinii pneumonia (PCP), Kaposi's sarcoma (a form of cancer), toxoplasmosis of the brain (an infection of parasites), or Herpes simplex with chronic ulcers. As HIV/AIDS progresses, the individual grows thinner and more fatigued. If left untreated, HIV/AIDS almost always kills within a few years.

HIV can be transmitted by contaminated blood, semen, vaginal secretions, or breast milk. The first three of these may enter the body through vaginal, anal, or oral–genital sex with an infected partner. Other avenues of infection include sharing a hypodermic needle with an infected person, transfusion with contaminated blood (rare today!), transplants of infected organs, artificial insemination with infected semen, being stuck by a needle used previously on an infected person, and childbirth.

Table 12-6 shows estimates for the means of transmission of HIV infection among adults in the United States. Diagnosis and treatment are described in Table 12-5. For the latest information on HIV/AIDS, call the government AIDS hotline: 1-800-342-AIDS. The call is free and anonymous.

Genital Herpes

Genital herpes is caused by the Herpes simplex virus type 2 (HSV-2 virus). Genital herpes is a common STI, affecting about one in six people in the 14- to 29-year-old age range.[20] Women are nearly twice as likely to contract genital herpes as men.[21] Most HSV-2 infections are transmitted by people who are not aware they are infected or are between flare-ups of symptoms. Although some people have mild infections, the virus produces painful sores and blisters on the genitals of others. After the initial attack, recurrent outbreaks may happen at the most inconvenient times, as around final exams. This is because stress can depress the immune system.

Another herpes virus, Herpes simplex virus type 1 (HSV-1 virus) causes oral herpes, which is characterized by cold sores or fever blisters on the lips or mouth. Both strains can be transmitted sexually.

Although genital herpes is most contagious during active flare-ups, it can also be transmitted when the person is asymptomatic.

Genital herpes raises the risk of miscarriage in pregnant women. Passage through the birth canal of an infected mother can infect babies with genital herpes, damaging or killing them. Obstetricians thus often perform cesarean sections if the mother has sores or blisters at the time of delivery.

Viruses do not respond to antibiotics. Antiviral drugs can relieve pain and speed healing. Oral administration of antiviral drugs may reduce the severity of the initial episode and, if taken regularly, the frequency and duration of flare-ups.

Viral Hepatitis

Hepatitis B can be transmitted sexually through anal, vaginal, or oral intercourse with an infected partner; through transfusion with contaminated blood supplies; by sharing contaminated needles, razors, and toothbrushes; and by contact with contaminated saliva, menstrual blood, nasal mucus, or semen. Hepatitis C and hepatitis D can also be transmitted sexually or through contact with contaminated blood.

Most people with hepatitis have no symptoms. When symptoms do appear, they often include jaundice, feelings of weakness and nausea, loss of appetite, abdominal discomfort, whitish bowel movements, and brownish or tea-colored urine.

Table 12-6 Cumulative Estimated Number of AIDS Diagnoses

TRANSMISSION CATEGORY	ADULT AND ADOLESCENT MALES	ADULT AND ADOLESCENT FEMALES	TOTAL
Men who have sex with men	529,908	—	529,908
Injecting drug use	186,318	87,126	273,444
Men who have sex with men and inject drugs	77,213	—	77,213
Heterosexual contact	72,183	126,637	198,820
Other*	12,744	7,032	19,776
Totals	878,366	220,795	1,099,161

*Includes hemophilia, blood transfusion, perinatal exposure, and risk not reported or not identified.

Source: Centers for Disease Control and Prevention. (2011, February 28). *Basic statistics*. Retrieved from http://www.cdc.gov/hiv/topics/surveillance/basic.htm#exposure

There is no cure for hepatitis. Bed rest and fluids are usually recommended until the acute stage of the infection subsides, generally in a few weeks. Full recovery may take months. A vaccine provides protection against hepatitis B and D.

HPV Infection/Genital Warts

HPV is the world's most common STI, affected an estimated 20 million people in the United States.[22] Another 6 million become infected each year. Most sexually active people will contract HPV at some time. It is estimated that nearly 60% of sexually active college women in the United States are infected with HPV.[23] However, they may never know it because HPV usually causes no symptoms.

Although most cases of HPV infection clear up on their own, HPV can progress to cause genital warts. But HPV infection can also progress to cause precancerous growth and cancers, especially cervical cancer in women. Cancer often takes years to develop after HPV infection.

HPV can be transmitted sexually through skin-to-skin contact during vaginal, anal, or oral sex. It can also be transmitted by touching infected towels or clothing. The incubation period may vary from a week to a couple of years.

Though genital warts may appear in visible areas of the genital region, they are more often found in other areas, such as on the cervix or in the urethra in men. Within a few months following infection, the warts are usually found in the genital and anal regions. Women who initiate sex prior to the age of 18 and who have many sex partners are particularly susceptible to infection. However, vaccines are now available that can protect females against the types of HPV that cause most cervical cancers. The American Cancer Society recommends routine HPV vaccination for girls 11 to 12 years old.[24] Another vaccine protects males from genital warts.

There are many ways to eliminate the warts, including freezing (*cryotherapy*), imiquimod cream, trichloroacetic acid (TCA), bichloroacetic acid (BCA), podophyllin, burning (by a doctor!), and surgery. But removal of the warts does not rid the body of HPV.

Other STIs

Other STIs are caused by fungal, protozoan, and parasitic pathogens. The pathogens, symptoms, methods of transmission, diagnosis, and treatment are described in Table 12-5.

HEALTH APPS: YOUR LINK TO ONLINE HEALTH APPLICATIONS

prevention — **Wash Those Hands!** Want to know one of the simplest and most effective ways to prevent contracting an infectious disease? It's hand washing. To learn more, read "Prevention 12-1."

diversity — **Children and Immunizations—Many Aren't Protected** Vaccination is one of the key tools for fighting infectious diseases, but children from certain minority groups in the United States are not receiving them. What is going on here, and why? For answers, go to "Diversity 12-1."

prevention — **Protecting Yourself from Lyme Disease** Have you decided that Lyme disease is not in your future? Good choice. "Prevention 12-3" has suggestions for your protection.

health skills — **Toward Safer Sex** Now that you have learned about sexually transmitted infections, what are you going to do about them? Read "Health Skills 12-2" to learn how to protect yourself and your partner from STIs.

Go to the CourseMate for HLTH at www.cengagebrain.com for additional resources including flashcards, games, self-quizzes, review exercises, web exercises, learning checks, and more.

Preventing Violence and Injury

"I never thought it would happen to me."

Anne is a first-year college student, away from home. She describes what happened when she met an upperclassman named Jim:

ANNE: I first met him at a party. He was really good looking and he had a great smile. I wanted to meet him but I wasn't sure how. I didn't want to appear too forward. Then he came over and introduced himself. We talked and found we had a lot in common. I really liked him. When he asked me over to his place for a drink, I thought it would be OK. He was such a good listener, and I wanted him to ask me out again.

When we got to his room, the only place to sit was on the bed. I didn't want him to get the wrong idea, but what else could I do? We talked for a while and then he made his move. I was so startled. He started by kissing. I really liked him so the kissing was nice. But then he pushed me down on the bed. I tried to get up and I told him to stop. He was so much bigger and stronger. I got scared and I started to cry. I froze and he raped me.

It took only a couple of minutes and it was terrible, he was so rough. When it was over he kept asking me what was wrong, like he didn't know. He had just forced himself on me and he thought that was OK. He drove me home and said he wanted to see me again. I'm so afraid to see him. I never thought it would happen to me.

Later Jim would say that he perceived Anne's protests as part of an adversarial sex game. Let's turn to his view of the situation:

Learning Outcomes

1 **Discuss crimes of violence in America and ways of avoiding becoming a victim.**

2 **Discuss crime on campus and its prevention**

3 **Explain what is meant by sexual coercion and discuss the problems of rape and sexual harassment**

4 **Discuss various kinds of unintentional injuries—injuries from accidents—and how to prevent them**

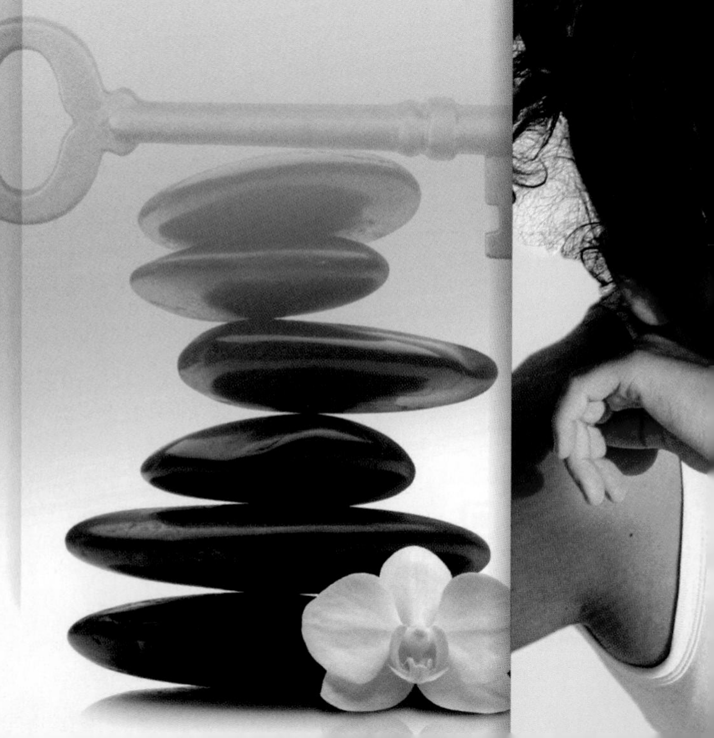

JIM: I first met her at a party. She looked really hot, wearing a sexy dress that showed off her great body. We started talking right away. I knew that she liked me by the way she kept smiling and touching my arm while she was speaking. She seemed pretty relaxed so I asked her back to my place for a drink. . . . When she said yes, I knew that I was going to be lucky!

When we got to my place, we sat on the bed, kissing. At first, everything was great. Then, when I started to lay her down on the bed, she started twisting and saying she didn't want to. Most women don't like to appear too easy, so I knew that she was just going through the motions. When she stopped struggling, I knew that she would have to throw in some tears before we did it.

She was still very upset afterwards, and I just don't understand it! If she didn't want to have sex, why did she come back to the room with me? You could tell by the way she dressed and acted that she was no virgin, so why she had to put up such a big struggle I don't know.

Despite his story, Jim is a date rapist. Date rapists may misperceive acceptance of a date as a sign of

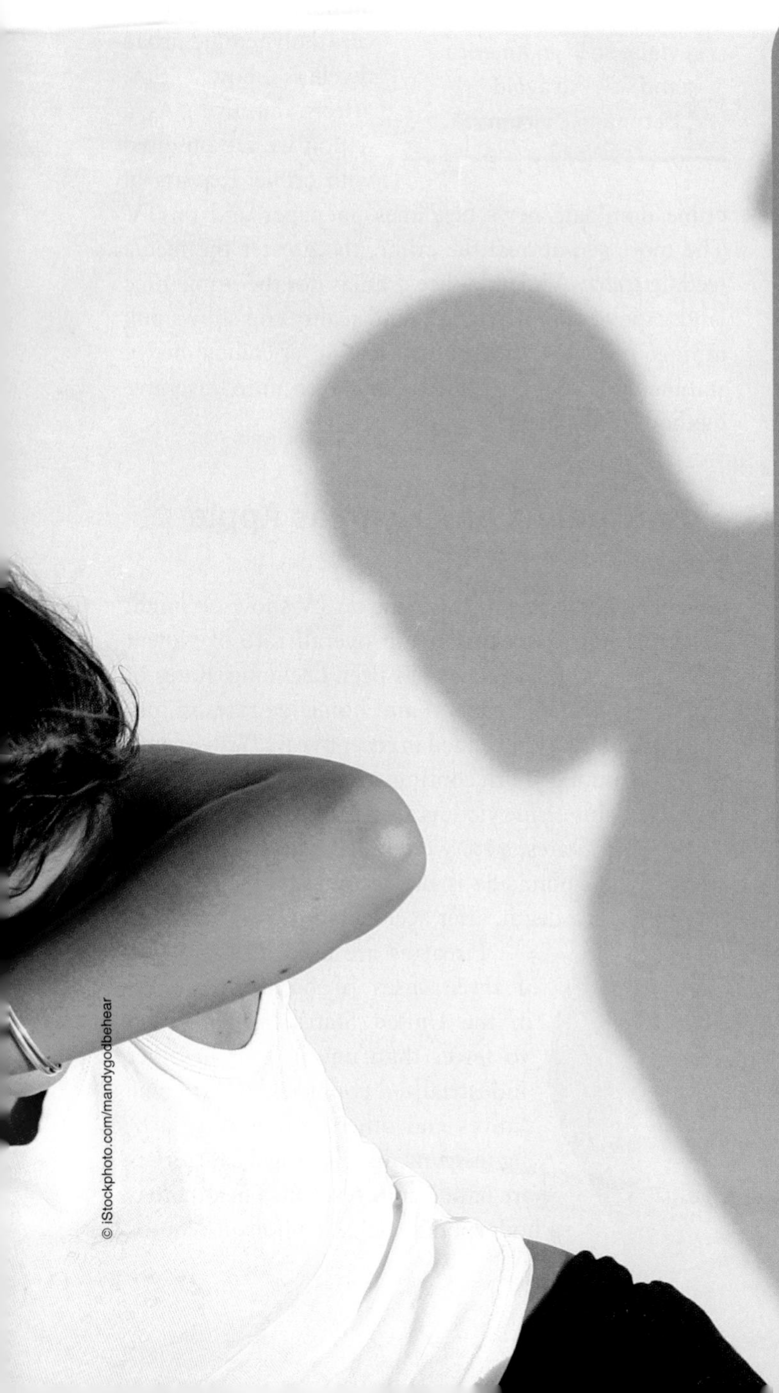

Did You Know That . . .

- Women who are raped are often blamed for what happened to them? (And some also blame themselves.) [p. 288]
- Homicide is the second leading cause of death among young people aged 10 to 24? (Do you know which is the first?) [p. 288]
- Neglect is the most common type of child abuse? [p. 291]
- Seven out of eight rapes of college women are perpetrated by people they know? [p. 295]
- It is dangerous, especially for a woman, to post pictures of themselves having fun at a drinking party? [p. 296]
- Sexual harassment has more to do with power and control than sex? [p. 299]
- Using a cell phone while driving is roughly the equivalent of driving drunk? [p. 301]

willingness to have sex, or they may believe that women should reciprocate with sex if they are taken to dinner or treated nicely. Other date rapists assume that women who frequent settings such as singles bars are expressing tacit agreement to have sex with men who show interest in them. Some date rapists believe that women who resist their advances are merely protesting so that they will not look easy—that "no" really means "maybe" and "maybe" really means "yes." They may interpret resistance as coyness—a ploy in the cat-and-mouse game that to them typifies the battle of the sexes. They may thus not see themselves as committing rape. But they are.

Women are not usually raped by strangers in dark alleyways. Like Anne, they are most often victimized by men they know. And that man may be a friend, a date, a boyfriend, or a former boyfriend.

Anne, like the great majority of women in her situation, did not report the rape to authorities. She was afraid nobody would believe her story, and she wondered if going back to Jim's place with him was some sort of signal that she was willing to have sex. Anne, like society at large, at least partly blamed the victim—herself. If you put Jim on the witness stand, you might find someone who thinks everything is getting blown out of proportion. He might admit to being sexually assertive, even a bit aggressive, but not all that different on a date from the other college men he knows.

And therein lie some of the problems: the tendency to blame the victim and the tendency to minimize the harm done by the perpetrator of a crime of violence.

Rape, as we will see, has become a part of college life. We'll also see that rape is a crime of violence that is committed more frequently in the United States than in any other developed nation. But rape is just one of many crimes that threaten us. In this chapter we look at the physical and psychological injuries that result from crime, especially crimes of violence, in the United States and on campus. We also discuss unintentional injuries—accidents. Much of our focus will be on preventing these injuries, but we'll also talk about what to do if you are victimized.

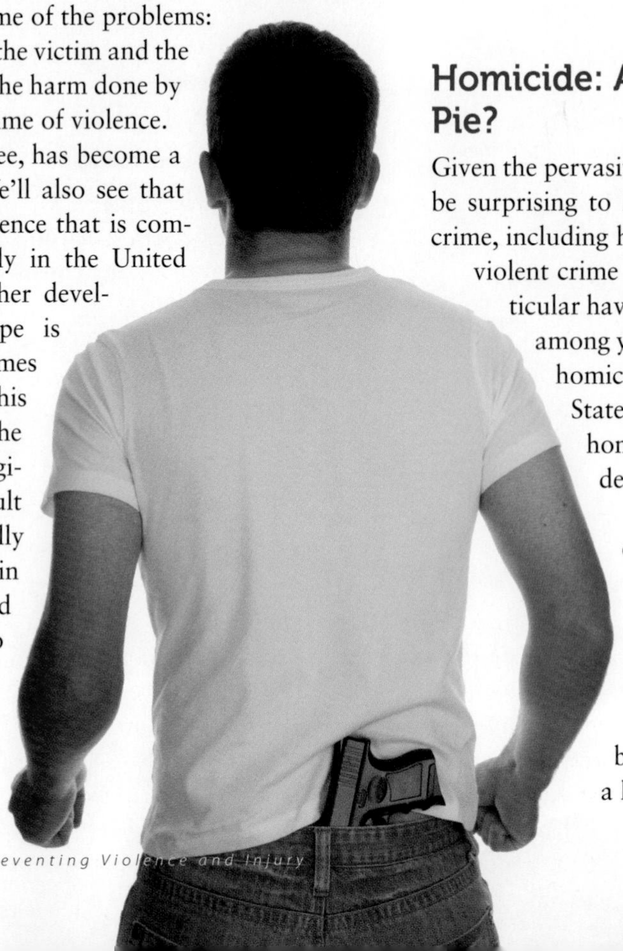

Crimes of Violence

America the beautiful? Yes, but also America the violent. Concerns about crime and violence have become a staple of American life. Many of us live behind triple-bolted doors, invest thousands in home security systems, and avoid parks at night. The wail of car alarms and the sirens on ambulances and police cars daily remind urban dwellers how crime affects our lives. As a nation we are obsessed with crime. Reports of crime dominate news headlines, in paper and on TV. The more sensational the crime, the greater the media feeding frenzy. Violent police dramas dot the prime-time landscape of commercial TV, and reality cop shows pull in huge revenues. Movies feature a never-ending diet of stabbings, slashings, bullets, and ever-more inventive methods of mayhem.

LEARNING OUTCOME 1

Discuss crimes of violence in in America and ways to avoid becoming a victim

Homicide: As American as Apple Pie?

Given the pervasiveness of crime on TV shows, it might be surprising to learn that the overall rate of violent crime, including homicide, has been declining. Rates of violent crime in general and homicide rates in particular have declined in recent years. Yet violence among youth continues to take its toll. Among homicide victims aged 10 to 24 in the United States, 84% were killed with firearms, and homicide is the second leading cause of death, after accidents.[1]

Firearms are used in about two of three cases of homicide overall in the United States, as compared to fewer than one in four in other industrialized countries.[2] Next come knives and other cutting and slashing instruments. The third category is bare hands and, yes, feet. Then there is a hodgepodge including poisons, motor vehicles, construction equipment, and whatever else you can think of.

Most murders occur among people who know each other and who are often members of the same family or household. The great majority occur among people of the same race.

Though no one factor accounts for the high rate of homicide in the United States, the availability of firearms is a contributing factor. Teenage boys are more likely to die from the use of firearms than from all natural causes combined. Overall, firearms account for more than 30,000 deaths in the United States annually as the result of homicide, suicide, and accidents.[3]

Roots of Violence

Violence usually has no single cause, but the major contributing factors are described next.

Violent Family of Origin

Being a member of a violent family exposes one to role models who may scream or punch first and discuss differences later—if at all. Being victimized by violence may also build reservoirs of hostility that may be tapped at unpredictable times.

Gangs

In many neighborhoods, especially impoverished neighborhoods, gangs harbor prestige among young people. They provide a source of social approval that can rival the approval of parents and schools, because youngsters see gang members as obtaining rewards and privileges that seem important to them. Gangs also protect their "turf" or "territories" from other gangs in ways that can give rise to explosive violence.

Stress

Stress is a major cause of violence because it can arouse people to a flight-or-flight response. Poverty and unemployment are key contributors to stress, and when impoverished people believe that their situation is unjust, they may lash out as well as seek political change through peaceful means.

Media Violence

Violent TV shows, books, and films do more than teach people how and when to act out violently; they may also work people up. Frequent exposure to violent TV shows, war footage, slasher movies, vampire movies, and so on can also give viewers the impression that the world is a violent place and that the best defense is to hurt someone else before he can hurt you. The flood of violent imagery also desensitizes viewers to violence; that is, they may come to assume that violence is a normal part of life and feel little sympathy for victims of violence.

Alcohol

Heavy use of alcohol and other drugs is also connected with many acts of violence, including domestic violence, homicide, and rape. Alcohol does not directly cause violence, but it has a number of effects that set the stage for violence. Before its depressive effects come into play, alcohol dilates blood vessels and works as a stimulant. Alcohol also loosens and impairs judgment, reducing our ability to weigh the consequences of our behavior. The setting in which people drink also plays a role. If students are drinking at a bar and arguing over the sports teams on the TV monitor, violence becomes a possible outcome.

Political Unrest

People may protest political regimes they find to be unjust or argue about differences in how to raise or reduce money for government functions. At the extreme, demonstrations and bickering can lead to violence.

Religious Differences

Many religions foster the view that theirs is the one true religion and that nonbelievers may be threats. Religious hatred turns violent on occasion throughout the world.

Terrorism

Both political and religious differences can give rise to terrorism, especially when groups with grievances do not possess the political power or weaponry of culturally dominant groups or of nations. Throughout its history, the United States was protected by the oceans that separated it from foreign enemies. World Wars I and II were generally fought overseas and not in the continental United States. The terrorist attacks of September 11, 2001, brought what seemed like a very new type of violence to the United States and gave many Americans a sense of vulnerability they had not experienced before. During the early years of the 21st century, there have been numerous terrorist attacks throughout the world with a variety of aims.

There is also the occasional (but all too common!) instance of terrorism by disturbed individuals in the United States, such as the Virginia Tech massacre of 2007, which killed thirty-three people, and the 2011 shootings in Tucson, Arizona, which left six people dead and fourteen wounded, including Congresswoman Gabrielle Giffords. In the case of the attack in Tucson, it appears that mental illness was involved.

Anger and Frustration

Emotional states such as anger and frustration can serve as catalysts for aggressive responses, especially when alcohol is part of the picture. Aggression is a complex form of behavior that involves the interplay of multiple factors. (If you have problems managing your feelings of anger, read the online feature "Health Skills 13-1.")

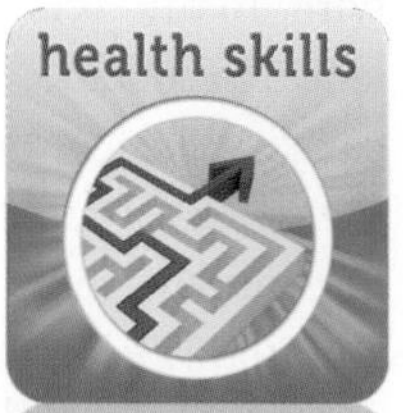

Access CourseMate for HLTH at www.cengagebrain.com.

Cultural Factors in Sexual Violence

Does our society breed rapists by socializing young men into socially and sexually dominant roles? American men are usually reinforced from an early age for aggressive and competitive behavior—for winning at all costs. As a result, some college athletes and other college men may see their roles with women as overcoming resistance.[4]

Sexual behavior and competitive sports are linked through common idioms. Friends may taunt a young man who has been on a date with such questions as "Did you score?" or more bluntly, "Did you get *in*?"

Violence at the Hands of Intimate Partners

Women's intimate partners subject them to nearly 5 million incidents of violence (also called *domestic violence*) annually in the United States.[5] Men too are victims—in nearly 3 million physical assaults by their intimate partners.

Women comprise about three-quarters of the victims of murders by intimate partners and about 90% of the victims of nonlethal intimate violence. More than 1,000 women die each year at the hands of their partners and husbands. To put these statistics in perspective, women are more likely to be beaten, raped, and killed by men they live with than by any other type of assailant.

Women also attack their male partners. In about one in two abusive relationships, the partners abuse each other. Women, however, are much more likely to sustain serious bodily harm at the hands of their partners, including broken bones, damage to internal organs, and death. Bruises and broken bones are the visible signs of abuse, but the psychological effects can linger and include post-traumatic stress disorder (PTSD), depression, low self-esteem, alcohol and substance abuse, and even suicide.

Batterers are found in every ethnic group and income bracket. However, partner abuse is more commonly reported among people in lower income groups, perhaps because of the added stress that financial hardship places on relationships that are already strained.

Many batterers have problems with anger control and are impulsive, antisocial, and hostile. Many have drug abuse problems and low self-esteem as well. They may feel personally inadequate, which leads them to feel threatened when they perceive their partners as growing distant, more independent, or developing interests of their own (such as school or work). Violence may then be triggered by criticism or rejection by their partner, and as in so many other instances of violence, the use of alcohol or other drugs heightens the risk.[6]

There is also an unequal power distribution between men and women in our society. Young men are socialized to play dominant roles and may expect women to bend to their wishes. Though battering may not be part of the male curriculum, men may enter relationships believing that force is appropriate when their needs are not met or their power is challenged.

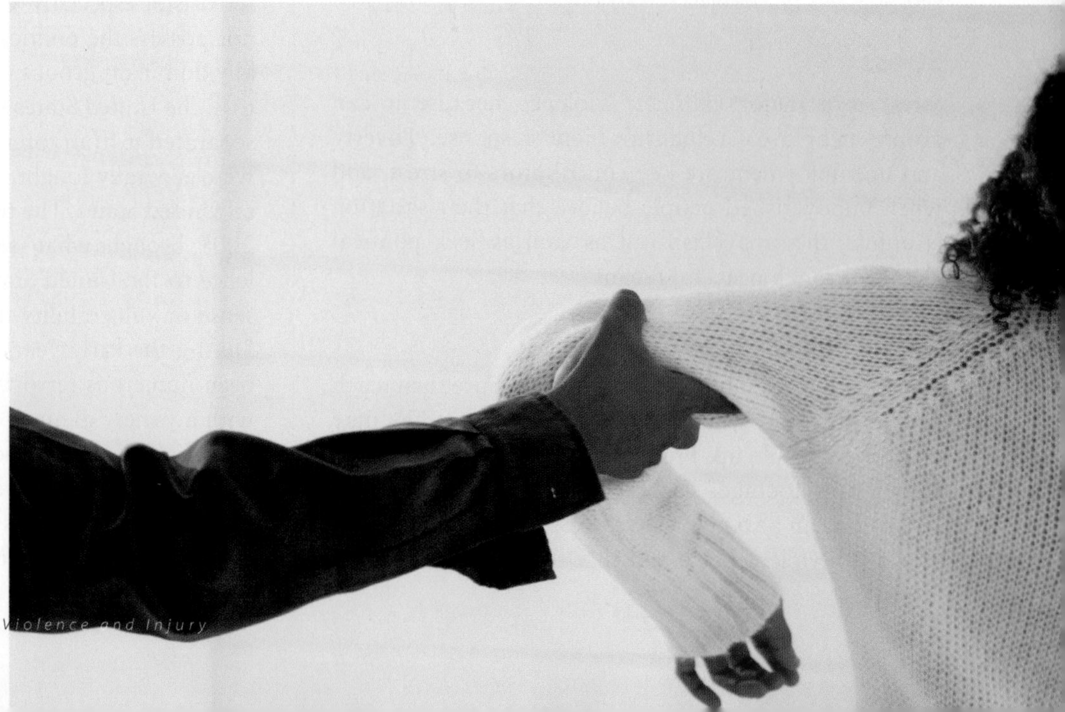

© Image Source/Jupiterimages

batterer
A person who inflicts violent physical abuse upon his or her intimate partner.

More than 3 million children in the United States witness partner abuse each year, and they too suffer psychological effects such as depression and anxiety.[7] Children with aggressive parents may be learning that violence is an acceptable means of solving conflicts. The lesson may "transmit" domestic violence from generation to generation.

How Does Society Respond to Violence by Intimate Partners?

How do police react when they are called to stop domestic violence? Too often they take the batterer aside and have a talk with him rather than arrest him. Even if the man is arrested, he may only receive a "slap on the wrist"—a lesser sentence than he would have received if he had attacked a stranger.

To end domestic violence parents must demonstrate zero tolerance of the behavior. Young men should be encouraged to respond to conflict with their heads, not their fists. The criminal justice system must deal with domestic violence as it deals with other acts of violence and not make exceptions because the victim lives with the assailant.

Hate Crimes

Violent crimes are motivated by many factors—revenge, profit, or sexual jealousy, to name a few. But hate crimes are motivated by pure hatred.

Hate crimes target people on the basis of their race, religion, sexual orientation, ethnicity/national origin, or physical or mental disability. These crimes can range from destruction or desecration of property (for example, drawing swastikas on the walls of synagogues) to assaults (for example, gay bashings) to rapes and murders. The Federal Bureau of Investigation (FBI) reported 8,336 hate crimes in the United States in a recent year.[8] The actual numbers are surely much higher, as many violent acts aren't recorded as hate crimes but are classified instead as simple assaults, rapes, or murders. Figure 13-1 shows the targets of these crimes.[9] Seven in 10 victims of race-related hate crimes were African Americans; seven in 10 victims of religious bias were Jews (see "Diversity 13-1" on the next page).

Most people who commit hate crimes are otherwise law-abiding citizens who may see little wrong with carrying out such acts. Hate crimes are rooted in extreme prejudice, clouding people's judgment of basic principles of morality. There are particularly strong legal sanctions for hate crimes, because legislators understand that hate crimes cannot be permitted to get out of hand.

*Figure 13-1 The Targets of Hate Crimes**

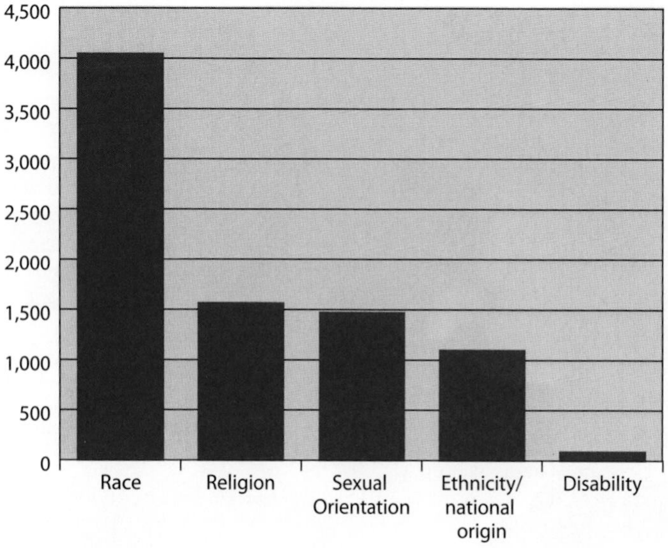

* Victims include individuals, businesses, institutions, and society as a whole.
Source: Federal Bureau of Investigation. (2010). *Latest hate crime statistics.*

Child Abuse and Neglect

More than 3.5 million children suffer from child abuse or neglect each year in the United States.[10] An estimated 1,760 children die each year as the result of abuse or neglect. These numbers are but the tip of the iceberg, because many, probably most, child abuse cases are not reported. Nearly half of the deaths from child abuse and neglect involve children younger than one year old. The great majority involve children younger than five years old. Boys and girls are about equally likely to be abused.

There are various forms of child abuse and neglect (see Figure 13-2 on the next page).

- *Neglect*, or failure to provide for a child's basic needs, is most common.
- *Physical abuse* involves punching, beating, kicking, biting, shaking, throwing, stabbing, choking, hitting, or burning a child.
- *Sexual abuse* includes fondling a child's genitals, penetration, incest, indecent exposure, and exploitation by means such as prostitution or creation of child pornography.
- *Emotional abuse* can involve constant criticism, threats, rejection, or withholding love, support, or guidance.

DIVERSITY 13-1

Race, Religion, and Violent Crime in America[11]

Among 10- to 24-year-olds, homicide is the leading cause of death for African Americans, the second leading cause of death for Latin Americans and European Americans, and the third leading cause of death for Asian Americans and Native Americans.

Homicide rates among African American males 10–24 years of age (60.7 per 100,000) exceed those of Latinos (20.6 per 100,000) and European Americans in the same age group (3.5 per 100,000).

African Americans account for 13% of the U.S. population but are the victims of about 15% of all nonfatal violent crime and about 49% of all homicides. In a recent year, African Americans were victims of an estimated 805,000 nonfatal violent crimes (rape, sexual assault, robbery, and assault).

> African Americans are the victims of nearly half of all U.S. homicides.

Since 2001, serious nonfatal violent victimization (rape, sexual assault, robbery, and aggravated assault) made up 48% of all nonfatal violent crime against African Americans, compared to 31% of violent crime against European Americans, 31% against Native Americans, 42% against Asian Americans, and about 40% against Latin Americans.

Seven in 10 victims of race-related hate crimes are African Americans. Seven in 10 victims of crimes based on religious bias are Jews.

© iStockphoto.com/mwojtan

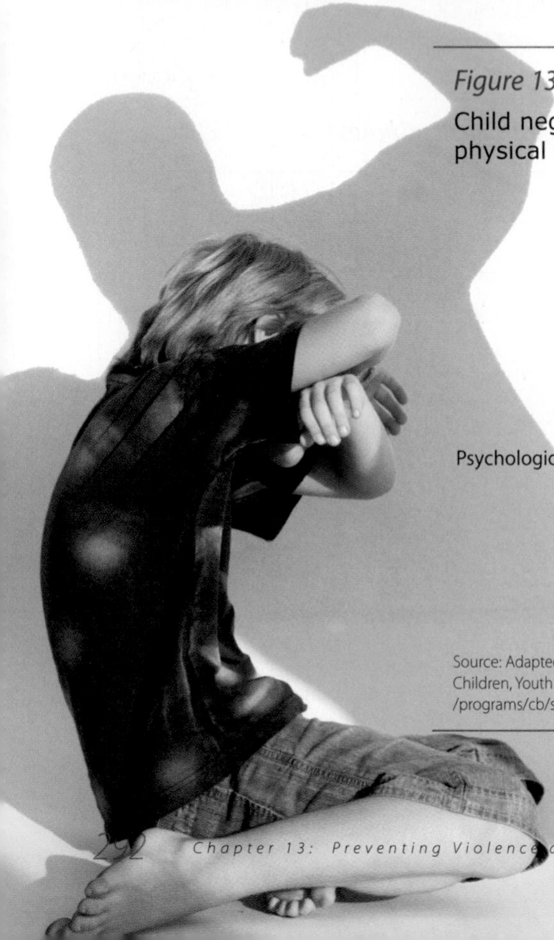

Figure 13-2 Cases of Child Maltreatment by Type

Child neglect is the most frequent type of child maltreatment, followed by physical abuse.

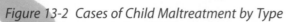

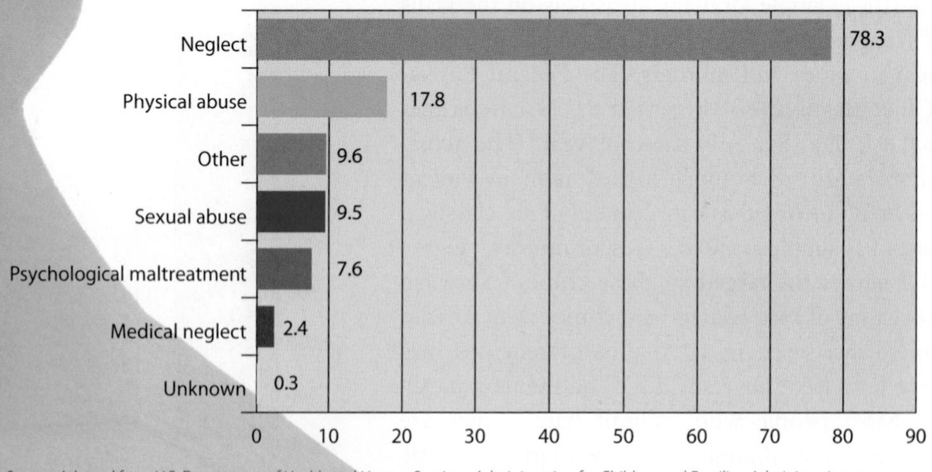

Source: Adapted from U.S. Department of Health and Human Services, Administration for Children and Families, Administration on Children, Youth and Families, Children's Bureau. (2010). *Child Maltreatment 2009: Table 3-13*. Retrieved from http://www.acf.hhs.gov /programs/cb/stats_research/index.htm#can.

© iStockphoto.com/mandygodbehear

Though child abuse cuts across all segments of our society, the abusive parent is often young, has limited parenting skills, is under stress, and resorts to force to control his or her children's behavior. A history of child abuse in the abuser's family of origin is also quite common. Abusive parents tend to lack parenting skills and fail to form strong attachments to their children. As in other kinds of violence, lack of anger management skills plays a role, as may use of alcohol and other drugs. Child abusers also tend to hold rigid attitudes toward child rearing. They typically rely more on physical punishment and less on reasoning as ways of controlling children than other parents do.

Child abuse generally becomes more severe over time. Rationalizations, such as blaming the child for the abuse (for example, "If he didn't want to get hit, he shouldn't have left his clothes lying around"), serve to justify the abuse.

Public concerns about protecting children have led to the passage of mandatory reporting laws in all 50 states. These laws require many professionals, including physicians, social workers, marriage and family counselors, and psychologists, to notify authorities when they suspect or know of abuse. Nevertheless, many cases still go unreported.

Health Effects of Child Abuse

Child abuse can cause serious, sometimes life-threatening injuries, ranging from welts and bruises to broken bones and massive internal damage. As with battering, physical injuries are the visible signs of abuse, but emotional wounds can run deeper and last longer.[12]

Abused or neglected children may have difficulty establishing healthy attachments and peer relationships, may lack the capacity for empathy, and may fail to develop a sense of conscience. They may act out in ways that mirror the cruelty they have endured. They may act aggressively toward smaller, more vulnerable children, torture and kill small animals, or set fires. Child abuse and neglect are connected with failure to thrive in infants, bed-wetting and thumb-sucking in early childhood, and poor academic achievement in middle childhood. Abused children often assume that they deserved "what they got." Misplaced self-blame can lower self-esteem and set the stage for depression, self-hatred, and suicidal behavior.

What Can Be Done?

Although child abuse and neglect remain pervasive problems, one encouraging sign is the development of parent training programs that target abusive parents. They help abusive parents develop better parenting techniques, control anger, and manage the stress that can set the stage for abuse. It would be desirable to direct parent training programs toward new and expectant parents, especially teenagers. Perhaps such programs can be integrated within the school curriculum, much as we now offer driver's education.

Crime on Campus

LEARNING OUTCOME 2

Discuss crime on campus and its prevention

We'd like to think of the college campus as a cloistered environment that insulates us from the threat of violent crime, but statistics tell another story. As you can see in Table 13-1, the college campus is not immune to the problem of violent crimes—crimes like robberies, sexual assaults, hate crimes, even homicides. **Identity theft** has also become a major problem on campus, as it has in society at large. The Federal Trade Commission estimates that nearly 10 million Americans become victims of identity theft each year. Armed with your name and social security number, thieves can steal your identity to acquire phony credit cards in your name, which can cause havoc with your personal credit. Though we cannot immunize ourselves against violent crime, we

identity theft
Impersonating another person for criminal purposes by means of using the person's social security number, bank account information, or other personally identifying information.

Table 13-1 Crimes on Campus (2009)[13]

TYPE OF CRIME	NUMBER	PERCENTAGE OF TOTAL
Murder	55	0.10%
Manslaughter	5	0.01%
Forcible sexual offense	3,287	6.19%
Robbery	4,562	8.60%
Aggravated assault	5,026	9.47%
Burglary	31,851	60.01%
Motor vehicle theft	7,465	14.06%
Arson	825	1.55%

can take steps to protect our personal safety on campus (see "Health Skills 13-2").

The great majority of crimes on campus are crimes against property. Burglary is the most prevalent of these, followed by motor vehicle theft and arson. Burglary is the illegal entry of a building in order to commit a theft. It includes what is commonly called "breaking and entering." If someone breaks or sneaks into your room and takes your iPad or your laptop computer, he is committing burglary. Of the violent crimes reported on college campuses, the largest number are aggravated assaults, followed by robberies, forcible rapes, and murder. Aggravated assault is an unlawful attack intended to inflict severe bodily injury. Robbery is the taking of something of value from another person by force or by the threat of force. Despite the large numbers of crimes committed on campuses, college students aged 18 to 24 actually encounter less violence than people of the same age who do not attend college. And despite the incidences of assaults against women, including intimate partner violence and rape, male college students are actually twice as likely as female students to be victims of violence.[14]

Sexual Coercion

Sexual coercion, or use of force, brings us back to the case of Anne and Jim.[15] It also brings us back—in most cases—to victimization of women by men, to a society that often blames the victim for what happens to her, and to men who too often can't understand, or say they can't understand, why people are making such a fuss. In this section, we look at the topics of rape and sexual harassment on campus—and everywhere else.

LEARNING OUTCOME 3

Explain what is meant by sexual coercion and discuss the problems of rape and sexual harassment

forcible rape
Sexual intercourse with a nonconsenting person achieved by force or threat of force.

statutory rape
Sexual intercourse with a person who is below the age of consent, even if the person cooperates.

Rape

Rape is both a sexual assault and a crime of violence in which sex is used as an instrument of aggression, anger, control, and power. There are two general legal categories of rape. **Forcible rape** is the use of force or the threat of force to compel a person into having sex. **Statutory rape** refers to sex with a person who is unable to give consent because he or she is under the age of consent or is mentally disabled. It doesn't matter if a child cooperates. Any sexual contact with a child is considered coercive, because children are considered too immature to consent.

Young women aged 16 to 24 are two to three times more likely to be raped than younger or older females. The majority of rapes, about six out of 10, are committed against girls under 18 years of age.[16] Yet any woman, young or old, African American or European American, is at risk of being raped. Rape is more common in the United States than in other developed nations such as Canada, Great Britain, and Japan.

There are some 90,000 reported forcible rapes in the United States each year.[17] But the great majority of rapes go unreported because of problems such as mistrust of the criminal justice system, tendencies to blame the victim, and because of disputes a victim might encounter as to whether a rape has actually occurred.[18] The odds that a woman in the United States will be raped at some point in her life are about one in four.[19] About 10% of rapes involve rapes against males. On college campuses, 35 of 1,000 women are sexually assaulted each year.[20]

Did You Know That...

- **1** woman in **4** will be sexually assaulted during her lifetime?
- More than **75%** of rapes are committed by men acquainted with the victim?
- Fewer than **5%** of college students who are sexually assaulted report it to the police?
- **90%** of sexual assaults of college students involve the use of alcohol?
- The majority of rapes occur in the student's dorm or home?
- A college or university can expect about **35** sexual assaults per **1,000** female students in any given year?

Source: Reprinted from Koss, Mary P., Gidycz, Christine A., Wisniewski, Nadine. The scope of rape: Incidence and prevalence of sexual aggression and victimization in a national sample of higher education students. *Journal of Consulting and Clinical Psychology*, 55 (2), 162-170. © 1987, with permission from Elsevier.

HEALTH SKILLS 13-2

Preventing Becoming a Victim on Campus

Here are some tips on how to protect yourself from crime on campus:

- *Become familiar with your campus.* Take a survey of your campus, noting the locations of the academic buildings, administrative buildings, campus security offices, and health services. Take note of the lighting conditions along campus walkways and parking areas. Determine the pathways you need to take to get to and from classes and residence halls.
- *Stop identity theft!* Stop identity theft in its tracks by not revealing your personal information to anyone other than campus officials or academic advisors. Never give out your social security number or bank account information on a public website. Many public websites sell personal information to marketers; this information sometimes winds up in the hands of identity thieves. It is more difficult to control credit card information if you're shopping online, but at least be certain that you know the vendor and that the website looks legitimate.
- *Carry a cell phone with you for security purposes or learn where emergency phones are located.*
- *Share your academic and social schedule with your parents or buddies.* Make sure that someone knows where you are expected to be.
- *Whenever possible, travel in groups, especially late at night.* Avoid walking alone, especially in deserted areas of campus. Don't take any shortcuts that pass through isolated or poorly lit areas.
- *Check the security of your living arrangements, whether on campus or off campus.* Make sure that all exterior doors are secured by dead-bolt locks and have peepholes. Inspect the lighting around building entrances to ensure there are no darkened areas. Do not loan out your keys or place them under a mat or in a flower box. Make sure your windows are securely locked. If you have roommates and cannot lock the room or suite, place valuables and your laptop computer in a locked trunk or secure box tucked away somewhere. (Ask building security what to do.)
- *Voice your concerns.* Bring any safety concerns to the attention of school public safety officers. Be on the lookout for broken locks, unsecured doors, absent or defective lighting in common areas, or unrestricted access to dormitories.

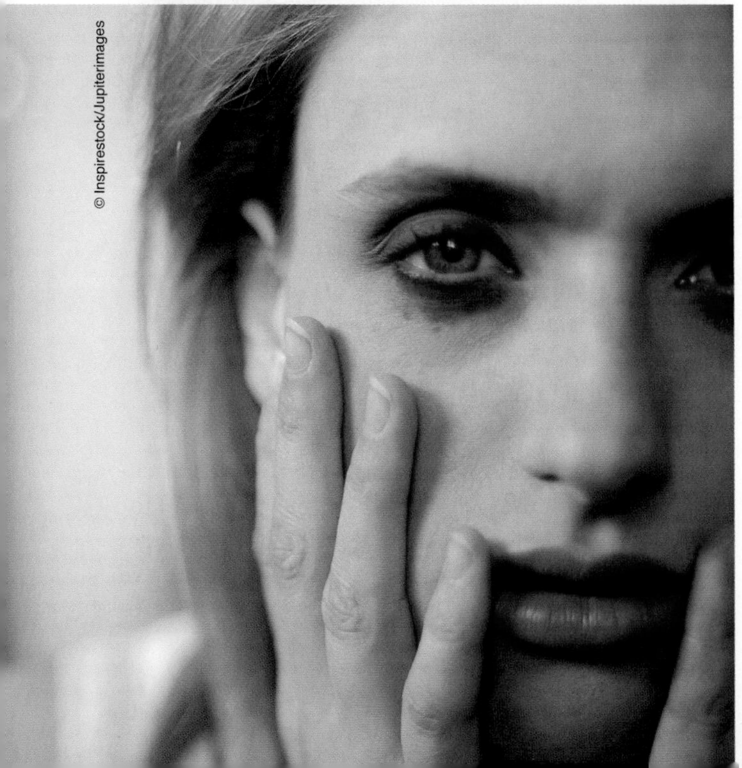

© Inspirestock/Jupiterimages

Rape on Campus

Rape on college campuses is a fact of life:[21]

- Three out of five college men admit that they might force women into sex under some circumstances. More than two out of five college men admit using force to have sex and ignoring a woman's protests. Virtually no college men who rape their dates or acquaintances think of what they did as rape.[22]
- Fraternity men are more likely than independents to use drugs and alcohol as a strategy to draw women into sex.
- The great majority of rapes of college women are perpetrated by someone they know. Seven of eight victims describe their rapist as a friend, acquaintance, or boyfriend. In one college study, most date rapes were not committed by recent acquaintances

Guidelines for Safe Social Networking in College[23]

Most college students not only e-mail and text their social acquaintances but also check out their photos and friends online. Social networking sites have greatly expanded students' opportunities for social interaction, but there are also some dangers connected with using them. Here are some safety precautions that will enable you to enjoy social networking while avoiding its pitfalls:

1. *Know how to set your privacy settings.* Everyone has the ability to edit their privacy settings and should set them accordingly. The safest option is to keep your pictures and statuses private, where only friends can see. Search settings are also important, and they fall into two categories: internal search listing and public search listing (which shows your public profile). Both of these can be turned off or adjusted to limit who can find you in a search. With this, be sure to add only people whom you know to your friends list, as it can lead to major consequences when strangers can access your personal information.
2. *Know your audience.* This is an important piece of advice, especially for college students. It is important to keep in mind whom you add to your friends list, such as family members, coworkers, bosses, and groups of people. If you are okay with adding them, be sure to keep in mind who your audience is when you post things. Posts and pictures can lead to everything from family disputes to problems at work or school. Keep in mind that simple posts such as "studying at Sarah's house" can let potentially dangerous people know you are not at home.
3. *Keep your page professional.* Although it may be tempting to post pictures of a fun drinking party or angry status updates about your teacher, these things can come back to haunt you. It has happened in the past. Even such comments such as "Bored at work" can end up with serious consequences as it did for Kimberly Swann, who got let go from her job after posting that as her Facebook status. Business and medical school admissions officers and potential employers have also been known to use social networking sites to get more background on potential hires. Keep in mind that photos posted on the Internet can hang around for years, even if you have deleted them. If friends download them and tag them, future employers and admissions officers can find them.
4. *Keep personal information private, or don't post it—period.* Keep addresses and phone numbers off Facebook completely. If people need your number or address, do not post it on their wall. Instead, send them a private message or call them.

Another tip is to manage your time when "Facebooking" and using other social networking sites. Leave yourself time to study and to actually interact with your friends—in the real world, that is.

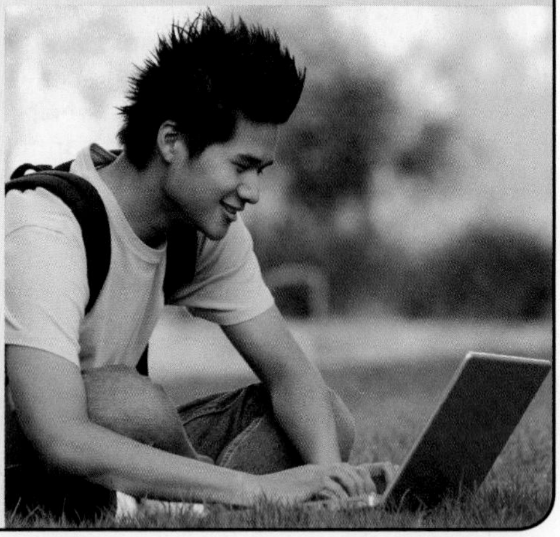

© Monkey Business Images/Shutterstock.com

or blind dates, but by men whom the women had known for a time.

- Nine out of 10 campus rapes take place under the influence of alcohol. Many college men assume that a woman who drinks on a date is willing to have sex, and 40% of men who believe this also think it's acceptable to force a woman who is drunk into sex. Binge drinking is a particularly strong predictor of being victimized by rape.[24]
- Nearly half of college rape victims are physically injured by the assault.
- Only one in four college women who are raped actually describe what happened as rape, and only one in 10 report the rape to authorities. Many women do not consider a sexual assault by an acquaintance to actually be rape.[25]
- College women, as in the case of Anne in the chapter opener example, are most likely to be raped before they get fully settled in to campus life—during the first weeks of their freshman or sophomore years.

Various cultural myths contribute to a social climate that legitimizes and increases the potential for rape. Many people believe that only bad girls get raped and that women "cry rape" only when they've been jilted. Another commonly held myth is that rapists are not responsible for their actions—that sexually provocative women unleash uncontrollable sexual urges in them. Some people even believe that deep down inside, women want to be raped. Though both men and women are susceptible to rape myths, college men show greater acceptance of them than do college women. What about you? How many rape myths do you believe? Complete "Health Check 13-1" to find out.

Health Effects of Rape

Depending on the brutality and amount of force, women may suffer grievous physical injuries, even death. Victims may also be infected with sexually transmitted infections or impregnated. The psychological effects may be deeper and longer lasting than the physical injuries.[26] Many rape survivors are distraught following the attack, and about half seek professional help.[27] They cry frequently and suffer insomnia, loss of appetite, cystitis and other gynecological problems, headaches, irritability, mood changes, and anxiety and depression. Many become withdrawn, sullen, and mistrustful. Because myths about rape tend to blame the victim, some survivors experience feelings of guilt and shame.

For some rape survivors, depression and anxiety last for many years. Future sexual and interpersonal relationships may be marred by sexual dysfunctions such as lack of sexual desire and mistrust. Many survivors also develop posttraumatic stress disorder (PTSD), as evidenced by intrusive memories and nightmares about the rape. Some survivors develop problems with alcohol and other drugs as well.

Rape Prevention

Rape prevention efforts should start at the broader societal level with socializing men to be respectful of women and better aware of the boundaries between consent and coercion. Rape prevention workshops that help promote more respectful attitudes toward women, like those offered in many colleges, need to be incorporated in the school curriculum in high schools and lower grades. Society at large needs to send a message

HEALTH CHECK 13-1

health check

Rape Myths: What Do You Believe?

Read each of the following statements and indicate whether you believe it to be true or false by selecting *T* or *F*. Then evaluate your beliefs.

T F 1. Women who dress provocatively in public places are just "asking for it."

T F 2. A woman who accompanies a man home from a club or a bar deserves whatever she gets.

T F 3. Women who claim they were raped are just looking for excuses for having had sex.

T F 4. Any physically healthy woman can resist a man's advances if she really wants to.

T F 5. If a woman allows a man to fondle her, it means she wants to have intercourse.

T F 6. Most women who are raped probably led the man on.

T F 7. If a woman initiates petting with a man, it's her own fault if things go too far.

T F 8. Women may not admit it, but they really want to be overpowered by men.

T F 9. If a woman has too much to drink at a party, it's her fault if men take advantage of her.

T F 10. Rape is often a misunderstanding that gets out of hand.

Each of these items represents a rape myth. For example, a rapist who believes that women truly desire to be overpowered by men may think he was just giving the woman what she wanted. But how can anyone know what someone else truly wants unless that person reveals it? Such beliefs are often used to rationalize unacceptable behavior. Let's be entirely clear about this: When it comes to sex, *no* means *no*. Not *maybe*. Not *sometimes*. Not *in a few minutes*. Just *no*. Moreover, consenting to one sexual act such as deep kissing or petting does not imply consent for any other sexual act. Anyone has a right to say *no* at any time or to place limits on what they are willing to do.

that sexual coercion, like any violent crime, will not be tolerated and will be punished to the fullest extent allowed by law.

However, society is not about to change tomorrow. It is prudent for women to take precautions to minimize their risk of being sexually assaulted. Are you wondering if even the listing of rape prevention measures is a subtle way of blaming the woman if she should fall prey to an attacker? No, providing the information does not blame the victim. The rapist is *always* responsible for the assault. Read the online feature "Prevention 13-1" to find out how to protect yourself from being raped.

prevention

Access CourseMate for HLTH at www.cengagebrain.com.

Treatment of Rape Survivors

Treatment of rape survivors typically involves a two-stage process of helping the victim through the crisis (see Health Skills 13-3) and then helping to foster long-term adjustment.[28] Crisis intervention services provide the survivor with support and information to help her express her feelings and develop strategies for coping with the trauma. Longer-term treatment can help the survivor cope with the emotional consequences of rape, avoid self-blame, improve self-esteem, and help her establish or maintain loving relationships. Family, friends, religious leaders, and health care specialists are all potential sources of help, so long as people who might blame the victim are not part of the circle. In major cities and many towns, rape crisis centers and hotlines, peer counseling groups, and referral agencies provide additional support. Phone numbers for these services can be obtained from women's organizations (for example, your local office of the National Organization for Women [NOW]), health centers, or the Rape, Abuse, and Incest National Network (http://rainn.org).

sexual harassment
Unwelcome comments, gestures, demands, overtures, or physical contact of a sexual nature.

Sexual Harassment

Sexual harassment is a form of sexual coercion that involves unwelcome sexual comments, jokes, overtures, demands for sexual favors, or outright physical contact. The great majority of cases are committed by men against women, although men too can be victimized.[29] Sexual harassment occurs everywhere—on high school and col-

HEALTH SKILLS 13-3

health skills

If You Are Raped . . .

Here are some suggestions about what to do in those terrible minutes and hours immediately after a sexual assault:[30]

- *Don't change anything about your body—don't wash or even comb your hair. Leave your clothes as they are.* Otherwise, you could destroy evidence.
- *Report the incident to police.* You may prevent another woman from being assaulted, and you will be taking charge, starting on the path from victim to survivor.
- *Ask a relative or friend to take you to a hospital if you can't get an ambulance or a police car.* If you call the hospital, tell them why you're requesting an ambulance, in case they are able to send someone trained to deal with rape cases.
- *Get help.* Seeking help is an assertive way to show your self-worth. Seek medical help to detect injuries of which you are unaware. Insist that a written or photographic record be made to document your condition. You may decide to file charges, and the prosecutor may need this evidence.
- *Ask questions.* You have medical rights. Ask what treatments are available to you. Ask for whatever will make you comfortable. Refuse what you don't want.
- *Call a rape hotline or rape crisis center for advice.* A rape crisis volunteer may be available to accompany you to the hospital and help see you through the medical evaluation and police investigation. It is not unusual for rape survivors to try to erase the details of the rape from their minds, but remembering details clearly will help you give an accurate description of the rapist to the police, including his clothing, type of car, and so on.

lege campuses, in our workplaces, in the military, and on the Internet.Examples of sexual harassment include:

- Verbal harassment or abuse
- Subtle pressure for sexual activity
- Remarks about a person's clothing, body, or sexual activities
- Leering or ogling at a person's body
- Unwelcome touching, patting, or pinching
- Brushing against a person's body
- Demands for sexual favors accompanied by implied or overt threats concerning one's job, opportunities for promotion or advancement, or student status
- Physical or sexual assault

Sexual harassment has more to do with the abuse of power than with sexual desire.[31] Relatively few cases of sexual harassment involve requests or demands for sexual favors. Most involve sexual taunts, unwelcome sexual gestures, or comments in which sex is used to humiliate, control, or frighten someone—usually a woman. The harasser usually abuses a dominant position to take advantage of the victim's vulnerability. Sexual harassment may also be used as a tactic of social control—a means of keeping women "in their place." This is especially true in traditional male preserves, such as the firehouse, the construction site, or the military academy or service unit.

Under the law, people subjected to sexual harassment can obtain a court order to have the harassment stopped, have their jobs reinstated (when they have lost them by resisting sexual advances), receive back pay and lost benefits, and obtain monetary awards for the emotional strain imposed by the harassment. However, proving charges of sexual harassment is generally difficult because there are usually no corroborating witnesses or evidence. As a result, relatively few women who are sexually harassed in the workplace report it. Like people subjected to other forms of sexual coercion, people who encounter sexual harassment often do not report the offense for fear that they will not be believed or will be subjected to retaliation. Some fear losing their jobs or being denied opportunities to advance in their careers.

Overall, about 25% to 30% of college students report at least one incident of sexual harassment, with males about twice as likely as females to be the harassers.[32] Sexual harassment on campus usually involves less severe forms of harassment, such as sexist comments and sexual remarks by faculty, as well as come-ons, suggestive looks, propositions, and light touching.[33] Relatively few acts involve direct pressure for sexual activity.

Sexual harassment may also occur between patients and doctors or between therapists and clients. These professionals may abuse their power and influence over clients to pressure them into having sexual relations. The harassment may be disguised, expressed in terms of its supposed "therapeutic benefits."

Sexual harassment is not just annoying or insensitive. People who are sexually harassed often report physical or emotional reactions such as anxiety, irritability, lowered self-esteem, and anger. Some find harassment on the job so unbearable that they feel forced to resign. College women have been forced to drop courses, switch majors, change graduate programs, or transfer to other colleges because of persistent sexual harassment. Learn how to deal effectively with sexual harassers in the online feature "Health Skills 13-4."

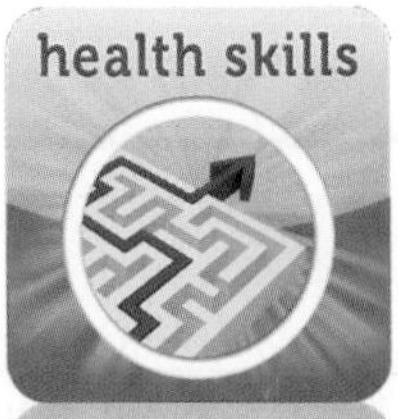

Access CourseMate for HLTH at www.cengagebrain.com.

Accidents

Accidents are the fifth leading cause of death in the United States, accounting for more than 100,000 deaths annually.[34] What is the most frequent type of fatal accident? If you guessed motor vehicle accidents, guess again. Number one on the list is accidents in the home, mostly from falls.

LEARNING OUTCOME 4

Discuss various kinds of unintentional injuries—injuries from accidents—and how to prevent them

Non-fatal accidents affect millions of people each year. Nearly four of 10 emergency room (ER) visits result from accidents. About one person in nine seeks medical attention for an accidental injury each year. Accidental falls account for one in four injury-related emergency room visits, while motor vehicle accidents account for one in eight. Accidentally being struck by people, objects, or falling objects accounts for another one in 10 accident-related visits, as do cuts or puncture wounds. Violent acts account for about one in 20.

Many people misjudge the risks of dying in natural disasters or from environmental causes. Are you more likely to die in a building fire or riding in a car? What really is the risk of dying from a lightning strike? How do the risks of death from natural disasters, such as floods and earthquakes, compare to those from accidental falls or crossing the street? The greatest risks involve the most ordinary life experiences, such as walking up or down stairs (deaths due to falls), taking a swim (accidental drowning), or crossing the street. We can compare relative risks by means of a "risk thermometer," as shown in Figure 13-3.[35]

Figure 13-3 Risk of Dying from . . . [36]

Here we see the relative size of risks from environmental hazards as well as human activity. Your personal risk of an accident also depends on the precautions you take to guard against risks.

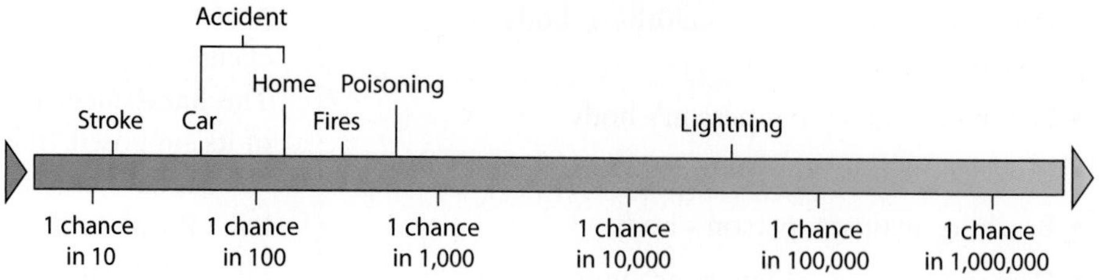

You stand a much greater chance of drowning in your bathtub than dying in a lightning strike. Yet the threat of lightning sends people scurrying for cover, as well it should, but few express any fears of taking a bath.

We're not suggesting living in fear of daily life experiences, but it would be logical to ensure that our homes and cars are safe and that we exercise some caution in driving, biking, swimming, and boating.

Let us start our search for safety where most of us get up in the morning—at home.

Playing It Safe at Home

"Home, sweet home," or so the expression goes. Our homes may be sweet but they are also places where we face the greatest risk of serious or disabling injuries. In fact, accidents in the home account for more than twice the number of disabling injuries from motor vehicle crashes. (See the online feature "Health Skills 13-5" for tips on making your home safer.) According to the latest available statistics, accidents in the home account for some 13 million disabling injuries and about 54,000 deaths annually in the United States.[37] By contrast, accidents in the workplace account for some 4,300 deaths and 3.2 million disabling injuries annually.

health skills

Access CourseMate for HLTH at www.cengagebrain.com.

More than 200 children die in the United States annually as the result of accidents involving firearms.[38] More than 750 Americans lose their lives each year as the result of accidental discharge of firearms, and thousands more are severely injured.[39]

Preventing Injuries on the Road

Think for a moment: What's the leading cause of death for young Americans 16 to 20 years old? Infectious diseases like HIV/AIDS? Suicide? Homicide? Cancer? Actually, the answer is motor vehicle crashes. Young, newly licensed drivers have the highest incidences of fatalities and injuries resulting from motor vehicle crashes.[40]

Preventing Repetitive Stress Injuries

Many college students complain of pain from using a keyboard. Continual keyboard use can lead to *carpal tunnel syndrome*, an inflammation of the tissue that covers nerves in the wrist. As the tissue becomes inflamed, it presses on nerves, causing pain and impairing functioning. Use of an ergonomically designed keyboard can help relieve stress on the wrists and hands, reducing the pain.

Other suggestions include:

- Adjust the height of the keyboard so that your forearms remain parallel to the floor.
- Adjust the height of your chair so that your thighs are also parallel to the floor.
- Keep your wrists parallel to the floor—don't rest them on the desk.
- Use your arms to move your fingers around the keyboard. Don't let your fingers do all the stretching.
- Sit straight up in your chair and avoid leaning toward the keyboard.
- Take frequent breaks to stretch and move about the room or office.

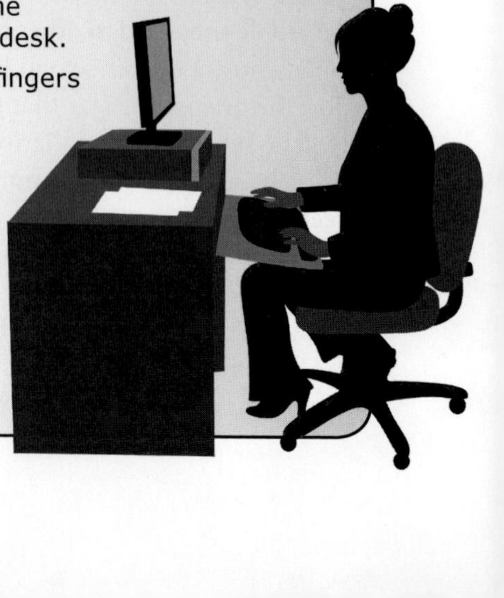

The National Highway Traffic Safety Administration (NHTSA) compiles and analyzes information about crashes to determine how best to make the nation's vehicles and the roads on which they travel safer. These efforts are paying off, as the numbers of motor vehicle fatalities have been declining, from 43,510 in 2005 to 33,963 in 2009.[41] Another 3 million suffer injuries as the result of motor vehicle accidents, a number that is also declining.[42]

Much of the credit for saved lives and declining numbers of injuries goes to increased use of seat belts and the construction of more crashworthy vehicles. Seat belts alone account for more than half of these saved lives[43] (see Figure 13-4). Seat belt use has been increasing, up to about 84% of all car occupants, but is lower among people in the 16- to 24-year-old age range than among older groups.[44]

The NHTSA estimates that seat belts in cars and trucks prevent more than 15,000 deaths and more than 300,000 serious injuries every year. On the other hand, use of alcohol is implicated in half of the nation's motor vehicle fatalities.

Although we have made much progress in promoting safety on the nation's roads, more than 30,000 Americans still die each year in motor vehicle accidents. Many of these deaths could be prevented. Table 13-2 on the next page offers some facts about the toll of motor vehicle accidents among young people.

What can *you* do to avoid becoming another statistic? A number of things:

- *Buckle up.* Use your seat belt and make sure children are securely buckled or, if young enough, placed in a children's car safety seat.
- *Obey the speed limit.* Each month more than 1,000 Americans are killed in crashes involving speeding.[46]
- *Stay sober.* Impairment of driving skills begins with the first drink and increases with each drink.

Let's also consider the dangers of driving while distracted, driving while drowsy, driving under the influence of alcohol or drugs, and road rage.

Driving while Distracted

Nineteen-year-old Aaron was driving home from a weekend with his girlfriend at 75 miles an hour when he felt he had to express his love by sending her a text message. He wound up pinned beneath a truck with two broken legs and injured his kidney, liver, and spleen.[47] Twenty percent of crashes resulting in injuries are due to distracted driving. The main risk faced by driving and phoning is loss of concentration, not fumbling with the phone.[48] According to Dr. Amy Ship of Harvard Medical School, "Driving while distracted is roughly equivalent to driving drunk."[49]

The U.S. government website for distracted driving, distraction.gov,[50] lists the following distractions:

- Texting
- Talking on a cell phone
- Eating and drinking
- Talking to passengers
- Grooming
- Reading, including maps

Figure 13-4 Top 10 Lifesavers on the Road[45]

This list identifies the 10 innovations in automotive safety that have saved the most lives over the last four decades.

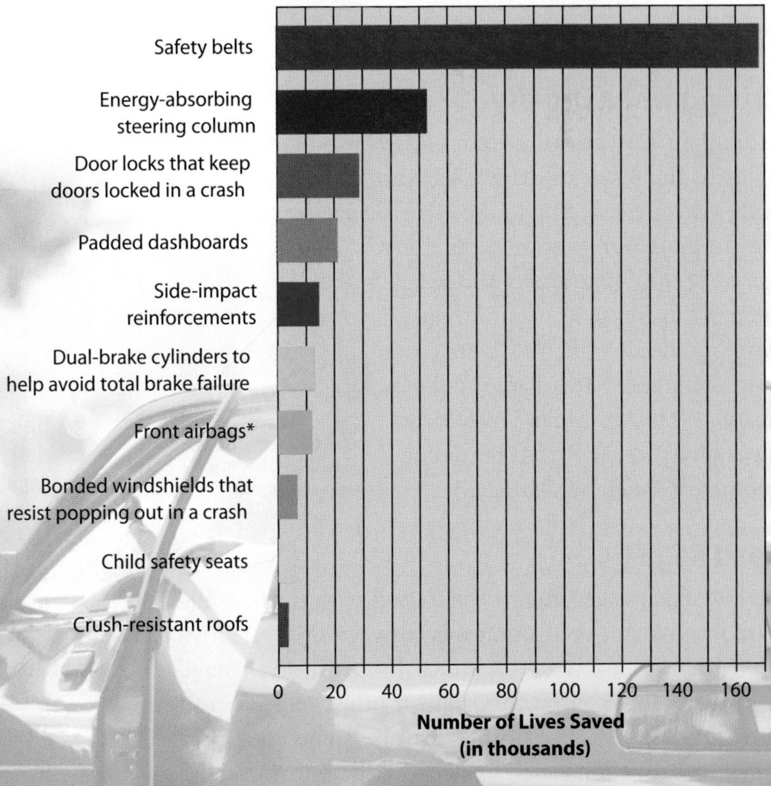

*Required only since 1990.

Table 13-2 Young People and Motor Vehicle Fatalities[51]

- Motor vehicle crashes are the leading cause of death for young adults 16 to 20 years of age.
- Drivers 16 to 20 years of age have the highest involvement rates for fatalities and injuries in passenger vehicle crashes, especially so for male drivers in this age range.
- Young drivers comprise about 6% of all licensed drivers but account for 12% of all drivers involved in fatal crashes and 15% of all drivers involved in police-reported injury crashes.

- Resetting a GPS unit
- Watching a video
- Changing the radio station, CD, or mp3 player

Fussing with a child in the back seat is also distracting. Although all forms of eating are distracting, foods that spill or ooze are a special problem (see the list of the worst offenders in the online feature "Prevention 13-2"). Table 13-3 shows the costs of distracted driving.

prevention

Access CourseMate for HLTH at www.cengagebrain.com.

Driving while Drowsy

More than 1,500 deaths occur each year on the nation's roads as the result of drivers who are drowsy or asleep at the wheel. According to the NHTSA, accidents involving sleepy drivers also account for some 71,000 injuries.[52] Accidents are most likely to occur in the early morning hours when drivers are most fatigued. (Read the online feature "Health Skills 13-6" for suggestions to keep from becoming another sleepy driver statistic.)

health skills

Access CourseMate for HLTH at www.cengagebrain.com.

Road Rage (!)

In road rage, anger due to frustration with traffic spills over into violent confrontations between drivers. Drivers with low levels of tolerance for frustration have come to blows, chased cars, cut off other vehicles, and even taken potshots at other drivers, sometimes over minor provocations such as beeping the horn or being passed. Cases of road rage may start with beeping the horn but escalate into exchanges of obscene gestures, tailgating, or even bumping into the other vehicle.

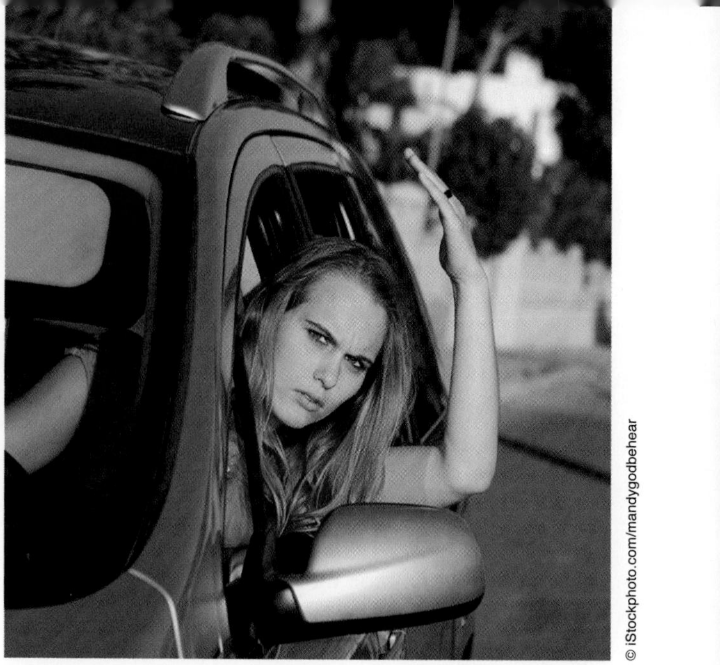

© iStockphoto.com/mandygodbehear

Road rage may lead to criminal acts in which a driver uses a motor vehicle as a weapon or pulls out another weapon to assault a driver or a passenger in another vehicle. Here are some tips to avoid becoming either a perpetrator or victim of road rage:

- *Never use your vehicle as a weapon or means of threatening other drivers.*
- *Be aware of glare.* Be aware of the potential consequences of glaring at another driver.
- *Don't get steamed.* Control your own anger. Don't respond to an aggressive or inconsiderate driver. Don't feel you need to teach him or her a lesson.

Table 13-3 Driving while Distracted[53]

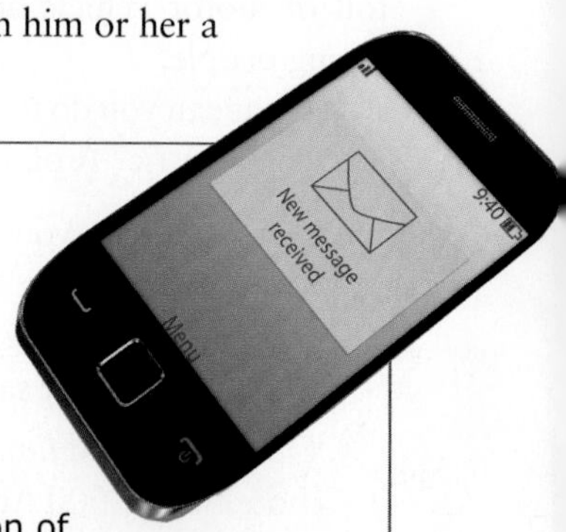

© iStockphoto.com/Alex Slobodkin

- Distracted driving is involved in one in six fatal automobile crashes.
- The under-20 age group has the highest proportion of distracted drivers involved in fatal crashes (16%). The age group with the next greatest proportion of distracted drivers is the 20- to 29-year-old age group—13% of all 20- to 29-year-old drivers in fatal crashes are reported to have been distracted.
- Cell phone distraction is reported for 24% of the 30- to 39-year-old distracted drivers in fatal crashes.
- Twenty-eight percent of the total number of crashes each year result from drivers talking on their cell phones or texting.

- *Keep a distance.* Maintain a safe distance from the car ahead of you on the road.
- *Don't drive aggressively.* Aggressive driving can easily escalate into a dangerous confrontation.
- *Don't beep.* Use your horn only to prevent an accident, not to express frustration or anger.
- *Do not respond to provocations.* If a hostile driver provokes you, don't respond and don't make eye contact. Let it pass.
- *Do not swear at or give another driver the finger.*
- *Keep your cool.* Don't let situations get out of hand.
- *Learn to control your anger.* Learn how to control the thoughts that make you angry before they lead to rage.
- If your community has a witness tip line, report dangerous drivers, or dial 911.

Cycling, Rollerblading, and Skateboarding

Driving a car has its risks, but they do not compare to the hazards of riding motorcycles. More than 5,000 people are killed in motorcycle accidents each year and some 96,000 are injured.[54] Mile for mile, motorcyclists are about 37 times more likely to die in a crash than are occupants of passenger cars. Motorcycles lack many of the safety features of cars and trucks. Unlike occupants of four-wheeled vehicles, the motorcyclist has no protective barrier of steel and padding. But motorcyclists can take steps to minimize their chances of being included in these statistics. According to the NHTSA, the helmet is the motorcyclist's most important piece of safety equipment. Helmets do not prevent crashes, but they reduce the risk of death by more than a third (37%).[55]

The NHSTA also recommends that motorcyclists participate in motorcycle safety programs, which include rider training and motorist awareness. Aggressive driving and use of alcohol figure prominently in many motorcycle crashes, as they do in automobile and boating accidents.

The value of wearing a helmet also applies to bicycling, rollerblading, and skateboarding. Wearing a bicycle helmet reduces the risk of suffering serious injuries to the head and brain injury by 85%.[56] Bicycle safety also includes obeying traffic signals, signaling before turning, using reflectors, and wearing brightly colored reflective clothing at night.

HEALTH APPS: YOUR LINK TO ONLINE HEALTH APPLICATIONS

health skills

Anger Management Are you a person who heats up under the collar at the slightest provocation? Your anger might pose a risk to others and to yourself. If you have problems managing your hostile feelings, "Health Skills 13-1" will show you how you can cope by identifying and correcting anger-inducing thoughts.

prevention

Rape Prevention How can you minimize your risk of being sexually assaulted? (Remember: By providing prevention information, we are not placing any blame on the victim. The rapist is always responsible for the assault.) Read "Prevention 13-1" for suggestions on how to protect yourself.

health skills

Combating Sexual Harassment Harassers often claim the charges against them are exaggerated or the person bringing charges "overreacted." The woman who assertively protects her rights may be branded a "troublemaker." Fair? No; abuse never is. For suggestions on how to deal effectively with sexual harassers, read "Health Skills 13-4."

health skills

Making Your Home a Safer Place The great majority of household accidents are preventable. The question is, how can we make our homes safer? Go to "Health Skills 13-5" for suggestions.

prevention

Eating while Driving? Really? Eating or drinking while driving distracts your attention from the road, but foods that drip, spill, and ooze are most likely to divert our attention. "Prevention 13-2" lists the top 10 food offenders.

health skills

How NOT to Sleep when Driving You can protect yourself from becoming another sleepy driver statistic by becoming better aware of the signs of drowsiness at the wheel and by following the suggestions in "Health Skills 13-6."

Go to the CourseMate for HLTH at www.cengagebrain.com for additional resources including flashcards, games, self-quizzes, review exercises, web exercises, learning checks, and more.

Managing Your Health Care

"The responsibility for managing your health care does not lie with physicians, government programs, or insurance carriers. It lies with you."

Laurie was 35. Her physician found a small lump in her breast and recommended follow-ups with scans and a biopsy. Laurie wouldn't have it. Instead she turned to a fierce regimen of exercise and dieting—eating only organic foods and wolfing down bottles of dietary supplements. She went for massages and Qigong, a form of "energy therapy." She chanted regularly before her Buddhist shrine. She meditated. Her chiropractor urged her to get the lump "worked up" and have whatever her physicians recommended—surgery, chemotherapy, radiation, hormone therapy. Still Laurie would have none of it. Nearly three years after the lump was discovered, she died from metastatic breast cancer.

Laurie rejected the health care system, and in her case, by doing so, she rejected life. Other people may not reject the system, but they have a difficult time navigating it.

Old movies still show the family doctor as a solo practitioner and someone who makes house calls. Today health care is more often a complex mix of medicine and big business. We are in an age of **managed care**, in which one hand is on the stethoscope and the other in the pocketbook. There is a bewildering array of health care plans and a sadder array of millions of people who cannot obtain any of them. We'll chart your way through the health care maze, deciphering acronyms such as HMOs, PPOs, and POS plans. We'll suggest ways you can protect yourself from *mis*managed care.

We'll also venture into complementary and alter-

managed care
A system of controlling health care costs by eliminating waste and unnecessary medical procedures.

Learning Outcomes

1 Discuss ways of managing your own health care

2 Describe the health care system in the United States

3 Discuss the benefits of health care insurance along with its drawbacks and inequities

4 Discuss complementary and alternative medicine (CAM)

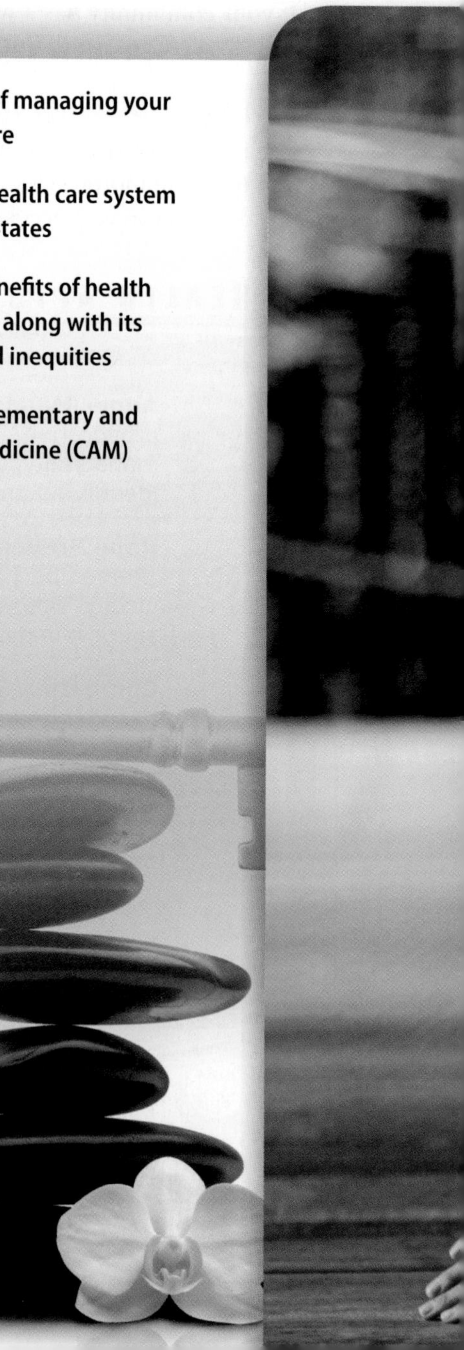

native medicine (CAM), as Laurie did—everything from acupuncture and aromatherapy to massage and meditation. We'll see that some people, like Laurie, use CAM rather than treatments prescribed by medical doctors. We'll also see that others use CAM as a supplement to conventional medical treatment.

But more broadly, this chapter is about you, the health care consumer. The responsibility for managing *your* health care does not lie with physicians, government programs, or insurance carriers. It lies with *you*. We each have a responsibility to become an active, informed health care consumer. We can take an active role in managing our health care by educating ourselves about our health care options, choosing our health care providers (HCPs), and weighing treatment alternatives carefully.

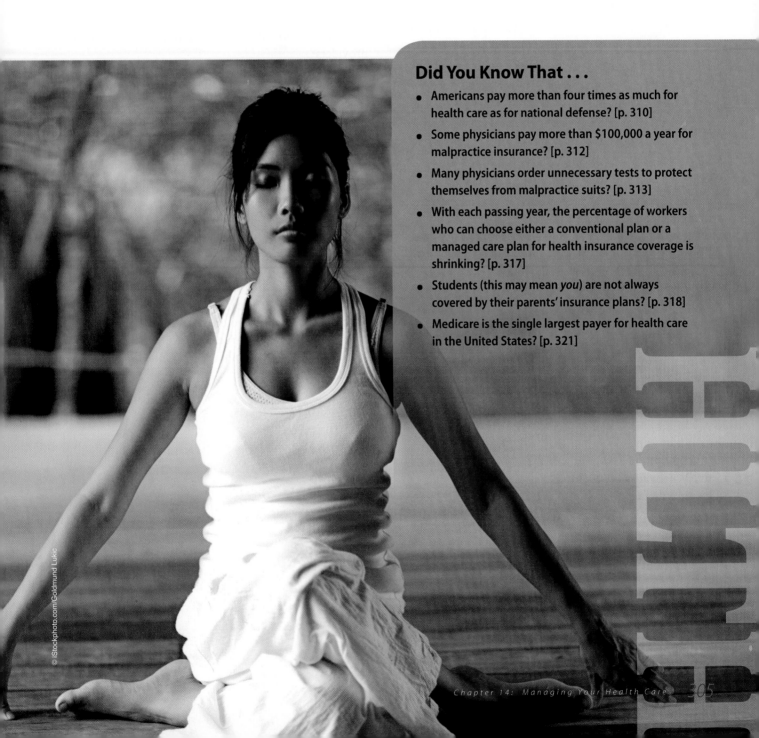

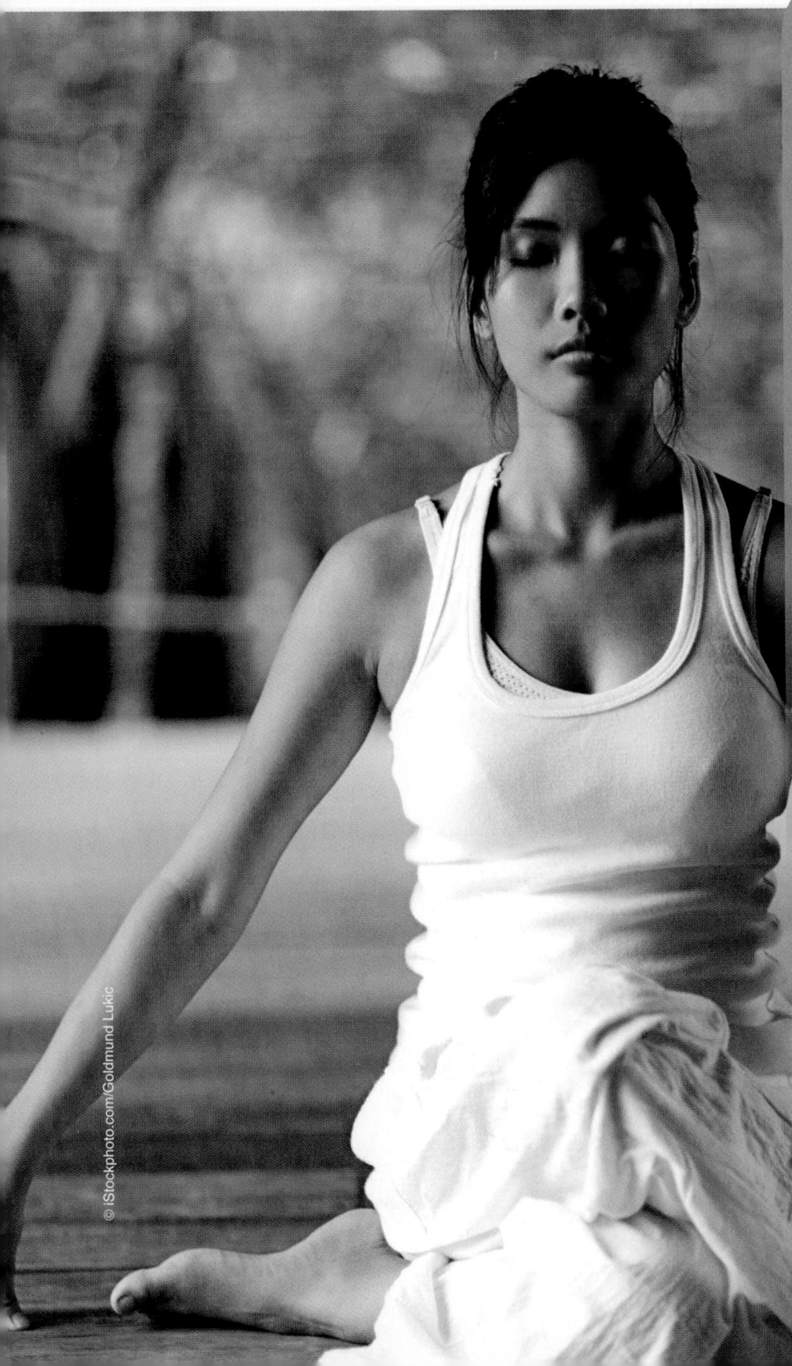

Did You Know That . . .

- **Americans pay more than four times as much for health care as for national defense? [p. 310]**
- **Some physicians pay more than $100,000 a year for malpractice insurance? [p. 312]**
- **Many physicians order unnecessary tests to protect themselves from malpractice suits? [p. 313]**
- **With each passing year, the percentage of workers who can choose either a conventional plan or a managed care plan for health insurance coverage is shrinking? [p. 317]**
- **Students (this may mean *you*) are not always covered by their parents' insurance plans? [p. 318]**
- **Medicare is the single largest payer for health care in the United States? [p. 321]**

Managing Your Own Health Care

You have probably heard the phrase "managed care." What you may not realize is that you are responsible for managing your own health care—wisely.

Some people are passive health care consumers. They wait until they get sick to seek health care or learn about health care options. They may carry an insurance card but know little about the services covered by their plan. Passive health care consumers typically do not get the best health care. They do not obtain regular physical examinations that might prevent the development or reduce the severity of serious and costly medical conditions.

☒ LEARNING OUTCOME 1

Discuss ways of managing your own health care

Passive health care consumers may see the health care system as too complicated to understand. Their attitudes and beliefs undercut their motivation to manage their own health care—"I prefer to leave medical matters in the hands of my doctor," "I do not really care what it costs, my insurance will cover it anyway," and, "I assume that all health care providers are competent and have my best interests at heart."

In contrast, people who take an active role in managing their health care ask their health care providers questions—plenty of them—to assure they get the best quality care. They see themselves, and not their HCPs or their insurance carriers, as ultimately responsible for managing their own health care. They take steps to protect themselves from mismanaged care.

What about you? Are you an active or a passive health care consumer? Evaluate whether you actively manage your own health care by completing "Health Check 14-1" on pages 308 and 309. Then ask yourself what changes you can make in your attitudes and behavior to get the most out of your health care.

Now let's see how you can choose a primary care physician, how you decide to call or see her or him, and how you can reap the most benefit from your interactions.

Choosing a Primary Care Physician

Many people spend more time picking out a new flat-screen TV than selecting a primary care physician. They may assume (wrongly) that all physicians are equally competent. Or they may not think they have the knowledge or competence needed to make an informed choice. True enough, the average consumer may not be able to judge medical competence. And medical boards do not routinely evaluate physicians' skills. Even well-informed patients may not know whether their doctors' skills are sharp or whether they keep abreast of the latest medical developments.

Despite the difficulty of judging medical competence, health consumers can do much toward making better-informed decisions about their health care providers:

Get recommendations. Ask around. Seek recommendations from friends and family members, especially people whose opinions you trust. Be aware, however, that what is important to one person, such as a physician's availability during weekend hours, may be relatively unimportant to another. It may be helpful to ask other medical professionals whom they would use themselves or to whom they would refer a sick relative. Another suggestion: Call your local medical center or medical school and ask for the unit or department in the area of specialty that you are inquiring about, such as pediatrics, internal medicine, or OB/GYN. Ask to speak to the head nurse on the unit. Explain that you are seeking a primary care physician and would like a recommendation for two or three doctors in your area. Nurses interact with a large number of doctors and may be able to give you an unbiased recommendation. Once

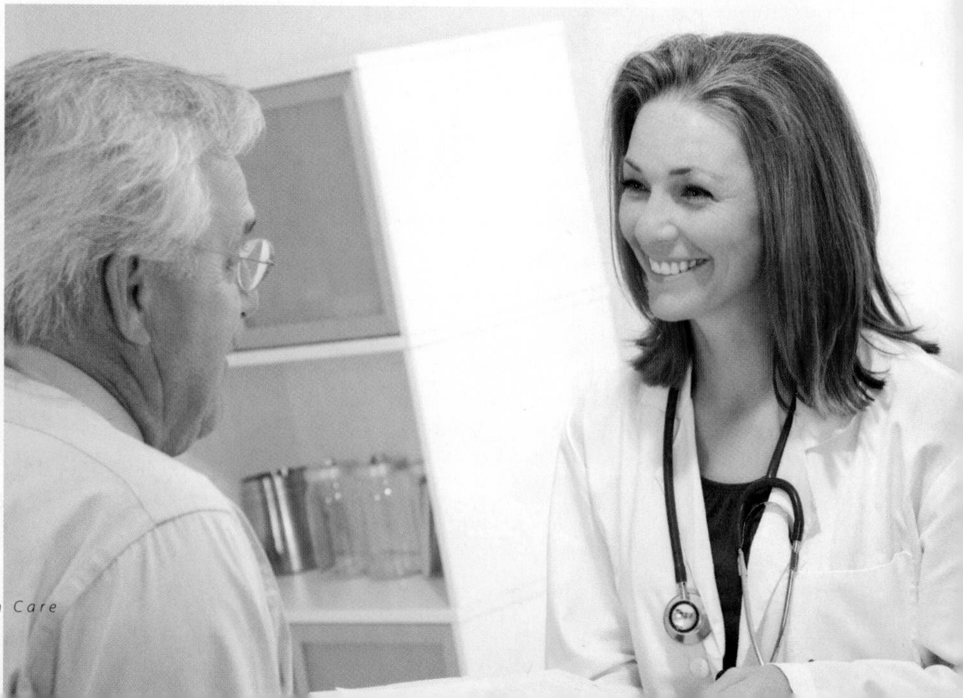

© iStockphoto.com/Steve Debenport

you have established a relationship with a primary care physician, use this person as a resource to check out the skills of any specialists you may need.

Set up an appointment. Selecting a primary care physician is one of the most important health care decisions you may ever make. This is the person in whom you place your trust for overseeing your health care and monitoring changes in your health status from year to year. Before making a choice, take a "test drive." Make an appointment for a brief interview or for a routine physical exam or consultation for a relatively minor medical problem. Then consider whether the physician makes the grade on the following key factors:

- ☑ *Empathy*. Empathic physicians relate to their patients in a warm and supportive manner. They express understanding and concern for their problems and complaints. They have what used to be called a "good bedside manner." Ask yourself the following questions:
  - Does the physician seem genuinely interested in me as a person, or do I seem to be just another case?
  - Does the physician take the time to get to know something about my background and health concerns? Or does the physician seem impatient or curt in his or her responses?
  - Does the physician seem to be the kind of person who will be available to me in times of medical need?
- ☑ *Availability.* Ask about office hours, coverage for medical emergencies, weekend and evening availability, and backup coverage during vacations. Ask whether he or she offers opportunities for phone consultation and how quickly you can expect a return call.
- ☑ *Ability to communicate medical information in language you can understand.* Steer clear of a doctor who speaks only in "doctorese." Likewise, avoid someone who is vague in giving answers or doesn't take the time or have the ability to explain medical information in a way that you can clearly understand. You can't make informed choices regarding your medical treatment if you don't understand the options available to you.
- ☑ *Credentials.* Don't be shy about asking the doctor about his or her professional background. Pose questions such as the following:
  - What medical school did you graduate from?
  - Where did you complete your residency training, and in what area or areas?
  - In which specialty areas are you board certified?

  Check out whether your doctor is board certified. Increasingly, board certification is becoming a minimum standard that doctors must meet to obtain hospital privileges and be accepted in managed care plans. Studies demonstrate that board certified doctors tend to provide better care than noncertified physicians. Also inquire about the hospitals with which the doctor is affiliated to check on the doctor's standing in the hospital and to make sure the hospital itself is accredited by the national accrediting body, the Joint Commission on Accreditation of Healthcare Organizations. More-prestigious hospitals tend to weed out doctors with questionable records. You may also want to select a doctor who practices in a hospital in your area that has a good reputation.

  You can check your doctor's credentials by using the American Medical Association's *Directory of Physicians in the United States*, a book that contains information about each doctor's medical and residency training, hospital affiliations, teaching positions, and board certification. Many public libraries have copies of the directory. You can also find out whether your doctor is board certified in his or her specialty area by calling the American Board of Medical Specialties at 1-866-ASK-ABMS (or www.abms.org). Don't be misled by the designation "board eligible." This means that the doctor has completed the required residency training in a specialty area but has not yet taken the required exam to become certified or may have flunked it.

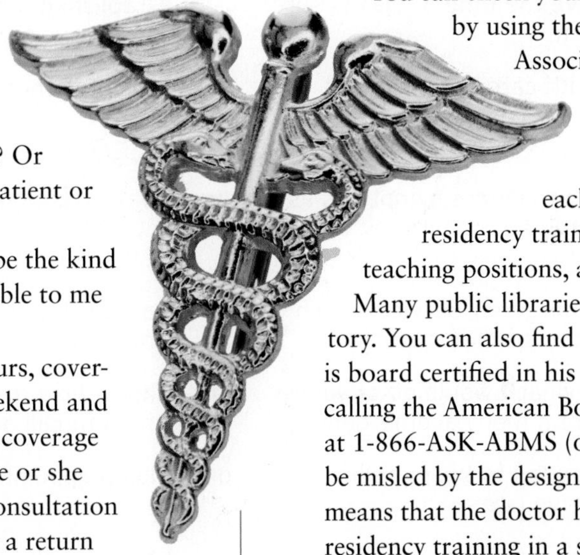

© Fuse/Jupiterimages

Now that you have a primary care physician, how do you decide when to see her or him?

Deciding When to Seek Help

Being a rugged individual is fine—as long as you remain rugged. Part of responsible management of your health is knowing when *not* to go it alone. Here are some suggestions for when to seek help:

- If you experience sudden pain that doesn't fade quickly.

Are You an Active Health Care Consumer?

Are you an active or passive health care consumer? Circle the statement that best represents your beliefs and attitudes concerning your health care and then consult the key that follows:

I put off thinking about my health care until a health care need arises.	or	I regularly consider my health care needs and plan ahead to meet them.
I don't know how to locate a personal physician and other health care providers (HCPs) in my area.	or	I have established a relationship with a primary HCP and other HCPs, such as a dentist and (if I'm female) a gynecologist.
I'm not aware of the major hospitals and clinics in my area or what services they provide.	or	I know the major health care facilities in my area, what services they offer, and how to get to them in case of emergency.
I don't have a list of phone numbers for hospitals and doctors I can call for help.	or	I keep handy a list of phone numbers and know whom to call for medical needs.
I have skipped regular medical exams because I didn't have the time or wasn't sure how to arrange them.	or	I have regular medical exams and have established a relationship with a primary HCP who knows my health history.
I cannot afford health care and have not made arrangements in case I need medical services.	or	I maintain health care coverage.
To be honest, I tend to ignore symptoms as long as possible in the hope that they will disappear.	or	I pay attention to any changes in my body and bring symptoms to the attention of my HCP in a timely manner.
I sometimes use emergency services, such as emergency rooms, for minor problems.	or	I always try to work through my primary HCP when I am in need of care.
I really don't know what I would do or where I would go in case of a medical emergency.	or	I know how to handle a medical emergency—whom to call and where to go.
I sometimes or often fail to keep medical appointments or arrive late.	or	I keep appointments and arrive on time.
I sometimes or often fail to call to cancel appointments ahead of time.	or	I always call to cancel appointments when necessary.

continued

- If you have symptoms you don't understand that do not go away on their own, such as a persistent burning sensation when you urinate, a rash that does not fade, or any kind of unexplained pain.
- If you experience unexplained pain in the chest or in an arm or a shoulder, especially when accompanied by shortness of breath.
- If you have had an accident—or have been assaulted!—and you are experiencing loss of blood, sizeable lacerations (cuts) of the skin, difficulty breathing, difficulty moving, loss of consciousness, or difficulty remaining awake and alert.
- If you are having persistent or recurrent diarrhea.

HEALTH CHECK 14-1, continued

I sometimes hold back information from my HCP or believe that doctors should be able to figure problems out by themselves.	or	I readily offer information to my HCP and describe my symptoms as clearly as possible.
I sometimes or often omit information on medical histories due to embarrassment, forgetfulness, or carelessness.	or	I give complete information and do not withhold, embellish, or distort information about my health.
I sometimes or often fail to pay attention to the doctor's instructions.	or	I listen carefully to instructions and ask for explanations of my condition and treatment.
I generally don't ask my physician to explain medical terms I don't understand.	or	I always ask my doctor to explain technical terms I don't understand.
I generally accept what my doctor tells me without questioning.	or	I ask questions when I don't understand or agree with the diagnosis or treatment plan.
Sometimes I don't fill prescriptions or take medications according to schedule.	or	I follow instructions and call the doctor or pharmacist for clarification when necessary.
I sometimes fail to keep follow-up appointments or neglect to update my HCP on my condition.	or	I reliably keep follow-up appointments and make update calls when indicated.
I simply stop following a treatment that has troubling side effects or no apparent effects and don't inform my HCP.	or	If a treatment doesn't appear to be working or produces negative effects, I call my HCP before making changes in the treatment plan.
I don't examine medical bills carefully, especially those that are paid by my insurance company.	or	I carefully examine bills for any errors or duplication of services and bring discrepancies to the attention of my HCP.
I don't question charges for medical services, even if they seem excessive or inappropriate.	or	I question my HCPs about charges that seem excessive or inappropriate.
I generally neglect filling out insurance claim forms for as long as possible.	or	I promptly complete insurance forms and send them in.
I generally don't keep records of my medical treatments and insurance claims.	or	I keep complete records of my medical visits and copies of insurance claim statements.

Interpreting Your Score. Statements in the left-hand column reflect a passive approach to managing your health care. Statements in the right-hand column represent an active approach. The more statements you circled in the right-hand column, the more active a role you are taking in managing your health care. For statements circled in the left-hand column, consider whether it is to your advantage to change your behavior to become an active rather than a passive health care consumer.

- If you are experiencing an unexplained loss of weight or unexplained changes in your sleeping habits.
- If your nail beds, lips, mouth, or skin take on a bluish color.
- If you are experiencing unexplained bleeding or a discharge from a body opening.
- If your temperature spikes up to 103°F, or if you have a persistent or recurrent fever.
- If you feel a lump under your skin, or swelling, or a sore that grows or does not fade away.
- If you believe that you are pregnant, or if an over-the-counter test kit shows that you are pregnant.

- If a health care provider recommends a schedule for certain kinds of check-ups and the time has come.
- If a health care provider recommends further workup of a symptom or a condition. Laurie's fatal mismanagement of her breast cancer began with refusal to follow her doctor's recommendation for further workup.

Throughout this book you have seen that early diagnosis and treatment of problems is most likely to lead to a cure or, depending on what is wrong, control of an unhealthful condition or a disease. You have also seen that men are generally more reluctant than women to seek help. Many men see themselves as being take-charge kinds of guys—but not necessarily when it comes to being active about their health care.

Now that you have decided to seek help, let's see how you can make the most of your visit.

Being Seen *and* Being Heard by Your Doctor

Hearing "The doctor will see you now" is not only an invitation to be seen. It is also an invitation to be *heard*. People who take an active role in managing their health care let their doctors know what is ailing them and gather the information they need to make informed decisions about treatment. Consumers' biggest complaint about health care is that they feel rushed by their physicians. Though your doctor's time may be valuable, you have the right to ask your doctor to take the time to explain your condition and recommended treatment in language you understand. When communicating with your doctor:

- *Describe your symptoms and complaints as clearly and as fully as possible.* Don't hold back, cover up, or distort your symptoms. By the same token, don't embellish your symptoms or repeat yourself. If your doctor interrupts you, say something like, "Doctor, if I may just finish. I'd like you to have the full picture . . ." If your doctor seems more interested in ushering you out the door than in hearing you out, find another doctor.
- *Don't accept a treatment recommendation that you don't want.* If your doctor's rationale for treatment leaves you shaking your head, get another opinion. Laurie wasn't happy with her doctor's recommendation for medical workup of the lump in her breast, but she didn't go for a second opinion. Instead, she made the unwise choice of deciding not to follow the recommendation.
- *Insist on explanations in plain language.* Another patient complaint is that the doctor does not explain things clearly—in language they understand. You can't make informed choices about treatment options if your doctor does not help you understand them.
- *Don't be swayed by a doctor who says your problems are "in your head."* Doctors may not take complaints seriously when there are no findings upon physical examination or from laboratory tests, especially if symptoms seem vague, like feelings of fatigue. If your doctor is stumped, you may need to consult another doctor.

Health Care, U.S.A.

LEARNING OUTCOME 2

Describe the health care system in the United States

The health care system isn't a system as much as it is a loosely coordinated network of health care providers, government programs, and health insurance and managed care companies. The system is based on the altruistic motives of preventing and caring for people with health problems, but it is also big business. Very big business. Health care is the second largest industry in the United States, exceeded only by retailing. Americans spend more than four times on health care what they spend for the national defense.[1] Yet despite these expenditures, one American in six remains uninsured.[2]

Change may be in the offing. The 2010 health care reform act provides additional health care protection and benefits to consumers and extends health care insurance to the previously uninsured. The health care act, called the Affordable Care Act, will be implemented gradually. When fully implemented, it will extend insurance benefits to an estimated 32 million people, providing insurance coverage to 95% or more of all Americans.[3] The health care act also focuses on prevention and wellness services so that diseases can be prevented or treated at the earliest possible stages. One of the law's provisions—if it withstands legal challenges—will require most Americans to obtain or purchase health care insurance.[4] Table 14-1 provides a summary of key aspects of the health care reform act.

The health care reform act also creates a competitive health insurance marketplace, scheduled to begin in

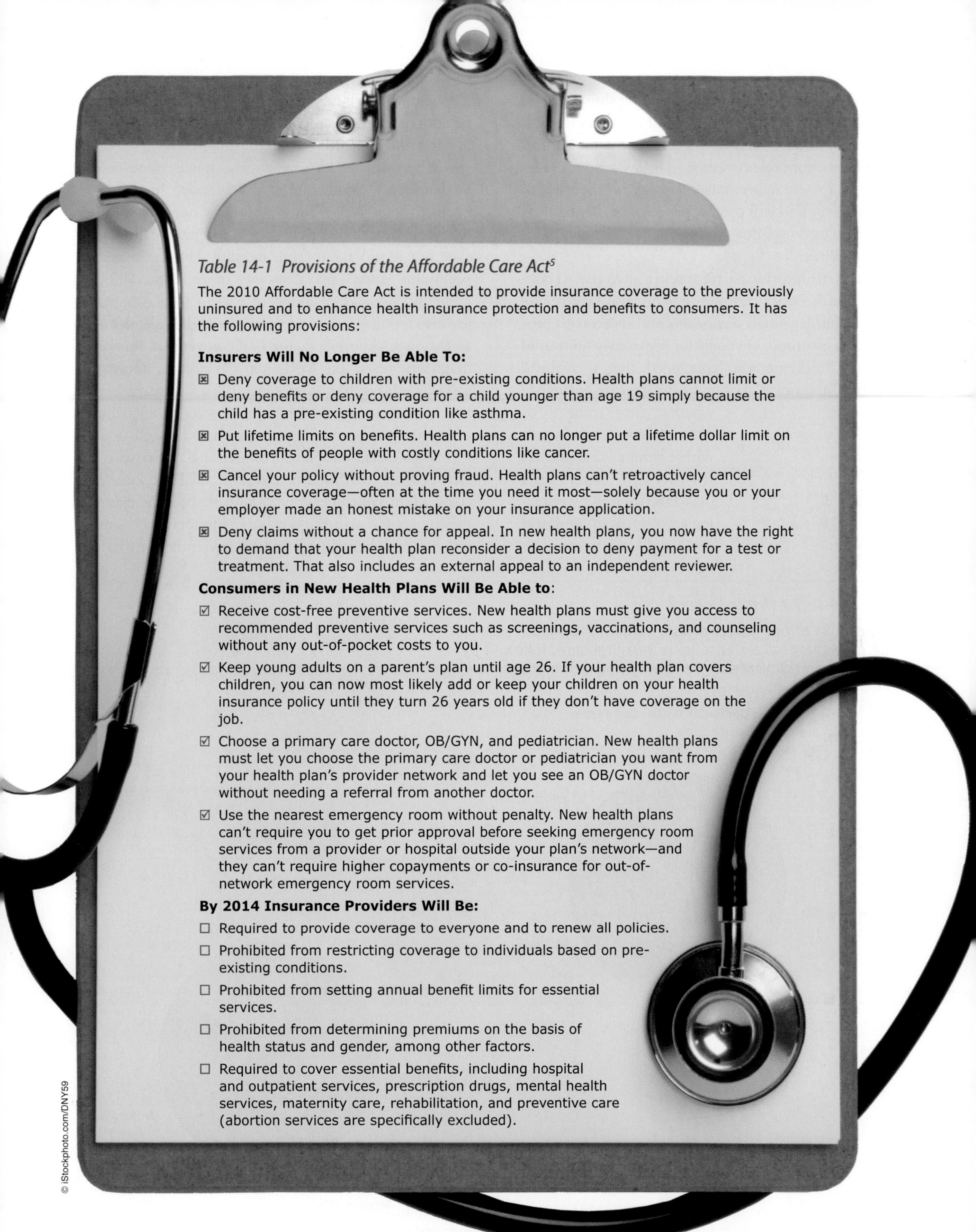

Table 14-1 Provisions of the Affordable Care Act[5]

The 2010 Affordable Care Act is intended to provide insurance coverage to the previously uninsured and to enhance health insurance protection and benefits to consumers. It has the following provisions:

Insurers Will No Longer Be Able To:

- ☒ Deny coverage to children with pre-existing conditions. Health plans cannot limit or deny benefits or deny coverage for a child younger than age 19 simply because the child has a pre-existing condition like asthma.
- ☒ Put lifetime limits on benefits. Health plans can no longer put a lifetime dollar limit on the benefits of people with costly conditions like cancer.
- ☒ Cancel your policy without proving fraud. Health plans can't retroactively cancel insurance coverage—often at the time you need it most—solely because you or your employer made an honest mistake on your insurance application.
- ☒ Deny claims without a chance for appeal. In new health plans, you now have the right to demand that your health plan reconsider a decision to deny payment for a test or treatment. That also includes an external appeal to an independent reviewer.

Consumers in New Health Plans Will Be Able to:

- ☑ Receive cost-free preventive services. New health plans must give you access to recommended preventive services such as screenings, vaccinations, and counseling without any out-of-pocket costs to you.
- ☑ Keep young adults on a parent's plan until age 26. If your health plan covers children, you can now most likely add or keep your children on your health insurance policy until they turn 26 years old if they don't have coverage on the job.
- ☑ Choose a primary care doctor, OB/GYN, and pediatrician. New health plans must let you choose the primary care doctor or pediatrician you want from your health plan's provider network and let you see an OB/GYN doctor without needing a referral from another doctor.
- ☑ Use the nearest emergency room without penalty. New health plans can't require you to get prior approval before seeking emergency room services from a provider or hospital outside your plan's network—and they can't require higher copayments or co-insurance for out-of-network emergency room services.

By 2014 Insurance Providers Will Be:

- ☐ Required to provide coverage to everyone and to renew all policies.
- ☐ Prohibited from restricting coverage to individuals based on pre-existing conditions.
- ☐ Prohibited from setting annual benefit limits for essential services.
- ☐ Prohibited from determining premiums on the basis of health status and gender, among other factors.
- ☐ Required to cover essential benefits, including hospital and outpatient services, prescription drugs, mental health services, maternity care, rehabilitation, and preventive care (abortion services are specifically excluded).

2014, which will offer a one-stop online shopping site that will allow consumers and small businesses to compare prices, benefits, and health plan performance and to purchase affordable coverage.[6] The law also provides tax credits to help many consumers pay for their health care insurance and will protect people from losing their health care coverage due to job loss, job changes, relocation, or illness.

The 2010 health care reform act gave rise to controversy, with critics claiming it will raise health care costs and burden small companies and insurers to provide health insurance coverage for previously uninsured persons. Critics are also concerned that it requires individual Americans to obtain health care insurance whether they want it or not. Advocates counter with estimates that the act will actually lower costs over time (in part by reducing enrollment in Medicaid costs and use of expensive emergency health care services by previously uninsured persons) and that the nation is responsible for providing affordable health care to all Americans.

malpractice
Failure of a professional to render proper treatment, especially when injury or harm occurs as a result.

Why does health care cost so much? One reason is that many doctors practice defensive medicine to protect themselves from **malpractice** suits. They order tests and procedures that may not be medically necessary but shield them from liability. Higher insurance premiums (some specialists pay more than $100,000 annually) are passed along in patient fees. Americans are also living longer, and people need more health care as they age. Another factor is the advent of expensive diagnostic tests, like MRIs and CAT scans, and medical procedures like angioplasty and coronary artery bypass surgery. Figure 14-1 shows where your trillions of health dollars come from and where they go.

Still another reason for rising health care costs is the lack of incentives for consumers or HCPs to constrain costs. Many consumers do not directly bear the brunt of these costs. Costs are largely borne by employers as medical insurance premiums and by government programs

Figure 14-1 Our Health Dollars[7]

About 40% of our health dollars come from private sources. The single largest expense is for hospital care, followed by physician and clinical services and prescription drugs.

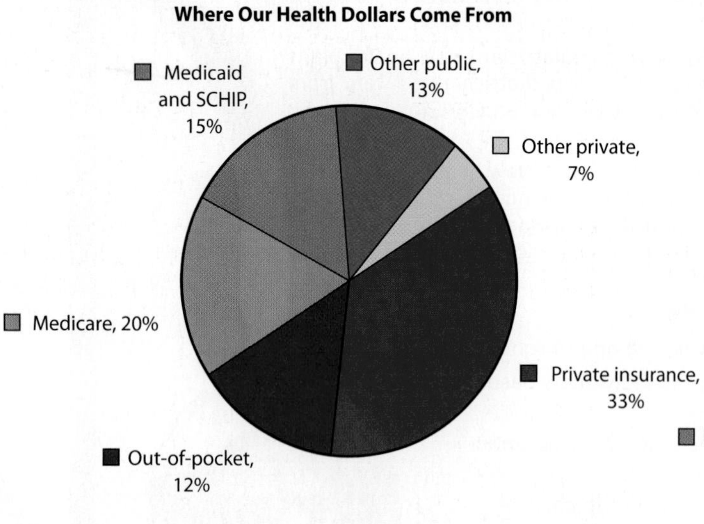

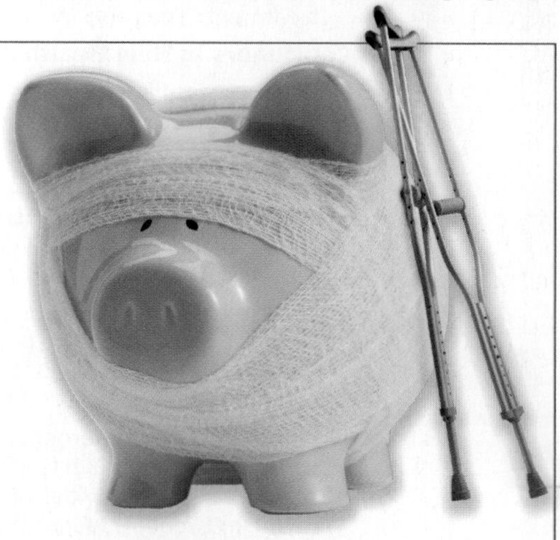

© iStockphoto.com/DNY59

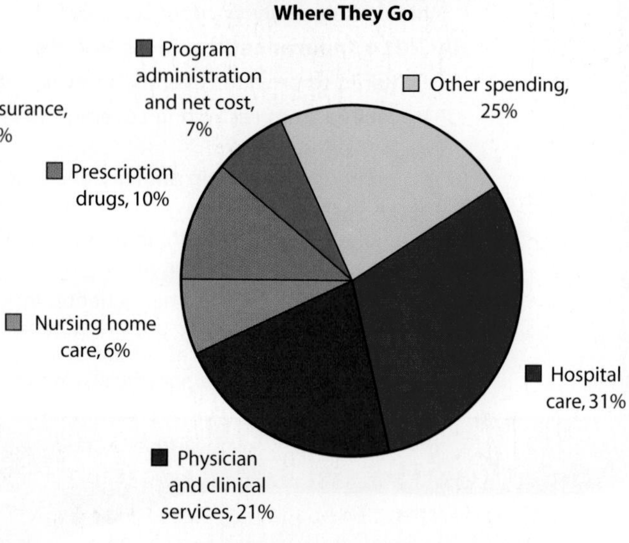

like Medicaid and Medicare, which provide care for older people, the disabled, and the poor. The lack of incentives to curtail costs results in unnecessary procedures, duplication of services, and inefficiency.

The health care system is in flux. Large employers, joined by state and federal governments, are balking at footing the ever-rising health care bill. General Motors has been referred to, tongue-in-cheek, as an HCP that happens to also make cars. Employers are turning to managed care companies that promise to contain costs while providing quality health care. Managed care may cost a bit less but, as we will see, it deprives consumers of certain choices.

Worries about health care run deep and are not limited to concerns about managed care. People worry about whether they will be able to obtain health insurance or keep it if they are laid off. The uninsured include nearly one in seven young people under the age of 18 and more than one in four 18- to 24-year-olds. Figure 14-2 shows that the problem is worse among ethnic minorities.[8]

Figure 14-2 Percentage of Persons without *Health Insurance Coverage, by Race/Ethnicity—United States*[9]

Latin Americans and Native Americans have the highest percentages of uninsured persons. Latin Americans are nearly three times as likely to lack health insurance as European Americans.

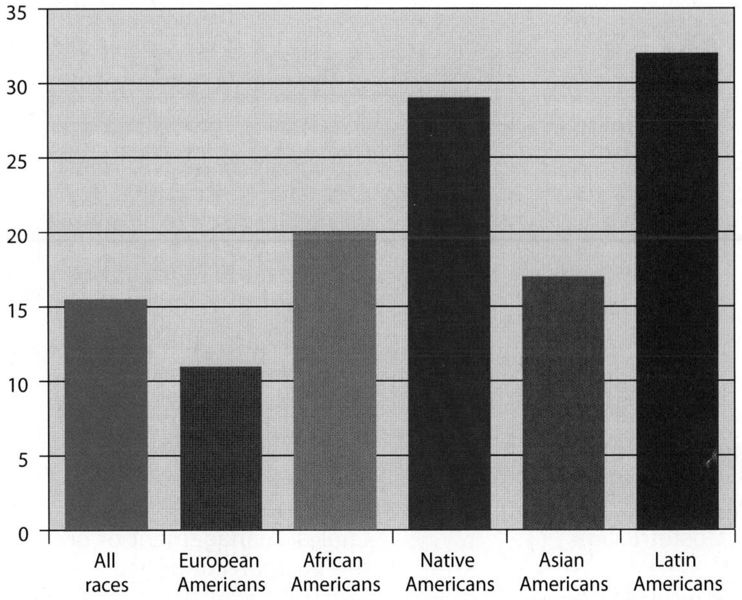

Let us review the types of HCPs and facilities available today. Then we look at various health care plans and what they may mean for you.

Types of Health Care Providers (HCPs)

Though we typically think of a health care provider as a physician, many HCPs perform other roles. There are physicians, nurses, and technicians as well as *allied health professionals* such as dentists, psychologists, optometrists, and pharmacists.

Physicians

Physicians hold either a Doctor of Medicine (MD) or a Doctor of Osteopathy (DO) degree. (Osteopaths make up 5% of the physicians in the United States.) Physicians complete a four-year postgraduate medical curriculum followed by an internship and residency. Training for MDs and DOs is similar except that osteopathy places somewhat greater emphasis on the musculoskeletal system. Physicians are licensed by the states in which they practice to diagnose health problems and treat them by methods such as medicine, radiation, and surgery.

Most physicians were once family doctors or general practitioners (GPs). Today, most are specialists (see Table 14-2 on the next page). Physicians become specialists through residency training. They become board certified by passing a formal examination in their specialty. Practitioners of internal medicine, general pediatrics, and family medicine provide the bulk of primary care. The percentage of medical students intending to specialize has been increasing because of the expansion of medical knowledge and complex medical technologies. On the other hand, the growth of managed care, which uses primary care physicians as gatekeepers for specialists to control costs, is increasing demand for generalists.

Nurses

Nurses are the largest professional group in health care. Yet the demand for their services appears to continually outstrip the supply.[10] As a result of this escalating demand, nurses' salaries are expected to increase significantly.

The majority (about 75%) of registered nurses (RNs) work in hospitals, but about one in four works in independent practice, private duty, public health, occupational health, nursing education, student health, extended care, and ambulatory care. RNs vary in their educational backgrounds and duties:

Table 14-2 Types of Medical Specialists

Allergists	Diagnose and treat allergies
Anesthesiologists	Administer anesthetics and monitor the condition of patients under anesthesia
Cardiologists	Diagnose and treat heart disease
Dermatologists	Diagnose and treat skin diseases
Emergency physicians	Diagnose and treat conditions resulting from trauma or sudden illness
Endocrinologists	Diagnose and treat conditions and diseases of the glands of internal secretion
Family physicians	Diagnose and treat a wide variety of conditions affecting all family members
Geriatricians	Diagnose and treat conditions affecting older people
Gynecologists	Diagnose and treat conditions affecting the female reproductive organs
Internists	Diagnose and treat conditions involving anatomy and physiology of internal body organs
Nephrologists	Diagnose and treat conditions involving the kidneys
Neurologists	Diagnose and treat conditions involving the central nervous system
Obstetricians	Clinical management of pregnancy, labor, delivery, and the postpartum period
Oncologists	Diagnose and treat cancer
Orthopedists	Diagnose and treat conditions involving the musculoskeletal system
Pathologists	Examine bodily tissues for presence of disease or abnormalities
Otolaryngologists	Diagnose and treat diseases of the ear, nose, and throat
Pediatricians	Diagnose and treat diseases of children
Proctologists	Diagnose and treat conditions involving the rectum and anus
Psychiatrists	Diagnose and treat nervous or mental disorders
Urologists	Diagnose and treat diseases of the urinary system in females and the genitourinary system in males

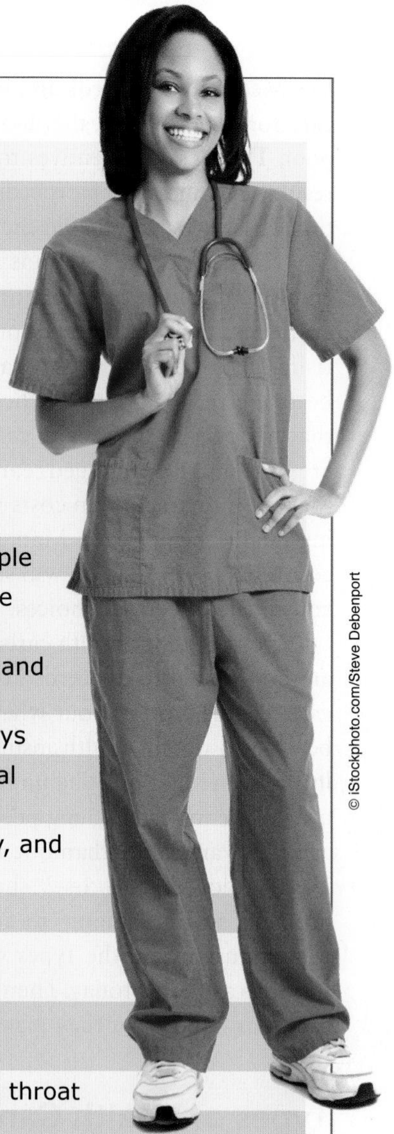

1. *RN, Associate Degree*: Has completed a two-year program earning an associates degree (AD). The majority of these RNs are employed in hospitals.
2. *RN, Diploma*: Has completed a three-year program usually affiliated with a hospital.
3. *RN, Bachelor of Science Degree*: Has completed a four-year program in a college or university and earned a Bachelor of Science in Nursing (BSN) degree. Professional options are greater than for an RN with an AD or diploma.
4. *RN, Nurse Practitioner*: Has completed a bachelor's and master's program in nursing (or a practitioner program). Nurse practitioners work in different capacities, including *family nurse practitioners*, who specialize in treating families, and *obstetrics-gynecology nurse practitioners*, who specialize in women's health.
5. *RN, Clinical Nurse Specialist*: Has completed a bachelor's and master's degree in nursing while specializing in a field such as cardiovascular disease, pulmonary disease, pediatrics, gerontology, or psychiatry. Roles for the clinical nurse specialists are broader and include clinician, manager, educator, consultant, and researcher in their specialty fields.
6. *RN, Certified Nurse-Midwife:* Has been educated in both nursing and midwifery in either a master's degree or certification program. May be

self-employed, work in birthing centers, nurse–physician practices, or hospitals.

7. *RN, Nurse Researcher and/or Nurse Educator*: Has completed at least a bachelor's and master's degree and possibly a doctoral degree in nursing. These RNs may teach in nursing programs in universities, colleges, or hospital-affiliated programs.

Many other health care professionals serve in allied fields, such as dentistry. They work cooperatively with physicians and nurses to provide comprehensive health care.

Dentists

Dentists complete a bachelor's degree and four years of dental school, earning either a Doctor of Medical Dentistry (DMD) or Doctor of Dental Surgery (DDS) degree. Dentists diagnose and treat diseases of the teeth, gums, and oral cavity and provide preventive dental care. They may prescribe drugs and perform surgery as needed in the treatment of dental conditions.

Technicians

Medical technicians serve many functions, such as drawing blood, taking X-rays or MRIs, doing laboratory work, or assisting dentists as oral hygienists. Depending on their positions and where they live, they have various kinds of education, training, and college degrees.

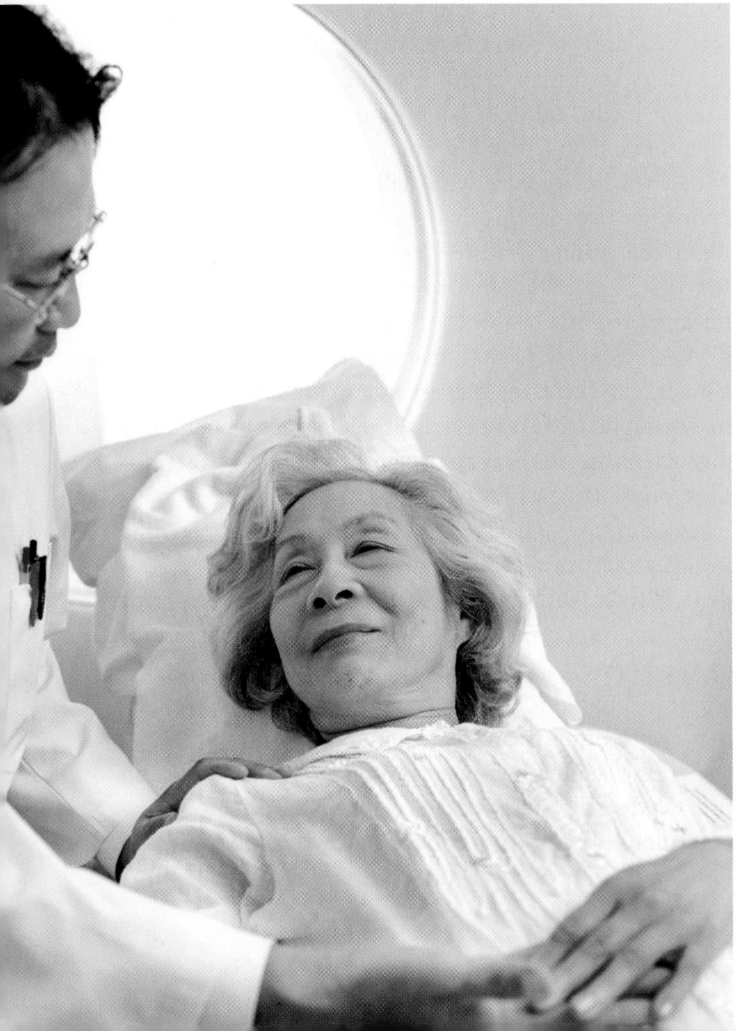

Physicians' Assistants

Physicians' assistants (PAs) are typically trained in university settings at the bachelor's level and take a state test for licensure. They work under a physician's supervision and perform certain medical procedures, such as suturing superficial wounds. PAs typically practice in hospitals, clinics, or physicians' offices.

Pharmacists

Pharmacists complete at least a bachelor's degree in pharmacy and may have additional training at the master's or doctoral levels. Pharmacists dispense medications and advise patients concerning proper use of medications and possible complications, including side effects.

Psychologists

Psychologists typically hold a doctoral degree—PhD, PsyD, or EdD. Psychologists use psychological tests to help diagnose mental disorders and they treat these disorders by means of psychotherapy.

Optometrists

Optometrists obtain the Doctor of Optometry (OD) degree. They are qualified to perform vision tests and prescribe and fit corrective glasses and contact lenses. Medical conditions affecting the eyes are treated by *opthamologists*, medical doctors who specialize in diseases of the eye.

Health care consumers need to be acquainted with the backgrounds and roles of HCPs. When in doubt, ask your HCPs to discuss the scope of their practices and the types of services they can provide in meeting your health care needs.

Types of Health Care Facilities

Health care is delivered in many different kinds of facilities ranging from doctor's offices to hospitals.

Hospitals

There are community and municipal hospitals, Veterans Administration hospitals, and long-term care facilities, such as psychiatric hospitals and rehabilitation centers. Hospitals vary in their services and capacities to house patients. A small rural or community hospital may be able to provide inpatient care for fewer than 25 patients, employ only a few nurses and ancillary staff, and limit their services to the basics, such as medical-surgical, labor and delivery, caring for the newborn, laboratory work, and pharmaceutical services.

Larger hospitals are typically located in metropolitan areas and may be affiliated with schools of medicine and nursing. In addition to direct care, larger hospitals often have teaching and research functions. They may have hundreds of beds and employ thousands of professionals (for example, nurses, doctors, and laboratory technicians) and ancillary staff (for example, secretaries, administrators, aides, and maintenance workers). They may have coronary care and intensive care units, specialized clinics and diagnostic services, trauma units, social services, and rehabilitation and long-term care facilities.

With increasing pressures on hospitals to contain costs, many carry out elective surgery on an outpatient or ambulatory care basis whenever feasible. Advances in surgical procedures have enabled many patients to go home on the same day or on the day following surgery. Minimizing hospital stays reduces costs and appeals to patients who prefer to recuperate at home.

Extended Care Facilities

Hospitals have increasingly become intensive care facilities that provide acute treatment for trauma and disease. The reasons for this are largely economic. Hospitals are labor intensive and expensive to operate. Insurance companies and government payers seek lower-cost alternatives to extended stays, such as extended care facilities, hospices, and home health care.

Extended care facilities include nursing homes and convalescent homes. These institutions provide long-term medical, nursing, or custodial care for patients with chronic physical illness and disability that prevents them from living independently. **Rehabilitation centers** treat patients suffering from stroke, spinal cord injuries, degenerative diseases, and other disabling conditions. They seek to restore patients to their maximal level of functioning and independence. Psychiatric hospitals provide long-term care to people with severe mental disorders, such as schizophrenia. **Hospices** provide care that respects the dignity of the terminally ill.

rehabilitation center
Health care facility that provides comprehensive medical, physical therapy, occupational therapy, and mental health services to help people with disabilities achieve a maximum level of functioning.

hospice
Interdisciplinary health care program that provides services to terminally ill patients, either in the home or in a hospice facility, that address the medical, spiritual, emotional, and economic needs of patients and their families.

Home Health Care

Many people with severe or prolonged health problems receive home health care. Home health care enables infirm older people to remain at home rather than be moved to a nursing home or other institution. Home health care typically costs far less than comparable treatment in hospitals or residential facilities. The types of home health care services offered vary with the needs of the patient. They may include visits by a registered nurse who is needed to perform such procedures as catheterizations, injections, and changes of dressings; regular visits by trained home care aides who provide custodial care, such as bathing, eating, and dressing; and visits by physical therapists.

Outpatient Facilities

Most health care services are offered on an outpatient basis and housed in a hospital, clinic, or medical office. In medical centers affiliated with medical schools, clinics may function as part of the school and participate in training medical students and residents.

Many colleges and universities operate outpatient student health centers. These centers provide services to students and in some cases to faculty members, staff members, and their families. Some student health centers also provide inpatient care. (To actively manage your own health care, you will of course get regular medical exams. Read the online feature "Prevention 14-1" to learn what to expect during a routine health checkup.)

prevention

Access CourseMate for HLTH at www.cengagebrain.com.

Groups of physicians may form an outpatient clinic. Clinics may offer diagnosis and treatment services in one or more areas of specialization. Clinics may include physicians, nurses, nurse specialists and nurse practitioners, physician assistants, and support staff.

Community health centers (CHCs) are public health clinics that serve traditionally underserved residents. Private physicians in these areas may be scarce or unwilling to accept patients without private insurance or the ability to pay themselves. CHCs treat patients who are eligible for Medicaid and Medicare, as well as those with other forms of coverage.

A physician who practices alone or in a small group practice usually specializes in a particular area of practice, such as pediatrics, gynecology, or family practice. Physicians in group practices may use outside support services such as labs and X-ray facilities, or have their own. They may also employ RNs or form partnerships with nurse practitioners or certified nurse midwives.

Health Insurance

A doctor's visit can cost hundreds of dollars, even more for a specialist. In addition to the doctor's fee, there are lab tests and sophisticated diagnostic tests, such as the MRI, which can cost several hundred dollars or more. The costs of hospitalization and surgery can quickly exceed the reach of all but the wealthiest among us. Were it not for medical insurance, quality medical care might be limited to the wealthiest few. A variety of programs are presently available to help Americans afford health care: (1) private health insurance, including traditional insurance ("fee-for-service") plans and managed care plans, (2) government insurance such as Medicaid and Medicare, and (3) public health programs, such as well-baby clinics (WBCs) and family planning clinics.

LEARNING OUTCOME 3

Discuss the benefits of health care insurance along with its drawbacks and inequities

Medical care is shifting from traditional fee-for-service insurance plans to managed care. About three of four workers belong to a managed care plan. The rise in the utilization of managed care is fueled by the rise in conventional, fee-for-service insurance premiums—paid largely by employers. Managed care plans promise to constrain rising costs.

The percentage of workers given a choice about their health care coverage has been shrinking. Employees are being forced to enroll in managed care plans or to use physicians from a designated provider list. Many are asked to pay more for doctor visits, to contribute more to annual premiums, and to pay larger **deductibles**.

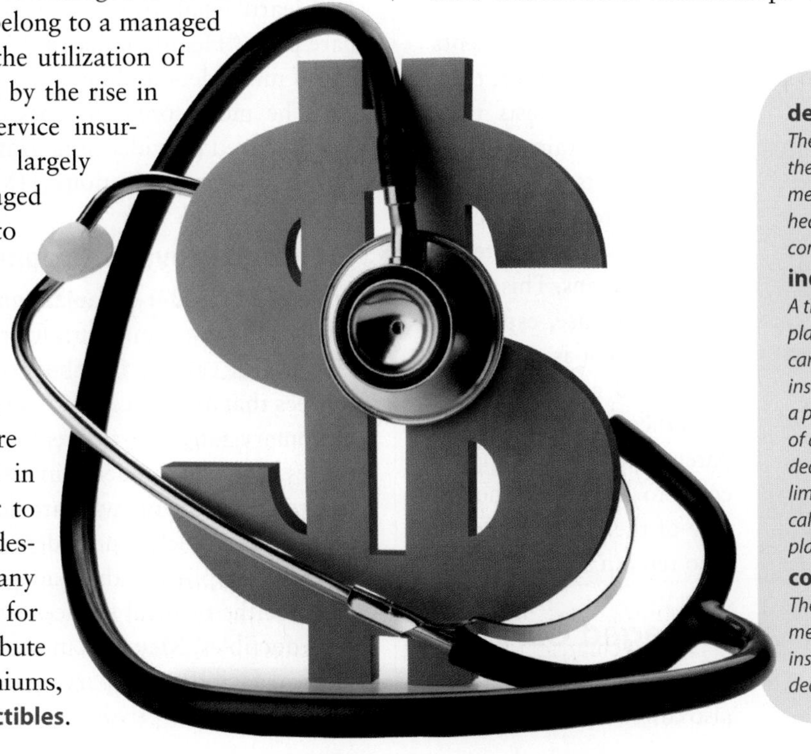
© iStockphoto.com/DNY59

Let us take a closer look at the two major types of health insurance plans: indemnity insurance plans ("fee-for-service" plans) and managed care plans. Knowing these plans' advantages and disadvantages helps us to make informed decisions regarding our health care. (Learn more about this important decision by reading the online feature "Health Skills 14-1.")

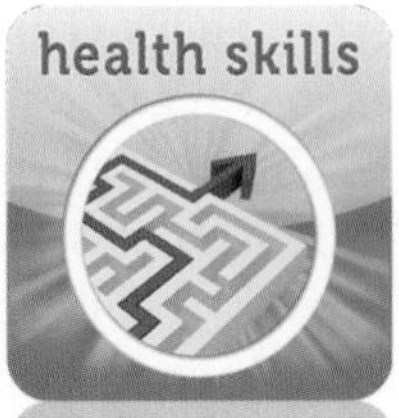

Access CourseMate for HLTH at www.cengagebrain.com.

Indemnity Insurance Plans (Fee-for-Service Plans)

Indemnity, or fee-for-service (FFS), plans offered by such carriers as Blue Cross/Blue Shield and other large insurance companies were once the standard form of private health insurance. Today, however, only about one in four working Americans who receive health insurance through their jobs is covered by one of them. Under an FFS plan, you can use any licensed physician or other HCP (such as a podiatrist), or use the services of any accredited hospital, and the plan will pay for a certain proportion—usually 80%—of the charges once an annual deductible is met. **Coinsurance** is the percentage of the bill that the insured person must pay, or co-pay.

Some plans also impose an *annual* or a *lifetime cap*. These are the maximum amounts they will cover for a particular condition within a given year or the person's lifetime. Under an indemnity plan, insurance carriers have nonexclusive relationships with physicians and

deductible
The annual amount that the individual must pay for medical expenses before the health insurance plan starts contributing its share.

indemnity
A traditional type of insurance plan in which the insurance carrier or employer (for self-insured employers) pays for a predetermined percentage of all medical bills after deductibles and barring any limitations or exclusions. Also called fee-for-service (FSS) *plan.*

coinsurance
The percentage of costs for medical services that the insured person must pay after deductibles are met.

other HCPs. This means that HCPs are free to treat anyone regardless of their insurance coverage.

In this traditional "unmanaged" plan, the insurance carrier processes claims and pays bills for services rendered by HCPs at rates that reflect customary and reasonable charges. Charges imposed by doctors in excess of charges that the insurance company deems reasonable are not covered. For this reason, it is prudent to check with your insurance carrier to determine the limits on their coverage before undergoing expensive medical procedures, such as elective surgery. You may be able to find health care practitioners, including surgeons, whose charges fall within the plan's guidelines. Or you might ask your HCPs whether they are willing to reduce their fees to the level set by your insurance company. Don't be hesitant about asking for a fee reduction if you fear that the costs may exceed your insurance coverage or ability to pay. Plans also vary with respect to their restrictions and limitations, so check the fine print. Such services as dental work and vision tests and eyeglasses are commonly not covered. Plans also limit coverage to treatments they deem medically necessary and effective.

Indemnity plans are usually purchased by employers for their employees as part of a benefits package. The broader the coverage, the greater the cost. In some cases, employees are required to contribute a portion of the annual premiums. Individuals or families may also purchase health insurance for themselves, though usually at higher cost than the comparable plans offered to large employers.

Colleges and universities may provide students with opportunities to purchase health insurance, typically at lower costs than they could obtain on their own. Students may assume that they are automatically covered by their parents' insurance plans. This is not always the case, especially if the student is no longer considered a minor. Some insurance companies offer parents an option (at higher cost) to cover the health care of their adult children who remain students.

capitated
In the context of managed care, a fixed dollar amount that the individual or the employer must pay for membership in the plan, regardless of how much medical services the individual uses.

copayment
A predetermined set amount the individual must pay for medical services.

preferred provider organization (PPO)
A group of health care providers who agree to provide health care services to members of a managed care plan for a discounted rate.

Managed Care

A managed care plan is also called a *prepaid health insurance plan*. In such plans, a group of doctors or hospitals, or more typically, a health benefits company, agrees to provide health care services to individuals or groups of employees for a prepaid amount of money. Premiums are usually **capitated**. That is, the managed care company gets a certain amount of money for each member (enrollee) in the plan, regardless of how much medical care the member requires. Large employers usually foot the bill for these annual premiums, though individuals may pay a fixed annual fee plus a modest **copayment** (typically $5 or $10) for each doctor's visit, with few if any deductibles. If members choose to see a doctor who is not on the list of approved HCPs, they can expect to pay more or all of the bill.

The assumption underlying managed care is that it is possible to reduce costs while maintaining quality care by cutting unnecessary or unduly expensive medical tests and procedures. A managed care plan might more accurately be described as a *managed costs* plan, since it attempts to provide health care while containing costs. Managed care companies employ case managers and health care professionals as "gatekeepers" who oversee referrals for consultation with specialists, use of expensive diagnostic tests (such as MRI), and medical procedures. Managed care companies also monitor the referral practices of doctors in their networks. In some cases, the plans reward doctors for limiting their use of outside specialists and medical tests, and penalize those they see as wasteful. (As an active health care consumer, you must ask questions and learn what you can expect from your managed care plan. "Health Skills 14-2" coaches you on how to avoid misunderstandings.)

The most common types of managed care plans are preferred provider organizations (PPOs) and health maintenance organizations (HMOs).

Preferred Provider Organizations (PPOs)

Preferred provider organizations (PPOs) are groups of HCPs who agree, in return for patient referrals, to provide health care to members of a managed care plan for fees that are typically 15% to 20% lower than their customary rates. Physicians treat patients in their own offices as they do under conventional FFS plans and are free to treat patients who are not members of the plan. Plan members select providers from the preferred provider list supplied by the managed care company, which pays for the medical services less required copayments or deductibles. Members may also select doctors or use medical facilities not participating in the plan but will pay more for the privilege.

HEALTH SKILLS 14-2

Avoid *Mis*managed Care

Successful managed care is a two-way responsibility. Managed care organizations should provide quality medical care and disclose service limitations and incentives for limiting patient care. Active health care consumers can protect themselves against *mis*managed care by:

- *Discussing coverage for hospital stays.* If you're planning major surgery, find out in advance what costs your managed care company will cover and how long a period of hospitalization you'll be permitted.
- *Insisting on your right to see a specialist.* Ask whether your doctor participates in any incentive program or feels pressured to minimize referrals to specialists. If your doctor doesn't provide straightforward answers, shop around for another doctor. If you feel that your condition calls for a specialist and one is not available to you as a member of the managed care plan, demand one. If you must go outside your plan to obtain a specialist's services, have the specialist cite the medical findings that justify the need for these services.
- *Learning what to do in case of emergencies.* If you are faced with a medical emergency, your first concern is to get proper care, not to haggle over costs with your managed care company. But before an emergency arises, you should take the time to learn about the provisions in your plan for obtaining emergency care.
- *Appealing refusal of coverage.* If you are refused coverage for services not covered by your plan, file an appeal. (The appeal process is typically laid out in the plan's handbook.) Document the need for services. Include supporting documents from physicians who referred you or provided the services. If an appeal doesn't succeed, your employer's benefits manager may be able to help. You may also file a formal complaint with your state department of insurance, which establishes a paper trail supporting your case. You can also consult a lawyer.

Health Maintenance Organizations (HMOs)

A **health maintenance organization (HMO)** is a prepaid medical service plan that offers medical and surgical services through affiliated doctors and hospitals or freestanding clinics. More than half of all employees in company-sponsored health insurance plans belong to HMOs (see Figure 14-3 on the next page).

As the managed care field continues to evolve, the structure of HMOs and their relationships with participating HCPs are growing more complex. HMOs vary in terms of where services are provided (individual doctor's offices, group practices, or staffed medical care settings) and the type of contractual relationship with participating doctors (exclusive versus nonexclusive; employee versus independent contractor).

The traditional HMO is a **staff model HMO** in which the company operates a community-based clinic or health facility that offers a range of services from primary care to specialty clinics. The physicians on staff treat only HMO members. The basic drawback of the staff model HMO is that many patients are reluctant to give up their usual doctors or the choice of doctors in their communities. Consequently, HMOs have been moving toward models that allow members greater flexibility.

In the **point-of-service (POS)** plan, members of the HMO can use HCPs within an approved network of HCPs or go outside the network for a higher per-visit charge. HCPs in the network may have an exclusive or nonexclusive relationship with the HMO.

Managed Care: Pros and Cons

Managed care companies are typically for-profit business ventures. When outlays for medical expenses fall below the capitated (per subscriber) level, the managed care company makes money. When outlays exceed the capitated level, the company may lose

health maintenance organization (HMO) *A prepaid type of managed care plan in which the costs are usually capitated according to a fixed amount of money per enrollee.*

staff model HMO *A type of HMO that offers comprehensive health care services within a free-standing clinic or health center that employs its own doctors, nurses, and allied health professionals.*

point-of-service (POS) *A type of HMO that offers its members the choice of using doctors within its network of providers or choosing their own doctors at higher cost.*

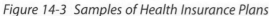

Figure 14-3 Samples of Health Insurance Plans

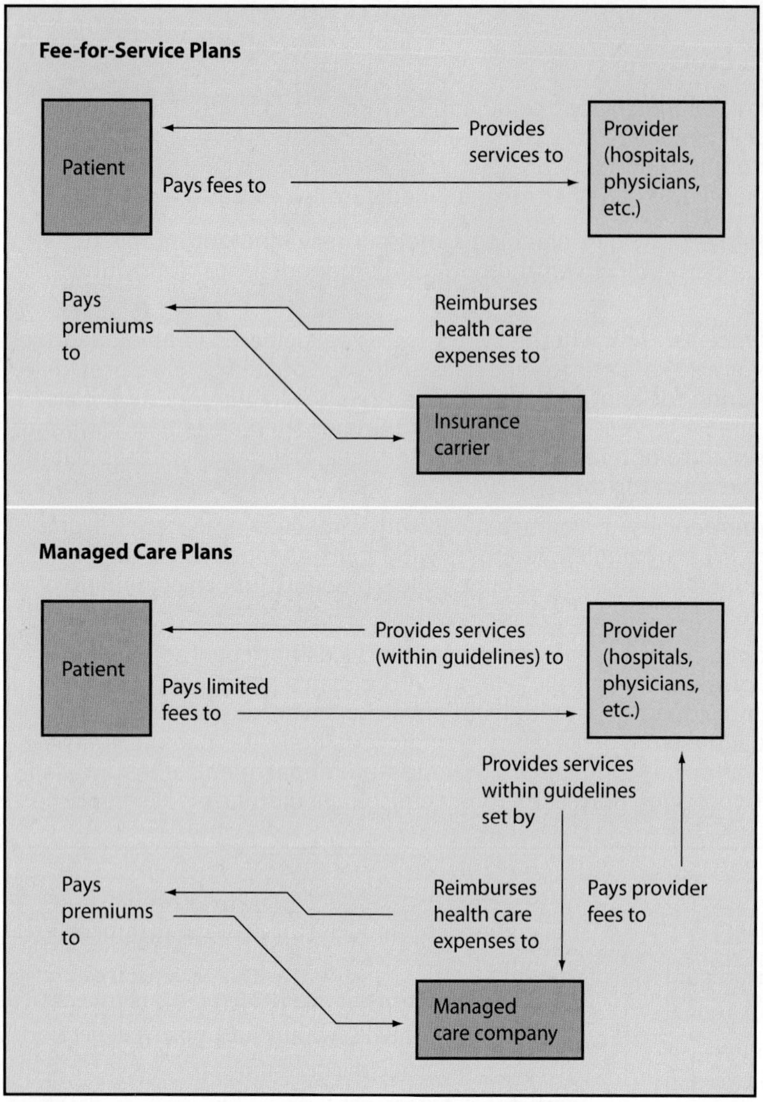

money. Since the company seeks to maximize profits, it strives to contain medical expenses. Many people are rightly concerned that the profit motive may lead companies to cut corners in providing medical care. Critics contend that managed care companies restrict the range of medically necessary services in various ways, as in denying benefits for some services, making other services less accessible, excluding expensive drugs, and making members and primary care physicians jump through hoops to get certain services approved. Adjusting to the constraints of managed care has left many consumers angry and confused.

Critics also contend that managed care systems may compromise the integrity of the physician–patient relationship. Plans may reward physicians for limiting their use of expensive diagnostic tests and referrals to specialists or other ancillary services. Plans may also drop doctors who refer too many patients for expensive tests or procedures. For these reasons, doctors may have conflicting loyalties between their own self-interests and the patient's best interests. Physicians are bound by the ethics of their profession to put the patient's interests first. But even so, the need for many procedures falls within gray areas, and physicians may now and then opt for a bonus rather than the highest level of patient care.

Patients, of course, may not know that available procedures and treatments are being withheld. Critics argue that physicians should divulge potential conflicts of interests to their patients, to state regulators, or both. In fact, some states now require such disclosure. The federal government has also placed limits on the bonuses that HMOs can pay doctors for controlling costs for services to Medicare and Medicaid patients. Patients should not hesitate to ask their HCPs for full disclosure of financial incentives that might pose a conflict of interest. If the HCP asks why you want to know, or appears evasive, you may want to find another HCP.

Supporters of managed care plans argue that they offer a wider range of services, including preventive care (for example, annual checkups, well-baby care, and mammograms) and vision examinations, than typical FSS plans do. They also offer low or no deductibles and lower out-of-pocket expenses for medical visits (typically a $5 or $10 copayment rather than a 20% contribution under an FSS plan). Many plans now offer a wider choice of HCPs, including opportunities for members to use outside HCPs, albeit at a higher cost. Since managed care companies do not receive higher fees for providing more services under capitation, they stand to gain by emphasizing preventive services. Supporters of managed care also argue that sufficient controls exist to ensure that necessary medical care is provided, including medical ethics, fear of malpractice suits, and oversight by state regulators. With an eye toward improving quality of care, some companies conduct surveys of patients and reward doctors for achieving higher ratings by patients.

Table 14-3 A Health Care Bill of Rights for Managed Care Patients[11]

- The health care provider is required to place the patient's interests first.
- The health care provider is required to push for care that will benefit the patient's health.
- The health care provider is required to discuss all treatment options, even options not covered by the plan. The patient can then decide whether or not to appeal for coverage of an uncovered option or to go outside the plan.
- There should be established adequate means for appealing disputes.
- Plans should disclose limitations of restrictions in coverage to prospective members deciding whether or not to join.
- Plans should not encourage or permit substandard care.
- Plans should disclose incentives to health care providers that limit care.
- Plans should limit the incentives health care providers receive for limiting care.

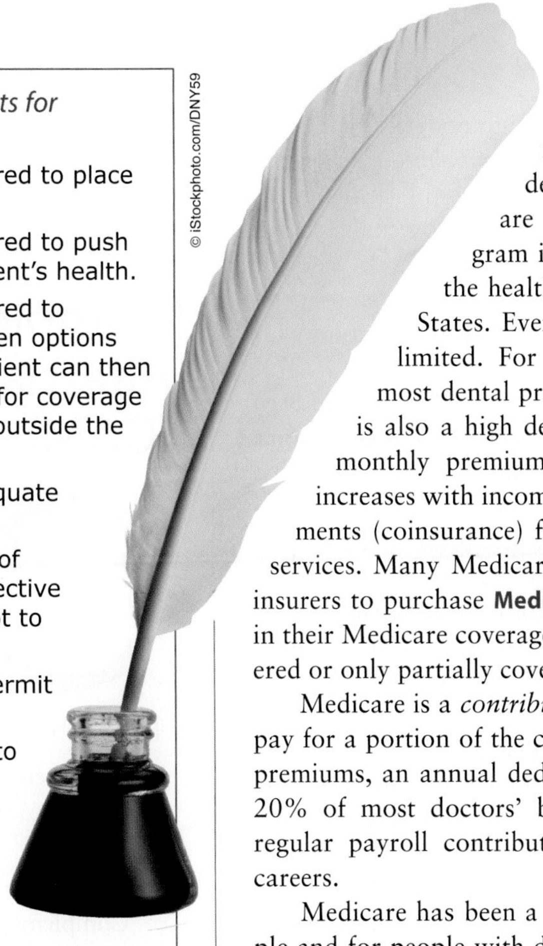
© iStockphoto.com/DNY59

The American Medical Association has issued a bill of rights for members of HMOs and other managed care plans. Though the bill of rights doesn't carry the force of law, it does govern what is expected of physicians who participate in these plans (see Table 14-3).

Americans are clearly worried about their health insurance. Many people fear that their health benefits will be reduced or that their health care will become unaffordable. They fear having a more limited choice of physicians and being forced by their employers to join managed care plans. Will the health care delivery system appease these concerns or add fuel to the fire?

Government-Sponsored Health Care Programs

Two major government programs, Medicare and Medicaid, provide health care services to the poor, to people with disabilities, and to older people.

Medicare

Medicare is the nation's health care program for older people and people with disabilities. The program pays for most medical expenses and prescription drug costs for eligible individuals (after deductibles and copayments are met). The Medicare program is the single largest payer in the health care system in the United States. Even so, Medicare coverage is limited. For example, it doesn't cover most dental procedures or dentures. There is also a high deductible for inpatient care, monthly premiums for outpatient care that increases with income level, and required copayments (coinsurance) for most outpatient medical services. Many Medicare recipients turn to private insurers to purchase **Medigap policies** to fill the gaps in their Medicare coverage for services either not covered or only partially covered by Medicare.

Medicare is a *contributory program.* Beneficiaries pay for a portion of the costs in the form of monthly premiums, an annual deductible, and copayments of 20% of most doctors' bills. Employees also make regular payroll contributions during their working careers.

Medicare has been a great benefit for older people and for people with disabilities, but concerns are mounting about the financial security of the program. Costs for maintaining the program have been rising steadily. Though some costs are offset by contributions from beneficiaries, most are borne by current workers through payroll deductions and from matching contributions from employers. The Medicare system faces a financial shock wave as millions of baby boomers reach retirement age and become eligible for benefits.

One effort to control Medicare costs ties hospital reimbursement to criteria based on *diagnostic related groups (DRGs).* The DRG is a classification system based on patient's age, diagnosis, and the procedures used. It is used to predict the use of hospital services, including length of stay, for patients with specific medical conditions. It sets fixed fees that hospitals can collect for these patients. If costs exceed those called for by the designated DRG, the hospital must accept the shortfall. If costs are less than the allowable costs, the hospital can bring in more money.

Medicare
A federally sponsored program that provides health care coverage for older Americans and people with disabilities.

Medigap policy
An insurance policy with a private carrier that fills gaps in Medicare coverage.

Medicaid

Medicaid provides medical care to poor people. Unlike Medicare, Medicaid is a *noncontributory program.* People do not pay premiums to receive benefits. Medicaid is funded by federal and state governments. The federal government funds most of the costs, and the states contribute the balance. Teaching hospitals, community health centers, and inner-city physicians provide the bulk of services to Medicaid patients.

Like Medicare, the costs for Medicaid have been rising rapidly. In an attempt to curtail rising costs, some states have cut Medicaid benefits. Others have moved Medicaid beneficiaries into managed care plans, typically HMOs. HMOs package health care programs for Medicaid recipients on a fixed per-person basis, which promises to reduce the costs for medical services. However, as HMOs expand into Medicaid, concerns have been raised that they will simply sign up Medicaid recipients but withhold needed care to minimize their costs. This is especially threatening to the most vulnerable populations, such as the disabled and chronically ill, who consume the lion's share of medical services under Medicaid. These fears may be well-founded, since older people and poor people with chronic medical conditions like diabetes and hypertension fare more poorly under managed care than under conventional insurance plans.

Public Health Programs

Public health programs emphasize preventive health care. They are relatively poorly funded in this country, because most medical resources are focused on treatment rather than prevention (read the online feature "Prevention 14-2" to learn more about that). Examples of public health programs include child health clinics (CHCs), family planning clinics, programs providing supplemental food for low-income women and their children, and immunization programs. Many public health programs offer services on a **sliding scale**. Fees are based on ability to pay. Public health programs probably do more to decrease human suffering and with less state and federal support than any other sector of the health care system (see "Diversity 14-1" on pages 324 and 325).

Medicaid
A federal program that provides health care benefits to the poor.

sliding scale
A system for adjusting fees according to the patient's income level.

complementary medicine
Health care practices and products that are used along with conventional medicine.

alternative medicine
Health care practices and products that are used instead of conventional medicine.

prevention

Access CourseMate for HLTH at www.cengagebrain.com.

Complementary and Alternative Medicine (CAM)

Complementary and alternative medicine (CAM) refers to medical and health care practices and products that are not part of conventional medicine. Although some CAM approaches have at least some scientific support, important questions remain as to whether CAM therapies are safe and effective preventatives or remedies for the diseases or conditions they target.

LEARNING OUTCOME 4

Discuss complementary and alternative medicine (CAM)

Complementary medicine and alternative medicine are not the same thing. **Complementary medicine** is used along with conventional medicine, as in the use of aromatherapy to increase a patient's comfort after surgery. **Alternative medicine** is used instead of conventional medicine, as in the use of diet rather than surgery, radiation, or chemotherapy to treat cancer. *Integrative medicine* combines conventional medical therapies with CAM methods for which there is some scientific support.

Medicine is evolving, and some nontraditional techniques of today may enter the mainstream of medical practice tomorrow if they are shown to be effective. The National Center for Complementary and Alternative Medicine (http://nccam.nih.gov/health/whatiscam/) is the government agency charged with assessing the effectiveness and safety of CAM.

Complementary and alternative medicine includes many specific techniques and practices, such as those shown in Table 14-4 on pages 326 and 327, as well as alternative medical systems of theory and practice to those in conventional American medical practice. Some of these systems were developed in Western cultures but stand apart from standard medical practice, such as homeopathic medicine and naturopathic medicine. Other systems were developed in non-Western cultures, such as Ayurvedic medicine and traditional Chinese medicine. Most people who use CAM to treat them-

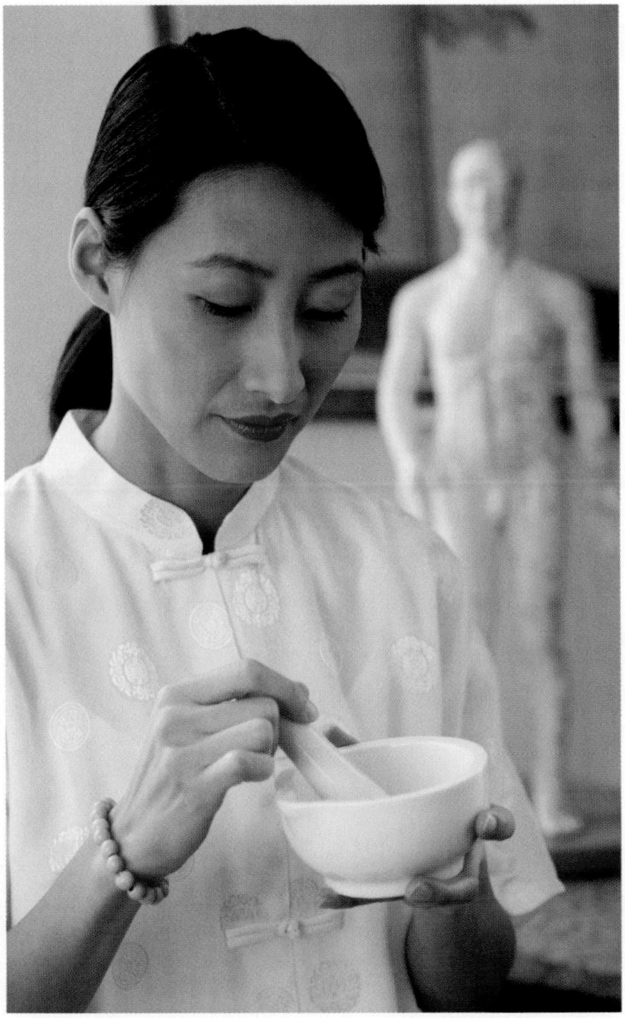
© Jon Feingersh/Blend Images/Jupiterimages

selves; relatively few seek care from a licensed CAM practitioner.

Who Uses Complementary and Alternative Medicine?

Use of CAM is not limited to a few patients on the fringe. Americans spend billions of dollars each year on CAM. More than one of three Americans (38%) use some form of CAM.[12] People of all backgrounds use CAM, but some groups are more likely to use it than others, including:

- Women
- People with higher educational levels
- People who have been hospitalized in the past year
- Former smokers, compared with current smokers or those who have never smoked

The common thread is likely that the four groups mentioned are more likely than others to have health on their minds. CAM use also varies across different racial and ethnic groups, as shown in Figure 14-4 on page 327. When we exclude prayer and megavitamin therapy, Asian Americans are most likely to use CAM, perhaps because of ancient Asian traditions. Reasons people use CAM are shown in Figure 14-5 on page 328.

Should *You* Use Complementary and Alternative Medicine?

Your decisions about your health care are important—including decisions about whether to use complementary and alternative medicine (CAM). The NCCAM has developed this fact sheet to assist you in your decision making about CAM. It includes frequently asked questions, issues to consider, and a list of sources for further information.

- Become an informed consumer. Laurie was not informed; she believed that CAM could prevent or cure breast cancer. It cannot. Find out what scientific studies have been done on the safety and effectiveness of the CAM treatment you are considering. Your primary physician will have this type of information available. You can ask the manufacturer of a CAM product or a CAM practitioner for scientific articles or the results of studies. They should be willing to share this information, if it exists. For additional information on CAM, go to http://www.nccam.nih.gov, the government website for the National Center for Complementary and Alternative Medicine. Ignore personal stories (anecdotes).
- Visit the FDA online at http://www.fda.gov to check for information about the product or practice. Information specifically about dietary supplements can be found on the FDA's Center for Food Safety and Applied Nutrition website at http://www.fda.gov/Food/DietarySupplements. Or visit the FDA's web page on recalls and safety alerts at http://www.fda.gov/Safety/Recalls.
- Make your decisions about CAM in consultation with your primary HCP and based on your own condition and needs.
- Let your primary HCP know about your use of CAM therapy so that she or he can point out possible benefits and pitfalls and develop a comprehensive treatment plan.
- If you use a CAM practitioner, such as an acupuncture provider, choose the practitioner with care. Check with your insurer to see if the services will be covered.

DIVERSITY 14-1

Serving the Underserved

Many groups in the United States have limited access to medical care, especially poor people, ethnic minority groups, and people living in inner cities or remote areas. For the very poor, the Medicaid program ordinarily picks up the tab for medical services. But barriers such as transportation problems, language differences, unwillingness of providers to treat Medicaid patients, and perceptions of callous treatment from providers limit access to health care. Many Medicaid recipients face long waiting periods for appointments and long lines in waiting rooms.

Access to health care services for the working poor is also limited. Low-paid workers might not be financially eligible for Medicaid, but they may also lack private health insurance because it is not offered by their employers and they cannot afford it on their own. Largely because of disparities in health insurance coverage, low-income families pay a higher percentage of their family income for health care than do high-income families. Recent immigrants, migrant workers, and the working poor employed in small business concerns are at greatest risk of being uninsured or underinsured.

Not only uninsured or underinsured people have problems obtaining care. Most people who are unable to obtain care actually do *have* health insurance. The major barrier to obtaining care for people with and without insurance is clear—cost. To the insured, factors such as deductibles, copayments, and restrictions on medical services block access.

People living in remote areas may have to travel 75 miles or more to see a doctor, and further if they require specialists or hospitalization. Many Native Americans are eligible for free health care through the Indian Health Service (IHS), but they live in rural areas in which there are few providers.[13] Many are also poor and cannot afford to travel to obtain care.

Poverty and race are large factors in access to health care. African Americans are less likely than European Americans to carry private health insurance.[14] Greater unemployment among African Americans figures prominently into this disparity, because health insurance is often tied to employment. Disparities also exist in the quality of care. Even when health insurance or government programs like Medicare and Medicaid are available, African Americans and poor people tend to receive lower-quality care than European Americans and affluent people do. Low-income Americans, racial and ethnic minorities, and other underserved populations often have higher rates of disease, fewer treatment options, and reduced access to care. They are also less likely to have health insurance than the population as a whole.

The 2010 health care reform legislation expanded health care services to groups that have traditionally lacked access to quality health care services. The health care reform act may not put an end to health care disparities, but hopefully will reduce these health disparities by expanding health care services and disease prevention programs to traditionally disadvantaged groups.

Health Care Reform: Reducing Health Care Disparities

The 2010 health care reform law, called the Affordable Care Act, seeks to reduce health care disparities by providing the following:

- ***Preventive care.*** Medicare and some private insurance plans will cover recommended preventive services like regular check-ups, cancer screenings, and immunizations at no additional cost to eligible people.

continued

- ***Coordinated care.*** The law calls for new investments in community health teams to manage chronic disease. This is important, because minority communities experience higher rates of illness and death for chronic diseases such as diabetes, kidney disease, heart disease, and cancer. Because infant mortality and post-birth complications are also higher in minority and low-income groups, the law includes new funds for home visits for expectant mothers and newborns.
- ***Diversity and cultural competency.*** The Affordable Care Act expands initiatives to increase racial and ethnic diversity in the health care professions. It also strengthens cultural competency training for all health care providers. Health plans will be required to use language services and community outreach in underserved communities. Improving communications between providers and patients will help address health disparities, particularly in Hispanic communities, which currently have high numbers of uninsured people.
- ***Health care providers for underserved communities.*** The Affordable Care Act expands the health care workforce and increases funding for community health centers, which provide comprehensive health care for everyone, no matter how much they are able to pay. Health centers serve an estimated one in three low-income people and one in four low-income minority residents. The new resources will enable health centers to double the number of patients they serve. Combined with investments made by the American Recovery and Reinvestment Act, the new law will support 16,000 new primary care providers.
- ***Ending insurance discrimination.*** Insurance discrimination will be banned, so people who have been sick can't be excluded from coverage or be charged higher premiums. Women will no longer have to pay higher premiums because of their gender. New funding will be available to collect information on how women and racial and ethnic minorities experience the health care system, leading to improvements that will benefit these groups.

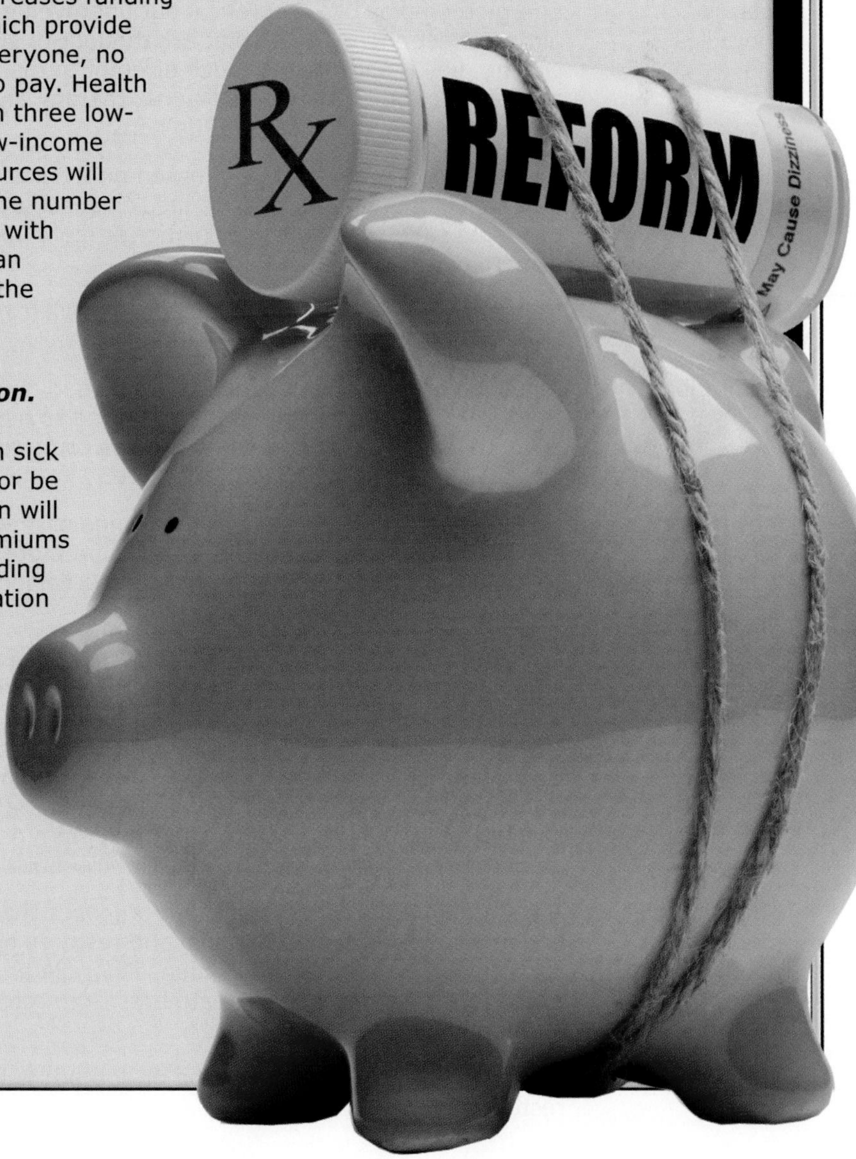

Table 14-4 Examples of Complementary and Alternative Medicine[15]

METHOD	ABOUT . . .
Acupuncture	Developed in ancient China, acupuncture stimulates anatomical points on the body. American acupuncture incorporates medical traditions from China, Japan, Korea, and other countries. The acupuncture technique that has been most studied scientifically involves penetrating the skin with thin metallic needles that are manipulated by the hands or transmit electrical stimulation.
Aromatherapy	Use of oils (extracts or essences) from flowers, herbs, and trees to promote health and well-being.
Ayurveda	An alternative medical system that has been practiced on the Indian subcontinent for 5,000 years. Ayurveda includes diet and herbal remedies and emphasizes the integration of body, mind, and spirit.
Chiropractic	An alternative medical system that focuses on the relationship between bodily structure (primarily the spine) and function. Chiropractors use manipulative therapy as a treatment tool.
Energy therapies	Energy therapies use theoretical but unproven energy fields. Biofield therapies aim to affect energy fields that are thought to surround and penetrate the body. Qigong, Reiki, and healing touch attempt to manipulate biofields by pressure on, or manipulation of, the body. Magnet therapy and light therapy attempt to affect electromagnetic fields around the body.
Homeopathic	An alternative medical system based on a belief that "like cures like," meaning that small, diluted quantities of medicinal substances can cure symptoms, whereas the same substances given at higher or more concentrated doses would cause the symptoms.
Massage	Manipulation of muscle and connective tissue to enhance function of those tissues and promote relaxation and well-being.
Meditation	Induction of relaxation by focusing attention on some activity, object, or image. In Eastern cultures, meditation is believed to help people achieve spiritual enlightenment. Traditional medicine has come to accept meditation as a means to combat stress and high blood pressure.
Movement therapies	Movement therapies include a wide range of practices that draw upon Eastern and Western traditions and are used to promote physical, mental, emotional, and spiritual well-being. Examples include the Feldenkrais method, the Alexander technique, pilates, and Rolfing.
Natural products and dietary supplements	Products taken orally and intended to supplement the diet. Ingredients include vitamins, minerals, herbs or other botanicals, amino acids, enzymes, organ tissues, and metabolites. They come in many forms, including extracts, concentrates, tablets, capsules, gel caps, liquids, and powders. Under the Dietary Supplement Health and Education Act (DSHEA), dietary supplements are considered foods, not drugs, but they have special requirements for labeling. Some dietary supplements, such as multivitamins used to meet minimum daily nutritional requirements or calcium used to promote bone health, are mainstream—not CAM.
Naturopathic medicine, or naturopathy	An alternative medical system that proposes that there is a healing power in the body that establishes, maintains, and restores health. Practitioners use treatments such as nutrition and lifestyle counseling, dietary supplements, medicinal plants, exercise, homeopathy, and treatments from traditional Chinese medicine to strengthen the power.
Prayer	Making a reverent petition to God or another object of worship to promote or restore health.

continued

Table 14-4 (continued)

METHOD	ABOUT . . .
Qigong ("chee-gung")	A traditional Chinese medicine that combines movement, meditation, and regulation of breathing to enhance the flow of "qi" (believed to be vital energy) in the body, improve circulation, and enhance immune function.
Reflexology	Manipulation of pressure points on the hands and feet to relieve stress and pain.
Reiki	A traditional Japanese method based on the belief that when spiritual energy is channeled through a Reiki practitioner, the patient's spirit is healed, which in turn heals the body.
Therapeutic touch	Also called "laying-on of hands," a method based on the belief that the healing force of the therapist affects the patient's recovery; healing is promoted when the body's energies are in balance; and, by passing their hands over the patient, healers can identify energy imbalances.
Traditional Chinese medicine	This ancient system of health care is based on a concept of balanced qi (pronounced "chee"), or vital energy, that is believed to flow through the body. Qi is proposed to regulate a person's spiritual, emotional, mental, and physical balance and to be influenced by the opposing forces of yin (negative energy) and yang (positive energy). Disease is proposed to result from an imbalance of yin and yang. Methods include herbal and nutritional therapy, physical exercises, meditation, acupuncture, and massage.

Figure 14-4 CAM Use by Race/Ethnicity[16]

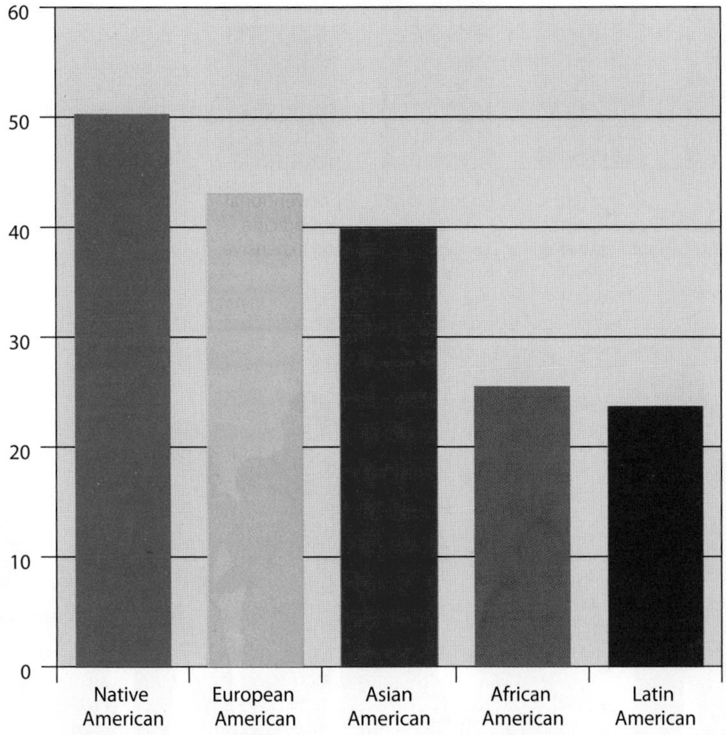

- For a CAM product that is sold over the counter (without a prescription), such as a dietary supplement, check out the components or ingredients that make up the product, where they come from, and the quality of the manufacturing process. Be aware that the FDA cannot require testing of dietary supplements prior to marketing. The FDA can only remove products from the marketplace if they are known to be dangerous. Fortunately, marketers cannot claim that dietary supplements can treat, cure, or prevent disease without scientific proof.

NCCAM offers some useful suggestions about the safety and effectiveness of complementary and alternative medical practices and therapies (see Table 14-5 on page 329).

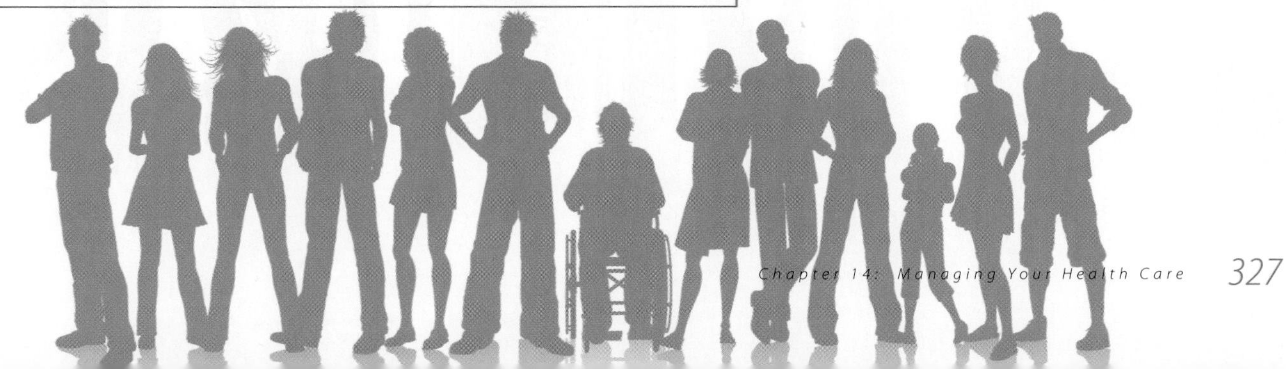

Figure 14-5 Reasons People Use CAM (%)[17]

Most people (55%) who used CAM also used conventional medicine (see Figure 14-4). But they believe CAM offers something extra. About half used CAM because it sounded interesting. In one in four cases (25.8%), a conventional HCP actually suggested it. About 28% believed that conventional medicine would do them no good; among these are people who did not believe in conventional medicine and those who had run out of treatment options. One in six, unfortunately, simply could not afford conventional treatment.

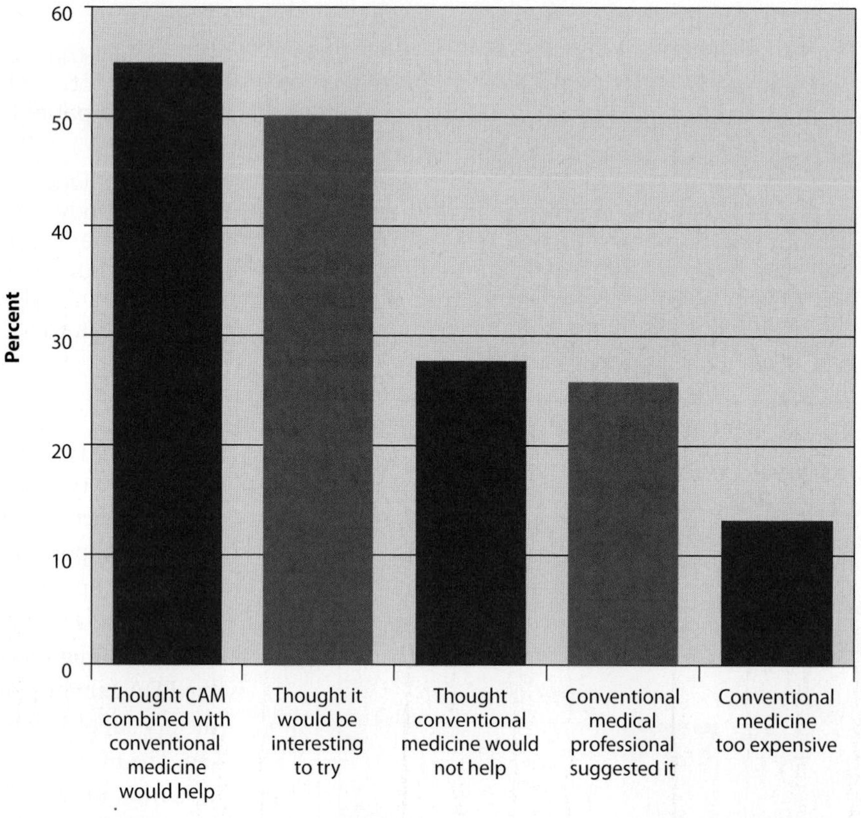

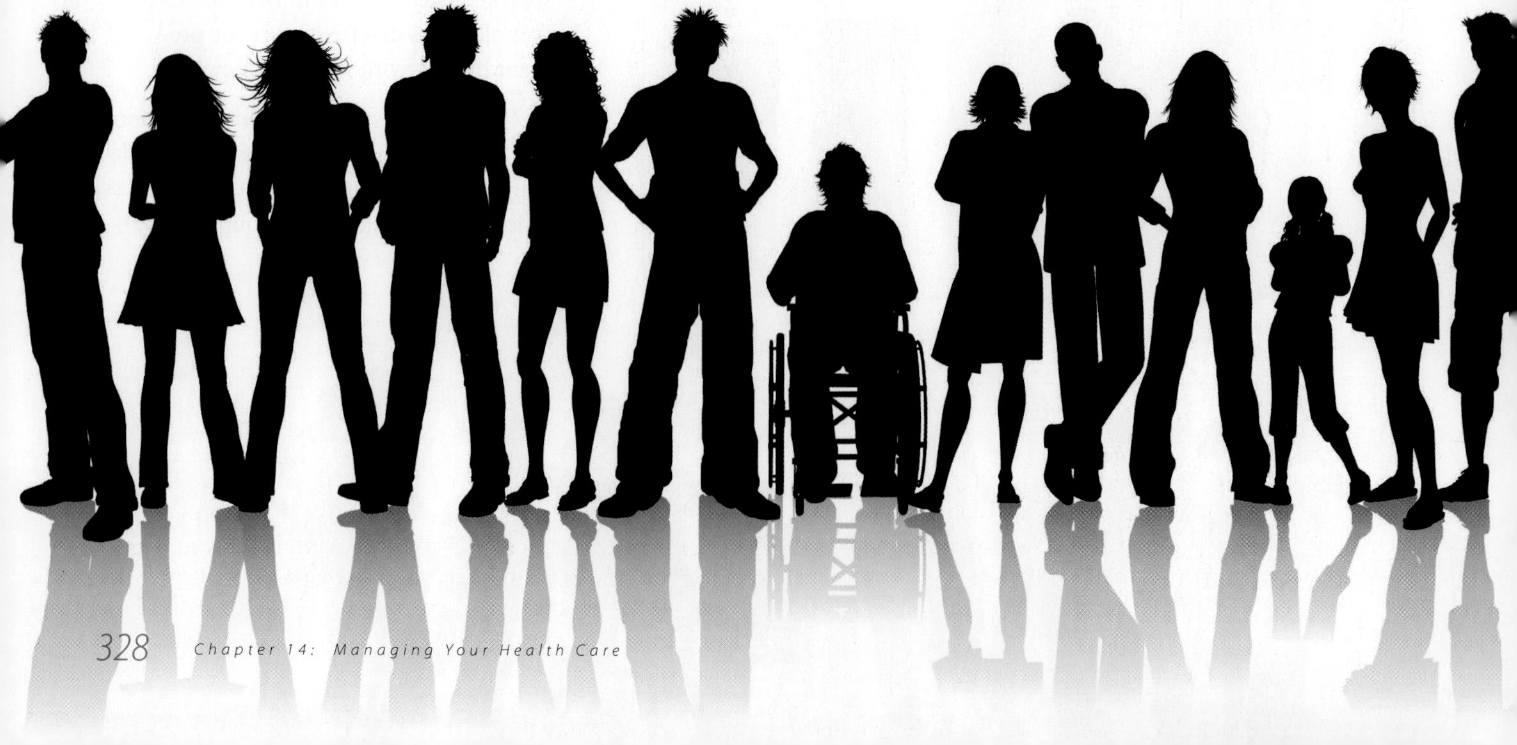

Table 14-5 A Note about Safety and Effectiveness[18]

Rigorous, well-designed clinical trials for many CAM therapies are often lacking; therefore, the safety and effectiveness of many CAM therapies are uncertain. NCCAM is sponsoring research designed to fill this knowledge gap by building a scientific evidence base about CAM therapies—whether they are safe, whether they work for the conditions for which people use them, and if so, how they work. As with any medical treatment, there can be risks with CAM therapies. These general precautions can help to minimize risks:

- Select CAM practitioners with care. Find out about the practitioner's training and experience.
- Be aware that some dietary supplements may interact with medications or other supplements, may have side effects of their own, or may contain potentially harmful ingredients not listed on the label. Also keep in mind that most supplements have not been tested on pregnant women, nursing mothers, or children.
- Tell all your health care providers about any complementary and alternative practices you use. Give them a full picture of what you do to manage your health. This will help ensure coordinated and safe care.

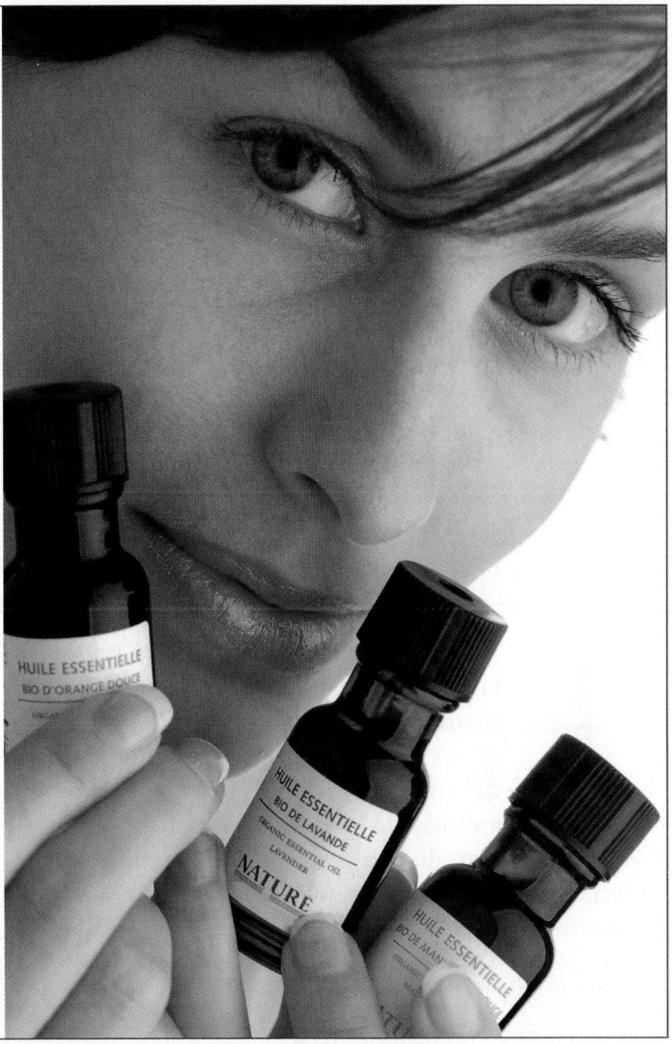

© PHANIE/Photo Researchers, Inc.

HEALTH APPS: YOUR LINK TO ONLINE HEALTH APPLICATIONS

prevention

Your Health Checkup—What Happens and Why People who actively manage their health care obtain regular medical checkups. They also educate themselves so they understand what happens during a physical exam, why it happens, and what is expected of them. "Prevention 14-1" is the place to learn what you can expect during a checkup and the types of common tests that may be ordered.

health skills

Choosing a Health Care Plan Selecting a health care plan is an important factor in meeting your health care needs. The *un*informed way of choosing is to be swayed by television commercials that show healthy, vigorous members of a particular plan enjoying the fullness of life. The informed way is to acquire information and carefully weigh the advantages and disadvantages of a variety of plans, which we help you sort out in "Health Skills 14-1."

prevention

Treatment Yes, Prevention Definitely One way to battle health care costs—as well as to remain healthy—is to use prevention. Have you had your recommended adult vaccinations? Do you even know what they are? Have you had screening tests for major diseases? Again, do you know what they are? Go to "Prevention 14-2" for answers to these questions and more.

Go to the CourseMate for HLTH at www.cengagebrain.com for additional resources including flashcards, games, self-quizzes, review exercises, web exercises, learning checks, and more.

Health and the Environment

"There may be no place like home, but hidden dangers may lurk there."

This book has already considered many environmental risks to our health, such as pathogens and carcinogens. Let's now broaden our perspective by focusing on environmental health problems such as toxic chemicals, radiation, pollution, and climate change. There are "big things" that can only be done by governments and corporations. But there are also things we can do ourselves, such as recycle, buy "greener" products, and vote for measures that protect the environment.

Learning Outcomes

1. Discuss health hazards in the home environment
2. Discuss health hazards in the community environment
3. Discuss the hazards of various kinds of radiation
4. Discuss the relationship between population growth and health
5. Discuss the health hazards of various kinds of pollution and what can be done about them
6. Discuss the relationship between climate change and health

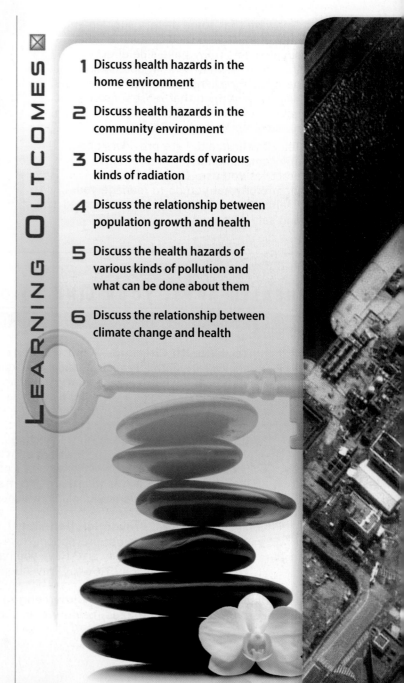

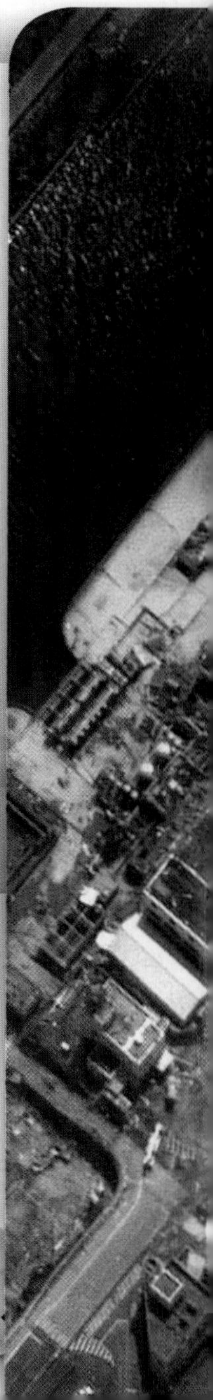

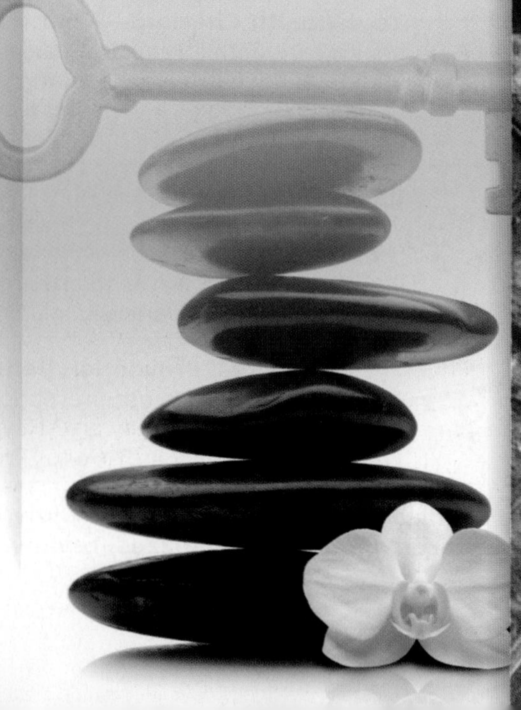

Environmental Issues Close to Home

There may be no place like home, but hidden dangers may lurk there. Let's talk about environmental threats we may face at home, beginning with the major risk many children face: lead poisoning.

LEARNING OUTCOME 1

Discuss health hazards in the home environment

Getting the Lead Out

Lead is a mineral found naturally in ore and soil. It enters our air and water via industrial emissions; from lead-based products, such as lead paint, found in many older buildings.

Lead poisoning, which occurs from ingestion of lead, is the major environmental health problem facing many U.S. children.[1] Inhaling or eating lead can have serious health consequences, especially when it continues over time. Although we all face potential risks of lead contamination, a young child's growing body absorbs as much as four times the levels of lead as an adult's. Exposure to lead can have damaging prenatal effects.[2] Maternal lead exposure can lead to miscarriage, premature birth, and low birthweight. It can also damage the nervous system of the fetus, leading to intellectual deficiency.[3] It also damages the kidneys and the blood-forming cells that make red blood cells.

We have already phased out lead in gasoline, reduced lead concentrations in drinking water and industrial chimney products, and banned or restricted lead in consumer products, including household paint. Yet potential exposure remains, especially from the chipping or flaking of old lead-based paint (see the online feature "Prevention 15-1"). Although blood levels of lead in American children have been declining, most still show some low-level exposure to lead.[4] Certain groups of children, especially poor children and children from minority groups, run a relatively higher risk of elevated blood levels of lead.

prevention

Access CourseMate for HLTH at www.cengagebrain.com.

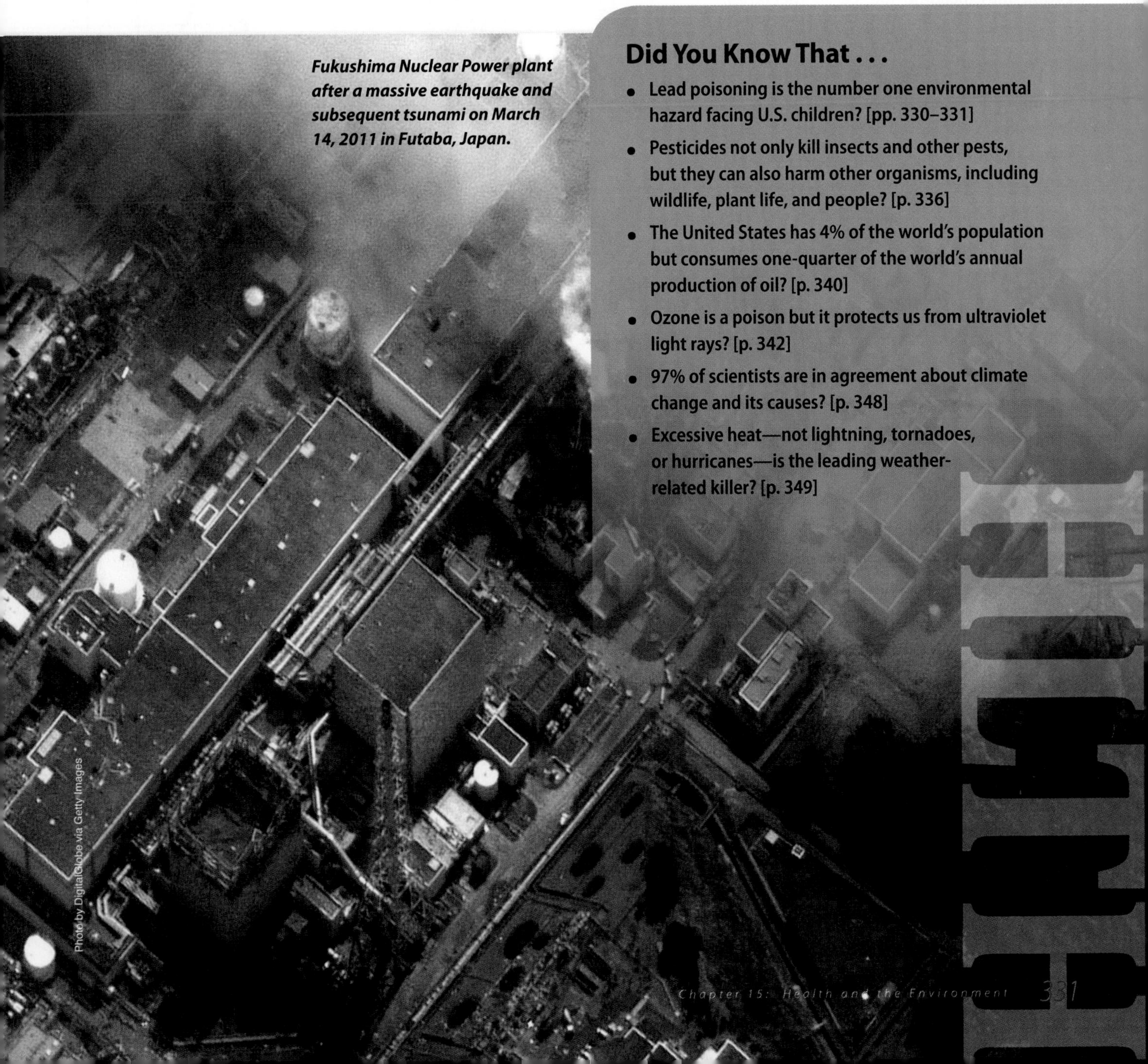

Fukushima Nuclear Power plant after a massive earthquake and subsequent tsunami on March 14, 2011 in Futaba, Japan.

Photo by DigitalGlobe via Getty Images

Did You Know That . . .

- **Lead poisoning is the number one environmental hazard facing U.S. children? [pp. 330–331]**
- **Pesticides not only kill insects and other pests, but they can also harm other organisms, including wildlife, plant life, and people? [p. 336]**
- **The United States has 4% of the world's population but consumes one-quarter of the world's annual production of oil? [p. 340]**
- **Ozone is a poison but it protects us from ultraviolet light rays? [p. 342]**
- **97% of scientists are in agreement about climate change and its causes? [p. 348]**
- **Excessive heat—not lightning, tornadoes, or hurricanes—is the leading weather-related killer? [p. 349]**

Radon

Radon is a radioactive gas emitted during the natural decay of the element *uranium*. Outdoors, radon presents little danger, except for underground miners exposed to high levels on the job. However, radon in the ground can enter our homes, schools, and office buildings through cracks or pores in concrete floors and walls, floor drains, sump pumps, joints, hollow-block walls, stone fireplaces, well water, and dirt floors (see Figure 15-1). Radon gas that becomes trapped in buildings may be inhaled. Tiny radioactive particles of radon may become lodged in the lungs, where they can accumulate and can cause lung cancer.[5] About 21,000 lung cancer deaths annually in the U.S are linked to radon, making it the second leading cause of cancer deaths, after smoking.[6] High levels of radon are found in parts of every state in the United States.

Because our senses do not detect radon, we need to have our homes inspected to ensure that we are not slowly being poisoned by it. Testing is relatively easy and inexpensive. EPA-approved "do-it-yourself" kits are available in local hardware stores. You can also hire EPA-qualified or state-certified radon testers.

Figure 15-1 How Radon Enters Your Home

Radon can seep into our homes from the soil through cracks in the floor or foundation, through exposed soil, and around pipe fittings. Radon can also enter the water supply in the home and pass into the household air whenever you turn on the shower or faucet.

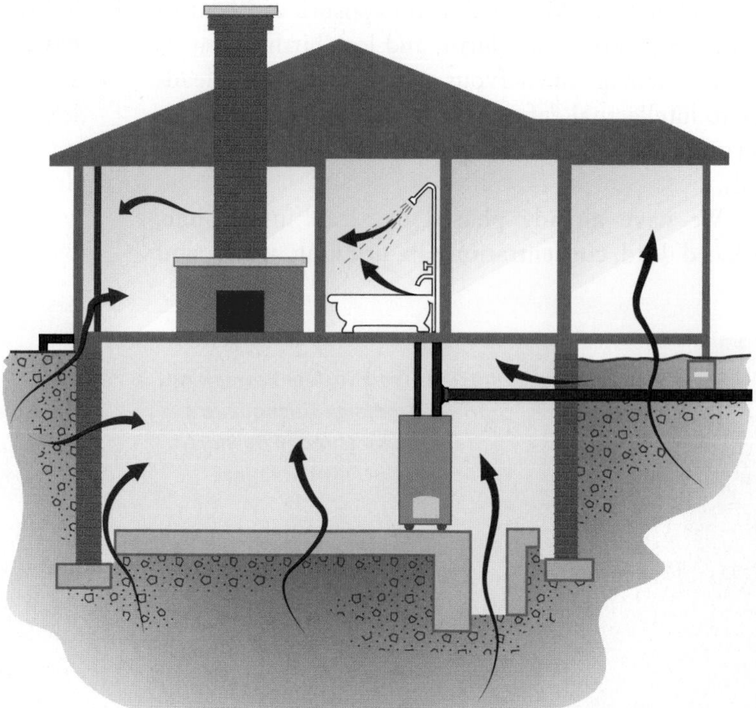

© Cengage Learning 2013

Ridding a home of radon may be as simple as opening basement and first-floor windows and vents, allowing the gas to escape. But the simple method may lead to loss of heat (or air-conditioning) and security concerns. Other procedures include installation of ventilation systems. Your state department of environmental protection can assist you in obtaining testing devices, interpreting results, and determining strategies for reducing radon levels in the home.

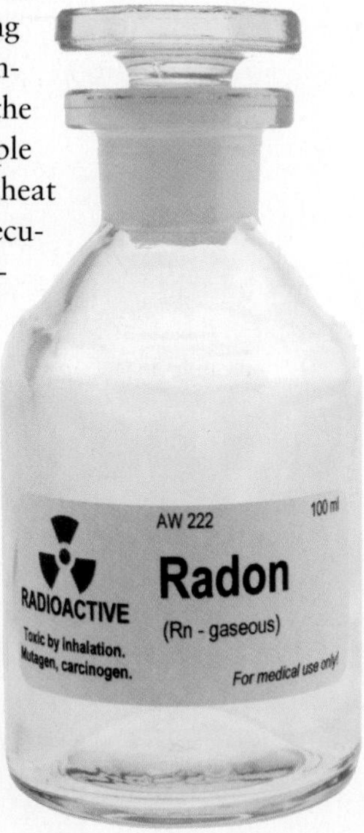

© iStockphoto.com/Zirafek

carbon monoxide
An odorless, colorless gas that is a major source of air pollution and is produced from the burning of carbon with insufficient air.

Carbon Monoxide

Another poisonous gas that can seep into our homes is **carbon monoxide** (CO). This odorless and colorless gas is formed from the incomplete combustion of fuels, wood, solid trash, and tobacco smoke. "Prevention 15-2" focuses on how we can protect ourselves from CO.

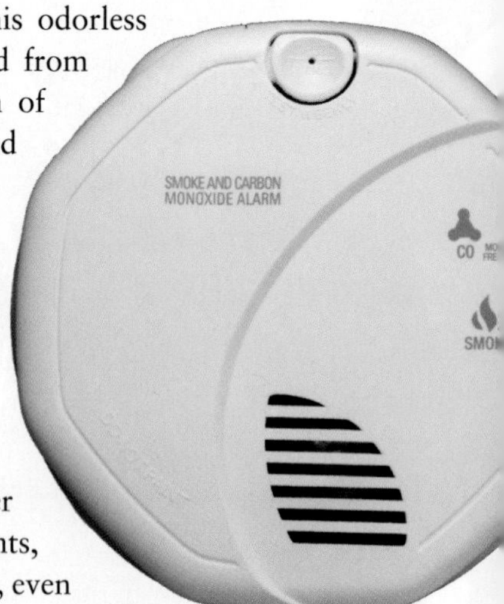

© iStockphoto.com/Kevin Visel

Household Chemicals

Laundry and dishwasher detergents, bleaches, solvents, and paint can be dangerous, even

PREVENTION 15-2

Keeping Our Homes Safe from Carbon Monoxide Poisoning

Carbon monoxide poisoning is the most common type of accidental poisoning in the United States, accounting for more than 15,000 emergency room visits annually and claiming nearly 500 lives.[7] Most people killed by carbon monoxide poisoning die in their sleep. One of the most common sources of carbon monoxide poisoning is a faulty or inefficient furnace, space heater, water heater, or wood stove. The gas can also seep into the home from the car exhaust when a car is left idling in an attached garage. Here are some tips to keep yourself and your home safe from carbon monoxide:

- *Maintain your home heating system to keep it in proper working condition.*
- *Adequately ventilate a fireplace or wood stove.*
- *Never build an enclosure around a household heating system that restricts the flow of air.*
- *Do not use a stove or oven to heat your home.* Also, never barbecue or burn charcoal indoors. Avoid using a kerosene heater indoors, unless you take special care to ensure it is properly vented to the outside.
- *Do not let your car idle in a closed garage.* Leaks from the exhaust system can usher carbon monoxide into the passenger compartment or the house. Make sure to keep your car's exhaust system in good working condition.
- *Install a carbon monoxide detector.* The peace of mind is worth the cost. *Consumer Reports* magazine rates different models.

deadly, when ingested or absorbed into the body. The dangers are greatest for children. Each year more than 1 million children in the United States are accidentally poisoned. More than 90% of poisonings occur in the home. Children are naturally inquisitive and may not realize that the colorful container under the sink isn't filled with fruit drink, but with a toxic detergent.

Here are some tips for keeping ourselves and our families safe from household chemicals:

- *Keep detergents, bleaches, cleansers, solvents, dishwashing liquid, and paint products out of reach of small children.* Don't store them under the sink, in the medicine cabinet, or anywhere children can reach.
- *Check product labels and follow instructions for use and storage.*
- *Never switch containers.* Never pour household chemicals into other containers.
- *Discard old or outdated products.*
- *Keep an eye on children, especially when they explore their surroundings.*
- *Keep the local poison control hotline number handy.* Check your phone directory for the telephone number. The national poison control telephone number is 1-800-222-1222. Or you can dial 911 and explain that the nature of the emergency is a possible poisoning.

800-222-1222

POISON HELP HOTLINE

Environmental Issues in the Community

Our environment extends from the home to our community, our region, our nation, our world. The air we breathe, the water we drink, and the food we eat sustain us. Yet they can also pose serious health threats, largely as the result of exposure to pollution and toxic wastes. What's the risk? Check out the online feature "Health Check 15-1."

☒ LEARNING OUTCOME 2

Discuss health hazards in the community environment

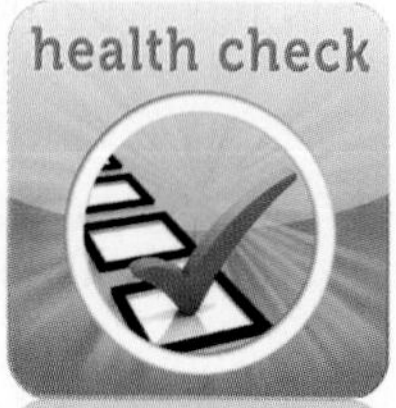

Access CourseMate for HLTH at www.cengagebrain.com.

Environmental Toxins

The environment contains countless naturally occurring toxins, and we humans have developed countless more (see Table 15-1). A toxin is a poisonous substance that is harmful to the body. Two major types of environmental toxins of concern to our health are (1) natural and synthetic chemicals, such as pesticides, and (2) radioactive substances, such as ultraviolet rays, X-rays, and radon. Environmental toxins enter the body through three major points of entry: the lungs, the skin, and the gastrointestinal (GI) tract (as the result of eating contaminated food or drinking contaminated water) (see Figure 15-3 on page 342).

neurotoxin
Poisonous substance that affects the brain and central nervous system (CNS).

mutagen
Substance that induces genetic mutations. Ionizing radiation and ultraviolet light are known mutagens.

Health Effects of Environmental Toxins

Pesticides not only kill insects but can also harm humans and other animals. **Neurotoxins** such as lead and mercury can damage the brain and central nervous system. Other toxins, including some chemicals and types of radiation, are **mutagens**. They change the genetic structure of the cell. Mutated cells may reproduce wildly, leading to cancer.

Although the body can break down (metabolize) certain toxins and excrete them without harmful consequences, other toxins accumulate, which can lead to chronic health problems. Some toxins travel through the bloodstream to wreak havoc on particular organs. For example, the metal *cadmium* is especially harmful to the kidneys. The lungs are susceptible to toxic particles in polluted air.

Certain groups of people are more susceptible to particular toxins. More vulnerable groups include infants and children, pregnant women, people with impaired immune systems, and older people. The health hazards of toxins are *dose dependent;* they are related to the amount of a toxin to which a person is exposed, the length of time the person is exposed, and how many times the person is exposed. The effects of toxins also depend on body weight; a child who consumes the same serving of contaminated fish as an adult faces a greater risk. Exposure to toxic chemicals during pregnancy can cause birth defects or problems after birth. Many toxins

Table 15-1 Types of Environmental Hazards

TYPES OF HAZARDS	EXAMPLES
Toxic chemicals	Chemical substances that are poisonous to organisms. There are thousands of harmful natural and synthetic (human-made) toxins, including heavy metals, petrochemicals, and pesticides.
Biological hazards	Viruses, bacteria, protozoa, and other pathogens. They are the chief cause of food-borne and waterborne diseases.
Physical hazards	Radiation; natural disasters (floods, earthquakes, and fires); violence and accidents in the home, workplace, or in transit; and noise (yes, noise).
Cultural/social hazards	Overpopulation, unhealthy learned habits (like smoking and excessive alcohol intake), lack of access to health care, and poverty. Violence is both a physical hazard and a cultural/social hazard. Poor people are more likely to work and live near environmental hazards and to suffer a disproportionate share of their ill effects. Agricultural workers may be forced into close contact with pesticides.

pass from the mother to the fetus across the placenta and enter the fetus's blood stream. Older adults have slower metabolism than young adults, so their bodies eliminate toxins less efficiently.

Types of Environmental Toxins

Many natural and synthetic substances found in our communities threaten our health. The soil is rich in minerals, which work their way into our food supply. We require small amounts of minerals, such as iron, selenium, and zinc, for good health, but excess amounts are toxic.

Here we focus on the health risks posed by metallic elements and by toxic chemicals, including those occurring naturally (for example, aflatoxin) and those manufactured by heavy industry.

Arsenic

Arsenic, a naturally occurring metal, is linked to skin, lung, bladder, and prostate cancers. It can also damage the heart, lungs, and immunological system. The federal government regulates levels of arsenic in drinking water, where trace amounts are found. Arsenic is also a constituent of tobacco smoke.

Aflatoxin

Aflatoxin is produced by certain kinds of molds. It can contaminate nuts and grains, especially when inadequate storage and drying methods are used in crop production. It can be found in corn and peanuts, including peanut butter. At high doses, aflatoxin can be a potent carcinogen, causing liver cancer and other liver diseases.[8] The Food and Drug Administration (FDA), the federal watchdog agency responsible for food safety, establishes regulatory limits for contamination to ensure that food is safe to eat.

Asbestos

Asbestos is a fibrous material occurring naturally and formerly used in commercial products such as roofing materials, brake pads, and insulation because of its resistance to heat, fire, and many chemicals. It is no longer used because inhaled asbestos fibers can become lodged in lung tissue and cause lung cancer and *mesothelioma*, a rare form of cancer that forms in the protective sac, called the mesothelium, that lines the chest and abdomen.[9] Asbestos exposure causes about 4,000 cancer deaths annually in the United States.[10]

Though the use of asbestos in commercial applications has greatly declined, the mineral is still found in many homes and work sites. Obtain a qualified asbestos-removal contractor to safely remove asbestos and avoid accidental release of the fibers into the air.

Heavy Metals

Even low levels of exposure to certain heavy metals, such as lead, mercury, and cadmium, are toxic. These metals are used in products ranging from paints to batteries. Most cases of toxic exposure to heavy metals involve lead poisoning, but other metals also pose significant risks. *Mercury* is a silver-white metal that becomes liquid at room temperatures (as in thermometers) and evaporates in air. Mercury has many industrial uses, including the manufacture of thermometers, dental fillings, and batteries. Mercury contamination generally comes from seepage of the metal from manufacturing plant sites into bodies of water where it is ingested by fish. Eating contaminated fish can damage the brain and kidneys, and cause visual impairment, learning disabilities, and hyperactivity in children.[11]

Fish are regularly inspected for levels of mercury. In the home, we need to handle products containing mercury such as thermometers and fluorescent light bulbs with care.

High continual exposure to the metal *selenium* can damage the kidneys, liver, circulatory system, and nervous system. Selenium is found in trace amounts in water supplies and in burning waste.

Cadmium, a metal found in the earth's crust, has widespread industrial applications, including battery manufacturing, metal soldering, and welding. Breathing high levels of cadmium can fatally damage the lungs. Cadmium can accumulate in the kidneys following long-term exposure to the metal in air, water, and food supplies. The long-term risks of exposure include kidney disease. Cadmium is also found in cigarette smoke and is suspected to be carcinogenic. Handle nickel-cadmium batteries and other cadmium-containing substances with care.

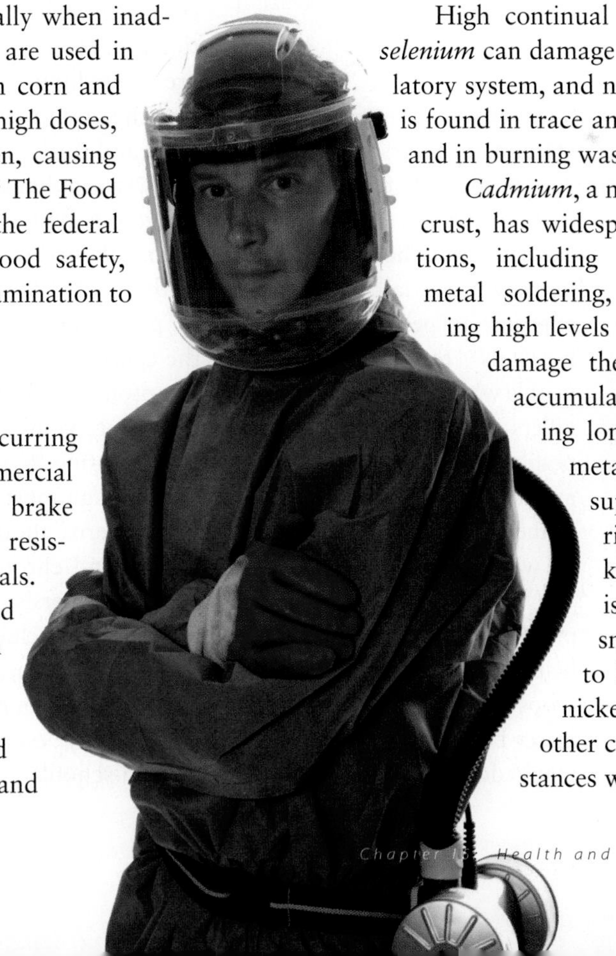

Petrochemicals

Petrochemicals are manufactured from crude oil and natural gas. Products including detergents, pesticides, pharmaceuticals, and cosmetics to plastics, paints, coatings, chemical solvents, fertilizers, and pesticides contain petrochemicals. Disposing of the hazardous wastes that arise from the manufacture of these products is an environmental challenge. They are a major source of air, water, and soil pollution. Many petrochemical products, including plastic shopping bags, are **nonbiodegradable**, which means they are not broken down naturally like other waste products. They are better recycled than tossed into landfills. Exposure to petrochemicals, especially pesticides, poses health risks.

One of the most widely used—and risky—petrochemicals is benzene. Benzene is a raw material used in manufacturing glues, paints, and marking pens, as well as pharmaceutical and agricultural chemicals. Leakage of benzene from industrial wastes and landfills contaminates food and water supplies. Continual exposure to benzene can lead to cancer, especially leukemia, and damage the circulatory and nervous systems.

Many people assume that "organically grown" fruits and vegetables are free of pesticides and chemical additives. But many contain traces of pesticides and other chemicals. Some unscrupulous growers misrepresent use of pesticides. In other cases, pesticides used on neighboring farms may wash over into the soil used for organically grown crops.

Pesticides

Pesticides are intended to exterminate insects, rodents, and weeds. They allow farmers to produce more plentiful crops on smaller acreages. Yet each year, thousands of farm workers fall ill from exposure to pesticides, and hospitals routinely treat people who mishandle weed killers and other household pesticides. In addition, we are all exposed to pesticides in the foods we eat and the air we breathe.

petrochemical
Chemical substance derived from petroleum or natural gas.

nonbiodegradable
Substances that do not decay naturally in the environment.

organochlorines
A class of petrochemicals, including some pesticides and other toxic substances, that is used widely in industrial settings.

organophosphates
A class of potentially dangerous chemical compounds used as pesticides and sometimes as chemical weapons.

The use of pesticides presents hard choices. They help prevent devastation of crops by insects and control insect-borne plagues. But many do not discriminate between pests and "good" insects and other wildlife. Pesticides contaminate the soil, air, and water and can be absorbed by animals via skin contact, inhalation, or ingestion. Agricultural workers and people living near farms bear the greatest risk of exposure.

Some of the better known but more dangerous pesticides are **organochlorines** (also called *chlorinated hydrocarbons*). These pesticides include DDT, heptachlor, chlordane, and lindane. Lindane (brand name *Kwell*) is used to kill head lice and pubic lice. The FDA advises parents not to overuse lindane because of possible toxic effects.

The other three organochlorines (DDT, heptachlor, chlordane) are banned for most uses in the United States. Until the health risks of DDT became known, it was widely used to control insects on agricultural crops and those carrying diseases such as malaria and typhus. DDT (dichlorodiphenyltrichloroethane) is now banned by the U.S. government because of its harmful effects on the environment and possible health risks, including its possible role as a carcinogen.[12] But traces of DDT remain in the environment. Many other countries also ban the use of DDT with the exception of public health efforts to control mosquitoes that serve as vectors for the transmission of malaria.

Some banned pesticides manufactured by U.S. companies are exported to other countries, (usually poorer countries), where they are used in agricultural production and enter meat, milk, and other food products that are then shipped back to the United States and other wealthy countries. Environmentalists have dubbed this back and forth as the "Circle of Poison."[13]

Organophosphates are another class of potentially dangerous pesticides. One example is the highly toxic chemical *methyl parathion*, which is used in farming in the United States, even though it is a leading cause of poisoning of farm workers. The chemical affects the central nervous system, producing potentially fatal symptoms including dizziness, headache, difficulty breathing, vomiting, diarrhea, tremors, blurred vision, and sweating.[14]

Though most household pesticides have low toxicity, concerns about potential health risks from overexposure and chronic exposure to lower levels of these chemicals persist, especially for children. Symptoms of exposure include a cough, shortness of breath, nausea, vomiting, headaches, and eye irritation. Medical authorities encourage school officials to protect schoolchildren by establishing pesticide-free buffer zones around schools.

Radiation

Radiation ("radiant energy") is energy that is transmitted in the form of waves or particles. The waveform of radiation includes visible light that we see, as well as radiation we can't detect with our eyes, including ultraviolet light, X-rays, radio waves, and microwaves. All forms of radiation fall within the *electromagnetic spectrum*, only a small portion of which consists of visible light. Shorter wavelength radiation, which includes X-rays, is more powerful and poses more potential health risks than longer wavelength radiation, such as radio waves. *Cosmic rays* are bursts of high-energy particles that originate in outer space.

☒ LEARNING OUTCOME 3

Discuss the hazards of various kinds of radiation

Some elements, such as uranium and radium, are naturally radioactive. They continuously emit energy-release waves or particles. Nuclear reactors and accelerators manufacture artificial radioactive substances. These substances are used in medicine, agriculture, food preservation, and in consumer products such as smoke detectors.

The word *radiation* may conjure up images of weapons of mass destruction or nuclear reactor accidents, but many lives have been saved by medical use of radiation in the form of *radiotherapy*. However, radioactive substances continue emissions long after they have run through their useful phases, which is why we have the problems of safely disposing radioactive waste products used in radiotherapy and in the production of nuclear energy.

Ionizing versus Nonionizing Radiation

Ions are electrically charged atoms and molecules. Atoms become positively charged when they lose electrons and negatively charged when they gain electrons.

Ionizing radiation is powerful, high-energy radiation that is capable of causing atoms to become ionized or electrically charged. Sources of ionizing radiation include X-rays, cosmic rays, radiation emitted from nuclear power plant accidents, and radiation emitted naturally from radioactive substances such as uranium and radium. Ionizing radiation is dangerous at high levels, so we need to control our exposure. It can alter the DNA structure within a cell's chromosomes, which can

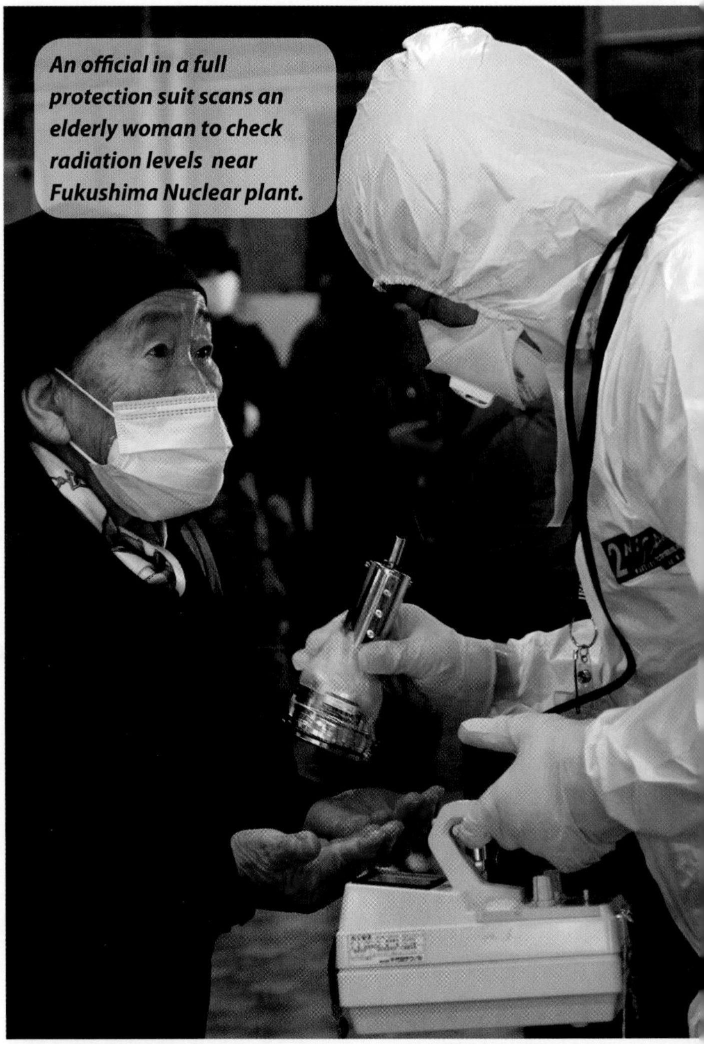

An official in a full protection suit scans an elderly woman to check radiation levels near Fukushima Nuclear plant.

destroy the cell's ability to replicate. It can also lead to the development of cancer. The risk of cancer depends upon the intensity and length of exposure.

Exposure to radiation is measured in **rads** (units of doses of radiation). The average person is exposed to perhaps 300 to 400 mrads (an mrad is 1/1000 of a rad) of ionizing radiation a year. Most of the radiation to which we are exposed comes from natural sources—rocks and soil, radon, and cosmic rays. X-rays account for about a 10th of the average person's exposure to radiation.

Acute exposure levels as low as 50 rads can induce *radiation sickness*, which can cause health problems such as nausea, fatigue, anemia, bleeding from the mouth and gums,

ion
Atom or molecule having a positive or negative electrical charge.

ionizing radiation
Powerful, high-energy radiation that is capable of causing atoms to become ionized or electrically charged.

rad
Short for radiation absorbed dose, *a measure of exposure to radiation.*

hair loss, and immune system disorders. Higher doses have more severe effects, including death. A dose of 800 rads is fatal to humans, though some deaths occur with as little as 200 rads. There is no agreed-upon "safe" level of exposure to radiation. Long-term exposure to higher-than-average levels of radiation may cause serious health problems, including cancer.

Nonionizing radiation does not have high enough energy to ionize matter with which it comes into contact. Common sources of nonionizing radiation include ultraviolet light (sunlight) and energy emitted by electrical appliances, radios, computers, televisions, and high-voltage power lines. Nonionizing radiation is less dangerous than ionizing radiation but can still be harmful. The most plentiful source of nonionizing radiation is sunlight, which can damage the skin, leading to premature wrinkling and skin cancer. The evidence of health risks is mixed and inconclusive for other forms of nonionizing radiation, such as the energy emitted from electrical equipment and electric power lines.

Use of Radiation in Dentistry and Medicine

The use of radiation in diagnostic medical procedures, such as X-rays, computed tomography scans (CT or CAT scans), and other imaging techniques, allows health professionals to probe inside the body without surgery. Mammograms are specialized breast X-rays that can detect breast tumors before they can be felt. Dental X-rays reveal tooth and bone decay.

nonionizing radiation
Radiation that lacks sufficient energy to cause atoms to become ions.

nuclear medicine
The branch of medicine that uses forms of radiation in the diagnosis and treatment of illness.

radioisotope
Radioactive material used in medical diagnosis and treatment.

X-ray
Ionizing radiation that can penetrate most solid objects and is used to project images of the body on photographic film.

electromagnetic fields (EMFs)
Energy fields resulting from the movement of electrical charges and that represent a source of nonionizing radiation.

Nuclear medicine uses radiation to diagnose and treat disease. Ionizing (X-ray) radiation is used in radiotherapy to treat certain forms of cancer, including breast cancer. Nonionizing radiation, such as infrared light, has helped speed recovery from muscle injuries. Physicians also inject small amounts or "chemical tracers" of radioactive chemical substances, called **radioisotopes**, into the patient's bloodstream and then follow their movements in the body via specialized equipment to detect tumors and other abnormalities. Radioisotopes are also used in the treatment of thyroid disorders and other health problems. Physicians also use injectable radioactive substances to detect blockages in blood vessels in and around the heart.

Let us take a closer look at the effects of a common source of ionizing radiation—X-rays—and two common sources of nonionizing radiation—electromagnetic fields and extremely low frequency electromagnetic radiation.

X-Rays

X-rays are waves of electromagnetic radiation of very short wavelengths. They penetrate the body and project images of internal structures onto photographic film to reveal abnormalities, such as broken bones, tumors, and tooth decay. The computed tomography scan (CT scan) combines the X-ray with computer imaging. The CT scan beams X-rays at the body at different angles. The computer analyzes the results to project a three-dimensional computerized image of the inner structures of the body. The amount of radiation emitted by X-ray machines is fairly small and the risk of harm very low. However, X-rays are not entirely risk-free, especially if the procedure is repeated often. Repeated X-rays can increase the risk of cancer and genetic damage. X-rays are especially risky to pregnant women and should be avoided unless they are essential. Some cautions are outlined in "Health Skills 15-1."

Electromagnetic Fields (EMFs)

Electromagnetic fields (EMFs) are forms of nonionizing electromagnetic radiation emitted from electric power lines and electrical appliances and consumer products found in homes and offices. Toasters and televisions, electric blankets and hair dryers, microwave ovens and computer monitors all produce electromagnetic fields. EMFs are strongest at their source and weaken with distance.

How significant is the health threat posed by EMFs? Based on careful review of the scientific evidence, the World Health Organization (WHO) concluded that there is no evidence that exposure to low-level electromagnetic fields from electric power lines or household appliances causes cancer or other health problems.[15]

But what about cell phones? Cell phones emit radiofrequency (RF) energy, which is a form of nonionizing radiation, like FM radio waves and visible light.[16] Most studies find no links between cell phone use and health problems. But an expert panel from the

HEALTH SKILLS 15-1

health skills

Practicing X-ray Safety[17]

These guidelines can help you ensure that X-rays are used appropriately and safely:

1. **Inquire about the need for an X-ray.** Chest X-rays are no longer considered routine. X-rays should only be taken when the results might affect medical treatment or outcomes.
2. **Don't refuse to have a vital X-ray taken because of concerns about exposure to radiation.** Not having an X-ray when it is medically needed may pose a much greater risk to your health than the small exposure to radiation.
3. **Inform your doctor or medical technician if you are pregnant or suspect you might be.** X-rays may harm the fetus.
4. **Make sure that your reproductive organs are covered or shielded from X-ray beams.** However, shielding cannot be used when your doctor needs an X-ray of your reproductive organs for medical purposes.
5. **Make sure a copy of your X-ray is kept safely on file.** Keeping a set of X-rays in your medical records or in your doctor's files will allow doctors treating you in the future to examine changes in your internal organs over time.

WHO recently classified cell phone radiation as "possibly carcinogenic," based on statistical evidence showing an increased risk of a rare form of brain cancer among heavy cell phone users.[18]

While we lack definitive evidence linking cell phone use to cancer or other health problems, people who are concerned about RF energy from cell phones can take steps to limit their exposure, especially to the head, such as by using a hands-free cell phone that works with an earpiece.[19] The earpiece creates more distance between the head and the phone's antenna, which reduces the amount of RF energy reaching the head. People can also limit their overall cell phone use, and use by their children, by reducing the number and length of calls.

Extremely Low Frequency (ELF) Electromagnetic Radiation

Computer monitors, TVs, radios, microwave ovens, and other home and office appliances emit **extremely low frequency (ELF) electromagnetic radiation**. Since many of us (your authors included) spend hours each day in close contact to ELF-producing equipment, concerns about health risks are understandable. Though no one has demonstrated a causal link between exposure to ELFs and health problems, research continues. In the meantime, one can reduce exposure to EMFs (including ELFs) by not sitting or standing too close to the TV, microwave oven, computer monitor, or other appliances when they are on; by avoiding or limiting use of electric blankets; and by placing one's alarm clock at least three feet from one's head.

Microwaves are forms of electromagnetic radiation used in radar, radio and television transmitters, and microwave ovens. In microwave ovens, microwaves cause water molecules in food to vibrate very fast. The vibrations produce heat, which cooks the food. (Glass and ceramic cookware do not vibrate, so they stay cool. But be careful. The heat from the cooked food can radiate to the cookware, which can heat up—ouch!). Microwave-cooked food is not radioactive, and, when used and maintained properly, microwave ovens pose no health risks. Still, microwave ovens may leak radiation, so check the seal on the door regularly. They all produce ELFs, as do other electrical appliances, so stand at least three feet away when using them.

extremely low frequency (ELF) electromagnetic radiation
A source of nonionizing radiation emitted by computer monitors, TVs, radios, and other appliances that is characterized by extremely low frequency electromagnetic waves.

microwave
A form of nonionizing radiation consisting of very high frequency electromagnetic waves that cause molecules to vibrate rapidly, thereby producing heat that can rapidly cook food or boil water.

Population Growth

Where will we put all the people? Better yet, how will we feed them? The population of planet Earth, which currently stands at about 6.9 billion people, has doubled in the past 40 years (see Figure 15-2).

LEARNING OUTCOME 4

Discuss the relationship between population growth and health

More than 1 billion people live in poverty worldwide—about one person in four. If population projections for 2050 come to pass, the world faces the prospect of widespread famine and epidemics, which in part are spread by contaminated water supplies and inadequate health care.

Developing countries in Asia, Africa, and Latin America account for about 95% of the world's population growth. They also contain the world's greatest share of poor people. Industrialized nations, the United States and Canada included, are also growing, but at much slower rates. Industrialized nations may account for but a minority of the world's population, but they are voracious consumers of the world's natural resources—its oil, timber, and mined minerals. The United States, which has a bit more than 4% of the world's population, uses more than one-quarter of the world's oil supply.

Health Threats of Overpopulation

As the world's human population continues to rise, so does the demand for food and shelter. The need for food and shelter leads to human encroachments into wilderness areas. Forested areas are cleared to provide the timber for housing and to make room for the roads and houses needed by an ever-expanding human population. One result of encroachment of natural environments is the extinction of thousands of plant and animal species.

Pollution from industrial plants and emissions from fossil-burning vehicles and homes also contributes to deforestation and damages other wilderness areas. In developing countries, people are caught between two worthy goals: feeding their ever-growing numbers and protecting the natural environment.

With increased human population comes the growing need for housing and food, paving of new roads, and the clearing of wilderness land for new developments and industrial uses, all of which contribute to the reduction of forests and other undeveloped areas. Expanding populations pose a threat of famine as well as increased risk of disease from overtaxed water and sanitation systems.

Zero Population Growth?

Although population growth worldwide continues to rise, the rate of increase has slowed in recent years. Widespread use of contraceptives has curbed fertility rates. Increased family income ironically leads couples to have fewer children because each one makes a measurable difference in the standard of living for the family. Zero population growth (ZPG) would be achieved if birth rates matched death rates, resulting in no net change in the population. ZPG has been achieved in some developed countries, including some countries in Western Europe where many couples are opting for fewer children. But zero population growth in developing nations remains an elusive goal that would require changes in cultural values and an increased standard of living.

Figure 15-2 World Population: 1950–2050[20]

The world population increased from 3 billion in 1959 to 6 billion by 1999, a doubling that occurred over 40 years. The Census Bureau's latest projections imply that population growth will continue into the 21st century, although more slowly. The world population is projected to grow from 6 billion in 1999 to 9 billion by 2044, an increase of 50% in only 45 years.

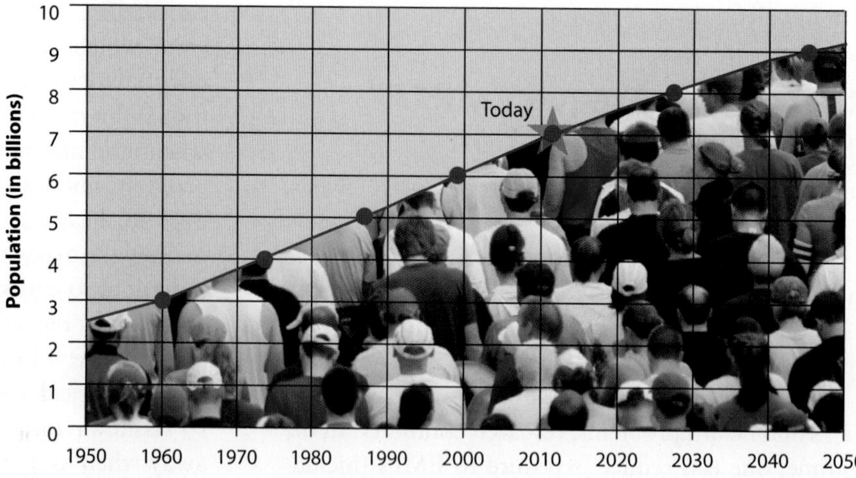

© iStockphoto.com/Lawrence Sawyer

Pollution

Pollution is contamination of the environment by poisonous substances. Some forms of pollution come from natural sources, such as the spewing of ash and gases into the air from volcanic eruptions. Human activity creates other pollutants such as exhaust from motor vehicles and from the burning of coal, fuel oil, and wood in homes, buildings, and factories. Pollution in any form, whether natural or human-made, can harm the environment and our health.[21]

LEARNING OUTCOME 5

Discuss the health hazards of various kinds of pollution and what can be done about them

Outdoor Air Pollution

Air pollution irritates the lungs and eyes and causes respiratory symptoms such as shortness of breath, coughing, and sore throat. Chronic exposure can weaken the immune system and damage the lungs, which can lead to or aggravate lung disorders such as bronchitis and emphysema. Air pollution is also linked to an increased risk of cancer and heart disease. A study of more than 150 metropolitan areas in the United States linked exposure to high levels of air pollution to increased mortality—not as significant a factor in mortality as smoking, but a significant link nonetheless. Even low levels of air pollution can be harmful, impairing lung function and leading to respiratory symptoms. Pollutants can also literally choke the life out of plants, which, through photosynthesis, manufacture the oxygen we need to survive.

Air is a mixture of oxygen (about 20%) and other gases, mostly nitrogen. Breathing (inhaling) pollutants increases the risks of health problems. Once a pollutant enters the body through inhaling, it can become embedded in the lungs (like asbestos) or travel through the bloodstream to other body parts, causing damage to bodily organs and systems (see Figure 15-3 on the next page).

The greatest source of outdoor air pollution is emissions from the burning of **fossil fuels**, the gasoline we use to power our cars, and the burning of oil, natural gas, and coal to heat our homes and provide electrical power. We draw most of the energy we use in this country from burning fossil fuels. The remainder comes from nuclear, solar, and wind power.

When we analyze the chemical makeup of pollutants, we find various toxic substances and gases, including carbon monoxide, sulfur dioxide, nitrogen dioxide, hydrocarbons, and suspended particles called *particulates* or *particulate matter.* Carbon monoxide is spewed from the exhausts of motor vehicles, especially those with inefficient engines and faulty exhaust systems, as well as from the burning of fossil fuels and trash. *Sulfur dioxide* and *nitrogen dioxide* are gaseous pollutants that come largely from coal-burning electric power plants and exhausts from motor vehicles. When these gases enter the body, they not only irritate the respiratory tract and lungs but over time can also lead to serious respiratory diseases such as bronchitis and pneumonia. *Hydrocarbons* are volatile organic compounds consisting of carbon and hydrogen. They are found in cigarette smoke and spewed from the exhaust pipes of motor vehicles and from the evaporation of solvents and fuels into the atmosphere.

Acid rain is precipitation (rain, fog, or snow) containing acids derived from industrial uses and car exhausts.[22] Acid rain illustrates that problems of pollution do not respect national or regional boundaries. Prevailing winds can carry the pollutants across both state and national borders. Sulfur dioxide and nitrogen oxides are the principal pollutants in acid rain. About two-thirds of the sulfur dioxide, and about one-fourth of the nitrogen oxides in acid rain come from electric power plants that rely on burning fossil fuels, such as coal. Motor vehicles also discharge sulfur dioxide and nitrogen dioxide into the atmosphere, where these gases react with water, oxygen, and other chemicals to form the acidic compounds found in acid rain. Acid rain also contains other pollutants, including such toxic substances as aluminum, cadmium, lead, and methyl mercury.

The pollutants in acid rain affect humans and other living organisms. They contaminate forests and soil, as well as lakes and other bodies of water. They also kill fish and make their way into our food supply. In people, the gases in acid rain are inhaled deeply in the lungs, where they can damage lung tissue and lead over time to increased risks of heart and lung disorders (including asthma and bronchitis) as well as premature death.

fossil fuels
Carbon-based sources of energy derived from deposits in the Earth, including oil, natural gas, and coal. These are considered nonrenewable sources of energy because they cannot be replenished.

acid rain
Polluted precipitation that results when pollutants such as sulfur dioxide and nitrogen oxide combine with water molecules in the atmosphere.

Figure 15-3 Health Effects of Pollution

Pollution of the air, water, and land can affect our health in many ways. Some of these effects occur shortly after exposure; others, such as cancer, take months or years to develop. Some effects are relatively minor, such as watery eyes. Others are more serious, including life-threatening lung damage.

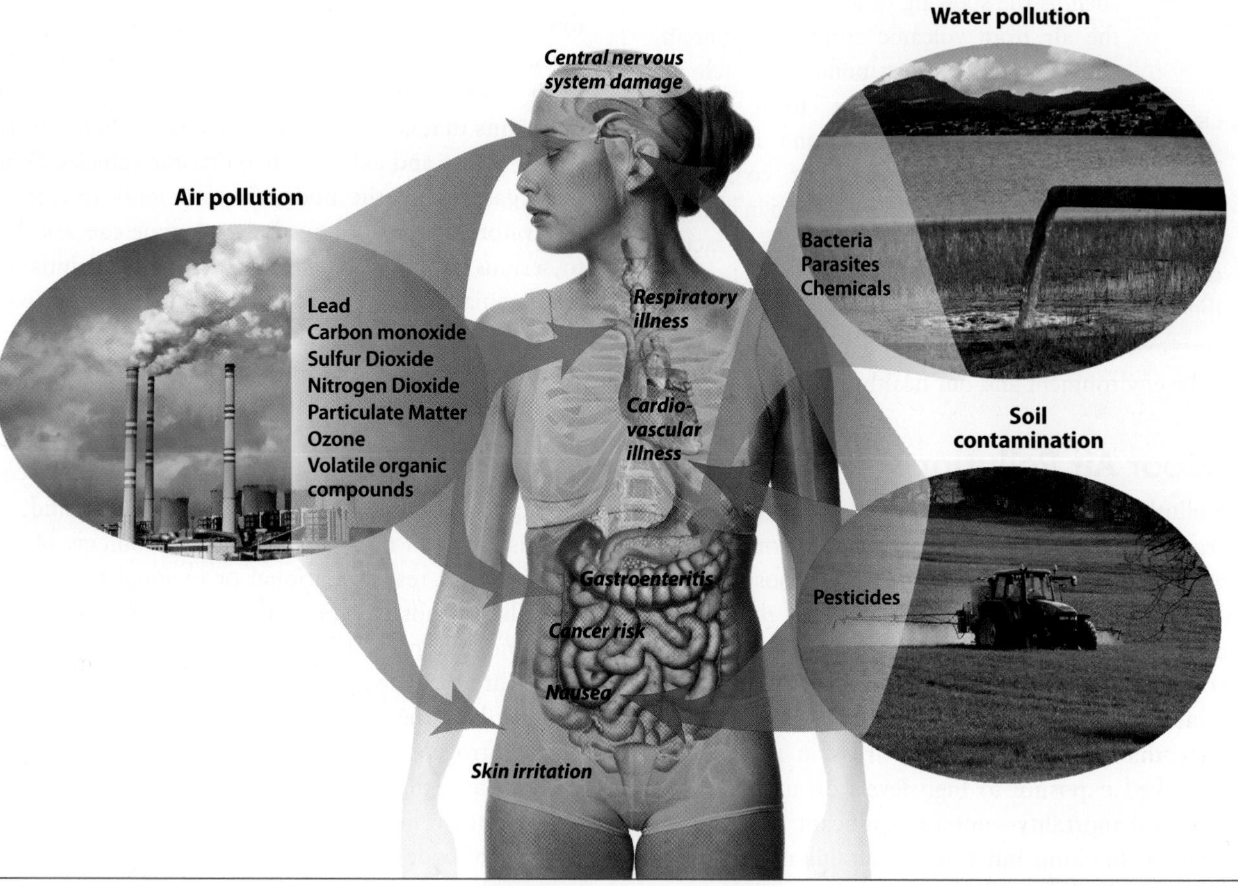

Particulate matter, consisting of dust, soot, ash, and other tiny solid particles, is another major source of air pollution. Particulate matter irritates our respiratory tract and poses yet more serious health risks because it contains known toxins, including pesticides, asbestos, and lead particles.

secondary air pollution *Pollution produced by chemical interactions involving primary pollutants, such as sulfur dioxide, hydrocarbons, and nitrogen oxide.*

ozone *An extremely reactive form of oxygen that is harmful to humans when inhaled and forms a major constituent of smog.*

When hydrocarbons are released into the atmosphere, they interact with sunlight and other pollutants, including sulfur dioxide and nitrogen oxides, to produce **secondary air pollution** in the form of **ozone** and other pollutants (see Figure 15-3). These secondary pollutants descend to ground level, combining with particulate matter, carbon monoxide, and smoke and chemical gases spewed from auto exhausts and industrial plants to form the unhealthy, foggy haze called *smog*. Smog pollutes the air of many of our major cities. The major constituent of smog is ozone.

Ozone

Ozone (O_3) is a highly reactive form of oxygen that occurs naturally in the stratosphere (upper atmosphere) as a result of sunlight acting on normal oxygen (O_2). (Instead of the two oxygen atoms that form breathable oxygen, a molecule of ozone contains three oxygen atoms). The high concentration of ozone in the upper atmosphere protects living things from the most dangerous forms of ultraviolet radiation from the sun. Without this protective ozone layer (about 12 to 30 miles above the earth), plants and animals would not be able to survive on land. It is ironic that the same ozone that preserves life when it is in the upper atmosphere is toxic even in low concentrations when we inhale it at ground level.

Ozone interferes with the lung's ability to defend itself against invading microorganisms, increasing the chances of lung and respiratory infections. It also dampens the body's immune response, which increases susceptibility to pathogens. The people most affected by smog are children, older people, and people with asthma, chronic bronchitis, or emphysema. Yet even robust, healthy people who seem unaffected by high ozone levels may suffer lung damage. Health officials are concerned that breathing smog on a regular basis early in life may lead to the development of chronic lung problems.

The ozone layer of the atmosphere has been thinning, so much so that a hole about the size of North America forms seasonally in the ozone layer over the South Pole. Ozone holes have also appeared above Canada and the northern parts of the United States and Europe. In other areas, the ozone layer has thinned to a lesser but still dangerous degree.

The release of petrochemicals called **chlorofluorocarbons**, or **CFCs**, is a primary cause of thinning of the ozone layer. CFCs are gases composed of carbon, chlorine, and fluorine. They are used mostly as coolants in refrigerators and air conditioners, as aerosol propellants, and in the manufacture of foam insulation. CFCs release chlorine molecules that literally eat ozone molecules. CFCs in aerosols are now banned in the United States, and refrigerator manufacturers have switched to another coolant, *hydrochlorofluorocarbons*, or HCFCs. These too deplete ozone, but not as much as CFCs.

Health officials fear that the thinning of the ozone layer may increase the risk of skin cancer and immune system disorders in humans. The phasing out of ozone-depleting chemicals should lead the ozone layer to thicken, but skin cancers usually develop decades after exposure. Skin damage caused by depletion of ozone during the latter part of the twentieth century may continue to produce skin tumors for many years.

Indoor Air Pollution

Nearly all of us are aware of the dangers of outdoor air pollution, but what about the air in your own home? Might it be too dangerous to breathe?

Many types of pollutants can poison the air we breathe in our home, including radon, lead particles, mercury fumes, and fumes and gases from petrochemical and pesticide products, to name a few. In fact, indoor pollutants are more of an immediate health threat than are outdoor pollutants.

Carbon monoxide, a colorless and odorless gas, is both an indoor and outdoor pollutant. But it poses a greater immediate threat indoors since it is not as easily dispersed. It can kill without warning. You cannot detect it with your senses. Yet we can safeguard the air we breathe in the home in many ways, such as by following the steps described earlier for minimizing the risks of radon, pesticides, and lead contamination. "Prevention 15-2" on page 333 describes how to protect oneself from carbon monoxide, the silent killer. Here's another rather simple, but useful, suggestion: Airing out the home once or twice a day during times of the year when windows are usually shut can help remove residues from cleaning sprays, pesticides, and other chemicals used around the house.

Water Pollution

Water makes up more than 70% of the Earth's surface, but nearly all of it (97%) is undrinkable saltwater. Of the 3% of the Earth's water that is fresh, only about 1% is drinkable. Still, this 1% would be enough to serve the needs of the world's population were it not for water pollution. As it stands, however, millions of people, mostly in developing nations but also in the United States and other industrialized nations, do not have clean water to drink. Water pollution comes from many sources, including municipal, agricultural and industrial wastes. These wastes can include toxic chemicals that are not broken down by natural processes in the environment and that can enter the body in the air we breathe, the food we eat, and the water we drink.

Nearly all of the Earth's freshwater (95%) comes from **groundwater**, which is found in natural rock formations called **aquifers**.[23] The rest comes from **surface water**, which is found in ponds, lakes, rivers, streams, and reservoirs. About half of the U.S. population draws its drinking water from groundwater, whereas the other half relies on surface water.

Is America's water supply fit to drink? The answer is yes, but it's a qualified yes. Though the great majority of Americans can safely drink water directly

chlorofluorocarbons (CFCs)
Organochlorine chemicals used as coolants, aerosol propellants, and solvents; the primary culprit in the depletion of the ozone layer.

groundwater
Water below the land surface from snow and rain that collects in porous rock formations.

aquifer
Geological formation that holds water.

surface water
Water found in aboveground bodies such as ponds, lakes, rivers, streams, and reservoirs.

from the tap, we still have a long way to go to meet the goal of providing clean drinking water to all Americans. The Centers for Disease Control and Prevention reports that more than 7,000 Americans each year become sick from drinking tap water. This figure represents but the tip of the iceberg, since in most cases people don't realize that it is their drinking water that is making them sick.

To protect our water supplies, public water systems undergo extensive purification and treatment processes. (People who depend upon private wells for their drinking water need to hire inspectors to check for contaminants and should do so annually.) Water purification involves several steps, beginning with filtration through sand beds, addition of chemicals that attract suspended particles, filtration to remove the particles, and—finally—disinfection and fluoridation. Chlorine is used widely as a disinfectant to kill harmful microbes. Chlorination of water supplies is not a health hazard, but the risks of typhoid and cholera from drinking contaminated water are very real health hazards and can even be deadly. Fluoridation is used in about half of the nation's public water supply to prevent tooth decay.

The provision of safe drinking water is one of the great success stories in public health in the United States in this century. The elimination of epidemics spread by contaminated water supplies, such as cholera, typhoid, and dysentery, has saved an incalculable number of lives and is a major contributor to the increase in life expectancy that has occurred over the past 100 years.

A major problem with America's water supply is that many of our water systems depend on outdated water-treatment systems. More than 90% of major water systems in the United States rely on chemical removal systems that were installed more than 50 years ago. These systems were not designed to filter out many of the chemical contaminants produced today, including many pesticides and industrial waste products. Some systems fail to meet EPA standards intended to safeguard against disease-causing organisms. Another problem is that many water systems fail to safeguard the watershed, the system of aquifers and streams that provide source water for the system. Polluted discharges or runoffs from farms, lawns, and city streets contaminate the watersheds that service many communities. Go online to read "Prevention 15-3" to learn what you and your neighbors can do to ensure your water is safe to drink.

hazmats
Industrial wastes that are considered hazardous (ignitable, corrosive, reactive, or toxic) and pose risks to health and environment.

prevention

Access CourseMate for HLTH at www.cengagebrain.com.

Land Pollution

Where does all the garbage go? We Americans produce more than 250 million tons of solid waste—commonly called *trash* or *garbage*—annually.[24] That amounts to about 4.5 pounds of stuff per person that we throw out every day. This monumental pile of waste includes food scraps, discarded paper products, clothing, furniture, cans and bottles, plastic bottles and containers, old appliances, and piles of newspapers and magazines. Figure 15-4 shows the composition of the enormous pile of garbage we Americans throw in the trash every year.

The largest contributor to our solid waste is paper, underscoring the need for community recycling programs that put paper waste and other recyclables to good use. Yet despite massive recycling efforts, several factors cause the total waste produced in the United States to continue to rise:

1. Huge increase in single-person households, each of which is equipped with household products that larger family units typically share.
2. Rise in the use of throwaway products that make cooking and cleaning more convenient but produce more waste.
3. Growth of an "information economy," which is increasingly dependent on paper products—from computer paper to junk mail.

We discard two kinds of solid waste. *Municipal solid waste* (MSW) is ordinary household waste and waste produced by light industry. This includes virtually anything that individuals and small business owners toss into the trash. *Industrial solid waste* is waste material produced by heavy industry, government, agriculture, sewage, and mining, among other sources. About 200 million tons of industrial wastes produced each year are hazardous materials ("hazmats"). **Hazmats** are ignitable, corrosive, reactive, or toxic. They pose risks to health and to the environment.

Where does all the garbage go? Most solid wastes are buried in underground disposal facilities called *landfills*. These facilities are lined with plastic to keep wastes from leaking into the ground and possibly contaminating groundwater and soil. When filled, landfills are capped over with asphalt or other materials. In many cases, however, landfills have seeped contaminants into soil and water. Though newer landfills are generally better designed to prevent leaks, the resistance of local residents to having landfills in their communities—the "Not in My Backyard," or NIMBY, syndrome—has prevented many new sites from opening (learn more by reading "Diversity 15-1" on page 347). Other barriers to creating new landfills include the high costs of both building and operating them, as well as the diminishing supply of potential sites

Many U.S. landfills have already run out of room; many others are nearing capacity. Recycled waste doesn't meet its final resting place in landfills but is recovered and used to make new products. Yet other waste is sometimes dumped illegally in open dumps on water and land, producing not merely an unsightly mess but potential contamination of groundwater and soil by seepage of toxic or hazardous substances. Other waste may be incinerated or burned under carefully controlled conditions. Incineration remains a controversial topic in waste management because the ash produced by burning solid waste is a source of air pollution and may contain toxic substances such as heavy metals and acid gases. The installation of specially designed pollution-control devices, such as scrubbers, helps to reduce the problem but doesn't eliminate it. Lacking any major new developments in waste management technology, *waste prevention* will surely become a watchword in the years ahead.

Let us end this section on a positive note. Despite the fact that the amount of solid waste continues to rise, the rate of increase has slowed in recent years. Recycling efforts are clearly making a dent in lessening the waste crisis we face. Go online to read "Health Skills 15-2" to learn how you can do your part in protecting the environment.

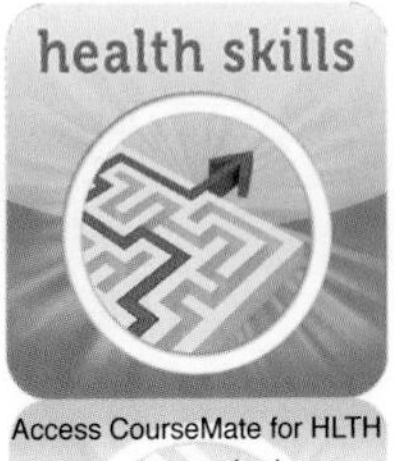

Access CourseMate for HLTH at www.cengagebrain.com.

Noise Polution: Living Loud

Noise is not just annoying. It is a health hazard that can lead to hearing problems, even hearing loss, as well as elevated blood pressure, learning problems, and other health problems.

Noise is any sound that is loud, discordant, or disagreeable. The loudness of sound is measured in decibels (dBA) (see Figure 15-5 on the next page). Our threshold for hearing begins at around 1 dBA. Any sound over 35 to 45 dBA can disturb sleep. Sound becomes noise at about 60 dBA.

Figure 15-4 What Makes Up Our Garbage?[25]

Here we see the contributions in percentage terms of different kinds of discarded trash and garbage that make up America's solid waste on an annual basis.

Total Annual Waste Generation in the United States (before recycling)

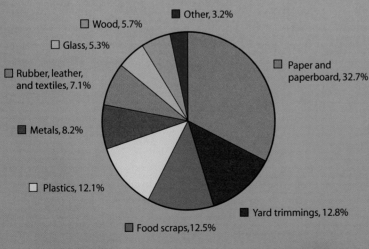

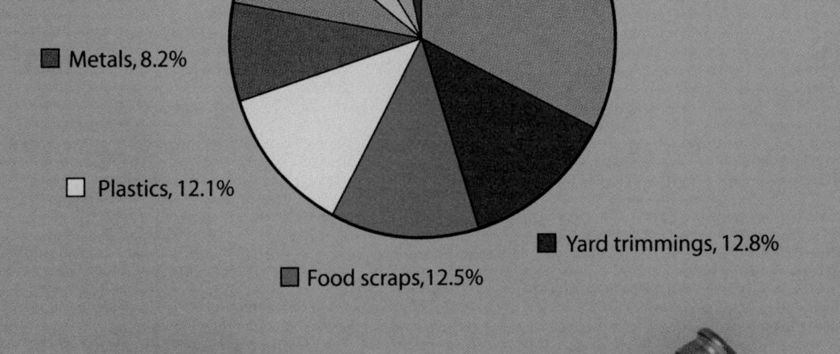

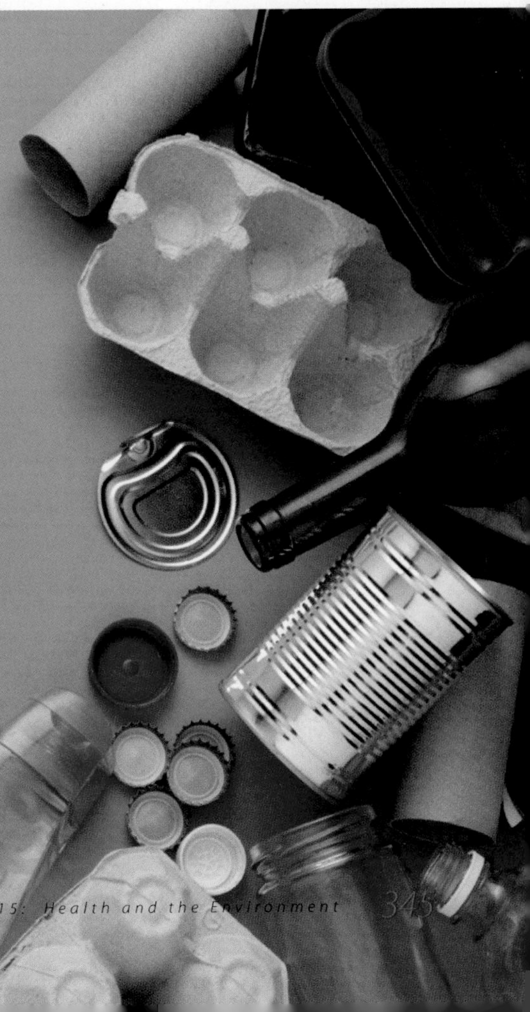

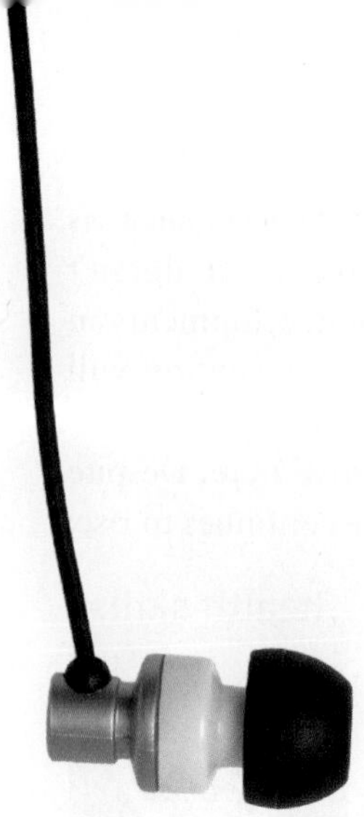

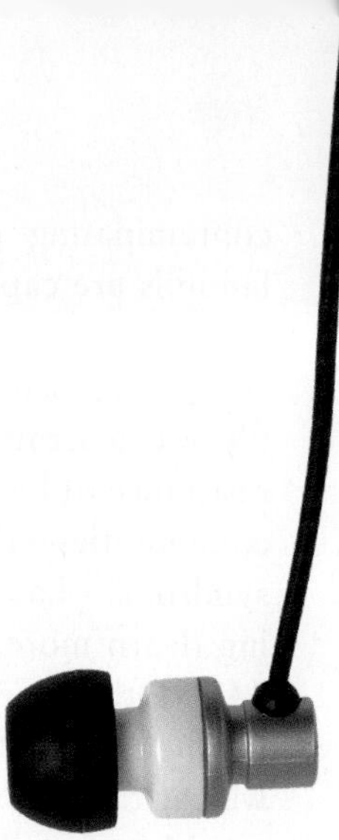

Figure 15-5 Sounds and Decibels

Permanent hearing loss may occur from prolonged exposure to sound over 85 dBA. The threshold level of human hearing is just above 0 dBA.

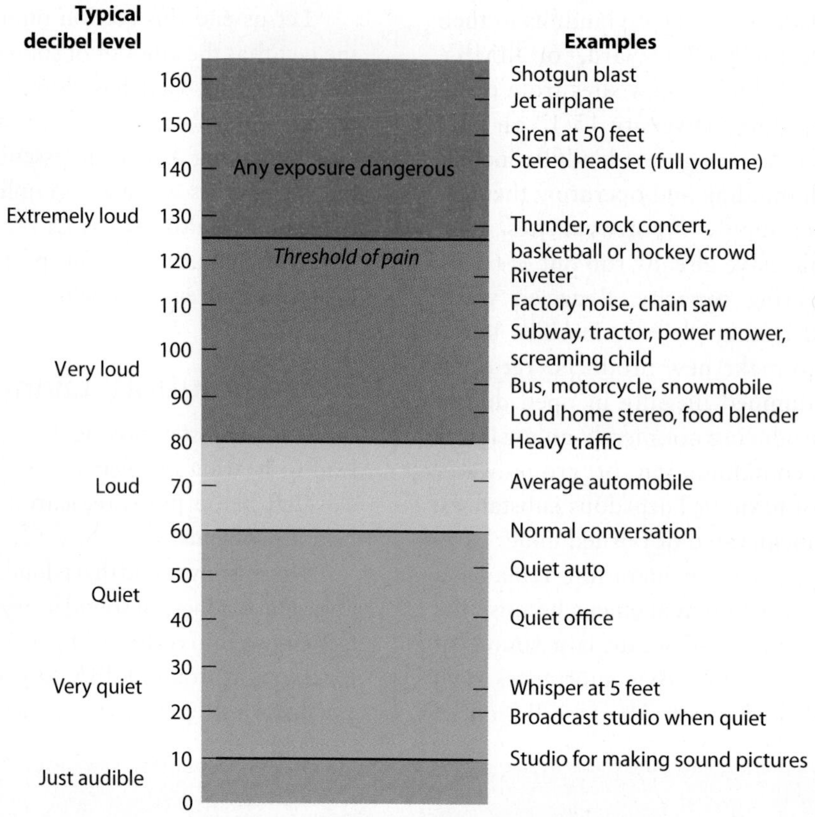

At levels of 85 dBA or higher, noise can trigger the body's stress response, inducing elevated blood pressure and indigestion. At about 125 dBA and beyond, noise becomes physically painful. But bear in mind that hearing loss can occur before pain sets it, such as from prolonged exposure to noise at 85 dBA or higher or exposure to brief bursts of noise of 120 dBA or louder.

How loud is 120 dBA? The noise level at most bars and clubs registers 110 to 120 dBA. People who work at nightclubs or frequent them often have ear damage. The clamor at rock concerts typically exceeds 100 dBA, subjecting musicians and frequent concert-goers to the risk of hearing loss.[26] Unmindful of the dangers, many young people play personal music players at similarly dangerous volumes day after day. Nearly 20% of teens already show evidence of some hearing loss.[27]

Though some cases of extreme noise (like explosions) can instantly rupture the eardrum, most cases of hearing loss occur gradually. The numbers of people with hearing impairment are expected to mushroom to 78 million by 2030, largely as the result of years of living loudly.[28]

You may not realize the damage you are doing to your ears by listening to loud music until many years afterwards. Though hearing loss is common among older people in our society, it is not inevitable. Older people in less technologically advanced societies often retain good hearing. Hearing loss in later life in our society is due largely to years of prior abuse from loud music and noise. "Health Check 15-2" on page 348 helps you evaluate the steps you are taking (or could be taking) to protect your hearing.

Occupational noise is a serious health problem in the workplace. The Occupational Health and Safety Administration (OSHA) requires employers to monitor noise levels and provide annual hearing tests for employees who are exposed to noise levels of 85 dBA or above. OSHA also mandates that employees be encouraged to wear hearing protection devices.

DIVERSITY 15-1

Toxic Communities: A Form of Environmental Racism?

The nation is littered with toxic waste sites where heavy industry has dumped chemicals and other hazardous wastes into the ground or discharged them into canals, rivers, and streams. To protect human health and the environment, the federal government has undertaken efforts to clean up hazardous waste sites. To date, more than half of the 1,500 priority sites identified by the government have been cleaned up.[29]

Millions of Americans live within a few miles of these priority sites. Yet the placement of toxic waste facilities is not color-blind. A disproportionate number of toxic waste facilities are located in areas with high concentrations of people of color. *Environmental racism* refers to racial bias in policy-making and enforcement efforts that leads to the disproportionate placement of waste sites and other environmental hazards in neighborhoods populated by poor people and people of color. Ethnic minorities, including African Americans and Latin Americans, are more likely than European Americans to live in areas with poor air quality. Though race and income are often intertwined, these differences are not explained simply by income or socioeconomic status. Though poor people are more likely than affluent people to live in areas of substandard air quality, even among poor people, African Americans and Hispanic Americans are more likely to breathe polluted air than poor European Americans are. Why? Largely because air-polluting facilities, such as industrial plants and electric generating facilities, are disproportionately placed in areas with high percentages of minority residents. Again, race is a more important factor in accounting for the placement of these environmental hazards than income. Terms such as *environmental racism* and *environmental justice* parallel concerns for justice and equality in other spheres of life, including housing and education.

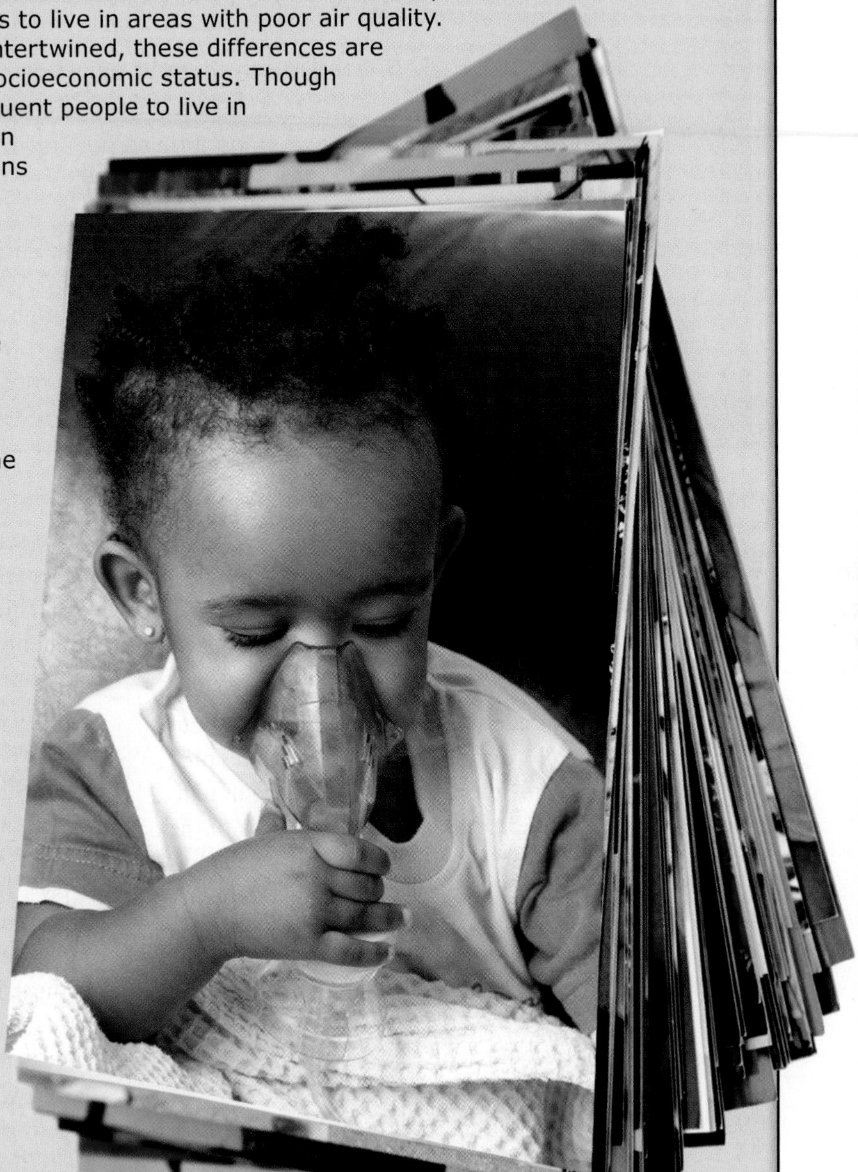

Nobody wants environmental hazards in their backyard (the NIMBY syndrome). Industries therefore typically place these facilities in communities with the least political clout. These are typically poorer communities and minority communities. The residents may be less well organized than members of more affluent communities. They may lack the resources of time, money, and contacts to affect policy decisions. Or they may be at a disadvantage because they are underrepresented on governing or regulatory bodies.

HEALTH CHECK 15-2

Preventing Noise-Induced Hearing Loss

What steps are you taking (or could you be taking) to protect your hearing from excessive noise?

YES	NO	DO YOU . . .
____	____	1. Turn down the volume on your personal music player and avoid playing it at the highest level?
____	____	2. Avoid attending ear-splitting concerts?
____	____	3. Take steps to soundproof your home if you live in a noisy environment, such as installing thick carpeting and double-paned windows?
____	____	4. Wear hearing protectors or soft foam or silicone-type earplugs when you can't avoid excessive noise, such as while at construction sites?
____	____	5. Get together with your neighbors if you live in a particularly noisy area to pressure government officials to seek remedies?
____	____	6. Avoid becoming a noise polluter by not honking your horn except in cases of emergency and by keeping your music system at a level that won't bother your neighbors?
____	____	7. Use your fingers (carefully) as earplugs in a noise emergency, such as when exposed to the siren of a nearby fire engine or ambulance or the screeching sounds of a passing subway train?

If you answered "Yes" to many of these steps, good for you; you are doing what you can to protect yourself against hearing loss. If you answered "No" to most of the protective practices listed here, you could very well be in danger of suffering noise-induced hearing loss in your future.

Climate Change

Global warming—the increasing average temperature in the Earth's atmosphere—has become one of the most controversial issues of our time. The average global temperature rose about 1 °F during the twentieth century. This may not seem like much, but the difference in temperature between the Earth today and the depths of the last ice age is only 5° to 9°. At the heart of the debate is whether the Earth's atmosphere is warming and whether humans are contributing to it. Although the debate over climate change has been highly politicized, a poll of the world's leading climate scientists showed that 97% agree that the atmosphere is warming, and that we humans are contributing to it through emissions of *greenhouse gases*.[30] Just as a greenhouse shields plants from cold temperatures outside but lets in natural sunlight, the atmosphere serves a natural function of shielding the Earth from the cold of outer space while letting the warmth of the sun shine through. Without this **greenhouse effect**, the Earth's temperature would be about 0°F. The problem is that human activities are increasing this natural greenhouse effect, leading to the gradual warming of the Earth's global temperature.

The greenhouse effect results from the trapping of heat in the Earth's lower atmosphere of greenhouse gases, such as carbon dioxide, methane, and nitrous oxide. The emission of greenhouse gases makes the Earth warmer by trapping energy in the atmosphere. These gases are released through the burning of fossil fuels (for example, coal, oil, and natural gas) by our motor vehicles, by furnaces in buildings, and by industry and agriculture.

global warming
The gradual increase in global temperatures.

greenhouse effect
The rise in atmospheric temperature resulting from the release of heat-trapping gasses produced by the burning of fossil fuels.

LEARNING OUTCOME 6

Discuss the relationship between climate change and health

Effects of Global Warming

Why should we be concerned about global warming? Increasing temperatures on Earth affect changes in climate, which can lead to rising sea levels, changes in rainfall patterns, and more severe weather patterns, causing more floods and droughts and reducing crop yields. Higher temperatures may spread tropical diseases such as malaria, yellow fever, and dengue to previously cooler areas. We can also expect more deaths from killer heat waves. Excessive heat is today's leading weather-related killer—not lightning, tornadoes, or hurricanes.

What Can Be Done?

Taking action may help slow the process of global warming. We can reduce our dependence on fossil fuels, especially coal and petroleum products like gasoline and home heating oil. Knowing what to do is one thing. Doing it is quite another. Some progress has been made in reducing fossil fuel consumption. For example, government regulations require higher mileage and lower emissions on motor vehicles as the years go on.

We can contribute by relying on more energy-efficient modes of transportation, as by using public transportation rather than private automobiles and by using more foot power (bicycling and walking) in place of motorized vehicles. The additional exercise will also be healthful. Trees "inhale" carbon dioxide and "exhale" oxygen, so reforestation of cleared regions would be of help. The online feature "Health Skills 15-3" promotes alternatives to our reliance on fossil fuels, such as hydropower, wind energy, solar energy, geothermal energy, and biomass energy.

health skills

Access CourseMate for HLTH at www.cengagebrain.com.

HEALTH APPS: YOUR LINK TO ONLINE HEALTH APPLICATIONS

prevention — **Protecting Our Families from Lead Poisoning** Although lead paint in homes has been banned, many older homes still have it on their walls. Lead is found in drinking water, even in dust we inhale. What can we do to protect our families from lead poisoning? Go to "Prevention 15-1" to find out.

health check — **Rating Environmental Hazards—What's the Risk?** Do your perceptions of the risks posed by environmental hazards square with those of environmental experts? Complete "Health Check 15-1" to find out.

prevention — **Protecting Our Drinking Water** Is your tap water safe to drink? Does your community's water supply meet clean water standards? Read "Prevention 15-3" to learn what you and your neighbors can do to ensure that your water is safe to drink.

health skills — **Doing Your Part to Make the Environment Safer and Healthier** A half century ago, the effects of pollution of our environment may have been a nuisance. Today, they are a global crisis. But governments alone cannot save the Earth. Go to "Health Skills 15-2" to learn how you can do your part.

health skills — **Renewable Sources of Energy in the United States** As gasoline prices and your awareness of global warning and its consequences both shoot up, you may switch to a smaller car or one with hybrid power. But there are also broader measures we can take, such as helping move the nation—and the world—in the direction of renewable energy. To learn more about alternatives to reliance on fossil fuels and nuclear power, go to "Health Skills 15-3."

Go to the CourseMate for HLTH at www.cengagebrain.com for additional resources including flashcards, games, self-quizzes, review exercises, web exercises, learning checks, and more.

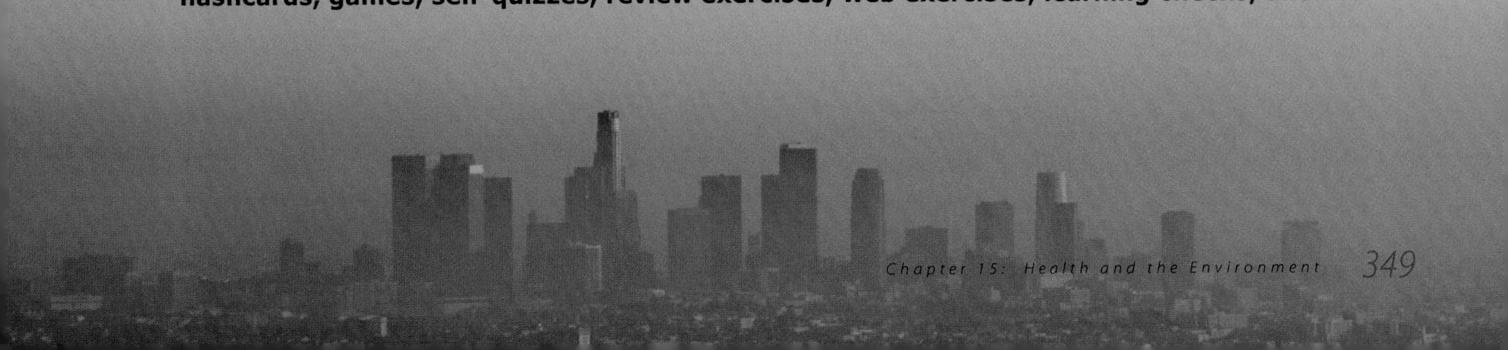

Health across the Life Span

"So far, everyone who has lived has aged—which may not be a bad fate, considering the alternative."

Learning Outcomes

1 Discuss physical changes in late adulthood

2 Compare programmed and cellular damage theories of aging

3 Identify common health concerns associated with late adulthood

4 Define *death* and discuss the process of dying

5 Discuss various kinds of euthanasia and controversies about them

6 Discuss ways of coping with death

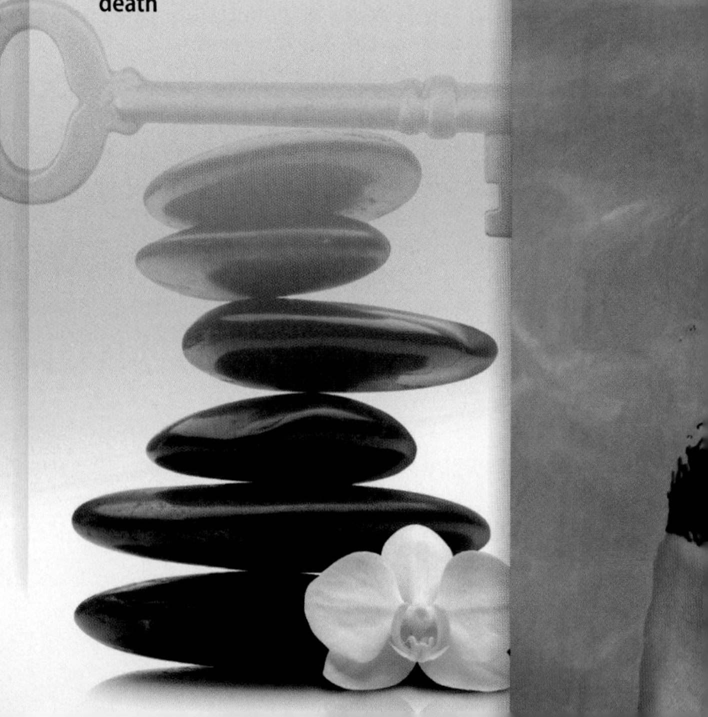

Longevity and Life Expectancy

In 1900, only one person in 25 was over the age of 65. Today, that figure has more than tripled, to one in eight. By midcentury, more than one in five Americans will be 65 years of age or older, and we expect to see the percentage of Americans over the age of 75 double. To put these numbers in historical context, consider that through virtually all of human history, until the beginning of the 19th century, only a small fraction of humans lived to the age of 50.

LEARNING OUTCOME 1

Discuss physical changes in late adulthood

One's **life span**, or **longevity**, is the length of time one can live under the best of circumstances. The life span of a species, including humans, depends on its genetic programming. With the right genes and environment, and with the good fortune to avoid serious injuries or illnesses, people have a maximum life span of about 115 years.

One's **life expectancy** refers to the number of years a person in a given population group can actually expect to live. The average European American child born 100 years ago in the United States could expect to live 47 years. The average African American could expect a shorter life of 35.5 years.[1] Since then, great strides have been made in increasing life expectancy. High infant mortality rates

life span (longevity)
The maximum amount of time a person can live under optimal conditions.

life expectancy
The amount of time a person can actually be expected to live in a given setting.

due to diseases such as German measles, smallpox, polio, and diphtheria contributed to the lower life-expectancy rates of a century ago. These diseases have been brought under control or eradicated. Other major killers, including bacterial infections such as tuberculosis, are now largely controlled by antibiotics. Factors that have contributed to increased longevity include public health measures such as safer water supplies, improved dietary habits, and health care. On the next page, "Diversity 16-1" examines gender differences in life expectancy, and Table 16-1 shows the life expectancy of males and females born today in various regions and countries of the world.

Although life expectancy has been increasing for both African Americans and White Americans in the United States, Whites still hold an advantage (see Chapter 1). However, racial differences have begun to narrow in recent years.

Physical Changes

No two people age in the same way or at the same rate. But whatever individual differences may exist, physiological aging is defined by changes in the body's integumentary system (the body's system of skin, hair, and nails), senses, reaction time, and lung capacity. These

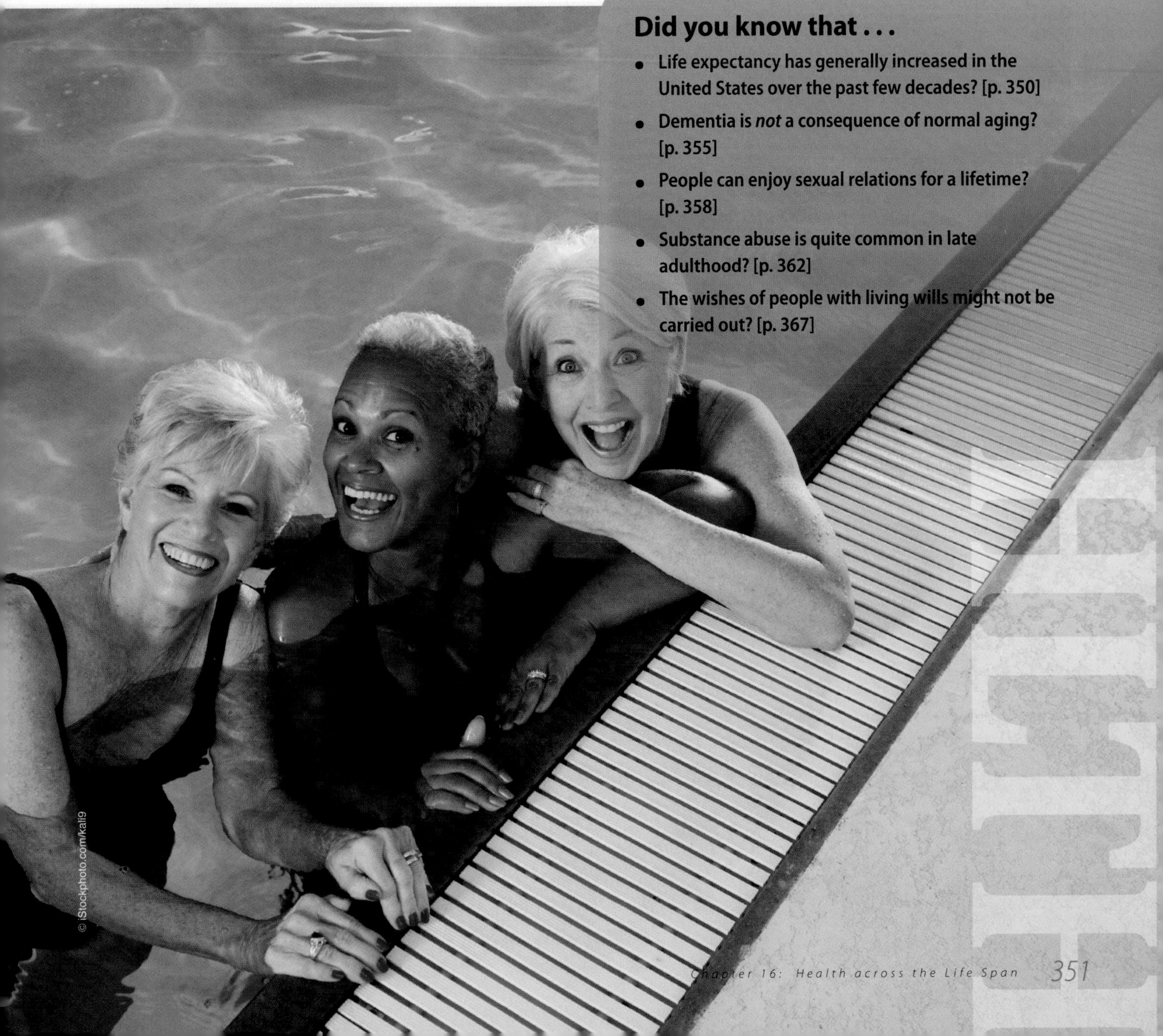

Did you know that . . .

- **Life expectancy has generally increased in the United States over the past few decades? [p. 350]**
- **Dementia is *not* a consequence of normal aging? [p. 355]**
- **People can enjoy sexual relations for a lifetime? [p. 358]**
- **Substance abuse is quite common in late adulthood? [p. 362]**
- **The wishes of people with living wills might not be carried out? [p. 367]**

DIVERSITY 16-1

Gender Differences in Life Expectancy

Life expectancy among men trails that among women by about five years (76 years for men versus 81 years for women).[2]

Why the gap? For one thing, heart disease typically develops later in life in women than in men, as estrogen provides women some protection against it. Also, men are more likely to die from accidents, cirrhosis of the liver, strokes, suicide, homicide, HIV/AIDS, and some forms of cancer. Many of these causes of death reflect unhealthful habits that are more typical of men, such as drinking, reckless behavior, and smoking.

Many men are also reluctant to have regular physical examinations or to talk over health problems with their doctors. Many men avoid medical attention until problems that could have been easily prevented or treated become serious or life-threatening. For example, women are more likely to examine themselves for signs of breast cancer than men are to examine their testicles for unusual lumps.

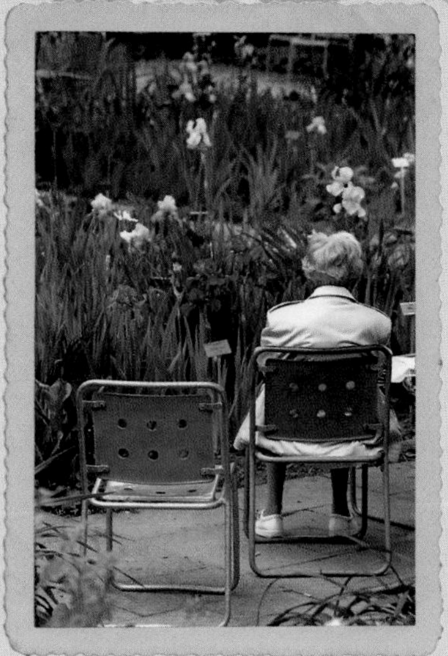

Table 16-1 Life Expectancy at Birth by Region, Country, and Gender

	MALES	FEMALES
AFRICA		
Mozambique	51	53
Egypt	70	75
ASIA		
Afghanistan	45	45
China	73	77
India	66	68
Japan	79	86
South Korea	76	82
LATIN AMERICA		
Brazil	69	76
Cuba	75	80
Jamaica	72	75
Mexico	74	79
EUROPE		
France	78	85
Germany	78	82
Italy	79	85
Poland	72	80
Russia	60	73
Sweden	79	84
United Kingdom	78	82
NORTH AMERICA		
Canada	79	84
United States	76	81

Source: Central Intelligence Agency. (2011). *World factbook*. Retrieved from https://www.cia.gov/library/publications/the-world-factbook/

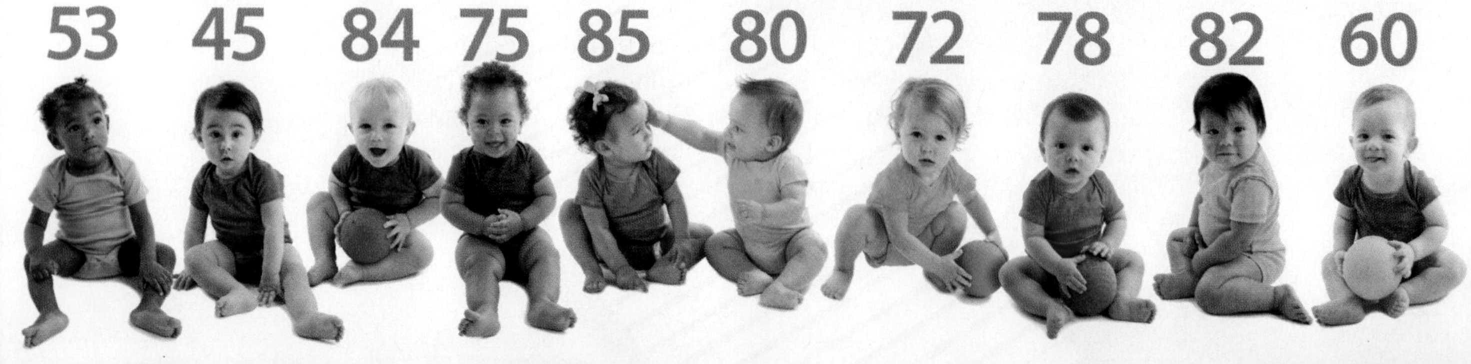

HEALTH CHECK 16-1

Ten Ways to Recognize Hearing Loss

The following questions will help you determine if you need to have your hearing evaluated by a medical professional:

YES	NO	
Y	N	Do you have a problem hearing over the telephone?
Y	N	Do you have trouble following the conversation when two or more people are talking at the same time?
Y	N	Do people complain that you turn the TV volume up too high?
Y	N	Do you have to strain to understand conversations?
Y	N	Do you have trouble hearing in a noisy background?
Y	N	Do you find yourself asking people to repeat themselves?
Y	N	Do many people you talk to seem to mumble (or not speak clearly)?
Y	N	Do you misunderstand what others are saying and respond inappropriately?
Y	N	Do you have trouble understanding the speech of women and children?
Y	N	Do people get annoyed because you misunderstand what they say?

If you answered "yes" to three or more of these questions, you might want to see an ear, nose, and throat specialist or an audiologist for a hearing evaluation.

Source: National Institute on Deafness and Other Communication Disorders (NIDCD). (2011, February 9). *Ten ways to recognize hearing loss.* Retrieved from http://www.nidcd.nih.gov/health/hearing/10ways.asp

changes may well be unavoidable. Changes in metabolism, muscle mass, strength, bone density, aerobic capacity, blood-sugar tolerance, and ability to regulate body temperature may be moderated and sometimes reversed through exercise and diet.

Skin and Hair

Hair usually begins to gray in middle adulthood as the production of *melanin*, the pigment responsible for hair color, decreases. Hair loss also accelerates with aging, especially in men. Much wrinkling associated with aging is actually caused by exposure to ultraviolet (UV) rays.

Beginning gradually in early adulthood, the body produces fewer proteins that give the skin its elasticity. The body also produces fewer *keratinocytes*—the cells in the outer layer of the skin that are regularly shed and renewed, leaving the skin dryer and more brittle.

Sensory Functioning

Normal age-related changes in vision begin to appear by the mid-30s and assert themselves as significant problems in middle adulthood. **Presbyopia** (Latin for "old vision") refers to loss of elasticity in the lens that makes it harder to focus on, or accommodate, nearby objects or fine print. Cataracts, glaucoma, and hearing loss are usually problems of late adulthood. Cataracts cloud the lenses of the eyes, reducing vision. Today, outpatient surgery for correcting cataracts is routine. If performed before the condition progresses too far, the outcome for regained sight is excellent. Glaucoma is a buildup of fluid pressure inside the eyeball. Glaucoma can lead to tunnel vision (lack of peripheral vision) or blindness. Glaucoma rarely occurs before age 40 and affects about one in 250 people over the age of 40, and one in 25 people older than 80. Rates are higher among African Americans than among European Americans, and higher among diabetics than among nondiabetics. Glaucoma is treated with medication or surgery.

The sense of hearing, especially the ability to hear higher frequencies, also declines with age. **Presbycusis** is age-related hearing loss that affects about one person in three over the age of 65.[3] Hearing ability tends to decline more quickly in men than in women. ("Health Check 16-1" will help you determine whether you need to have your hearing evaluated.) Hearing aids magnify

presbyopia
Gradual, age-related loss of elasticity of the lens of the eye, making focusing on close objects or fine print difficult.

presbycusis
Loss of acuteness of hearing due to age-related degenerative changes in the ear.

sound and can compensate for hearing loss. Taste and smell become less acute as we age.

Our sense of smell decreases almost ninefold from youth to advanced late adulthood. We also lose taste buds in the tongue with aging. As a result, foods must be more strongly spiced to yield the same flavor.

Reaction Time

Reaction time—the amount of time it takes to respond to a stimulus—increases with age, mainly because of changes in the nervous system. At around age 25, we begin to lose neurons, which are responsible for sensing signals such as sights and sounds and those involved in coordinating muscular responses to them.

Lung Capacity

Lung tissue stiffens with age, diminishing capacity to expand, such that breathing capacity may decline by half between early and late adulthood. Regular exercise can offset much of this loss, and beginning to exercise regularly in middle adulthood can expand breathing capacity beyond what it was earlier in life.

Lean-Body Mass and Body Fat

Beginning at age 20, we lose nearly seven pounds of lean-body mass with each decade. The rate of loss accelerates after the age of 45. Fat replaces lean-body mass, which includes muscle. Consequently, the average person's body mass index (BMI) rises.

Muscle Strength

Loss of muscle lessens strength. However, the change is gradual, and in middle adulthood, exercise can readily compensate by increasing the size of remaining muscle cells. Exercise will not restore the prowess of the athlete from early adulthood, but it will contribute to vigor, health, and a desirable body shape.

Metabolism

Metabolism is the rate at which the body processes or "burns" food to produce energy. The resting metabolic rate—also called the *basal metabolic rate (BMR)*—declines as we age. Fatty tissue burns fewer calories than muscle, and the decline in BMR is largely attributable to the loss of muscle tissue and the corresponding increase in fatty tissue. Since we require fewer calories to maintain our weight as we age, middle-aged people (and older adults) are likely to gain weight if they eat as much as they did as young adults.

osteoporosis
A disorder in which bones become more porous, brittle, and subject to fracture, due to loss of calcium and other minerals.

Bone Density

Bones begin to lose density in middle adulthood, becoming more brittle and vulnerable to fracture. Bones in the spine, hip, thigh, and forearm lose the most density as we age. **Osteoporosis** is a disorder in which bones lose so much calcium that they become dangerously prone to breakage. An estimated 10 million people in the United States over the age of 50 have osteoporosis of the hip.[4] Osteoporosis results in more than 1 million bone fractures a year in the United States, the most serious of which are hip fractures (that is, breaks in the thigh bone, just below the hip joint). Hip fractures often result in hospitalization, loss of mobility, and, as is often the case in people in advanced late adulthood, death from complications. Between 15% and 20% of older people who sustain a hip fracture die within a year.

Osteoporosis can shorten one's stature by inches and deform one's posture, causing the curvature in the spine known as "dowager's hump." Both men and women are at risk of osteoporosis, but it poses a greater threat to women. Men typically have a larger bone mass, which provides them with more protection against the disorder. Following the decline in bone density that women experience after menopause, women stand about twice the risk of hip fractures and about eight times the risk of spine fractures that men do. But older women who regularly walk for exercise are less likely than their sedentary counterparts to suffer hip fractures. What can you do now to protect your future bone health? Read "Prevention 16-1" for some suggestions.

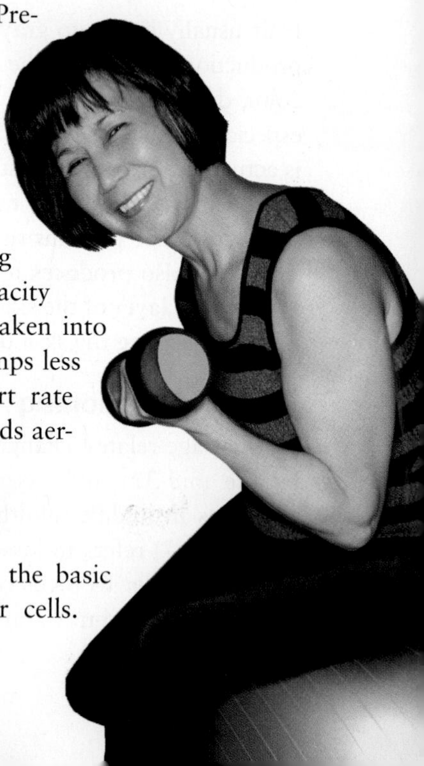

Aerobic Capacity

As we age, the cardiovascular system becomes less efficient. Heart and lung muscles shrink. Aerobic capacity declines as less oxygen is taken into the lungs and the heart pumps less blood. The maximum heart rate declines, but exercise expands aerobic capacity at *any* age.

Blood Sugar Tolerance

Blood sugar, or glucose, is the basic fuel and energy source for cells.

PREVENTION 16-1

Preventing Osteoporosis: Key Messages from the U.S. Surgeon General

There is much that individuals can do to promote their own bone health, beginning in childhood and continuing into late adulthood. These activities also contribute to overall health and vitality.

- Eat a well-balanced diet.
- Get the recommended daily requirements for calcium. Three eight-ounce glasses of low-fat milk each day combined with the calcium from the rest of a normal diet is enough for most individuals.
- If one cannot get enough vitamin D from sunshine, changes in diet and vitamin supplements can help make up the difference.
- In addition to meeting recommended guidelines for physical activity (at least 30 minutes a day for adults and 60 minutes for children), specific strength and weight-bearing activities help build and maintain bone mass throughout life.

Source: Adapted from *Bone health and osteoporosis: A report of the Surgeon General*, 2005.

The energy from glucose supports cell activities and maintains body temperature. Glucose circulates in the bloodstream and enters cells with the help of insulin, a hormone secreted by the pancreas.

As we age, the tissues in our body become less capable of taking up glucose from the bloodstream. Body tissues lose their sensitivity to insulin; the pancreas must thus produce more of it to achieve the same effect. Therefore, blood sugar levels rise, increasing the risk of adult-onset diabetes.

Physical changes that occur with aging are summarized in Figure 16-1 on the next page.

Sleep

Older people need at least seven hours of sleep per night, yet sleep disorders such as insomnia and **sleep apnea** become more common in later adulthood. Sleep apnea sufferers stop breathing repeatedly during the night, causing awakenings. Apnea may be more than a sleep problem. For reasons that are not entirely clear, it is linked to increased risk of heart attacks and strokes.

Sleep problems in late adulthood may involve physical changes that bring discomfort. Sometimes they symptomize psychological disorders such as depression, anxiety, or dementia. Men with enlarged prostate glands commonly need to urinate during the night, causing awakening. Other contributing factors include loneliness, especially after the death of a close friend, spouse, or life partner.

Sleep medications are the most common treatment for insomnia.[5] Alternatives may include keeping a regular sleep schedule, challenging exaggerated worries about the consequences of remaining awake, using relaxation techniques, and exercise. Sleep apnea may be treated with surgery to widen the upper airways that block breathing or by the use of devices such as a nose mask that maintains air pressure to keep airway passages open during sleep.

Changes in Memory Functioning

We can expect some declines in mental abilities as we age. We may have greater difficulty recalling recent events, such as what we ate for dinner last night, as well as remembering names and telephone numbers or holding information in mind.[6] The good news is that apart from the occasional social embarrassment of forgetting people's names, the normal decline in memory most people encounter as they age does not typically impair daily functioning. More severe memory problems, such as memory lapses associated with *dementia*, are not normal or inevitable parts of the aging process. Dementia is caused by degenerative brain diseases, such as Alzheimer's disease, as we'll see next.

You may experience greater difficulty solving problems quickly or handling tasks that require visual–spatial skills, such

sleep apnea
The temporary suspension of breathing while asleep.

Figure 16-1 The Relentless March of Time

A number of physical changes occur during the later years. However, the reasons for aging are not yet completely understood. People can also affect the pace of their aging by eating properly, exercising, maintaining a positive outlook, and finding and meeting challenges that are consistent with their abilities.

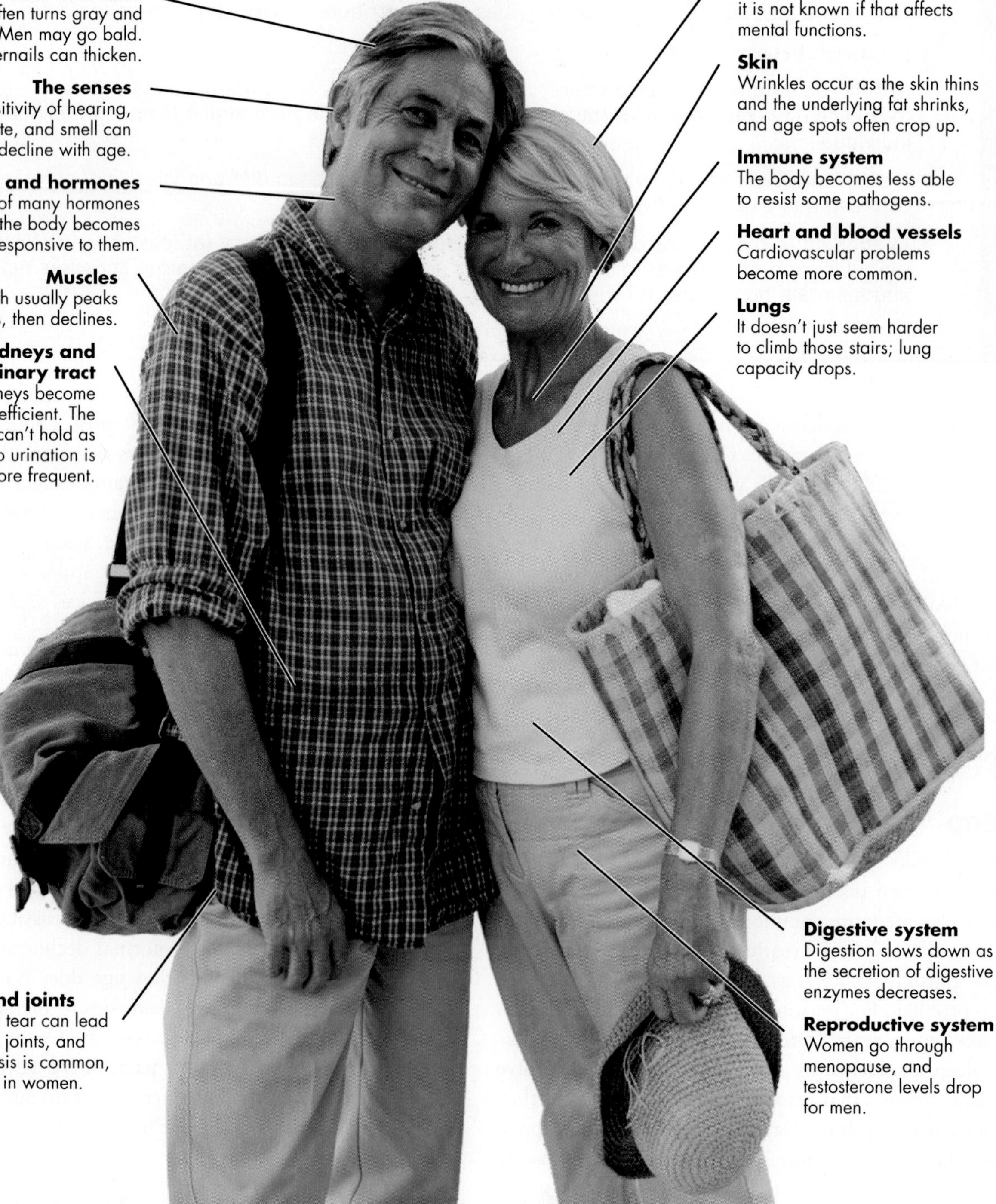

Hair and nails
Hair often turns gray and thins out. Men may go bald. Fingernails can thicken.
The senses
The sensitivity of hearing, sight, taste, and smell can all decline with age.
Glands and hormones
Levels of many hormones drop, or the body becomes less responsive to them.
Muscles
Strength usually peaks in the 20s, then declines.
Kidneys and urinary tract
The kidneys become less efficient. The bladder can't hold as much, so urination is more frequent.
Bones and joints
Wear and tear can lead to arthritic joints, and osteoporosis is common, especially in women.
Brain
The brain shrinks, but it is not known if that affects mental functions.
Skin
Wrinkles occur as the skin thins and the underlying fat shrinks, and age spots often crop up.
Immune system
The body becomes less able to resist some pathogens.
Heart and blood vessels
Cardiovascular problems become more common.
Lungs
It doesn't just seem harder to climb those stairs; lung capacity drops.
Digestive system
Digestion slows down as the secretion of digestive enzymes decreases.
Reproductive system
Women go through menopause, and testosterone levels drop for men.

as map reading. But most mental abilities, such as vocabulary, general knowledge, reasoning, and ability to recall important information, generally remain intact as we age.[7]

Dementia and Alzheimer's Disease

Dementia is a condition characterized by dramatic deterioration of cognitive abilities involving thinking, memory, judgment, and reasoning. Dementia is not a consequence of normal aging, but of disease processes that damage brain tissue. Some causes of dementia include brain infections such as meningitis, HIV, and encephalitis; and chronic alcoholism, infections, strokes, and tumors (see Figure 16-2). The most common cause of dementia is **Alzheimer's disease (AD)**, a progressive brain disease affecting 4 to 5 million Americans.

The risk of AD increases dramatically with age (see Figure 16-3). About one in 10 Americans over the age of 65 has AD, jumping to more than one in two among those 75 to 84 years old. AD is rare in people under the age of 65. Although some dementias may be reversible, especially those caused by treatable tumors or infections and those that result from depression or substance abuse, dementia resulting from AD is progressive and irreversible.

Figure 16-3 Rates of Alzheimer's Disease among Older Adults

The risk of Alzheimer's disease is greatest among people in the 75- to 84-year age range.

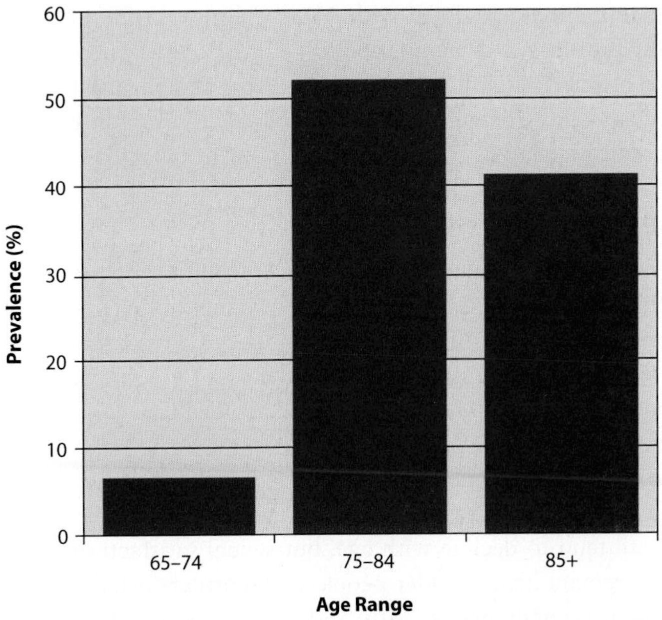

Source: Herbert, L. E., et al. (2003). Alzheimer's disease in the U.S. population: Prevalence estimates. *Archives of Neurology, 60,* 1119–1122. Copyright © 2003 American Medical Association. All rights reserved.

AD is the fifth leading killer of older Americans. It progresses in several stages. At first there are subtle cognitive and personality changes in which people with AD have trouble managing finances and recalling recent events. As AD progresses, people find it harder to manage daily tasks, select clothes, recall names and addresses, and drive. Later, they have trouble using the bathroom and maintaining hygiene. They no longer recognize family and friends or speak in full sentences. They may become restless, agitated, confused, and aggressive. They may get lost in stores, parking lots, even their own homes. They may experience hallucinations or paranoid delusions, believing that others are attempting to harm them. People with AD may eventually become unable to walk or communicate and become completely dependent on others.

Figure 16-2 Causes of Dementia

Alzheimer's disease is the leading cause of dementia.

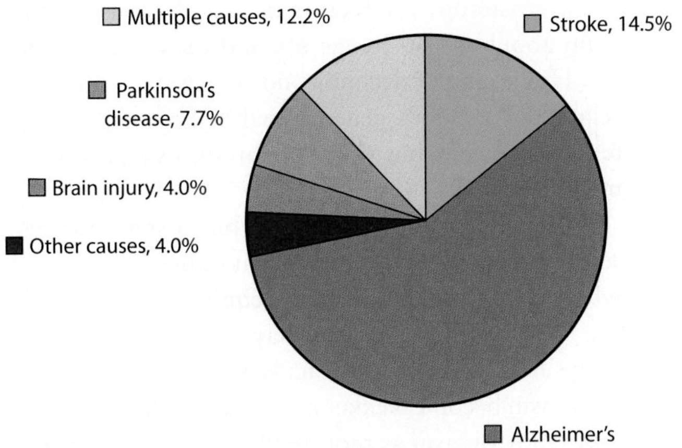

Source: Heron, M. P. (2007). *National Vital Statistics Reports, 56*(5). Centers for Disease Control and Prevention. Retrieved from www.cdc.gov/nchs/data/nvsr/nvsr56/nvsr56_05

Although the cause or causes of AD remain a mystery, scientists believe that both environmental and genetic factors are involved.[8] It is possible that the accumulation of plaque causes the memory loss and other symptoms of AD; however, experiments with non-humans suggest that memory deficits may precede the formation of significant deposits of plaque.[9]

dementia
A broad-based and significant deterioration of mental abilities such as memory, reasoning, language skills, and judgment.

Alzheimer's disease (AD)
A degenerative brain disease characterized by a progressive form of dementia.

Medicines can help improve memory functions in people with AD, but their effects are modest at best. Researchers are investigating whether regular use of anti-inflammatory drugs and antioxidants may lower the risk of developing AD by preventing the brain inflammation associated with AD.[10] Calorie restriction may prevent the accumulation of plaque.[11] Researchers are also investigating whether cognitive training that focuses on the enhancement of memory and processing speed can delay or prevent the development of AD.[12]

Sexuality

Even in the aftermath of the sexual revolution of the 1960s, many people still tie sex to reproduction. Therefore, they assume that sex is appropriate only for the young. There are unfounded cultural myths to the effect that older people are sexless and that older men with sexual interests are "dirty old men."

However, people do not lose their sexuality as they age.[13] Sexual daydreaming, sex drive, and sexual activity all tend to decline with age, but sexual satisfaction may remain high.[14] Older people with partners usually remain sexually active. Most older people report that they like sex. Sexual activity among older people, as among other groups, is influenced not only by physical structures and changes, but also by psychological well-being, feelings of intimacy, and cultural expectations.[15]

Although many older people retain the capacity to respond sexually, physical changes do occur.

Changes in Women

Many of the physical changes in older women stem from a decline in estrogen production. The vaginal walls lose much of their elasticity and grow paler and thinner. Thus, sexual activity may become painful. The thinning of the walls may also place greater pressure against the bladder and urethra during sex, sometimes leading to urinary urgency and a burning sensation during urination.

The vagina shrinks. The labia majora lose much of their fatty deposits and become thinner. The vaginal opening constricts, and penile entry may become difficult. Following menopause, women also produce less vaginal lubrication, and lubrication may take minutes, not seconds, to appear. Lack of adequate lubrication is a key reason for painful sex. Women's nipples still become erect as they are sexually aroused, but the spasms of orgasm become less powerful and fewer in number. Thus, orgasms may feel less intense, even though the experience of orgasm may remain just as satisfying. Despite these changes, women can retain their ability to reach orgasm well into their advanced years. Nevertheless, the uterine contractions that occur during orgasm may become discouragingly painful for some older women.

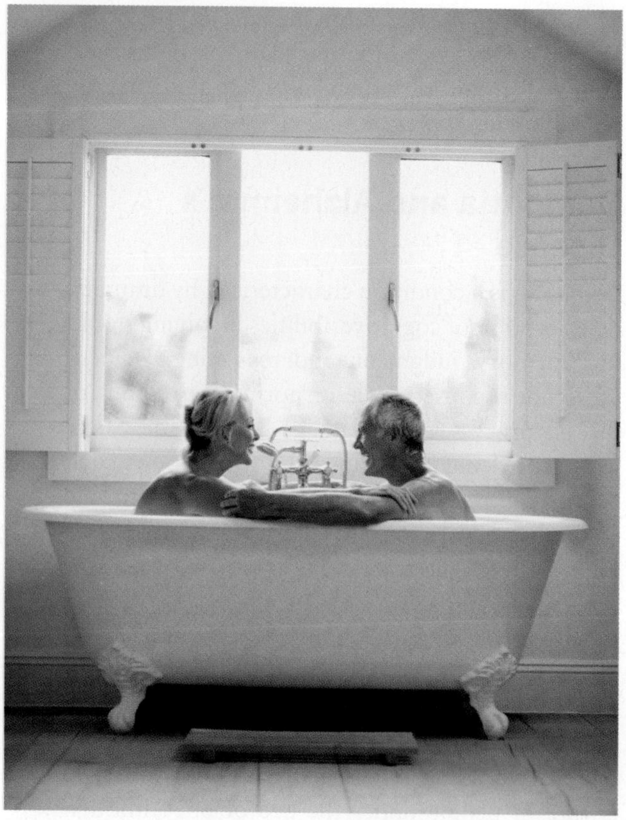

© iStockphoto.com/kupicoo

Changes in Men

Age-related changes tend to occur more gradually in men than in women and are not clearly connected with any one biological event. Male adolescents may achieve erection in seconds. After about age 50, men take progressively longer to achieve erection. Erections become less firm, perhaps because of lowered testosterone levels.

Testosterone production usually declines gradually from about age 40 to age 60, and then begins to level off. However, the decline is not inevitable and may be related to a man's general health. Sperm production tends to decline, but viable sperm may be produced by men in their 70s, 80s, and 90s.

An adolescent may require but a few minutes to regain erection and ejaculate again after a first orgasm, whereas a man in his 30s may require half an hour. Past age 50, regaining erection may require several hours. Older men produce less ejaculate, and the contractions of orgasm become weaker and fewer. Still, an older male may enjoy orgasm as thoroughly as he did at a younger age. Following orgasm, erection subsides more rapidly than in a younger man.

Patterns of Sexual Activity

Despite decline in physical functions, older people can lead fulfilling sex lives. Years of sexual experience may more than compensate for any lessening of physical response. Frequency of sexual activity tends to decline with age because of hormonal changes, physical problems, boredom, and cultural attitudes. Many older people engage in sexual activity as often as or more often than when younger; some develop an aversion to sex; others lose interest.

Couples may adapt to the physical changes of aging by broadening their sexual repertoire to include more diverse forms of stimulation. The availability of a sexually interested and supportive partner may be the most important determinant of continued sexual activity.[16]

Theories of Aging

So far, everyone who has lived has aged—which may not be a bad fate, considering the alternative. Although we can make lengthy lists of the things that happen as we age, we don't know exactly why they happen. Theories of aging fall into two broad categories:

- *Programmed theories* see aging as the result of genetic instructions.
- *Cellular damage theories* propose that aging results from damage to cells.

LEARNING OUTCOME 2

Compare programmed and cellular damage theories of aging

Programmed Theories of Aging

Programmed theories of aging propose that aging and longevity are determined by a biological clock that ticks at a rate governed by genes. That is, the seeds of our own demise are carried in our genes. Evidence supporting a genetic link to aging comes in part from studies showing that longevity tends to run in families. For example, the siblings of centenarians are more likely than members of the general population to live to be 100 themselves.[17]

But why should organisms carry "suicidal" genes? Programmed aging theorists believe that it would be adaptive for species to survive long enough to reproduce and transmit their genes to future generations. From the evolutionary perspective, there would be no advantage to the species (and probably a disadvantage given limited food supplies) to repair cell machinery and body tissues to maintain life indefinitely.

Cellular clock theory focuses on the built-in limits of cell division. After dividing about fifty times, human cells cease dividing and eventually die.[18] Researchers find clues to the limits of cell division in **telomeres**, the protective segments of DNA at the tips of chromosomes. Telomeres shrink each time cells divide. When the loss of telomeres reaches a critical point after a number of cell divisions, the cell may no longer be able to function. The length of the telomeres for a species may determine the number of times a cell can divide and survive.

Hormonal stress theory focuses on the endocrine system, which releases hormones into the bloodstream. Hormonal changes foster age-related changes such as puberty and menopause. As we age, stress hormones, including corticosteroids and adrenaline, are left at elevated levels following illnesses, making the body more vulnerable to chronic conditions such as diabetes, osteoporosis, and heart disease. The changes in production of stress hormones over time may be preprogrammed by genes.

Immunological theory holds that the immune system is preset to decline by an internal biological clock. For example, the production of antibodies declines with age, rendering the body less able to fight off infections. Age-related changes in the immune system also increase the risk of cancer and may contribute to general deterioration.

Cellular Damage Theories of Aging

Programmed theories assume that internal bodily processes are preset to age by genes. **Cellular damage theories of aging** propose that internal bodily changes

programmed theories of aging
Views of aging based on the concept that the processes of aging are governed, at least in part, by genetic factors.

cellular clock theory
A theory of aging focusing on the limits of cell division.

telomeres
Protective segments of DNA located at the tips of chromosomes.

hormonal stress theory
A theory of aging that hypothesizes that stress hormones, left at elevated levels, make the body more vulnerable to chronic conditions.

immunological theory
A theory of aging that holds that the immune system is preset to decline by an internal biological clock.

cellular damage theories of aging
Views of aging based on the concept that internal bodily changes and external environmental insults, such as carcinogens and poisons, cause cells and organ systems to malfunction, leading to death.

Is Calorie Restriction the Fountain of Youth?

Restricting calories by approximately 30% may trigger anti-aging responses that evolved to increase the chances of survival when food is scarce. For example, calorie restriction in humans, non-human primates, and other mammals lowers blood pressure, cholesterol, and blood sugar and insulin levels. It strengthens the immune system and lowers the fat mass.[19] Calorie restriction also fends off Alzheimer's-like symptoms in rhesus monkeys.

In laboratory experiments, mice were fed a diet that was 30% to 40% lower in calories than normal but contained all necessary nutrients. The development of chronic diseases and cancers was retarded, and the mice lived 50% beyond their normal life spans.[20]

Raising levels of the hormone DHEAS (dehydroepiandrosterone sulfate) may be one way that calorie restriction reduces the risk of cancer and improves immune system functioning. DHEAS production usually begins to decline after approximately age 30. DHEAS levels are relatively higher in long-lived people and in monkeys with calorie-restricted diets.[21]

It remains to be seen whether calorie restriction extends the life span of people who have access to modern health care. Moreover, it is difficult enough for many people to keep their weight within normal limits. How willing would we be to lower our calorie intake further? Researchers are therefore also seeking alternate ways of triggering the anti-aging responses caused by calorie restriction.

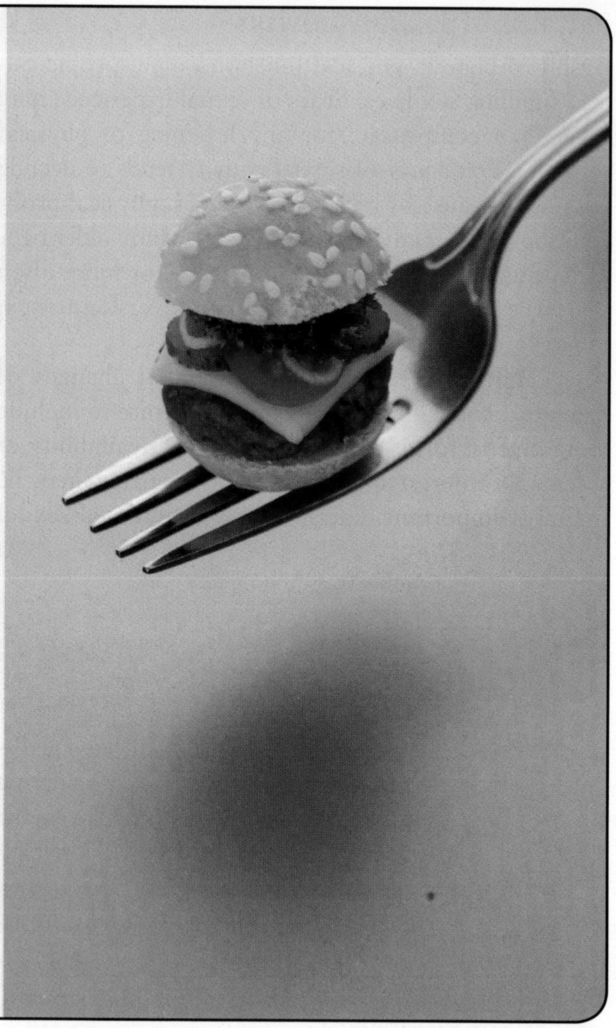

and external environmental assaults (such as carcinogens and toxins) cause cells and organ systems to malfunction, leading to death. For example, the **wear-and-tear theory** suggests that over the years our bodies—as machines that wear out through use—become less capable of repairing themselves.

wear-and-tear theory
A theory of aging that suggests that over time our bodies become less capable of repairing themselves.

free-radical theory
A theory of aging that attributes aging to damage caused by the accumulation of unstable molecules called free radicals.

cross-linking theory
A theory of aging that holds that the stiffening of body proteins eventually breaks down bodily processes, leading to aging.

The **free-radical theory** attributes aging to damage caused by the accumulation of unstable molecules called *free radicals*. Free radicals are produced during metabolism by oxidation, possibly damaging cell proteins, membranes, and DNA.[22] Most free radicals are naturally disarmed by nutrients and enzymes called *antioxidants*. Most antioxidants are either made by the body or found in food. As we age, our bodies produce fewer antioxidants. People whose diets are rich in antioxidants are less likely to develop heart disease and some cancers.

As we age, cell proteins bind to one another in a process called *cross-linking*, thereby toughening tissues. Cross-linking stiffens collagen—the connective tissue supporting tendons, ligaments, cartilage, and bone. One result is coarse, dry skin. (Flavored animal collagen, or gelatin, is better known by the brand name Jell-O.) **Cross-linking theory** holds that the stiffening of body proteins accelerates and eventually breaks down bodily processes, leading to some of the effects of aging.[23] The immune system combats cross-linking, but becomes less able to do so as we age.

In considering the many theories of aging, we should note that aging is an extremely complex biological process that may not be explained by any single theory or cause. Aging may involve a combination of these and other factors.

Health Concerns and Aging

Although aging takes a toll on our bodies, disease is not inevitable. We can distinguish between *normal aging* and *pathological aging*. In normal aging, physiological processes decline slowly with age and the person is able to enjoy many years of health and vitality into late adulthood. In **pathological aging**, chronic diseases or degenerative processes, such as heart disease, diabetes, and cancer, lead to disability or premature death. Older people typically need more health care than younger people. Though people over the age of 65 make up about 12% of the population, they occupy 25% of the hospital beds.

LEARNING OUTCOME 3

Identify common health concerns associated with late adulthood

Most older adults do not require institutional care, such as nursing homes or residential care facilities. More than two of three adults age 65 and older live in their own homes. Less than 10% of older adults live in nursing homes or other long-term care facilities. The population of nursing homes is made up largely of people age 80 and older. Yet if older adults live long enough, nearly half will eventually require some form of nursing or home health care.

A century ago, older people were more likely to die from infectious diseases such as influenza and pneumonia than they are today. Today, older people are at greater risk of dying from chronic diseases such as heart disease and cancer. More than four out of five people over the age of 65 have at least one chronic health problem. Some, like varicose veins, are minor. Others, like heart disease, pose serious health risks. Figure 16-4 shows the percentages of people age 65 and older who are affected by common chronic health conditions. While longevity is increasing, so too is the number of years older persons are living with one or more chronic health problems.

Figure 16-4 Chronic Health Conditions among People Age 65 and Older

The leading chronic health conditions affecting people in late adulthood are hypertension, heart disease, and arthritis.

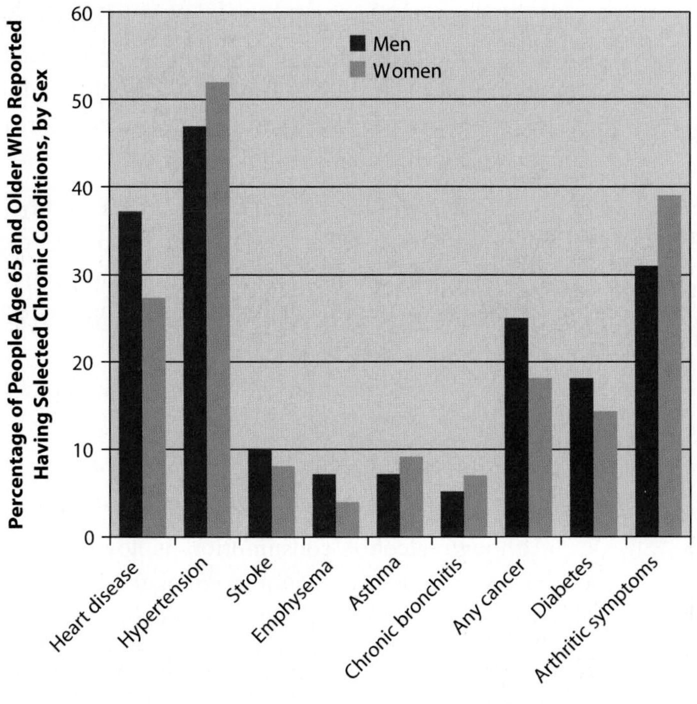

Source: Heron, M. P. (2007). *National Vital Statistics Reports, 50*(5). Centers for Disease Control and Prevention. Retrieved from www.cdc.gov/nchs/data/nvsr/nvsr56/nvsr56_05

Heart Disease, Cancer, and Stroke

The three major causes of death of Americans age 65 and older are heart disease, cancer, and stroke (see Table 16-2 on the next page). Cancer is the leading cause of death in women between the ages of 40 and 79, and men between the ages of 60 and 79, but heart disease is the nation's leading cause of death among both men and women beyond the age of 80. The risk of most cancers rises as we age because the immune system becomes less able to rid the body of precancerous and cancerous cells.

Among the top chronic conditions listed in Figure 16-4, several are also leading causes of death or pose significant risk factors for mortality. Hypertension, which affects about 50% of Americans over the age of 65, is a major risk factor for heart attacks and strokes. Diabetes, the fifth most common chronic illness, is also one of the leading causes of death among older adults. Other chronic conditions, such as cataracts, chronic sinusitis, visual impairment, and varicose veins, are rarely fatal but can lead to disability.

pathological aging
Aging in which chronic diseases or degenerative processes, such as heart disease, diabetes, and cancer, lead to disability or premature death.

Table 16-2 Ten Leading Causes of Death, All Races, Men and Women, 65 Years and Older

CAUSE OF DEATH	PERCENT OF TOTAL DEATHS (MALE)	PERCENT OF TOTAL DEATHS (FEMALE)
Heart disease	29.4	28.7
Cancer	25.4	19.3
Chronic respiratory diseases	6.4	5.3
Stroke	5.5	7.6
Diabetes	3.1	2.9
Influenza and pneumonia	2.7	2.9
Alzheimer's disease	2.6	5.2
Accidents	2.3	1.9
Kidney diseases	2.2	2.0
Blood poisoning	1.4	1.5

Source: Heron, M. P. (2010). *National Vital Statistics Reports, 58*(14). Centers for Disease Control and Prevention. Retrieved from http://www.cdc.gov/nchs/data/nvsr/nvsr58/nvsr58_14.pdf

Arthritis

Arthritis is joint inflammation that results from conditions affecting the structures inside and surrounding the joints. Symptoms progress from swelling, pain, and stiffness to loss of function. Children can also be affected by arthritis, but it is more common with advancing age. Arthritis is more common in women than in men and more common in African Americans than in European Americans. Osteoarthritis and rheumatoid arthritis are the two most common forms of arthritis.

Osteoarthritis is a painful, degenerative disease characterized by wear and tear on joints. By the age of 60, more than half of Americans show some signs of the disease. Among people over the age of 65, two of three have the disease. The joints most commonly affected are in the knees, hips, fingers, neck, and lower back. Osteoarthritis is caused by erosion of cartilage, the pads of fibrous tissue that cushion the ends of bones. As cartilage wears down, bones grind together, causing pain. Osteoarthritis is more common among overweight people because excess weight adds to the load on the hip and knee joints. Health professionals recommend anti-inflammatory drugs to help relieve pain and discomfort. In severe cases, joint replacement surgery may be needed. Exercises are also sometimes prescribed.

osteoarthritis
A painful, degenerative disease characterized by wear and tear on joints.

rheumatoid arthritis
A painful, degenerative disease characterized by chronic inflammation of the membranes that line the joints.

Rheumatoid arthritis is characterized by chronic inflammation of the membranes that line the joints because the body's immune system attacks its own tissues. The condition affects the entire body. It can produce unrelenting pain and eventually lead to severe disability. Bones and cartilage may also be affected. Onset of the disease usually occurs between the ages of 40 and 60. Anti-inflammatory drugs are used to treat it.

Substance Abuse

Abuse or misuse of medication (prescription and over-the-counter drugs), much of which is unintentional, pose a serious health threat to older Americans. Forty percent of all prescription drugs in the United States are taken by people age 60 and older, and more than half of them take two to five medications daily.[24] Among the most commonly used drugs are blood pressure medication, tranquilizers, sleeping pills, and antidepressants. Taken correctly, prescription drugs can be of help. If used incorrectly, they can be harmful.

Millions of older adults are addicted to, or risk becoming addicted to, prescription drugs, especially tranquilizers. About a quarter of a million older adults are hospitalized each year because of adverse drug reactions. Reasons include the following:[25]

1. *The dosage of drugs is too high.* Because bodily functions slow with age (such as the ability of the liver and kidneys to clear drugs out of the body), the same amount of drug can have stronger effects and last longer in older people.
2. *Some people may misunderstand directions or be unable to keep track of their usage.*
3. *Many older people have more than one doctor, and treatment plans may not be coordinated.*

Although alcohol consumption is lower overall among older people compared to younger adults, many older adults suffer from long-term alcoholism. However, the health risks of alcohol abuse increase with age. The slowdown in the metabolic rate reduces the body's ability to metabolize alcohol, increasing the likelihood of intoxication. The combination of alcohol and other drugs, including prescription drugs, can be dangerous

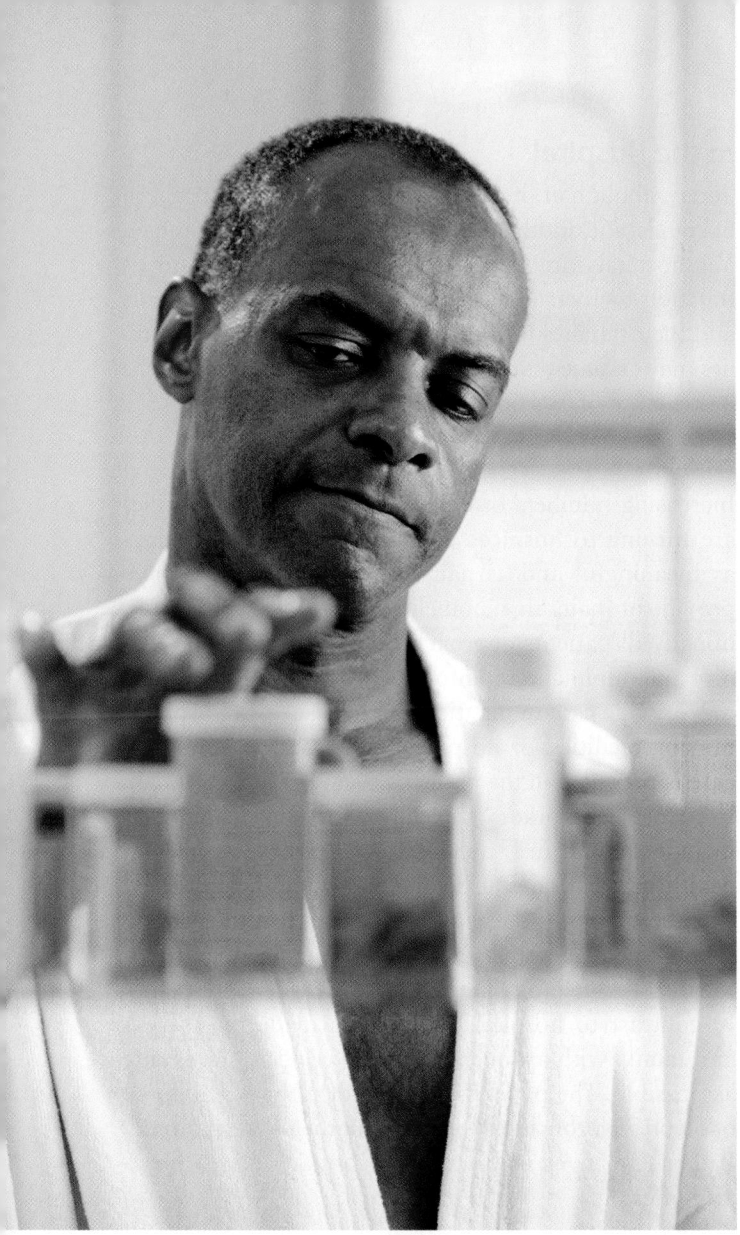

© iStockphoto.com/Christine Glade

or even lethal. Alcohol can also lessen or intensify the effects of prescription drugs.

Accidents

Although accidents can occur at any age, older people face greater risks of unintentional injuries from falls, motor vehicle accidents, residential fires, and nonfatal poisoning. Accidents are the ninth leading cause of death among older Americans. Falls are especially dangerous for older adults with osteoporosis because of the increased risks of fractures.

Many accidents involving older adults could be prevented by equipping the home with safety features such as railings and nonskid floors. Wearing proper glasses and using hearing aids can reduce the risk of accidents resulting from vision or hearing problems, including many motor vehicle accidents. Adherence to safe driving speeds is especially important among older drivers because they have slower reaction times than do younger drivers.

Death and Dying

Many people think of death as a part of life, but *death* is the termination of life and not a part of life. *Dying*, though, is a part of life. It is the end stage of life in which bodily processes decline, leading to death.

LEARNING OUTCOME 4

Define *death* and discuss the process of dying

Medical authorities generally use **brain death** as the basis for determining that a person has died. The most widely used standard for establishing brain death is absence of activity of the cerebral cortex, as shown by a flat electroencephalogram (EEG) recording. When there is no activity in the cortex, consciousness—the sense of self and all psychological functioning—has ceased. The broader concept of **whole brain death** includes death of the brain stem, which is responsible for certain automatic functions, such as reflexes like breathing. Thus a person who is brain dead can continue to breathe. On the other hand, in some cases people are kept alive, even though they are whole brain dead, by life-support equipment that takes over their breathing and circulation.

People whose hearts and lungs have ceased functioning but whose brains remain alive can often be revived with cardiopulmonary resuscitation (CPR).

Are There Stages of Dying?

Our overview of the process of dying has been influenced by Elisabeth Kübler-Ross.[26] From her observations of terminally ill patients, Kübler-Ross found some common responses to news of impending death. She hypothesized that there are five stages through which many dying patients pass:

1. *Denial.* In this stage, people think, "It can't be me. The diagnosis must be wrong." Denial can be flat and absolute, or it can fluctuate so that one minute the patient

brain death
Cessation of activity of the cerebral cortex.

whole brain death
Cessation of activity of the cerebral cortex and brain stem.

accepts the medical verdict, and the next, the patient starts chatting animatedly about distant plans.

2. *Anger*. Denial usually gives way to anger and resentment toward the young and healthy, and, sometimes, toward the medical establishment: "It's unfair. Why me?" or "They didn't catch it in time."
3. *Bargaining*. People may bargain with God to postpone death, promising to do good deeds if they are given another six months, or another year.
4. *Depression*. With depression come feelings of grief, loss, and hopelessness—grief at the prospect of leaving loved ones and life itself.
5. *Final acceptance*. Ultimately, inner peace may come as a quiet acceptance of the inevitable. This "peace" is not contentment; it is nearly devoid of feeling. The patient may still fear death but comes to accept it with a sense of peace and dignity.

There are critiques of the views of Kübler-Ross. For example, Kübler-Ross's case studies all involve people who receive a diagnosis of a terminal illness. Most people die because of advanced years with no specific terminal diagnosis. Moreover, the key factors that appear to affect the adjustment of the dying individual include the nature and extent of cognitive impairment, pain and weakness, age, the person's philosophy of life (and death), and prior experiences with crises.

Where People Die

A hundred years ago, most people died in their homes, surrounded by family members. Today, only a small minority of Americans—typically those who are in advanced old age or who are gravely or terminally ill—die in their own homes. The growing exception concerns those terminally ill patients who receive hospice care at home. According to the National Hospice and Palliative Care Organization, 74% of hospice patients die in a private residence, nursing home, or other residential facility.[27] Many people, of course, die suddenly wherever they happen to be at the time, either because of accidents, heart attacks, or other unanticipated events.

hospice
An approach to treating dying patients that focuses on support and understanding, rather than curative treatment; also refers to houses or facilities that provide palliative (supportive) care to dying patients.

palliative care
Treatment focused on the relief of pain and suffering rather than cure.

In the Hospital

Today, about half of deaths in the United States occur in hospitals, and another one in five occur in nursing homes. Yet hospitals are impersonal places to die. Hospitals function to treat diseases, not to help prepare patients and their families for death. Yet patients and their families may assume that going to the hospital gives them the best chance of averting death.

Hospice Care

Increasing numbers of dying people and their families are turning to **hospices** to help make their final days as meaningful and as pain-free as possible. Hospices provide or maintain a homelike atmosphere to help terminally ill patients approach death with maximal dignity and minimal discomfort. When necessary, hospices can provide care in inpatient settings such as hospitals, nursing facilities, or hospice centers, but most hospice care is provided in the patient's home.

Hospice workers typically work in teams that include physicians, nurses, social workers, mental health or pastoral counselors, and home health aides. Members support the entire family, not just the patient. Bereavement specialists assist the family to prepare for the loss and help them through grieving after the death. In contrast to hospitals, hospices provide the patient and family with as much control over decision making as possible. The patient's wishes not to be resuscitated or kept alive on life-support equipment are honored. Patients are given ample amounts of narcotics to alleviate suffering.

Hospices are less costly than hospital treatment, especially home-based care. Though the patient may be required to pay some of the costs, most of the costs are borne by insurance plans.

Hospice care has the following characteristics:

- Hospices offer **palliative care** rather than curative treatment. They control pain and symptoms to enable the patient to endure as fully and comfortably as possible.
- Hospices treat the person, not the disease. The hospice team addresses the medical, emotional, psychological, and spiritual needs of patients, family, and friends.
- Hospices emphasize quality rather than length of life, neither hastening nor postponing death.
- The hospice considers the entire family, not just the patient, to be the unit of care.
- Help and support is available to the patient and family around the clock.

Supporting a Dying Person

Hospice workers are trained in what to do to help people who are dying. Following are some things you can do: First of all, you must be there for the person. Put yourself at the same eye level and don't withhold touching. Be available to listen, to talk, and to share experiences. Give the person the opportunity to talk about death and to grieve, but don't be afraid to also talk about the ongoing lives of mutual acquaintances. People who are dying often need to focus on things other than impending death, and some enjoy humorous events. They may be comforted to hear about your life experiences—your concerns and worries as well as your joys, hopes, and dreams. But be aware of the person's emotional state on any given day. Some days are better than others. Don't attempt to minimize the person's emotional pain or need to grieve by changing the subject or refusing to acknowledge it. Be sensitive to the person's feelings, and offer consolation and support. People with cognitive impairment may repeat certain thoughts many times; you can go with it or gently guide the conversation in another direction. They may repeatedly ask whether certain tasks have been taken care of, and a simple yes may do each time.

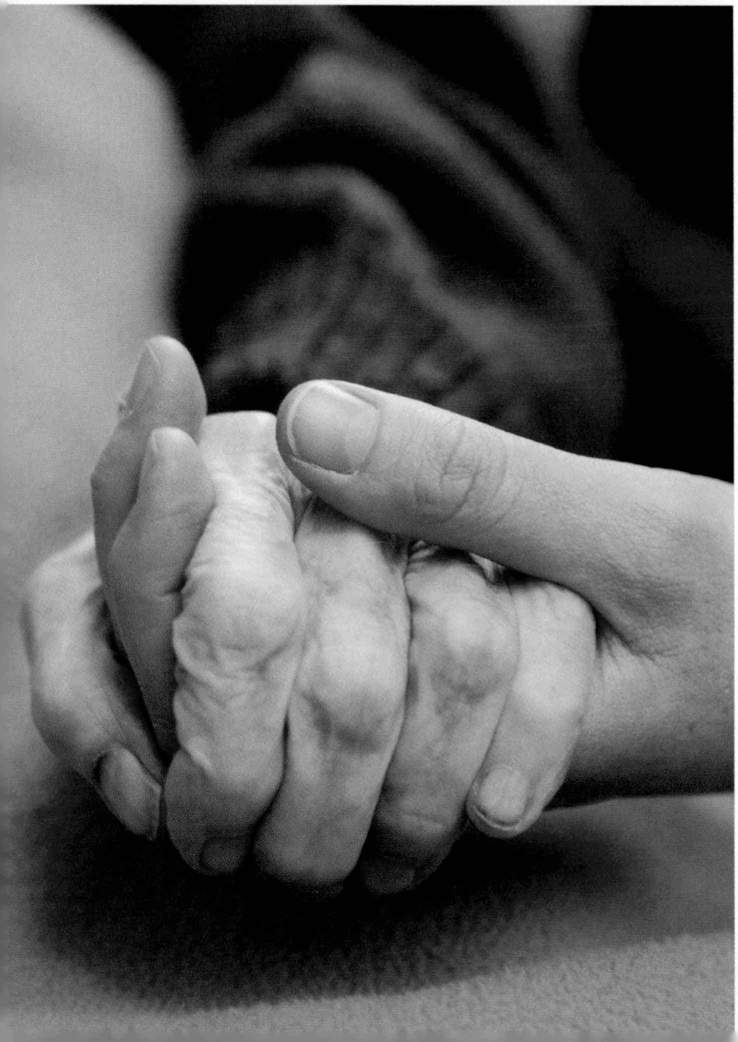

Euthanasia

The word **euthanasia**, literally meaning "good death," is derived from the Greek roots *eu* ("good") and *thanatos* ("death"). Also called *mercy killing*, it refers to the purposeful taking of a person's life through gentle or painless means to relieve pain or suffering.

LEARNING OUTCOME 5

Discuss various kinds of euthanasia and controversies about them

Active Euthanasia: Mercy Killing or Murder?

In **active euthanasia**, a lethal treatment (usually a drug) is administered to cause a quick and painless death. Usually a spouse or family member administers it.

Voluntary Active Euthanasia

When euthanasia is carried out with the patient's consent, it is called **voluntary active euthanasia**. Voluntary active euthanasia remains illegal throughout most of the United States, although legal challenges to state laws are working their way through the courts. It is not illegal in some other countries, such as the Netherlands.

Physician-Assisted Suicide

In some cases of active voluntary euthanasia, physicians have assisted patients with terminal or incapacitating illnesses who wished to die by providing them with lethal doses of drugs or sometimes by administering the drugs when the patients were too ill to administer them themselves. The best-known cases of such physician-assisted suicides have involved the late Dr. Jack Kevorkian, a pathologist dubbed "Dr. Death" by the press for having assisted in more than 35 patient suicides. Following an assisted suicide that was aired on *60 Minutes*, Kevorkian was convicted of second-degree homicide in Michigan and served eight years of a 10- to 25-year prison sentence. Unlike Kevorkian, most

euthanasia
The purposeful taking of life to relieve suffering.

active euthanasia
The administration of a lethal treatment (usually a drug) to cause a quick and painless death.

voluntary active euthanasia
The intentional administration of lethal drugs or other means of producing a painless death with the person's informed consent.

physicians who assist in patient suicides do so without publicity, for fear of legal prosecution and sanctions by medical societies, which remain ethically opposed to the practice.

Involuntary Active Euthanasia

Involuntary active euthanasia stands on shakier moral, ethical, and legal ground than voluntary euthanasia. In involuntary active euthanasia, a person causes the death of another person without that person's informed consent. Cases of involuntary euthanasia usually involve patients who are comatose or otherwise incapacitated and whose guardians believe they would have wanted to die if they had retained the capacity to make the decision. Still, in the eyes of the law, it is considered homicide.

Terminal Sedation

Terminal sedation is an alternative to euthanasia. It is the practice of relieving distress in a terminally ill patient in the last hours or days of his or her life, usually by means of a continuous intravenous infusion of a sedative drug, such as a tranquilizer. Terminal sedation is not intended to hasten death, although there is debate as to whether it has that effect.

Attitudes toward Physician-Assisted Suicide

The issue of physician-assisted suicide continues to be debated among physicians and in the lay community, even though the American Medical Association stands strongly against it. Physicians themselves are split on the question of whether this form of active euthanasia is ever justified. Physicians opposing assisted suicides often cite the belief that it goes against thousands of years of medical tradition of treating patients.

Euthanasia is legal in the Netherlands, but that does not mean that it is undertaken lightly. For example, when a patient or a patient's family requests euthanasia to relieve a terminally ill patient's suffering, many physicians suggest that it is may be possible to lessen patients' suffering without hastening their death.

Euthanasia, defined as performance of the death-inducing act by another person (such as a physician), is illegal nearly everywhere in the United States. Oregon and Washington have enacted Death with Dignity Acts which enable terminally ill patients to ask physicians to prescribe lethal doses of medication. The medication is then administered by patients themselves.

involuntary active euthanasia
The intentional administration of lethal drugs or other means of producing a painless death without the person's informed consent.

passive euthanasia
The withholding or withdrawal of life-sustaining treatment to hasten death.

living will
A document prepared when a person is well, directing medical care providers to terminate life-sustaining treatment in the event he or she becomes incapacitated and unable to speak.

Passive Euthanasia

Passive euthanasia hastens death by withholding potentially life-saving treatments, as in failing to resuscitate a terminally ill patient who stops breathing, or withdrawing medicine, food, or life-support equipment (such as a respirator) from a comatose patient. The legal status of passive euthanasia varies with the circumstances. One form of passive euthanasia that is legal throughout the United States and Canada is the withholding or withdrawing of life-sustaining equipment or techniques from terminally ill people who clearly specify their wish not to be kept alive by aggressive or "heroic" treatment. The declaration of these wishes may be in the form of a *living will*, which specifies the conditions under which the person desires to have life-sustaining treatment withdrawn or withheld.

The Living Will

The U.S. Supreme Court has ruled that individuals have a right to end life-sustaining treatment. The decision provided the legal basis for the **living will**, a legal document that people draft when well that directs health care workers not to use aggressive medical procedures or life-support equipment to prolong vegetative functioning in the event they became permanently

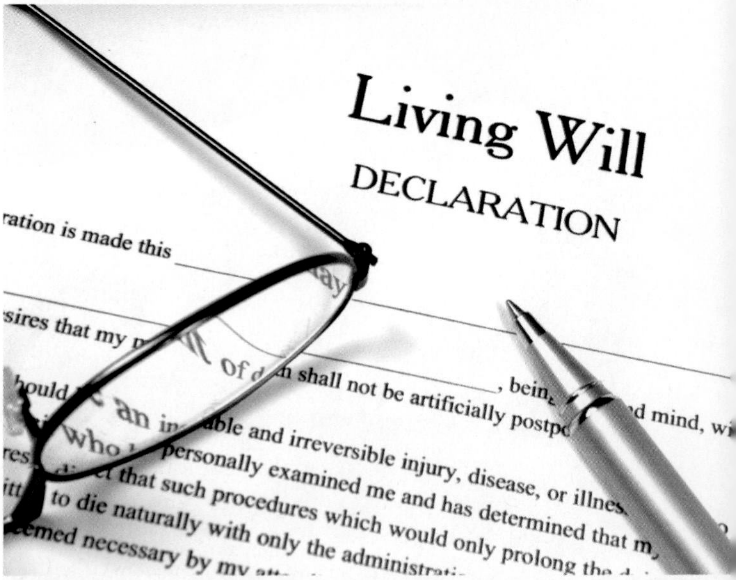

© iStockphoto.com/John Cooke

incapacitated and unable to communicate their wishes. Terminally ill patients can insist, for example, that "do not resuscitate" orders be included in their charts, directing doctors not to use CPR in the event they suffer cardiac arrest.

The withdrawal of life-sustaining treatment is a form of passive euthanasia. Unlike active euthanasia, death is not induced by administering a drug or assisting in the patient's suicide.

Living wills must be drafted in accordance with state laws. The living will only takes effect if people are unable to speak for themselves. For this reason, living wills usually identify a proxy such as the next of kin to make decisions in the event that the signer cannot communicate.

Still, many living wills are ignored. Some are disregarded by proxies, often because they don't judge the patient's wishes accurately, or if they do, because they can't bear the emotional burden of "pulling the plug." Physicians, too, might not comply with advance directives, perhaps because they weren't available when needed or they weren't clear. Physicians are more likely to follow specific advance directives (for example, "do not resuscitate") than general guidelines.

Without taking sides in what we might think of as a religious debate, we can note that many people believe in a form of spiritual reversibility in death.[28] Religious traditions inform them that the soul of the person who has passed on will dwell in heaven or in paradise forever, or that it will be reincarnated on Earth.

What to Do when Someone Dies

LEARNING OUTCOME 6

Discuss ways of coping with death

If you are present at someone's death, call the family doctor, the police, or 911. A doctor is needed to complete the death certificate and indicate the cause of death. If the cause of death is unclear, a coroner or medical examiner may become involved. Once the body has been examined by the doctor and the death certificate has been completed, a funeral director may be contacted to remove the body from the home or the hospital, and arrangements may be made for burial, cremation, or placement in a mausoleum. If death occurs unexpectedly or foul play is involved or suspected, an autopsy may be performed to determine the cause and circumstances of death. Sometimes an autopsy is performed, with the family's consent, if the knowledge gained from the procedure could benefit medical science.

Funeral Arrangements

Funerals provide an organized way of responding to death that is tied to religious custom and cultural tradition. They offer family and community a ritual that allows them to grieve publicly and say farewell to the person who died. Funerals grant a kind of closure that can help observers begin to move on with their lives.

Family members of the deceased decide how simple or elaborate they prefer the funeral to be, whether they want embalming (treating a dead body with chemicals in order to preserve it), and whether the deceased's body should be buried or cremated (reducing a dead body to ashes, by burning, usually as a funeral rite). Sometimes these matters are spelled out by religious or family custom. Sometimes family members fight over them.

After their homes, automobiles, and children's educations, funerals may be American families' next largest expense. Consider these guidelines to arrange a funeral that meets your needs and remains in your budget.

1. Have a good friend go with you to arrange the funeral. Bring someone who will be able to make decisions based on reason and good sense rather than emotions or guilt.
2. If a funeral home has not yet been selected, shop around; you can and should ask about services and costs.
3. Be aware that some cemeteries offer the plot for free but then make their profits from charging exorbitant maintenance fees, opening and closing fees, charges for monuments, and other fees.
4. Veterans are entitled to a free burial plot in a national cemetery, but the family will incur the costs of transporting the body.
5. Caskets are often the major burial expense and can range from $500 to $50,000 or more! Ask the funeral director to show you models that fall within your price range.

Legal and Financial Matters

Many legal and financial matters usually require attention following a death. There may be issues concerning estates, inheritance, outstanding debts, insurance, and amounts owed for funeral expenses. Family who find it

bereavement
The state of deprivation brought about by the death of a family member or close friend.

difficult to focus on these matters should seek legal counsel to answer questions concerning how to handle the deceased person's affairs and to protect their own financial interests. Usually an attorney will be needed to settle the estate, especially if the estate is sizeable or if complex matters arise in sorting through the deceased person's affairs.

Grief and Bereavement

The death of a close friend or family member can be a traumatic experience. It typically leads to a state of **bereavement**, an emotional state of longing and deprivation that is characterized by feelings of grief and a deep sense of loss. *Mourning* is synonymous with grief over the death of a person but also describes culturally prescribed ways of displaying grief. Different cultures prescribe different periods of mourning and different rituals for expressing grief. The tradition of wearing unadorned black clothing for mourning dates at least to the Roman Empire. In rural parts of Mexico, Italy, and Greece, widows are often still expected to wear black for the remainder of their lives. In England and the United States, the wearing of black is on the decline.

Coping with loss requires time and the ability to come to terms with the loss and move ahead with one's life. Having a supportive social network also helps. What can you do if you are faced with the death of someone who is close to you? The online feature "Health Skills 16-1" has some advice.

health skills
Access CourseMate for HLTH at www.cengagebrain.com.

Grieving

There is no one right way to grieve nor a fixed period of time for which grief should last. In some cases, especially for parents who have lost a child, grief never ends, although it does tend to lessen over time. People grieve in different ways. Some grieve more publicly,

© iStockphoto.com/Rubberball

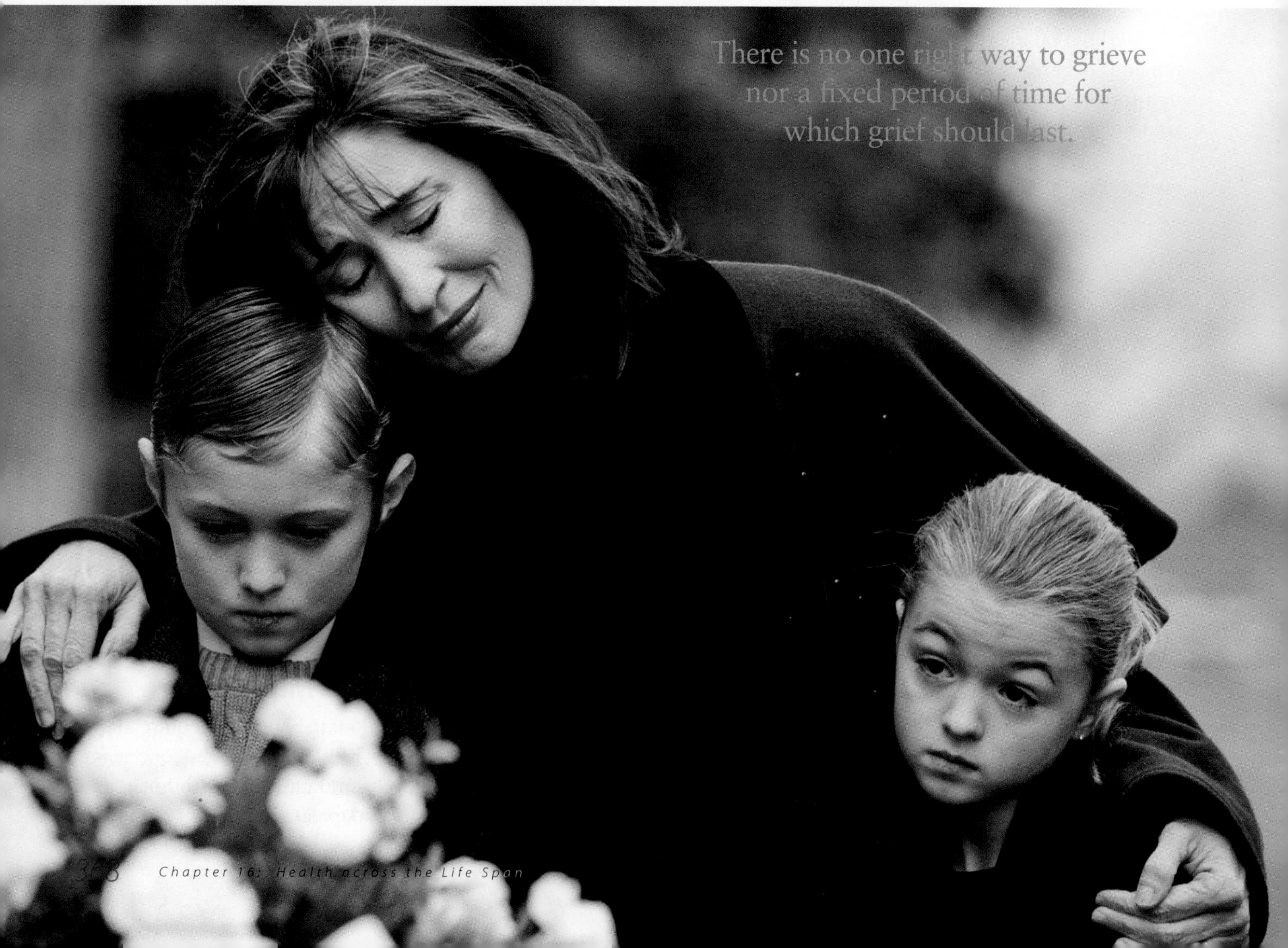
There is no one right way to grieve nor a fixed period of time for which grief should last.

while others reveal their feelings only in private. You may not always know when someone is grieving. Many cultures have festivals or holidays during which they celebrate the dead; to learn more, check out the online feature "Diversity 16-2."

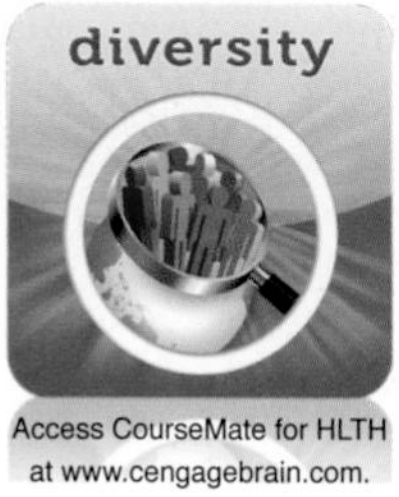

Stages of Grieving?

Selby Jacobs modified Kübler-Ross's stage theory of grief to include the following stages: numbness-disbelief, separation distress (yearning-anger-anxiety), depression-mourning, and recovery.[29] Researchers tested Jacobs' theory by using psychological tests to measure disbelief, yearning, anger, depression, and acceptance of death to 233 bereaved individuals from one to 24 months following their losses.[30] The results are shown visually in Figure 16-5. Disbelief was highest just after the loss and gradually waned over the course of two years. Acceptance of the loss shows the opposite course, being nonexistent at the outset, growing gradually, and peaking two years later. Yearning, anger, and depression rise suddenly in the predicted order and then each wanes gradually.

Figure 16-5 Indicators of Grief among Bereaved People

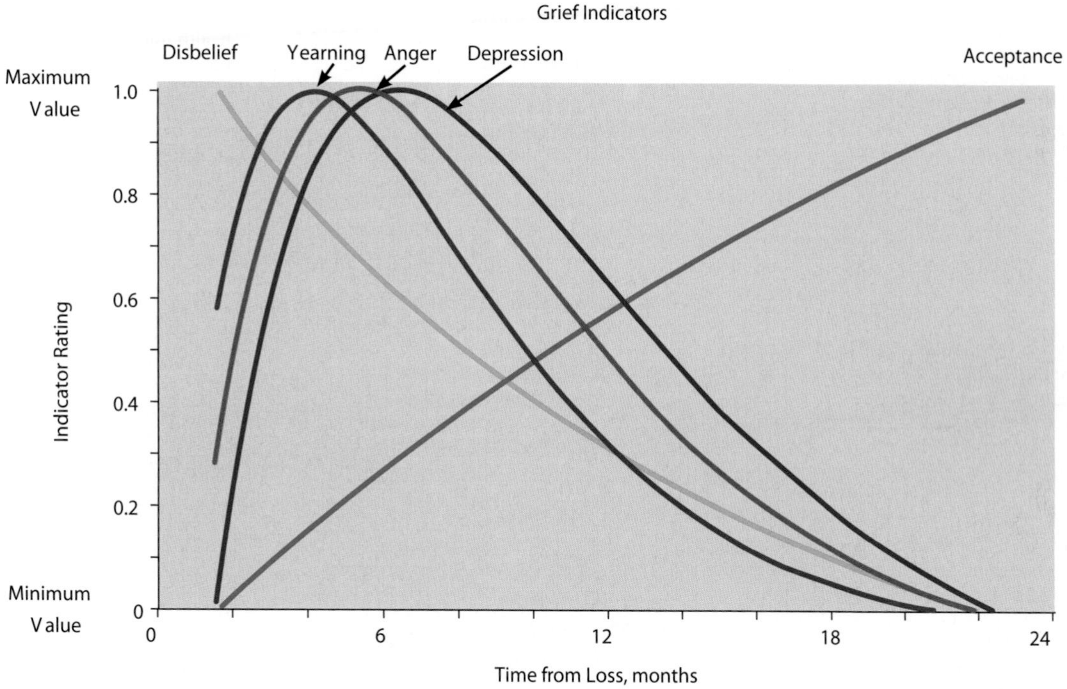

Source: Maciejewski, P. K., Zhang, B., Block, S. D., & Prigerson, H. G. (2007). An empirical examination of the stage theory of grief. *Journal of the American Medical Association, 297*, 716-723.

HEALTH APPS: YOUR LINK TO ONLINE HEALTH APPLICATIONS

health skills

Advice for Coping with a Death What can you do if you are faced with the death of someone who is close to you? "Health Skills 16-1" has some very helpful suggestions.

diversity

Death around the Globe—Festivals for the Dead? Around the globe, there are those who depart the world and those who are left behind to remember them and, often, to celebrate them. Many cultures have festivals or holidays during which they celebrate the dead. Read about them in "Diversity 16-2."

Go to the CourseMate for HLTH at www.cengagebrain.com for additional resources including flashcards, games, self-quizzes, review exercises, web exercises, learning checks, and more.

Endnotes

Chapter 1

1. Schroeder, S. A. (2007). We can do better—Improving the health of the American people. *New England Journal of Medicine, 357*, 1221–1228; Roberts, C. K., & Barnard, R. J. (2005). Effects of exercise and diet on chronic disease. *Journal of Applied Physiology, 98*, 3–30.
2. Benowitz, N. L. (2010). Nicotine addiction. *New England Journal of Medicine, 362*, 2295–2303; U.S. Department of Health & Human Services, Office of the Surgeon General. (2010, December). *How tobacco causes disease: The biology and behavioral basis for smoking-attributable disease: A report of the surgeon general.*
3. U.S. Census Bureau, Population Division. (2010, June). *Annual estimates of the resident population by sex, race, and hispanic origin for the United States: April 1, 2000 to July 1, 2009* (NC-EST2009-03).
4. Multiracial America is fastest growing group. (2009, May 28). *MSNBC.com*. Retrieved from http://www.msnbc.msn.com/id/30986649/
5. Arias, E. (2010, June 8). *National vital statistics reports, Vol. 58, No. 21. United States life tables*. Centers for Disease Control and Prevention, National Center for Health Statistics, National Vital Statistics System.
6. Siegler, I., Bosworth, H. B., & Poon, L. W. (2003). Disease, health, and aging. In R. M. Lerner, M. A. Easterbrooks, & J. Mistry (Eds.), *Handbook of psychology: Developmental psychology* (Vol. 6, pp. 423–442). New York: John Wiley and Sons.
7. Etchason, J., et al. (2001). Racial and ethnic disparities in health care. *Journal of the American Medical Association, 285*, 883.
8. Troxel, W. M. (2003). Chronic stress burden, discrimination, and subclinical carotid artery disease in African American and caucasian women. *Health Psychology, 22*, 300–309.
9. Fryar, C. D., et al. (2010, April). Hypertension, high serum cholesterol, and diabetes: Racial and ethnic prevalence differences in U.S. adults, 1999–2006. *NCHS Data Brief*, Number 36.
10. Brown, M. J. Hypertension and ethnic group. (2006). *British Medical Journal, 332*; American Heart Association, 2009.
11. Chen, J., et al. (2001). Racial differences in the use of cardiac catheterization after acute myocardial infarction. *New England Journal of Medicine, 44*, 1443–1449.
12. National Cancer Institute, National Institutes of Health. (2008, March). *Cancer health disparities*. Retrieved from http://www.cancer.gov/cancertopics/factsheet/cancer-health-disparities; National Cancer Institute, National Institutes of Health. (2010, July). *Cancer snapshots: Disease focused and other snapshots*. Retrieved from http://www.cancer.gov/Templates/doc.aspx?viewid=868242CD-C444-4CFD-B03F-24EE1320D2DB
13. Bach, P. B., et al. (2002). Survival of blacks and whites after a cancer diagnosis. *Journal of the American Medical Association, 287*, 2106–2113.
14. U.S. Department of Health & Human Services, National Partnership for Action to End Health Disparities. (2010, February). *Health disparities*. Retrieved from http://minorityhealth.hhs.gov/npa/templates/browse.aspx?lvl=1&lvlid=
15. Arias, 2010.
16. Doctors tie male mentality to shorter life span. (1995, June 14). *The New York Times*. Retrieved from http://www.nytimes.com/1995/06/14/us/doctors-tie-male-mentality-to-shorter-life-span.html
17. Centers for Disease Control and Prevention. (2009, October). *Healthy People 2000*. Retrieved from http://www.cdc.gov/nchs/healthy_people/hp2000.htm
18. Centers for Disease Control and Prevention. (2009, October). *About Healthy People 2010*. Retrieved from http://www.cdc.gov/nchs/healthy_people/hp2010.htm
19. U.S. Department of Health and Human Services, Office of Disease Prevention and Health Promotion. (2009, November). *Healthy People 2020: The road ahead*. Retrieved from http://www.healthypeople.gov/hp2020/
20. Eysenbach, G., Powell, J., Kuss, O., & Sa, E.-R. (2003). Empirical studies assessing the quality of health information for consumers on the World Wide Web: A systematic review. *Journal of the American Medical Association, 287*, 2691–2700.

Chapter 2

1. Johnston-Brooks, C. H., Lewis, M. A., & Garg, S. (2002). Self-efficacy impacts self-care and Hba1c in young adults with Type I diabetes. *Psychosomatic Medicine, 64*, 43–51.
2. Gwaltney, C. J., Metrik, J., Kahler, C. W., & Shiffman, S. (2009). Self-efficacy and smoking cessation: A meta-analysis. *Psychology of Addictive Behaviors, 23*, 56–66; Motl, R. W., Dishman, R. K., Ward, D. S., Saunders, R. P., Dowda, M., Felton, G., et al. (2002). Examining social-cognitive determinants of intention and physical activity among black and white adolescent girls using structural equation modeling. *Health Psychology, 21*, 459–467.
3. Benight, C. C., & Bandura, A. (2004). Social cognitive theory of posttraumatic recovery: The role of perceived self-efficacy. *Behaviour Research and Therapy, 10*, 1129–1148; Bandura, A. (2006). Toward a psychology of human agency. *Perspectives on Psychological Science, 1*, 164–180.
4. Tindle, H. A., Chang, Y. F., Kuller, L. H., Manson, J. E., Robinson, J. G., Rosal, M. C., et al. (2009). Optimism, cynical hostility, and incident coronary heart disease and mortality in the women's health initiative. *Circulation, 120*, 656–662.
5. Carver, C. S., Scheier, M. F., & Segerstrom, S. C. (2010). Optimism. *Clinical Psychology Review*, 30, 879–889; Scheier, M. F., & Carver, C. S. (1985). Optimism, coping, and health: Assessment and implications of generalized outcome expectancies. *Health Psychology, 4*, 219–247.
6. Bjerklie, D. (2005, January 17). Can sunny thoughts halt cancer? *Time*, A14; Trunzo, J. J., & Pinto, B. M. (2003). Social support as a mediator of optimism and distress in breast cancer survivors. *Journal of Consulting and Clinical Psychology, 71*, 805–811; Shnek, Z. M., Irvine, J., Stewart, D., & Abbey, S. (2001). Psychological factors and depressive symptoms in ischemic heart disease. *Health Psychology, 20*, 141–145.
7. Carver, C. S., Scheier, M. F., & Segerstrom, S. C. (2010). Optimisim. *Clinical Psychology Review, 30*, 879–889; Lobel, M., DeVincent, C. J., Kaminer, A., & Meyer, B. A. (2000). The impact of prenatal maternal stress and optimistic disposition on birth outcomes in medically high-risk women. *Health Psychology, 19*, 544–553.
8. Scheier, M. F., Matthews, K. A., Owens, J. F., Magovern, G. J., Sr., Lefebvre, R. C., Abbott, R. A., et al. (1989). Dispositional optimism and recovery from coronary artery bypass surgery: The beneficial effects on physical and psychological well-being. *Journal of Personality and Social Psychology, 57*, 1024–1040.
9. Kesebir, P., & Diener, E. (2008). In pursuit of happiness: Empirical answers to philosophical questions. *Perspectives on Psychological Science, 3*, 117–125.
10. Corliss, R. (2003, January 20). Is there a formula for joy? *Time*, 44–46; Hsee, C. K., Hastie, R., & Chen, J. (2008). Hedonomics: Bridging decision research with happiness research. *Perspectives*

on Psychological Science, 3, 224–243; Kahneman, D., Krueger, A. B., Schkade, D., Schwarz, N., & Stone, A. A. (2006). Would you be happier if you were richer? A focusing illusion. *Science, 312*, 1908–1910.
11. Munsey, C. (2010, October). Does marriage make us happy? *Monitor on Psychology*, 20–21.
12. Ibid.
13. Lucas, R. E., Clark, A. E., Georgellis, Y., & Diener, E. (2003). Reexamining adaptation and the set point model of happiness: Reactions to changes in marital status. *Journal of Personality and Social Psychology, 84*, 527–539.
14. Seligman, M. E. P. (2003, August). *Positive psychology: Applications to work, love, and sports.* Paper presented at the meeting of the American Psychological Association, Toronto, CA.
15. See, for example, Derringer, J., Krueger, R. F., Dick, D. M., Saccone, S., Grucza, R. A., Agrawal, A., et al., Gene Environment Association Studies (GENEVA) Consortium. (2010). Predicting sensation seeking from dopamine genes: A candidate-system approach. *Psychological Science, 9*, 1282–1290; Harro, J. , Merenäkk, L., Nordquist, N., Konstabel, K., Comasco, E., Oreland, L. (2009). Personality and the serotonin transporter gene: Associations in a longitudinal population-based study. *Biological Psychology, 81*, 9–13; Lahey, B. B. (2009). Public health significance of neuroticism. *American Psychologist, 64*, 241–256.
16. Duric, V., Banasr, M., Licznerski, P., Schmidt, H. D., Stockmeier, C. A., Simen, A. A., et al. (2010). A negative regulator of map kinase causes depressive behavior. *Nature Medicine, 16*, 1328–1332; McClellan, J., & King, M. C. (2010). Genomic analysis of mental illness: A changing landscape. *Journal of the American Medical Association, 303*, 2523–2524; Walters, J. T., R., Corvin, A., Owen, M. J., Williams, H., Dragovic, M., Quinn, E. M., et al. (2010). Psychosis susceptibility gene ZNF804A and cognitive performance in schizophrenia. *Archives of General Psychiatry, 67*, 692–700.
17. Hsee, C. K., Hastie, R., & Chen, J. (2008). Hedonomics: Bridging decision research with happiness research. *Perspectives on Psychological Science, 3*, 224–243; Kesebir, P., & Diener, E. (2008). In pursuit of happiness: Empirical answers to philosophical questions. *Perspectives on Psychological Science, 3*, 117–125; Paul, P. (2005, January 17). The power to uplift. *Time*, A46–A48.
18. Braam, A. W., Schaap-Jonker, J., Mooi, B., de Ritter, D., Beekman, A. T. F., & Deeg, D. J. H. (2008). God image and mood in old age. *Mental Health, Religion, & Culture, 11*, 221–237; Korff, S. C. (2006). Religious orientation as a predictor of life satisfaction within the elderly population. *Dissertation Abstracts International, 67*(1-B), 550.
19. Park, N. S., Klemmack, D. L., Roff, L. L., Parker, M. W., Koenig, H. G., Sawyer, P., et al. (2008). Religiousness and longitudinal trajectories in elders' functional status. *Research on Aging, 30*, 279–298.
20. Marks, L., Nesteruk, O., Swanson, M., Garrison, B., & Davis, T. (2005). Religion and health among African Americans: A qualitative examination. *Research on Aging, 27*(4), 447–474.
21. O'Connor, P. J., Pronk, N. P., Tan, A., & Whitebird, R. R. (2005). Characteristics of adults who use prayer as an alternative therapy. *American Journal of Health Promotion, 19*(5), 369–375.
22. Kessler, R. C., Berglund, P., Demler, O., Jin, R., Merikangas, K. R., & Walters, E. E. (2005). Lifetime prevalence and age-of-onset distributions of *DSM-IV* disorders in the National Comorbidity Survey Replication. *Archives of General Psychiatry, 62*, 593–602.
23. Kessler, R. C., Demler, O., Frank, R. G., Olfson, M., Pincus, H. A., Walters, E. E., et al. (2005). Prevalence and treatment of mental disorders, 1990 to 2003. *New England Journal of Medicine, 352*, 2515–2523; Kessler, R. C., Chiu, W. T., Demler, O., Merikangas, K. R., & Walters, E. E. (2005). Prevalence, severity, and comorbidity of 12-month *DSM-IV* disorders in the National Comorbidity Survey Replication. *Archives of General Psychiatry, 62*, 617–627.
24. Druss, B. G., Miller, C. L., Rosenheck, R. A., Shih, S. C., & Bost, J. E. (2002). Mental health care quality under managed care in the United States: A view from the Health Employer Data and Information Set (HEDIS). *American Journal of Psychiatry, 159*, 567–572; Stewart W. F., Ricci, J. A., Chee, E., Hahn, S. R., & Morganstein, D. (2002). Cost of lost productive work time among U.S. workers with depression. *Journal of the American Medical Association, 289*, 3135–3144.
25. Barnett, J. H., & Smoller, J. W. (2009). The genetics of bipolar disorder. *Neuroscience,* 164, 331–343; Duric, V., Banasr, M., Licznerski, P., Schmidt, H. D., Stockmeier, C. A., & Simen, A. A. (2010). A negative regulator of map kinase causes depressive behavior. *Nature Medicine, 16*, 1328–1332; Smoller, J. W., Paulus, M. P., Fagerness, J. A., Purcell, S., Yamaki, L. H., Hirshfeld-Becker, D., et al. (2008). Influence of RGS2 on anxiety-related temperament, personality, and brain function. *Archives of General Psychiatry, 65*, 298–308; Uher, R., & Perroud, N. (2010). Probing the genome to understand suicide. *American Journal of Psychiatry, 167*, 1425–1427; Walker, E., Shapiro, D., Esterberg, M., & Trotman, H. (2010). Neurodevelopment and schizophrenia: Broadening the focus. *Psychological Science, 19*, 204–208.
26. Kessler, R. C., Borges, G., & Walters, E. E. (1999). Prevalence of and risk factors for lifetime suicide attempts in the National Comorbidity Survey. *Archives of General Psychiatry, 56*, 617–626.
27. Centers for Disease Control and Prevention. (2009, Summer). *Suicide: Facts at a glance*. National Center for Injury Prevention and Control.
28. Rawe, J., & Kingsbury, K. (2006, May 22). When colleges go on suicide watch. *Time*, 62–63.
29. Centers for Disease Control and Prevention. (2009, September 30). *Suicide rates among persons ages 10 years and older, by race/ethnicity and sex, United States, 2002–2006*. Retrieved from http://www.cdc.gov/violenceprevention/suicide/statistics/rates02.html; Miller, M., Azrael, D., & Hemenway, D. (2004). The epidemiology of case fatality rates for suicide in the Northeast. *Annals of Emergency Medicine, 43*, 723–730.
30. LaFromboise, T. D., Albright, K., & Harris, A. (2010). Patterns of hopelessness among American Indian adolescents: Relationships by levels of acculturation and residence. *Cultural Diversity and Ethnic Minority Psychology, 16*, 68–76; Garlow, S. J., Purselle, D., & Heninger, M. (2005). Ethnic differences in patterns of suicide across the life cycle. *American Journal of Psychiatry, 162*, 319–323; Gone, J. (2004). Mental health services for Native Americans in the 21st-century United States. *Professional Psychology: Research and Practice, 35*, 10–18; Meyers, L. (2007, February). A struggle for hope. *Monitor on Psychology, 38*(2), 30–31.
31. Ibid.
32. McGowan, S., Lawrence, A. D., Sales, T., Quested, D., & Grasby, P. (2004). Presynaptic dopaminergic dysfunction in schizophrenia: A positron emission tomographic [18f]fluorodopa study. *Archives of General Psychiatry, 61*, 134–142.
33. Medda, P., Perugi, G., Zanello, S., Ciuffa, M., & Cassano, G. B. (2009). Response to ECT in bipolar I, bipolar II and unipolar depression. *Journal of Affective Disorders, 118*, 55–59; Bailine, S., Fink, M., Knapp, R., Petrides, G., Husain, M. M., Rasmussen, K., et al. (2010). Electroconvulsive therapy is equally effective in unipolar and bipolar depression. *Acta Psychiatrica Scandinavica, 121*, 431.
34. Kennedy, S. H., Lam, R., Parikh, S. V., Patten, S. B., & Ravindran, A. V. (2009). Canadian Network for Mood and Anxiety Treatments (CANMAT) clinical guidelines for the management of major depressive disorder in adults: IV. Neurostimulation therapies. *Journal of Affective Disorders, 117*, S44–S53.

Chapter 3

1. Smith, T. W., & Gallo, L. C. (2001). Personality traits as risk factors for physical illness. In A. Baum, T. A. Revenson, & J. E. Singer (Eds.), *Handbook of health psychology* (pp. 139–174). Mahwah, NJ: Lawrence Erlbaum Associates.
2. Chida, Y., & Steptoe, A. (2009). The association of anger and hostility with future coronary heart disease: A meta-analytic review of prospective evidence. *Journal of the American College of Cardiology, 53*, 936–946; Denollet, J., & Pedersen, S. S. (2009). Anger, depression, and anxiety in cardiac patients: The complexity of individual differences in psychological risk. *Journal of the American College of Cardiology, 53*, 947–949.
3. Benson, H., Corliss, J., & Cowley, G. (2004, September 27). Scientists are mapping the pathways that link emotion to health. The challenge for the rest of us is to put the discoveries to work. *Newsweek Health Online*. Retrieved from http://www.msnbc.msn.com/id/6038621/site/newsweek.
4. Cutrona, C. E., et al. (2000). Direct and moderating effects of community context on the psychological well-being of African American women. *Journal of Personality and Social Psychology, 79*, 1088–1101.
5. LaFromboise, T. D., Albright, K., & Harris, A. (2010). Patterns of hopelessness among American Indian adolescents: Relationships by levels of acculturation and residence. *Cultural Diversity and Ethnic Minority Psychology, 16*, 68–76; Rodriguez, J., et al. (2009). Cultural processes in parenting and youth outcomes: Examining a model of racial-ethnic socialization and identity in diverse populations. *Cultural Diversity and Ethnic Minority Psychology, 15*, 106–111; Smith, C. O, et al. (2009). A developmental perspective of the relationship of racial–ethnic identity to self-construct, achievement, and behavior in African American children. *Cultural Diversity and Ethnic Minority Psychology, 15*, 145–157.
6. Gray-Little, B., & Hafdahl, A. R. (2000). Factors influencing racial comparisons of self-esteem: A quantitative review. *Psychological Bulletin, 126*, 26–54.
7. Anderson, L. P. (1991). Acculturative stress: A theory of relevance to black Americans. *Clinical Psychology Review, 11*, 685–702.
8. Aich, P., Potter, A. A., & Griebel, P. J. (2009). Modern approaches to understanding stress and disease susceptibility: A review with special emphasis on respiratory disease. *International Journal of General Medicine, 2*, 19–32.
9. Scott-Sheldon, L. A. J., Kalichman, S. C., Carey, M. P., & Fielder, R. L. (2008). Stress management interventions for HIV+ adults: A meta-analysis of randomized controlled trials, 1989 to 2006. *Health Psychology, 27*(2), 129–139.
10. Glaser, R., et al. (1993). Stress and the memory T-cell response to the Epstein-Barr virus. *Health Psychology, 12*, 435–442.
11. Coskun, O., et al. (2010). Stress-related Epstein-Barr virus reactivation. *Clinical and Experimental Medicine, 10*, 15–20.
12. Michael, Y. L., et al. (2009). Influence of stressors on breast cancer incidence in the women's health initiative. *Health Psychology, 28*, 137–146.
13. Sánchez-Ortuño, M. M., & Edinger, J. D. (2010). A penny for your thoughts: Patterns of sleep-related beliefs, insomnia symptoms and treatment outcome. *Behavior Research and Therapy, 48*, 125–133; Smith, M. T., & Perlis, M. L. (2006). Who is a candidate for cognitive-behavioral therapy for insomnia? *Health Psychology, 25*, 15–19; Dolan, D. C., Taylor, D. J., Bramoweth, A. D., & Rosenthal, L. D. (2010). Cognitive behavioral therapy of insomnia: A clinical case series study of patients with comorbid disorders and using hypnotic medications. *Behavior Research and Therapy, 48*, 321–327.

Chapter 4

1. Michael, R. T., Gagnon, J. H., Laumann, E. O., & Kolata, G. (1994). *Sex in America: A definitive survey.* Boston: Little, Brown.
2. Berscheid, E., & Regan, P. (2005). *The psychology of interpersonal relationships.* New York: Prentice-Hall; Strassberg, D. S., & Holty, S. (2003). An experimental study of women's Internet personal ads. *Archives of Sexual Behavior, 32*, 253–260.
3. Streeter, S. A., & McBurney, D. H. (2003).Waist–hip ratio and attractiveness: New evidence and a critique of a "critical test." *Evolution and Human Behavior, 24*, 88–98.
4. Pawlowski, B., & Koziel, S. (2003). The impact of traits offered in personal advertisements on response rates. *Evolution and Human Behavior, 23*, 139–149.
5. Sternberg, R. J. (1997). Construct validation of a triangular love scale. *European Journal of Social Psychology, 27*, 313–335.
6. Bramlett, M. D., & Mosher, W. D. (2002). *Cohabitation, marriage, divorce, and remarriage.* National Center for Health Statistics, Vital Health Statistics, 23. Retrieved from http://www.cdc.gov/nchs/data/series/sr_23/sr23_022.pdf
7. Whitehead, B. D., & Popenoe, D. (2006). *The state of our unions: The social health of marriage in America.* New Brunswick, NJ: Rutgers University.
8. Luo, S., & Klohnen, E. C. (2005). Assortative mating and marital quality in newlyweds: A couple-centered approach. *Journal of Personality and Social Psychology, 88*, 304–326; Rushton, J. P., & Bons, T. A. (2005). Mate choice and friendship in twins: Evidence for genetic similarity. *Psychological Science, 16*, 555–559
9. Reynolds, C. A., Barlow, T., & Pedersen, N. L. (2006). Alcohol, tobacco and caffeine use: Spouse similarity processes. *Behavior Genetics, 36*, 201–215.
10. Arnett, J. J. (2011). Emerging adulthood. In L. A. Jensen (Ed.), *Bridging cultural and developmental approaches to psychology: New syntheses in theory, research and policy* (pp. 255ff.). New York: Oxford University Press.
11. Doherty, W. J., Carroll, J. S., & Waite, L. J. (2007). Supporting the institution of marriage: Ideological, research, and ecological perspectives. In A. S. Loveless & T. B. Holman (Eds.), *The family in the new millennium, vol. 2: Marriage and human dignity* (pp. 21–51). Westport, CT: Praeger Publishers/Greenwood Publishing Group.
12. Grall, T. S. (2009). Custodial mothers and fathers and their child support: 2007. Retrieved from http://www.census.gov/prod/2009pubs/p60-237.pdf
13. Bertoni, A., et al. (2007). Stress communication, dyadic coping and couple satisfaction: A cross-sectional and cross-cultural study. *Età Evolutiva, 86*, 58–66.
14. Patrick, S., Sells, J. N., Giordano, F. G., & Tollerud, T. R. (2007). Intimacy, differentiation, and personality variables as predictors of marital satisfaction. *The Family Journal, 15*, 359–367
15. Perrone, K. M., Webb, L. K., & Jackson, Z. V. (2007). Relationships between parental attachment, work and family roles, and life satisfaction. *The Career Development Quarterly, 55*, 237–248.
16. Matthews, R. A., et al. (2006). Work-to-relationship conflict: Crossover effects in dual-earner couples. *Journal of Occupational Health Psychology, 11*, 228–240.
17. Kurdek, L. A. (2006). What do we know about gay and lesbian couples? *Current Directions in Psychological Science, 14*(5), 251; Kurdek, L. A. (2005). Differences between partners from hetersosexual, gay, and lesbian cohabiting couples. *Journal of Marriage and the Family, 68*, 509–528.
18. Marazziti, D., et al. (2003). Normal and obsessional jealousy: A study of a population of young adults. *European Psychiatry, 18*, 106–111.
19. Hetherington, E. M. (2006). The influence of conflict, marital problem solving and parenting on children's adjustment in nondivorced, divorced and remarried families. In A. Clarke-Stewart and J. Dunn (Eds.), *Families count: Effects on child and adolescent development* (pp. 203–237). Cambridge, UK: Cambridge University Press; Lansford, J. E. (2009). Parental divorce and children's adjustment. *Perspectives on Psychological Science, 4*, 140–152.
20. Troxel, W. M., & Matthews, K. A. (2004). What are the costs of marital conflict and dissolution to children's

physical health? *Clinical Child and Family Psychology Review, 7*, 29–57.
21. Kiesner, J. (2009). Physical characteristics of the menstrual cycle and premenstrual depressive symptoms. *Psychological Science, 20*, 763–770; Yonkers, K. A., O'Brien, P. M. S., & Eriksson, E. (2008). Premenstrual syndrome. *The Lancet, 371*, 1200–1210; Heinemann, L., et al. (2010). Explorative evaluation of the impact of severe premenstrual disorders on work absenteeism and productivity. *Women's Health Issues, 20*, 58–65.
22. Bäckström, T., et al. (2003). The role of hormones and hormonal treatments in premenstrual syndrome. *CNS Drugs, 17*, 325–342.
23. Chlebowski, R. T., et al. (2003). Influence of estrogen plus progestin on breast cancer and mammography in healthy postmenopausal women: The women's health initiative randomized trial. *Journal of the American Medical Association, 289*, 3243–3253.
24. Tobian, A. et al. (2009). Male circumcision for the prevention of HSV-2 and HPV infections and syphilis. *New England Journal of Medicine, 360*, 1298–1309.
25. Masters, W. H., & Johnson, V. E. (1966). *Human sexual response.* Boston: Little, Brown.
26. Mosher, W. D., Chandra, A., & Jones, J. (2005). *Sexual behavior and selected health measures: Men and women 15–44 years of age, United States, 2002. Advance data from vital and health statistics, No. 362.* Hyattsville, MD: National Center for Health Statistics.
27. Hyde, J. S. (2005). The genetics of sexual orientation. In J. S. Hyde (Ed.), *Biological substrates of human sexuality* (pp. 9–20). Washington, DC: American Psychological Association.
28. Långström, N., et al. (2010). Genetic and environmental effects on same-sex sexual behavior: A population study of twins in sweden. *Archives of Sexual Behavior, 39*, 75–80.
29. Fitzpatrick, K. K. (2005). Gender role, sexual orientation, and suicide risk. *Journal of Affective Disorders, 87*, 35–42; Mills, T. C., et al. (2004). Distress and depression in men who have sex with men: The urban men's health study. *American Journal of Psychiatry, 161*, 278–285.
30. Laumann, E. O., Gagnon, J. H., Michael, R. T., & Michaels, S. (1994). *The social organization of sexuality: Sexual practices in the United States.* Chicago: University of Chicago Press, Table 3.3, p. 86.
31. Herbenick, D., et al. (2010). Sexual behaviors, relationships, and perceived health status among adult women in the United States: Results from a national probability sample. *Journal of Sexual Medicine, 7*(Suppl 5), 277–290; Reece, M., et al. (2010). Sexual behaviors, relationships, and perceived health among adult men in the United States: Results from a national probability sample. *Journal of Sexual Medicine, 7*(Suppl 5), 291–304.
32. Herbenick, D., et al. (2010). Sexual behavior in the United States: Results from a national probability sample of men and women ages 14–94. *Journal of Sexual Medicine, 7*(Suppl 5), 255–265.
33. Herbenick et al., 2010
34. Nevid, J. S. Rathus, S. A., & Greene, B. (2011). *Abnormal psychology in a changing world* (8th ed.). Upper Saddle River, NJ: Prentice-Hall.
35. Rees, P. M., Fowler, C. J., & Maas, C. P. (2007). Sexual function in men and women with neurological disorders. *The Lancet, 369*, 512–525; Basaria, S., et al. (2010). Adverse events associated with testosterone administration. *New England Journal of Medicine, 363*, 109–122; Montorsi, F., et al. (2010). Summary of the recommendations on sexual dysfunctions in men. *Journal of Sexual Medicine, 7* (11), 3572–3588.

Chapter 5

1. Sanger, M. (1938). *Margaret Sanger: An autobiography*. New York: Norton.
2. American Fertility Association. (2010). *Age and female fertility*. Retrieved from http://www.theafa.org/library/article/age_and_female_fertility/
3. American Fertility Association. (2010). *Who's infertile? Us?* Retrieved from http://www.theafa.org/library/article/whos_infertile_us/
4. American Fertility Association. (2010). *A baby, maybe?* Retrieved from http://www.theafa.org/library/article/a_baby_maybe/
5. Frisch, R. E. (2004). *Female fertility and the body fat connection.* Chicago: University of Chicago Press.
6. Gnagy, S., et al. (2000). Declining ovarian cancer rates in U.S. women in relation to parity and oral contraceptive use. *Epidemiology, 11*, 102–105; Hatcher, R. A., et al. (2007). *Contraceptive technologies* (19th ed.). New York: Ardent Media.
7. American College of Obstetricians and Gynecologists (ACOG). (2006). Retrieved from http://www.acog.org
8. American College of Obstetricians and Gynecologists (ACOG). (2006). *The ABCs of oral contraceptives.* Retrieved from http://www.acog.org
9. Hofmeyr, D. G., & Greeff, A. P. (2002). The influence of a vasectomy on the marital relationship and sexual satisfaction of the married man. *Journal of Sex & Marital Therapy, 28*, 339–352.
10. Hatcher, et al., 2007.
11. Hatcher, et al., 2007.
12. Guttmacher Institute. (2010). *Facts on induced abortion in the United States.* Retrieved from http://www.guttmacher.org/pubs/fb_induced_abortion.html; Jones, R. K., et al. (2008). Abortion in the United States: Incidence and access to services, 2005. *Perspectives on Sexual and Reproductive Health, 40*, 6–16.
13. Flaxman, S. M., & Sherman, P. W. (2000). Morning sickness: A mechanism for protecting mother and embryo. *The Quarterly Review of Biology, 75*, 113–148.
14. Grady, D. (2010, March 23). Caesarean births are at a high in U.S. *The New York Times*, p. A13.
15. Hopkins-Golightly, T., Raz, S., & Sander, C. J. (2003). Influence of slight to moderate risk for birth hypoxia on acquisition of cognitive and language function in the preterm infant: A cross-sectional comparison with preterm-birth controls. *Neuropsychology, 17*, 3–13.
16. Nadeau, L., et al. (2003). Extremely premature and very low birthweight infants: A double hazard population? *Social Development, 12*, 235–248.
17. Anderson, P., et al. (2003). Neurobehavioral outcomes of school-age children born extremely low birth weight or very preterm in the 1990s. *Journal of the American Medical Association, 289*, 3264–3272; Nadeau, et al., 2003.
18. Fuentes-Afflick, E., & Hessol, N. A. (2000). Interpregnancy interval and the risk of premature infants. *Obstetrics & Gynecology, 95*, 383–390.
19. Friedman, S. H. (2009). Postpartum mood disorders: Genetic progress and treatment paradigms. *American Journal of Psychiatry, 166*, 1201–1204; Centers for Disease Control and Prevention. (2008). Prevalence of self-reported postpartum depressive symptoms—17 states, 2004–2005. *MMWR: Morbidity and Mortality Weekly Report, 57*, 361.
20. Munk-Olsen, T., et al. (2009). Risks and predictors of readmission for a mental disorder during the postpartum period. *Archives of General Psychiatry, 66*, 189–195; Mahon, P. B., et al. (2009). Genome-wide linkage and follow-up association study of postpartum mood symptoms. *American Journal of Psychiatry, 166*, 1229–1237; Phillips, J., et al. (2010). Subtypes of postnatal depression? A comparison of women with recurrent and de novo postnatal depression. *Journal of Affective Disorders, 120*, 67–75; Vesga-López, O., et al. (2008). Psychiatric disorders in pregnant and postpartum women in the United States. *Archives of General Psychiatry, 65*, 805–815.
21. American Academy of Pediatrics. (2006). Retrieved from http://www.aap.org/
22. American Academy of Pediatrics. (2007). *Children's health topics: Breastfeeding.* Retrieved from http://www.aap.org/breastfeeding/index.html

Chapter 6

1. Kalat, J. W. (2009). *Biological psychology*. Belmont, CA: Wadsworth.
2. Han, D. H., et al. (2007). Dopamine genes and reward dependence in adolescents with excessive internet video game

play. *Journal of Addiction Medicine, 1*, 133–138; Weinstein, A. M. (2010). Computer and video game addiction—A comparison between game users and non-game users. *The American Journal of Drug and Alcohol Abuse, 36*, 268–276.
3. Black, D. W. (2010). *A review of compulsive shopping and spending.* Paper presented to the Iowa Psychiatric Society Meeting, Iowa City, IA.
4. Barnes, G. M., et al. (2010). Comparisons of gambling and alcohol use among college students and noncollege young people in the United States. *Journal of American College Health, 58*, 443–452; Dixon, M. R., Newman, T. N., & Nastally, B. A . (2009). Comparison of and maintaining cause for pathological gambling in fraternity and non-fraternity members. *Analysis of Gambling Behavior, 3*, 21–25.
5. Stuhldreher, W. L., Stuhldreher, T. J., & Forrest, K.Y. (2007). Gambling as an emerging health problem on campus. *Journal of American College Health, 56*, 75–83.
6. Leung, K. S., & Cottler, L. B. (2009). Treatment of pathological gambling. *Current Opinion in Psychiatry, 22*, 69–74.
7. Aboujaoude, E. (2010). Problematic internet use: An overview. *World Psychiatry, 9*, 85–90.
8. Christakis, D. A. (2010). Internet addiction: A 21st century epidemic? *BMC Medicine, 8*, 61. doi: 10.1186/1741-7015-8-61
9. Aboujaoude, 2010.
10. Volkow, N. D., et al. (2006). Cocaine cues and dopamine in dorsal striatum: Mechanism of craving in cocaine addiction. *Journal of Neuroscience, 26*, 6583–6588; Voruganti, L. N. P., & Awad, A. G. (2007). Role of dopamine in pleasure, reward and subjective responses to drugs. In M. S. Ritsner & A. G. Awad (Eds.), *Quality of life impairment in schizophrenia, mood and anxiety disorders* (pp. 21–31). Netherlands: Springer; Whitten, L. (2009). Receptor complexes link dopamine to long-term neuronal effects. *NIDA Notes, 22*(4), 15–16.
11. Krantz, M. J., & Mehler, P. S. (2004). Treating opioid dependence: Growing implications for primary care. *Archives of Internal Medicine, 164*, 277–288.
12. Volkow, N. (2005, April 25). Methamphetamine abuse [Testimony before the Senate Subcommittee on Labor, Health and Human Services, Education, and Related Agencies]. Committee on Appropriations. National Institute on Drug Abuse.
13. Homer, B. D., et al. (2008). Methamphetamine abuse and impairment of social functioning: A review of the underlying neurophysiological causes and behavioral implications. *Psychological Bulletin, 134*, 301–310.
14. Adapted from USDA National Nutrient Database for Standard Reference, 2009.
15. Bakker, R., et al. (2010). Maternal caffeine intake from coffee and tea, fetal growth, and the risks of adverse birth outcomes: The generation R study. *The American Journal of Clinical Nutrition, 91*, 1691–1698.
16. American Dietetic Association. (2010). *The buzz on caffeine*. Retrieved from http://www.eatright.org/Public/content.aspx?id=6442452080andterms=caffeine
17. Cornelis, M. C., et al. (2006). Coffee, CYP1A2 genotype, and risk of myocardial infarction. *Journal of the American Medical Association, 295*, 1135–1141.
18. Winkelmayer, W. C., et al. (2005). Habitual caffeine intake and the risk of hypertension in women. *Journal of the American Medical Association, 294*, 2330–2335.
19. Collins, K. (2004, December 3). How much caffeine is too much? *MSNBC .com*. Retrieved from http://www .msnbc.com
20. National Institute on Drug Abuse. (2009, June). *NIDA InfoFacts: Hallucinogens - LSD, peyote, psilocybin, and PCP*. Retrieved from http://drugabuse .gov/infofacts/hallucinogens.html
21. National Institute on Drug Abuse. (2010, November). NIDA InfoFacts: Marijuana. Retrieved from http://www .drugabuse.gov/infofacts/marijuana.html
22. Budney, A. J., et al. (2004). Review of the validity and significance of cannabis withdrawal syndrome. *American Journal of Psychiatry, 161*, 1967–1977.
23. Puighermanal, E., et al. (2009). Cannabinoid modulation of hippocampal long-term memory is mediated by motor signaling. *Nature Neuroscience, 12*, 1152–1158; Yücel, M., et al. (2008). Regional brain abnormalities associated with long-term heavy cannabis use. *Archives of General Psychiatry, 65*, 694–701.
24. Singh, R., et al. (2009). Evaluation of the DNA damaging potential of cannabis cigarette smoke by the determination of acetaldehyde derived N2-ethyl-2-deoxyguanosine addicts. *Chemical Research in Toxicology, 22*, 1181–1188.
25. de Win, M. M. L., et al. (2008). Sustained effects of ecstasy on the human brain: A prospective neuroimaging study in novel users. *Brain, 131*, 2936; Eisner, R. Study suggests cognitive deficits in MDMA-only drug abusers. *NIDA Notes, 19*. Retrieved from http://www.nida.nih.gov/NIDA_notes /NNvol19N5/Study.html
26. Drug Policy Information Clearing House, Office of National Drug Control Policy. (2005, June). Rohypnol. Retrieved from http://www.whitehouse drugpolicy.gov/publications/factsht /rohypnol
27. Foster, S. E., et al. (2003). Alcohol consumption and expenditures for underage drinking and adult excessive drinking. *Journal of the American Medical Association, 289*, 989–995.
28. Centers for Disease Control and Prevention. (2010, January 18). *Fast stats: Illegal drug use.* Retrieved from http:// www.cdc.gov/nchs/fastats; Substance Abuse and Mental Health Services Administration (SAMHSA), USDHHS. (2010, September). *Results from the 2009 National Survey on Drug Use and Health: Volume I. Summary of National Findings.*
29. Johnston, L. D., et al. (2010, December 14). *Marijuana use is rising; Ecstasy use is beginning to rise; and alcohol use is declining among U.S. teens.* University of Michigan News Service: Ann Arbor, MI. Retrieved from http://www .monitoringthefuture.org
30. Substance Abuse and Mental Health Services Administration (SAMSHA). *Results from the 2008 National Survey on Drug Use and Health: National Findings, Updated 2010*, http://oas .samhsa.gov/NSDUH/2K8NSDUH /tabs/toc.htm
31. Johnston, L. D., O'Malley, P. M., Bachman, J. G., & Schulenberg, J. E. (2010). *Monitoring the future national survey results on drug use, 1975–2009: Volume II, College students and adults ages 19–50* (NIH Publication No. 10-7585) (pp. 250–252). Bethesda, MD: National Institute on Drug Abuse.
32. American Lung Association. (2004, November). *Smoking 101 fact sheet.* Retrieved from http://www.lungusa .com
33. Friedman, R. A. (2006). The changing face of teenage drug abuse—the trend toward prescription drugs. *New England Journal of Medicine, 354*, 1448–1450.
34. Blomeyer, D., et al. (2008). Interaction between CRHR1 gene and stressful life events predicts adolescent heavy alcohol use. *Biological Psychiatry, 63*, 146; Kendler, K. S., et al. Genetic and environmental influences on alcohol, caffeine, cannabis, and nicotine use from early adolescence to middle adulthood. *Archives of General Psychiatry, 65*, 674–682; Uhl, G. R., (2008). Genome-wide association for methamphetamine dependence: Convergent results from 2 samples. *Archives of General Psychiatry, 65*, 345–355.
35. Pierce, R. C., & Kumaresan, V. (2006). The mesolimbic dopamine system: The final common pathway for the reinforcing effect of drugs of abuse? *Neuroscience and Biobehavioral Reviews, 30*, 215–238; Whitten, L. (2009). Receptor complexes link dopamine to long-term neuronal effects. *NIDA Notes, 22*, 15–16; Voruganti, L. N. P., & Awad, A. G. (2007). Role of dopamine in pleasure, reward and subjective responses to drugs. In M. S. Ritsner & A. G. Awad (Eds.), *Quality of life impairment in schizophrenia, mood and anxiety disorders* (pp. 21–31). Netherlands: Springer.

36. Martinez, D., et al. (2009). Lower level of endogenous dopamine in patients with cocaine dependence: Findings from PET imaging of D2/D3 receptors following acute dopamine depletion export. *American Journal of Psychiatry, 166*, 1170–1177.
37. Cheetham, A., et al. (2010). The role of affective dysregulation in drug addiction. *Clinical Psychology Review, 30*, 621–634; Weiss, R. D., & Mirin, S. M. (1995). *Cocaine: The human danger, the social costs, the treatment alternative* (2nd ed.). New York: Ballantine Books.
38. Goldstein, A. *Addiction: From biology to drug policy.* New York: W. H. Freeman.
39. Kandel, D. B. (2003). Does marijuana use cause the use of other drugs? *Journal of the American Medical Association, 289*, 482–483.
40. Cunningham, J. A., & Breslin, F. C. (2004). Only one in three people with alcohol abuse or dependence ever seek treatment. *Addictive Behaviors, 29*, 221–223.
41. Veilleux, J. C., (2010). A review of opioid dependence treatment: Pharmacological and psychosocial interventions to treat opioid addiction. *Clinical Psychology Review, 30*, 155–166.
42. Krantz, M. J., & Mehler, P. S. (2004). Treating opioid dependence: Growing implications for primary care. *Archives of Internal Medicine, 16*, 277–288.
43. Anton, R. F. (2008). Naltrexone for the management of alcohol dependence. *New England Journal of Medicine, 359*, 715–721; Myrick, H., et al. (2008). Effect of naltrexone and ondansetron on alcohol cue–induced activation of the ventral striatum in alcohol-dependent people. *Archives of General Psychiatry, 65*, 466–475.

Chapter 7

1. Johnston, L. D., O'Malley, P. M., Bachman, J. G., & Schulenberg, J. E. (2010). *Monitoring the future: National survey results on drug use, 1975–2009. Volume II: College Students and Adults Ages 19–50* (NIH Publication No. 10-7585). Bethesda, MD: National Institute on Drug Abuse.
2. Johnston et al., 2010.
3. Hingson, R., et al. (2002). *A call to action: Changing the culture of drinking at U.S. colleges.* Washington, DC: National Institutes of Health: National Institute of Alcohol Abuse and Alcoholism.
4. McCauley, J. L., Calhoun, K. S., & Gidycz, C. A. (2010). Binge drinking and rape: A prospective examination of college women with a history of previous sexual victimization. *Journal of Interpersonal Violence, 25*, 1655–1668; Randolph, M. E., et al. (2009). Alcohol use and sexual risk behavior among college students. *American Journal of Drug and Alcohol Abuse, 35*, 80–84; Swartout, K. M., & White, J. W. (2010). The relationship between drug use and sexual aggression in men across time. *Journal of Interpersonal Violence, 29*, 1716–1735.
5. Naimi, T., Nelson, D., & Brewer, R. (2010). The intensity of binge alcohol consumption among U.S. adults. *American Journal of Preventive Medicine, 38*, 201–207.
6. Johnston et al., 2010.
7. Hingson et al., 2002; Hustad, J. T. P., Barnett, N. P., Borsari, B., & Jackson, K. M. (2010). Web-based alcohol prevention for incoming college students: A randomized controlled trial. *Addictive Behaviors, 35*, 183–189.
8. Johnston, L. D., O'Malley, P. M., Bachman, J. G., & Schulenberg, J. E. (2005). *Monitoring the future: National results on adolescent drug use: Overview of key findings* (NIH Publication No. 05 5726). Bethesda, MD: National Institute On Drug Abuse.
9. Johnston, L. D., et al. (2010). *Monitoring the future: National survey results on drug use, 1975–2009. Volume II: College students and adults ages 19–50* (NIH Publication No. 10-7585). Bethesda, MD: National Institute on Drug Abuse.
10. Slutske, W. S. (2005). Alcohol use disorders among U.S. college students and their non-college-attending peers. *Archives of General Psychiatry, 62*, 321–327.
11. Hingson, R. W., et al. (2009). Magnitude of and trends in alcohol-related mortality and morbidity among U.S. college students ages 18 to 24, 1998–2005. *Journal of Studies on Alcohol and Drugs, 16*, 12–20.
12. National Institute On Alcohol Abuse and Alcoholism, National Institutes of Health, 2010
13. Mitka, M. (2009). College binge drinking still on the rise. *Journal of the American Medical Association, 302*, 836–837.
14. Wechsler, H., & Nelson T. F. (2008). What we have learned from the Harvard School of Public Health college alcohol study. *Journal of Studies on Alcohol and Drugs, 69*, 481–490.
15. Singleton, R. A. Jr., & Wolfson, A. R. (2009). Alcohol consumption, sleep, and academic performance among college students. *Journal of Studies on Alcohol and Drugs, 70*, 355.
16. Buddie, A. M., & Testa, M. (2005). Rates and predictors of sexual aggression among students and nonstudents. *Journal of Interpersonal Violence, 20*, 713–724; Murphy, C. M., et al. (2005). Alcohol consumption and intimate partner violence by alcoholic men: Comparing violent and nonviolent conflicts. *Psychology of Addictive Behaviors, 19*, 35–42; Stith, S. M., et al. (2004). Intimate partner physical abuse perpetration and victimization risk factors: A meta-analytic review. *Aggression and Violent Behavior, 10*, 65–98.
17. The American College Health Association. (2005). The American College Health Association National College Health Assessment (Acha-Ncha), spring 2003 reference group report. *Journal of American College Health, 53*, 199–210.
18. Centers for Disease Control and Prevention. (2010, May 20). Deaths: Final data for 2007. *National Vital Statistics Reports, 58*(19).
19. Ting Kai L. (2005, March). National Institute On Alcohol Abuse and Alcoholism House Subcommittee On Labor HS Education Appropriations. Retrieved from http://www.hhs.gov/budget/06budget/documents/niaaa.doc
20. King, D. E., Mainous III, A. G., & Geesey, M. E. (2008). Adopting moderate alcohol consumption in middle age: Subsequent cardiovascular events. *American Journal of Medicine, 121*, 201–206; Di Castelnuovo, A., et al. (2006). Alcohol dosing and total mortality in men and women: An updated meta-analysis of 34 prospective studies. *Archives of Internal Medicine, 166*, 2437–2445; Harvard School of Public Health. (2005). *Possible health benefits of alcohol.* Retrieved from http://www.hsph.harvard.edu/nutritionsource/alcohol.html
21. National Institute of Alcohol Abuse and Alcoholism. (n.d.) *Alcohol liver disease.* Retrieved from http://www.niaaa.nih.gov/resources/graphicsgallery/liver/disease.htm.
22. National Institute On Alcohol Abuse and Alcoholism (NIAA), July 27, 2005.
23. National Institute on Alcohol Abuse and Alcoholism (NIAA), July 27, 2005.
24. Bischof, G., et al. (2005). Gender differences in temptation to drink, self-efficacy to abstain and coping behavior in treated alcohol-dependent individuals. *Addiction Research and Theory, 13*, 129–136.
25. Johnston, L. D., et al. (2010, December 14). *Marijuana use is rising; ecstasy use is beginning to rise; and alcohol use is declining among U.S. teens.* University of Michigan News Service: Ann Arbor, MI; http://www.Monitoringthefuture.org; Johnston, L. D., et al. (2010). *Monitoring the future: National survey results on drug use, 1975–2009. Volume I: Secondary School Students* (NIH Publication No. 10-7584). Bethesda, MD: National Institute on Drug Abuse; Johnston, L D., et al. (2010, May). *Monitoring the future: National survey results on drug use: Overview of key findings, 2009* (NIH Publication No. 10-7583). Bethesda, MD: National Institute on Drug Abuse.
26. Centers for Disease Control and Prevention (CDC). (2009, June 19). Alcohol and suicide among racial/ethnic populations —17 states, 2005–2006. *Morbidity and Mortality Weekly Report, 58*(23), 637–641.

27. Centers for Disease Control and Prevention (CDC). (2010, July). *Injury prevention and control: Motor vehicle safety: Impaired driving.* Retrieved from http://www.cdc.gov/motorvehiclesafety/impaired_driving/impaired-drv_factsheet.html
28. Deadly states for teen drivers. (2005, August 4). *CNN.* Retrieved from http://www.cnn.com/2005/Autos/07/19/Teen_Drivers.
29. Blomeyer, D., et al. (2008). Interaction between *Crhr1* gene and stressful life events predicts adolescent heavy alcohol use. *Biological Psychiatry, 63,* 146; Ming, D. L., & Burmeister, M. (2009). New insights into the genetics of addiction. *Nature Reviews Genetics, 10,* 225–231; Treutlein, J., et al. (2009). Genome-wide association study of alcohol dependence. *Archives of General Psychiatry, 66,* 773–784.
30. Eng, M. Y., Schuckit, M. A., & Smith, T. L. (2005). The level of response to alcohol in daughters of alcoholics and controls. *Drug and Alcohol Dependence, 79,* 83–93; Schuckit, M. A., Danko, G. P., & Smith, T. L. (2004). Patterns of drug-related disorders in a prospective study of men chosen for their family history of alcoholism. *Journal of Studies on Alcohol, 65,* 613–620.
31. Heinz, A., et al. (2004). Pharmacogenetic insights to monoaminergic dysfunction in alcohol dependence. *Psychopharmacology, 174,* 561–570.
32. Benowitz, N. L. (2010). Nicotine addiction. *New England Journal of Medicine, 362,* 2295–2303; Centers for Disease Control (CDC). (2009). Cigarette smoking among adults and trends in smoking cessation: United States, 2008. *Morbidity and Mortality Weekly Report, 58*(44), 1227–1232.
33. Benowitz, 2010; U.S. Department of Health and Human Services, Office of the Surgeon General. (2010, December). *How tobacco causes disease: The biology and behavioral basis for smoking-attributable disease: A report of the Surgeon General.*
34. World Health Organization. (2005, February 24). *Global tobacco treaty enters into force with 57 countries already committed* [Press release].
35. Centers for Disease Control (CDC), 2008.
36. Tobacco use in the USA. (2010, September 18). *The Lancet, 376,* 930; U.S. report details harm of even light smoking. (2010, December 10). *The New York Times,* A24.
37. Substance Abuse and Mental Health Services Administration. (2010). *Results from the 2009 National Survey on Drug Use and Health: National findings.* Office of Applied Studies, NSDUH Series H-38a, HHS Publication No. SMA 10-4586. Rockville, MD.
38. U.S. report details harm of even light smoking, 2010
39. Centers for Disease Control and Prevention, Office on Smoking and Health, National Center for Chronic Disease Prevention ahd Health Promotion. (2010, September 9). *Current cigarette smoking among adults aged ≥18 years—United States, 2009.*
40. Centers for Disease Control and Prevention, Office on Smoking and Health, 2010.
41. Surveillance, Epidemiology, and End Results (Seer) Program (n.d.). Seer*Stat database: Mortality—all COD, public-use with state, total U.S. (1969–2002). Retrieved from http://www.seer.cancer.gov; National Cancer Institute, DCCPS, Surveillance Research Program, Cancer Statistics Branch. (2005, April). Underlying mortality data provided by NCHS. Retrieved from http://www.cdc.gov/nchs
42. Henley, S. J., et al. (2004). Association between exclusive pipe smoking and mortality from cancer and other diseases. *Journal of the National Cancer Institute, 96,* 853–861; Substance Abuse and Mental Health Services Administration (SAMSHA), Office of Applied Studies. (2009, January 15). *The NSDUH report —Cigar use among young adults aged 18 to 25.* Rockville, MD: SAMSHA.
43. U.S. Department of Health and Human Services. (1992). *Smokeless tobacco or health: An international perspective.* Bethesda, MD: National Institutes of Health, National Cancer Institute.
44. Tobacco use in the USA, 2010.
45. National Center for Chronic Disease Prevention and Health Promotion, Office On Smoking and Health. (2010, September). *CDC reports provide vital info about smoking.*
46. Cigarette Smoking and Cancer: Questions and Answers, 2004.
47. Judge, D. E., (2002, March 5). You can quit smoking: Plan for success. *Journal Watch Women's Health.*
48. Why Do You Smoke? U.S. Department of Health and Human Services, Public Health Service, National Institutes of Health. (NIH Publication No. 87-1822). Bethesda, MD: National Cancer Institute, 1987.
49. *The health consequences of smoking: A report of the Surgeon General.* (2004). Washington, DC: Department of Health and Human Services, Centers for Disease Control National Center for Chronic Disease Prevention and Health Promotion, Office On Smoking and Health.
50. Doll, R., et al. (2004). Mortality in relation to smoking: 50 years' observations on male British doctors. *British Medical Journal, 328,* 1519–1529.
51. *How tobacco causes disease,* 2010.
52. *The health consequences of smoking* (2004).
53. *The health consequences of smoking* (2004).
54. Centers for Disease Control and Prevention, Office on Smoking and Health, National Center for Chronic Disease Prevention and Health Promotion. (2009, May). *Smoking and tobacco use.*
55. *Smoking among adults: Reproductive health—The health consequences of smoking, a report of the Surgeon General.* (2004). U.S. Department of Health and Human Services, Centers for Disease Control and Prevention, National Center for Chronic Disease Prevention and Health Promotion, Office On Smoking and Health.
56. *Smoking among adults: Reproductive health,* 2004.
57. American Lung Association. (2004, November). *Smoking 101 fact sheet.* Retrieved from http://www.lungusa.com
58. Neergaard, L. (2010, December 9). Even a bit of social smoking can trigger heart attack. *MSNBC.com.* Retrieved from http://www.msnbc.msn.com/Id/40576433/Ns/Health-Addictions/
59. FDA will regulate tobacco under new law. (2009, June 30). *NCI Cancer Bulletin.* Retrieved from http://www.cancer.gov/NCIcancerbulletin/063009/page2
60. *How tobacco causes disease,* 2010.

Chapter 8

1. The President's Council on Physical Fitness and Sports. (2010, December). *Physical activity facts.*
2. King, D. E., Mainous, A. G., 3rd, Carnemolla, M., & Everett, C. J. (2009). Adherence to healthy lifestyle habits in US adults, 1988–2006. *American Journal of Medicine, 122,* 528–534.
3. Alford, L. (2010). What men should know about the impact of physical activity on their health. *International Journal of Clinical Practice, 64,* 1731; The President's Council on Physical Fitness and Sports (2010, December). *Physical activity facts.*
4. Blumenthal, J. A., Sherwood, A., Babyak, M. A., Watkins, L. L., Waugh, R., Georgiades, A., et al. (2005). Effects of exercise and stress management training on markers of cardiovascular risk in patients with ischemic heart disease: A randomized controlled trial. *Journal of the American Medical Association, 293,* 1626–1634.
5. Kokkinos, P., Holland, J. C., Narayan, P., Colleran, J. A., Dotson, C. O., & Papademetriou, V. (1995). Miles run per week and high-density lipoprotein cholesterol levels in healthy, middle-aged men. *Archives of Internal Medicine, 155,* 415–420.
6. Davis, J. M., Murphy, E. A., Brown, A. S., Carmichael, M. D., Ghaffar, A., & Mayer, E. P. (2004). Effects of moderate exercise and oat beta-glucan on innate immune function and susceptibility to respiratory infection. *The American Journal of Physiology—Regulatory, Integrative and Comparative Physiology, 286,* R366–72.
7. Miles, M. P. (2002). The relationship of natural killer cell counts, perforin MRNA and CD2 expression to post-

exercise natural killer cell activity in humans. *ACTA Physiologica Scandinavica, 174*, 317–325.
8. National Cancer Institute. (2009, July). *Physical activity and cancer*; Wolin, K., Yan, Y., Colditz, G. A., & Lee, I. M. (2009). Physical activity and colon cancer prevention: A meta-analysis. *British Journal of Cancer, 100*, 611–616.
9. Lagerros, Y. T., Hsieh, S. F., & Hsieh, C. C. (2004). Physical activity in adolescence and young adulthood and breast cancer risk: A quantitative review. *European Journal of Cancer Prevention, 13*, 5–12.
10. *How to prevent or delay diabetes*. (2005). American Diabetes Association.
11. Harris, A. H. S., Cronkite, R., & Moos, R. (2006). Physical activity, exercise coping, and depression in a 10-year cohort study of depressed patients. *Journal of Affective Disorders, 93*, 79–85; Scarmeas, N., Luchsinger, J. A., Schupf, N., Brickman, A. M., Cosentino, S., Tang, M. X., et al. (2009). Physical activity, diet, and risk of Alzheimer disease. *Journal of The American Medical Association, 302*, 627–637; Weuve, J., Kang, J. H., Manson, J. E., Breteler, M. M., Ware, J. H., & Grodstein, F. (2004). Physical activity, including walking, and cognitive function in older women. *Journal of the American Medical Association, 292*, 1454–1461.
12. Adapted from Nevid, J. S., Rathus, S. A., & Rubenstein, H. (1998). *Health in the new millennium*. New York: Worth; Brody, J. E. (1990, January 25). Exercise can improve many aspects of a disabled person's life. *The New York Times*, p. B11; *Directors column: 2005-03 issue: Young athletes with disabilities grow into healthy adults*. (2005). NCPAD. Retrieved from http://www.ncpad.org/director/fact_sheet.php?sheet=295

Chapter 9

1. United States Department of Agriculture. (2011, June 2). *First Lady, Agriculture Secretary launch MyPlate icon as a new reminder to help consumers to make healthier food choices* [Press release].
2. *The burden of colorectal cancer*. (2005, October). National Center for Chronic Disease Prevention and Health Promotion, Centers for Disease Control. Retrieved from http://www.cdc.gov/nccdphp/burdenbook2004/Section02/colocancer.htm; Katcher, H. I., et al. (2008). The effects of a whole grain–enriched hypocaloric diet on cardiovascular disease risk factors in men and women with metabolic syndrome. *American Journal of Clinical Nutrition, 87*, 79–90.
3. Mente, A., et al. (2009). A systematic review of the evidence supporting a causal link between dietary factors and coronary heart disease. *Archives of Internal Medicine, 169*, 659–669; Park, Y., et al. (2005). Dietary fiber intake and risk of colorectal cancer. *Journal of the American Medical Association, 294*, 2849–2857.
4. Sinha, R., et al. (2009). Meat intake and mortality: A prospective study of over half a million people. *Archives of Internal Medicine, 169*, 562–571; Popkin, B. M. (2009). Reducing meat consumption has multiple benefits for the world's health. *Archives of Internal Medicine, 169*, 543–545.
5. Appleby, P. N., et al. (2002). Hypertension and blood pressure among meat eaters, fish eaters, vegetarians and vegans in EPIC-Oxford. *Public Health Nutrition, 5*, 645–654.
6. United States Department of Agriculture. (2011, January 31). *Dietary guidelines for Americans 2010: Executive summary*. Retrieved from https://docs.google.com/viewer?url=http://www.cnpp.usda.gov/Publications/DietaryGuidelines/2010/PolicyDoc/ExecSumm.pdf
7. *Dietary guidelines for Americans 2010: Executive summary*. (2011, January 31).
8. Eckel, R. H. (2008). Egg consumption in relation to cardiovascular disease and mortality: The story gets more complex. *American Journal of Clinical Nutrition, 87*(4), 799–800.
9. Are you vitamin D-deficient? (2009, June). *Tufts University Health & Nutrition Letter, 27*, 4–5; Ginde, A. A., Liu, M. C., & Camargo, C. A., Jr. (2009). Demographic differences and trends of vitamin D insufficiency in the U.S. population, 1988–2004. *Archives of Internal Medicine, 169*, 626–632; Vitamin D: Builds bones and much more. (2009, April 25). *ScienceDaily*. Retrieved from http://www.sciencedaily.com/releases/2008/07/080714162515.htm
10. Hooper, L., et al. (2006). Risks and benefits of omega 3 fats for mortality, cardiovascular disease, and cancer: Systematic review. *British Medical Journal, 332*, 752–760; Levitan, E. B., Walk, A., & Mittleman, M. A. (2009). Fish consumption, marine omega-3 fatty acids, and incidence of heart failure: A population-based prospective study of middle-aged and elderly men. *European Heart Journal, 30*, 1495–1500.
11. Eidelman, R. S., et al. (2004). Randomized trials of vitamin E in the treatment and prevention of cardiovascular disease. *Archives of Internal Medicine, 164*, 1552–1556; Sesso, H. D., et al. (2008). Vitamins E and C in the prevention of cardiovascular disease in men. *Journal of the American Medical Association, 300*, 2123–2133; Stanner, S. A., et al. A review of the epidemiological evidence for the "antioxidant hypothesis." *Public Health Nutrition, 7*, 407–422; American Association for Cancer Research. (2008, November 17). No protective effect on cancer from long-term vitamin E or vitamin C supplementation, trial shows. *ScienceDaily*.
12. Douglas, R. M., et al. (2001). Vitamin C for preventing and treating the common cold (Cochrane Review). In *The Cochrane Library, 3*, Oxford: Update Software; Audera, C., et al. (2001). Mega-dose vitamin C in treatment of the common cold: A randomised controlled trial. *The Medical Journal of Australia, 175*, 359–362.
13. Halliwell, B., Rafter, J., & Jenner, A. (2005). Health promotion by flavonoids, tocopherols, tocotrienols, and other phenols: Direct or indirect effects? Antioxidant or not? *American Journal of Clinical Nutrition, 81*(Suppl.), 268S–276S; MLA USDA/Agricultural Research Service. (2009, April 24). How plants protect us from disease. *ScienceDaily*. Retrieved from http://www.sciencedaily.com/releases/2009/04/090419202029.htm; Serafini, M., et al. (2003). Plasma antioxidants from chocolate: Dark chocolate may offer its consumers health benefits the milk variety cannot match. *Nature, 424*, 1013.
14. Mathews, T. J. (2009, May 4). *Spina bifida and anencephalus in the United States, 1991–2006*. Division of Vital Statistics Centers for Disease Control; U.S. Preventive Services Task Force. (2009). Folic acid for the prevention of neural tube defects: U.S. Preventive Services Task Force recommendation statement. *Annals of Internal Medicine, 150*, 626–631.
15. Clarke, R., et al. (2010). Effects of lowering homocysteine levels with B vitamins on cardiovascular disease, cancer, and cause-specific mortality: Meta-analysis of 8 randomized trials involving 37,485 individuals. *Archives of Internal Medicine, 170*, 1622–1631; Figueiredo, J. C., et al. Folic acid and risk of prostate cancer: Results from a randomized clinical trial. *Journal of the National Cancer Institute, 101*, 432–435.
16. U.S. Department of Agriculture (2011, January 31). *Dietary guidelines for Americans, 2010*. Retrieved from http://www.cnpp.usda.gov/DGAs2010-PolicyDocument .htm
17. *Dietary guidelines for Americans 2010: Executive summary*, 2011, January 31; Sodium intake among adults—United States, 2005–2006. (2010). *Journal of the American Medical Association, 304*, 738–740; U. S. Department of Agriculture. (2010). *What we eat in America*. Retrieved from http://www.ars.usda.gov/service/docs.htm?docid=15044
18. *Dietary guidelines for Americans 2010: Executive summary*, 2011, January 31; Chertow, G. M., Moran, A. E., Coxson, P. G., & Goldman, L. Consuming a little less salt could mean fewer deaths. American Heart Association. Retrieved from http://www.sciencedaily.com /releases/2009/03/090311162801.htm\

Chapter 10

1. Centers for Disease Control and Prevention. (2010, June). *Obesity and overweight.* Retrieved from http://www.cdc.gov/nchs/fastats/overwt.htm; Ryan, D. H., & Kushner, R. (2010). The state of obesity and obesity research. *Journal of the American Medical Association, 304*, 1835–1836.
2. Vastag, B. (2004). Obesity is now on everyone's plate. *Journal of the American Medical Association, 291*, 1186–1188.
3. Dying to eat: A graphical view of U.S. obesity. (2010, September 24). *Scientific American.* Retrieved from http://www.scientificamerican.com/article.cfm?id=dying-to-eat; Li, D., et al. (2009). Body mass index and risk, age of onset, and survival in patients with pancreatic cancer. *Journal of the American Medical Association, 301*, 2553–2562; Snowden, R. B. (2009, November 6). Over 100,000 cancers linked to excess body fat. *American Cancer Society*. Retrieved from http://www.acs.org; Centers for Disease Control. (2009, August). *Overweight and obesity: Health consequences.* Retrieved from http://www.cdc.gov/obesity/causes/health.html
4. Fontaine, K. R., et al. (2003). Years of life lost due to obesity. *Journal of the American Medical Association, 289*, 187–193; Flegal, K. M., et al. (2005). Excess deaths associated with underweight, overweight, and obesity. *Journal of the American Medical Association, 293*, 1861–1867.
5. Olshansky, S. J., et al. (2005). A potential decline in life expectancy in the United States in the 21st century. *New England Journal of Medicine, 352*, 1138–1145; Preston, S. H. (2003). Deadweight?—The influence of obesity on longevity. *New England Journal of Medicine, 352*, 1135–1137.
6. Flegal, K. M., et al. (2005). Excess deaths associated with underweight, overweight, and obesity. *Journal of the American Medical Association, 293*, 1861–1867.
7. Harp, J. B., & Hecht, L. (2005). Obesity in the National Football League. *Journal of the American Medical Association, 293*, 1061–1062.
8. Jacobs, E. J., et al. (2010). Waist circumference and all-cause mortality in a large U.S. cohort. *Archives of Internal Medicine, 170*, 1293; National Heart Lung and Blood Institute & National Institutes of Health. (n.d.). *Assessing your weight and health risk. Classification of overweight and obesity by BMI, waist circumference, and associated disease risks.* Retrieved from http://www.nhlbi.nih.gov/health/public/heart/obesity/lose_wt/risk.htm
9. Hu, G., et al. (2010). Joint effects of physical activity, body mass index, waist circumference, and waist-to-hip ratio on the risk of heart failure. *Circulation, 121*, 237–244.
10. Harvard School of Public Health. (2004). *Healthy weight.* Retrieved from http://www.hsph.harvard.edu/nutritionsource/weight.html; Pischon, T., et al. (2008). General and abdominal adiposity and risk of death in Europe. *New England Journal of Medicine, 359*, 2105–2120; Yusef, S., et al. (2005). Obesity and the risk of myocardial infarction in 27,000 participants from 52 countries: A case-control study. *The Lancet, 366*, 1640–1649.
11. Loos, R. J. F., et al. (2008). Association studies involving over 90,000 people demonstrate that common variants near to MC4R influence fat mass, weight and risk of obesity. *Nature Genetics, 40*, 768–775; Six newly discovered genes for obesity have a neural effect. (2009, April 24). *Science Daily*. Retrieved from http://www.sciencedaily.com/releases/2009/01/090108082908.htm
12. Rosenbaum, M., & Leibel, R. L. (2010). Adaptive thermogenesis in humans. *International Journal of Obesity, 34*, S47–S55.
13. Rosenbaum & Leibel, 2010.
14. Major, G. C., et al. (2007). Clinical significance of adaptive thermogenesis. *International Journal of Obesity, 31*, 204–212.
15. Levine, J. A., et al. (2005). Interindividual variation in posture allocation: Possible role in human obesity. *Science, 307*, 584–586.
16. Parloff, R. (2003, Februrary 3). Is fat the next tobacco? *Fortune*, 51–54.
17. National Eating Disorders Association. (2010). Retrieved from http://www.nationaleatingdisorders.org/information-resources/general-information.php
18. Nakanishi, S., et al. (2004). A comparison between Japanese-Americans living in Hawaii and Los Angeles and native Japanese: The impact of lifestyle westernization on diabetes mellitus. *Biomedical Pharmacotherapy, 58*, 571–577.
19. *Overweight and obesity—Statistics.* American Heart Association, based on data from NHANES (1999–2002), Centers for Disease Control, National Center for Health Statistics.
20. Flum, D. R., et al. (2005). Early mortality among medicare beneficiaries undergoing bariatric surgical procedures. *Journal of the American Medical Association, 294*, 1903–1908; Robinson, M. K. (2009). Surgical treatment of obesity—weighing the facts. *New England Journal of Medicine, 361*, 520–521.
21. *Well and good.* (2002). A publication of University of Iowa Health Care. Used by permission of University of Iowa Health Care.
22. Ackard, D. M., Fulkerson, J. A., & Neumark-Sztainer, D. (2007). Prevalence and utility of DSM-IV eating disorder diagnostic criteria among youth. *International Journal of Eating Disorders, 40*, 409–417.
23. Cobb, K. (2008). Eating disorders in athletes. In S. R. Bakere (Ed.), *Hot topics in sports and athletics* (pp. 17–50). Hauppauge, NY: Nova Science; Lock, J. (2009). Trying to fit square pegs in round holes: Eating disorders in males. *Journal of Adolescent Health, 44*, 99–100.
24. Striegel-Moore, R. H., et al. (2003). Eating disorders in white and black women. *American Journal of Psychiatry, 160*, 1326–1331.
25. Andersen, A. E., & Ryan, G. L. (2009). Eating disorders in the obstetric and gynecologic patient population. *Obstetrics and Gynecology, 114*, 1353–1367.
26. Gardini, G. G., et al. (2009). Respiratory function in patients with stable anorexia nervosa. *Chest, 136*, 1356–1363.
27. Papadopoulos, F. C., Ekbom, A., Brandt, L., & Ekselius, L. (2009). Excess mortality, causes of death and prognostic factors in anorexia nervosa. *British Journal of Psychiatry, 194*, 10–17.
28. Andersen & Ryan, 2009.
29. Hrabosky, J., et al. (2009). Multidimensional body image comparisons among patients with eating disorders, body dysmorphic disorder, and clinical controls: A multisite study. *Body Image, 6*, 155–163; Miyake, Y., et al (2010). Neural processing of negative word stimuli concerning body image in patients with eating disorders: An fMRI study. *NeuroImage, 50*, 1333–1339.
30. Costin, C. (1996). *Your dieting daughter*. New York: Psychology Press.
31. Bravender, T., et al. (2010). Classification of eating disturbance in children and adolescents: Proposed changes for the DSM-V. *European Eating Disorders Review, 18*, 79–89.
32. Cifani, C., et al. (2009). A preclinical model of binge eating elicited by yo-yo dieting and stressful exposure to food: Effect of sibutramine, fluoxetine, topiramate, and midazolam. *Psychopharmacology, 204*, 113–225; White, M. A., Masheb, R. M., & Grilo, C. M. (2009). Regimented and lifestyle restraint in binge eating disorder. *International Journal of Eating Disorders, 42*, 326–331.
33. Franco, K., et al. (2009). The role of perfectionism on eating behaviors among women with eating disorders. *Appetite, 52*, 832; Watson, H. J., et al. (2010). Mediators between perfectionism and eating disorder psychopathology: Shape and weight overvaluation and conditional goal-setting. *International Journal of Eating Disorders, 44*, 142–149.
34. Mendelsohn, F., & Warren, M. (2010). Anorexia, bulimia, and the female athlete triad: Evaluation and management. *Endocrinology and Metabolism Clinics of North America, 39*, 155–167.
35. Wilson, G. T., Wilfley, D. E., Agras, W. S., & Bryson, S. W. (2010). Psychological treatments of binge eating disorder.

Archives of General Psychiatry, 67, 94–101.
36. Wade, T. D., Bulik, C. M., Neale, M., & Kendler, K. S. (2000). Anorexia nervosa and major depression: Shared genetic and environmental risk factors. *American Journal of Psychiatry, 157*, 469–471.
37. Cooper, M., Galbraith, M., & Drinkwater, J. (2001). Assumptions and beliefs in adolescents with anorexia nervosa and their mothers. *Eating Disorders: Journal of Treatment and Prevention, 9*, 217–223; Crittenden, P. M., & Dallos, R. (2009). All in the family: Integrating attachment and family systems theories. *Clinical Child Psychology and Psychiatry, 14*, 389–409.
38. Leung, P., Curtis, R. L., Jr., & Mapp, S. C. (2010). Incidences of sexual contacts of children: Impacts of family characteristics and family structure from a national sample. *Children and Youth Services Review, 32*, 650–656.
39. Karwautz, A., et al. (2001). Individual-specific risk factors for anorexia nervosa: A pilot study using a discordant sister-pair design. *Psychological Medicine, 31*(2), 317–329.
40. Schick, V. R., Rima, B. N., & Calabrese, S. K. (2009). Evulvalution: The portrayal of women's external genitalia and physique across time and the current Barbie doll ideals. *Journal of Sex Research, 48*, 74–81.
41. University of Iowa Hospitals and Clinics. Department of Psychiatry. Retrieved from http://www.uihealthcare.com/depts/med/psychiatry/divisions/eatingdisorders/quiz.html [accessed March 24, 2011]. Used by permission of University of Iowa Health Care.
42. Lock, 2009.
43. Baker, J. H., et al. (2009). Genetic risk factors for disordered eating in adolescent males and females. *Journal of Abnormal Psychology, 118*, 576–586.
44. Altman, S. E., & Shankman, S. A. (2009). What is the association between obsessive-compulsive disorder and eating disorders? *Clinical Psychology Review, 29*, 638–646; Ansell, E. B., et al. (2010). The prevalence and structure of obsessive-compulsive personality disorder in Hispanic psychiatric outpatients. *Journal of Behavior Therapy and Experimental Psychiatry 41*, 275–281.
45. Walsh, B. T., et al. (2004). Treatment of bulimia nervosa in a primary care setting. *American Journal of Psychiatry, 161*, 556–561.

Chapter 11

1. American Heart Association. (2009). *Heart disease and stroke statistics—2009 update at-a-glance*. Dallas, Texas: American Heart Association; Centers for Disease Control and Prevention (CDC). (2010, October). *Heart disease: Fast stats; Deaths: Final data for 2007*. National Vital Statistics Reports, Centers for Disease Control (CDC). Retrieved from http://www.cdc.gov/NCHS/data/nvsr/nvsr58/nvsr58_19.pdf
2. Centers for Disease Control and Prevention, 2010, October.
3. Vital and Health Statistics. (2010, August). *Summary health statistics for U.S. adults: National health interview survey, 2009*. Series 10, No. 49.
4. National Cholesterol Education Program, National Heart, Lung, and Blood Institute, National Institutes of Health. (2004). *Live healthier, live longer*. Retrieved from http://www.nhlbi.nih.gov/chd
5. American Heart Association, 2009.
6. The Emerging Risk Factors Collaboration. (2010). C-reactive protein concentration and risk of coronary heart disease, stroke, and mortality: An individual participant meta-analysis. *The Lancet, 375*, 132–140.
7. Centers for Disease Control and Prevention. (2011). Vital signs: Prevalence, treatment, and control of hypertension—United States, 1999–2002 and 2005–2008. *Morbidity and Mortality Weekly Report, Journal of the American Medical Association, 305*, 531–534.
8. Franklin, S. S., et al. (2009). Single versus combined blood pressure components and risk for cardiovascular disease: The Framingham heart study. *Circulation, 119*, 119.
9. Chobanian, A. V., et al. (2003). The seventh report of the Joint National Committee on Prevention, Detection, Evaluation, and Treatment of High Blood Pressure: The JNC 7 report. *Journal of the American Medical Association, 289*, 2560–2567.
10. American Heart Association, 2009.
11. Centers for Disease Control and Prevention, 2011.
12. Egan, B. M., Zhao, Y., & Axon, R. N. (2010). U.S. Trends in prevalence, awareness, treatment, and control of hypertension, 1988–2008. *Journal of the American Medical Association, 303*, 2043–2050.
13. Forman, J. P., Stampfer, M. J, & Curhan, G. C. (2009). Diet and lifestyle risk factors associated with incident hypertension in women. *Journal of the American Medical Association, 302*, 40–41; Meyers, L. (2007). Building a strong heart. *Monitor on Psychology, 38*(1), 52–54; National Heart, Lung, and Blood Institute, National Institutes of Health. *Your Guide to Lowering High Blood Pressure*. (2005). Retrieved from http://www.nhlbi.nih.gov/hbp/index.html
14. American Heart Association. (2005). *Stroke facts*. Retrieved from http://www.americanheart.org/presenter.jhtml?identifier=1200026.
15. American Heart Association, 2009; Heart disease and stroke statistics 2009 update: A report from the American Heart Association Statistics Committee and Stroke Statistics Subcommittee. (2009). *Circulation, 119*, e121–e181.
16. American Heart Association. (2005). *Transient ischemic attack (TIA)*. Retrieved from http://www.americanheart.org/presenter.jhtml?identifier=4781.
17. Adapted from *Harvard Health Letter*, January 1996.
18. Blumenthal, J. A., et al. (2005). Effects of exercise and stress management training on markers of cardiovascular risk in patients with ischemic heart disease: A randomized controlled trial. *Journal of the American Medical Association, 293*, 1626–1634.
19. Adapted from Acting on warning signs of stroke is latest in treatment. (1997). *American Medical Association Science News*; National Stroke Association. (2010, May). *Women and stroke*.
20. Jones, D. W., et al. (2002). Risk factors for coronary heart disease in African Americans: The atherosclerosis risk in communities study, 1987–1997. *Archives of Internal Medicine, 162*, 2565–2571; Shields, A. E., et al. (2005). The use of race variables in genetic studies of complex traits and the goal of reducing health disparities: A transdisciplinary perspective. *American Psychologist, 60*, 77–103.
21. Centers for Disease Control and Prevention. (2010, May 20). Deaths: Final data for 2007. *National Vital Statistics Report, 58*(19).
22. Troxel, W. M., et al. (2003). Chronic stress burden, discrimination, and subclinical carotid artery disease in African American and caucasian women. *Health Psychology, 22*, 300–309.
23. American Heart Association. (2005). *What Are healthy levels of cholesterol?* Retrieved from http://www.americanheart.org/presenter.jhtml?identifier=183
24. National Cholesterol Education Program, & National Heart, Lung, and Blood Institute, National Institutes of Health. (2004). *Live healthier, live longer*. Retrieved from http://www.nhlbi.nih.gov/chd
25. National Heart, Lung, and Blood Institute, & National Institutes of Health. (2005). *Statins, cholesterol lowering medicines*.
26. Ford, E. S., et al. (2009). Hypertriglyceridemia and its pharmacologic treatment among U.S. adults. *Archives of Internal Medicine, 169*, 572–578; Freiberg, J. J., et al. (2008). Nonfasting triglycerides and risk of ischemic stroke in the general population. *Journal of the American Medical Association, 300*, 2142–2152.
27. American Heart Association. (2010). *Metabolic syndrome*. Retrieved from http://www.americanheart.org/presenter.jhtml?identifier=4756
28. National Institutes of Health, & National Heart, Lung, and Blood Institute. (2007, December 10). Heart attack symptoms in women—Are they different? *NIH News*; American Heart Association, 2009; National Heart Lung and Blood Institute, & National

Institutes of Health. (2009, November). *Heart disease in women*. Retrieved from http://www.nhlbi.nih.gov/health/dci/Diseases/hdw/hdw_whatis.html

29. Gopalakrishnan, P., Ragland, M. M., & Tak, T. (2009). Gender differences in coronary artery disease: Review of diagnostic challenges and current treatment. *Postgraduate Medicine, 121*(2).
30. Chida, Y., & Steptoe, A. (2009). The association of anger and hostility with future coronary heart disease: A meta-analytic review of prospective evidence. *Journal of the American College of Cardiology 53*, 936–946; Denollet, J., & Pedersen, S. S. (2009). Anger, depression, and anxiety in cardiac patients: The complexity of individual differences in psychological risk. *Journal of the American College of Cardiology, 53*, 947–949. Lampert, R., et al. (2009). Anger-induced T-wave alternans predicts future ventricular arrhythmias in patients with implantable cardioverter-defibrillators. *Journal of the American College of Cardiology, 53*, 779–781.
31. Frasure-Smith, N., & Lespérance, F. (2005). Depression and coronary heart disease: Complex synergism of mind, body, and environment. *Current Directions in Psychological Science, 14*, 39–43; Glassman, A. H., Bigger, T., Jr., & Gaffney, M. (2009). Psychiatric characteristics associated with long-term mortality among 361 patients having an acute coronary syndrome and major depression: Seven-year follow-up of SADHART participants. *Archives of General Psychiatry, 66*, 1022; Whooley, M. A., et al. (2008). Depressive symptoms, health behaviors, and risk of cardiovascular events in patients with coronary heart disease. *Journal of the American Medical Association, 300*, 2379–2388.
32. Heron, M. (2010, March 31). Deaths: Leading causes for 2006. *National Vital Statistics Reports, 58*(14). U.S. Department of Health and Human Services, Centers for Disease Control and Prevention, National Center for Health Statistics, National Vital Statistics System; Horner, J. M., et al. (Eds.). (2009). *SEER cancer statistics review, 1975–2006*. Bethesda, MD: National Cancer Institute; U.S. Department of Health and Human Services, National Institutes of Health, & National Cancer Institute. (2010, May). *2008–2009 Annual report: President's cancer panel: Reducing environmental cancer risk: What we can do now.*
33. Kochanek, K. D., et al. Centers for Disease Control and Prevention (CDC). (2011, March 16). Deaths: Preliminary data 2009. *National Vital Statistics Report, 59*(4).
34. American Cancer Society. (2010). *Oncogenes, tumor suppressor genes, and cancer*. Retrieved from http://www.cancer.org/cancer/cancercauses/geneticsandcancer/oncogenesandtumorsuppressorgenes/index
35. Altekruse, S. F., et al. (Eds). (2010, November). *SEER cancer statistics review, 1975-2007*. Bethesda, MD: National Cancer Institute. Retrieved from http://seer.cancer.gov/csr/1975_2007/; *SEER stat fact sheets*, 2010, November.
36. *SEER stat fact sheets*, 2010, November.
37. Jemal, A., et al. (2008). Annual report to the nation on the status of cancer, 1975–2005. *Journal of the National Cancer Institute, 100*, 1672–1694; Cutler, D. M. (2008). Are we finally winning the war on cancer? *Journal of Economic Perspectives, 22*, 3–26; Snowden, R. V. (2009, May 27). Cancer death rate steadily declining: Annual cancer statistics report shows progress in cancer fight. *American Cancer Society Publication.*
38. Godtfredsen, N. S., Prescott, E., & Osler, M. S. (2005). Effect of smoking reduction on lung cancer risk. *Journal of the American Medical Association, 294*, 1505–1510.
39. *SEER stat fact sheets*, 2010, November.
40. American Cancer Society. (2011). Retrieved from http://www.cancer.org/Search/index?QueryText=warning+signs&x=48&y=27
41. Trichopoulos, D., Li, F. P., & Hunter, D. J. (1996). What causes cancer? *Scientific American, 275*, 80–87.
42. *SEER cancer statistics review, 5-year relative survival by year*. Retrieved January 2011.
43. *The health consequences of smoking: A report of the surgeon general.* (2004). Rockville, MD: U.S. Department of Health and Human Services, Centers for Disease Control and Prevention, National Center for Chronic Disease Prevention and Health Promotion, Office on Smoking and Health; *Targeting tobacco use: The nation's leading cause of death.* (2003). Atlanta, GA: U.S. Department of Health and Human Services, Centers for Disease Control and Prevention.
44. Key, T. J., et al. (2002). The effect of diet on risk of cancer. *Lancet, 360*, 861–868.
45. Prentice, R. L., et al. (2006). Low-fat dietary pattern and risk of invasive breast cancer: The women's health initiative randomized controlled dietary modification trial. *Journal of the American Medical Association, 295*, 629–642; Beresford, S.A.A., et al. (2006). Low-fat dietary pattern and risk of colorectal cancer: The women's health initiative randomized controlled dietary modification trial. *Journal of the American Medical Association, 295*, 643–654; Howard, B. V., et al. (2006). Low-fat dietary pattern and risk of cardiovascular disease: The women's health initiative randomized controlled dietary modification trial. *Journal of the American Medical Association, 29*, 655–666.
46. Study links obesity to aggressive prostate cancer. (2005, May 31). *NCI Cancer Bulletin, 2*(22); Buzdar, A. U. (2006). Dietary modification and risk of breast cancer. *Journal of the American Medical Association, 295*, 691–692; Stolzenberg-Solomon, R. Z., et al. (2008). Physical activity, and pancreatic cancer in the National Institutes of Health-AARP diet and health cohort. *American Journal of Epidemiology, 167*, 586–597.
47. *Energy balance: The complex interaction of diet, physical activity, and genetics in cancer prevention and control* [Director's update]. (2004, January 30). National Cancer Institute, National Institutes of Health.
48. American Cancer Society. (2007). *Alcohol and cancer*. Retrieved from https://docs.google.com/viewer?url=http://www.cancer.org/acs/groups/content/%40healthpromotions/documents/document/acsq-017622.pdf; Key, T. J. (2010, in press). Fruit and vegetables and cancer risk. *British Journal of Cancer.*
49. Allen, N. E., et al. (2009). Moderate alcohol intake and cancer incidence in women. *Journal of the National Cancer Institute, 101*(5); Lauer, M., & Sorlie, P. (2009). Alcohol, cardiovascular disease, and cancer: Treat with caution. *Journal of the National Cancer Institute, 101*, 282–283; Snowden, R. V. (2009, February 25). Even moderate alcohol use increases risk of certain cancers in women [press release]. *ACS News.*
50. Zinzani, P. L. (2005). Lymphoma: Diagnosis, staging, natural history, and treatment strategies. *Seminars in Oncology, 32*, 4–10.
51. Adedayo, O. A., & Shehu, S. M. (2004). Human T-cell lymphotropic virus type 1 (HTLV-1) and lymphoid malignancies in Dominica: A seroprevalence study. *American Journal of Hematology, 77*, 336–339.
52. Chen, J., Odenike, O., & Rowley, J. D. (2010). Leukaemogenesis: More than mutant genes. *Nature Reviews: Cancer, 10*, 23–36; Piñol, V., et al. (2005). Accuracy of revised Bethesda guidelines, microsatellite instability, and immunohistochemistry for the identification of patients with hereditary nonpolyposis colorectal cancer. *Journal of the American Medical Association, 293*, 986–1994.
53. Martinez, M. E. (2005). Primary prevention of colorectal cancer: Lifestyle, nutrition, exercise. *Cancer Research, 166*, 177–211.
54. *SEER stat fact sheets*, 2010, November.
55. Snowden, R. V. (2009, September 30). *Breast cancer death rate declining, but not for all women, ACS report shows.* American Cancer Society.
56. National Cancer Institute, National Institutes of Health. (2010). *SEER stat fact sheets: Breast.*
57. Garber, J. E., & Offit, K. (2005). Hereditary cancer predisposition syndromes.

Journal of Clinical Oncology, 23, 276–292.
58. *Breast Cancer.* (2010, November). American Cancer Society; *American Cancer Society recommendations for early breast cancer detection.* (2010, September). Retrieved from http://www.cancer.org/healthy/toolsandcalculators/videos/mammograms-matter-video
59. Snowden, 2009, May 27.
60. Consortium modelers interpret U.S. trends in breast cancer mortality. (2005, November 8.) *National Cancer Institute Bulletin.* Berry, D. A., et al. (2005). Effect of screening and adjuvant therapy on mortality from breast cancer. *New England Journal of Medicine, 353*, 1784–1792.
61. *Breast cancer prevention.* (2010, March). National Cancer Institute; Lagerros, Y. T., Hsieh, S. F., & Hsieh, C. C. (2004). Physical activity in adolescence and young adulthood and breast cancer risk: A quantitative review. *European Journal of Cancer Prevention, 13*, 5–12.
62. *Breast cancer prevention*, 2010, March; Key, 2010; Lagiou, P., Olsen, J., & Trichopoulos, D. (2005). Consumption of vegetables and fruits and risk of breast cancer. *Journal of the American Medical Association, 293*, 2209; *The complete guide—Nutrition and physical activity*. (2008, March 19). American Cancer Society.
63. National Cancer Institute. (2008, March). *Tamoxifen: Questions and answers*; Fisher, B., et al. (2005). Tamoxifen for the prevention of breast cancer: Current status of the national surgical adjuvant breast and bowel project P-1 study. *Journal of the National Cancer Institute, 97*, 1652–1662.
64. American Cancer Society. (2010, November). *Ovarian cancer*. Retrieved from http://www.cancer.org/Cancer/OvarianCancer/index.
65. American Cancer Society. (2010, July). *Cervical cancer*. Retrieved from http://www.cancer.org/Cancer/CervicalCancer/index
66. American Cancer Society. (2009, October). *How is HPV related to cervical cancer?* Retrieved from http://www.cancer.org/Cancer/CancerCauses/OtherCarcinogens/InfectiousAgents/HPV/HumanPapillomaVirusandHPVVaccinesFAQ/hpv-faq-hpv-and-cervical-cancer
67. American Cancer Society. (2010, May). *Lycopene*. Retrieved from http://www.cancer.org/Treatment/Treatmentsand SideEffects/ComplementaryandAlternativeMedicine/DietandNutrition/lycopene
68. American Cancer Society. (2010, August). *What are the risk factors for endometrial cancer?* Retrieved from http://www.cancer.org/cancer/endometrialcancer/detailedguide/endometrial-uterine-cancer-risk-factors
69. National Cancer Institute, National Institutes of Health. (2010). *Colon and rectal cancer*. Retrieved from http://www.cancer.gov/cancertopics/types/colon-and-rectal
70. Levin, B., et al. (2008). Screening and surveillance for the early detection of colorectal cancer and adenomatous polyps, 2008: A joint guideline from the American Cancer Society, the U.S. Multi-Society Task Force on Colorectal Cancer, and the American College of Radiology. *CA: A Cancer Journal for Clinicians, 58*. Published online March 5, 2008.
71. European Association of Urology. (2009, March 24). PSA screening cuts deaths by 20 percent. *ScienceDaily*. Retrieved from http://www.sciencedaily.com /releases/2009/03/090318140524.htm
72. Gerrit, D., et al. (2009). Study methods influence estimates of lead time and overdiagnosis in prostate cancer. *Journal of the National Cancer Institute, 101*, 374–383.
73. National Cancer Institute, 2009.
74. National Cancer Institute. (2009, March 18). *Early prostate cancer*.
75. Jaroff, L. (1996, April 1). The man's cancer. *Time*.
76. American Cancer Society. (2010, May). *Lycopene*. Retrieved from http://www.cancer.org/Treatment/Treatmentsand SideEffects/ComplementaryandAlternativeMedicine/DietandNutrition/lycopene
77. American Cancer Society. (2008, November). *Green tea*. Retrieved from http://www.cancer.org/Treatment/TreatmentsandSideEffects/ComplementaryandAlternativeMedicine/HerbsVitaminsandMinerals/green-tea
78. National Cancer Institute, National Institutes of Health. (2010). *Skin cancer*. Retrieved from http://www.cancer.gov/cancertopics/types/skin; National Cancer Institute, National Institutes of Health. *Melanoma*. Retrieved from http://www.cancer.gov/cancertopics/types/melanoma
79. American Cancer Society. (Updated July 2010). *Skin cancer prevention and early detection*. Retrieved from http://www.cancer.org/Cancer/CancerCauses/SunandUVExposure/SkinCancerPreventionandEarlyDetection/index
80. American Melanoma Foundation. (2005–2006). *ABCD's of melanoma*.
81. American Cancer Society. (2010, August). *How is melanoma staged? Detailed guide: Skin cancer—Melanoma*. Retrieved from http://www.cancer.org/Cancer/SkinCancer-Melanoma/DetailedGuide/melanoma-skin-cancer-staging
82. National Cancer Institute, National Institutes of Health. (2010). *Leukemia*. Retrieved from http://www.cancer.gov/cancertopics/types/leukemia
83. American Cancer Society. (2010, October). *What are the risk factors for non-Hodgkin lymphoma?* Retrieved from http://www.cancer.org/cancer/non-hodgkinlymphoma/detailedguide/non-hodgkin-lymphoma-risk-factors
84. National Cancer Institute, National Institutes of Health. (n.d.) *Pancreatic cancer*. Retrieved from http://www.cancer.gov/cancertopics/types/pancreatic
85. National Institute of Diabetes and Digestive and Kidney Diseases (NIDDK), National Diabetes Information Clearinghouse (NDIC). (2011). *National Diabetes Statistics*. Retrieved from http://diabetes.niddk.nih.gov/dm/pubs/statistics/#hds
86. National Institute of Diabetes and Digestive and Kidney Diseases, 2011.
87. National Institute of Diabetes and Digestive and Kidney Diseases, 2011.
88. National Institute of Diabetes and Digestive and Kidney Diseases, 2011.
89. Nathan, D. M. (2010). Navigating the choices for diabetes prevention. *New England Journal of Medicine, 362*, 1477–1490.
90. Tinker, L. F., et al. (2008). Low-fat dietary pattern and risk of treated diabetes mellitus in postmenopausal women: The women's health initiative randomized controlled dietary modification trial. *Archives of Internal Medicine, 168*, 1500–1511; Li, G., et al. (2008). The long-term effect of lifestyle interventions to prevent diabetes in the China Da Qing diabetes prevention study: A 20-year follow-up study. *Lancet, 371*, 1783–1789; Scheen, A. J. (2009). Voglibose for prevention of Type 2 diabetes mellitus. *Lancet, 373*, 1579–1580.
91. National Institute of Diabetes and Digestive and Kidney Diseases, 2011.
92. National Heart, Lung, and Blood Institute. (2010, June). *What is COPD?*

Chapter 12

1. Bongaarts, J., Pelletier, F., & Gerland, P. (2010). How many more AIDS deaths? *Lancet, 375*, 103–104; Bongaarts, J., Pelletier, F., & Gerland, P. (2010). Global trends in AIDS mortality. In R. G. Rogers, & E. M. Crimmins (Eds.). (2010). *International handbook of adult mortality*. New York: Springer; Hall, H. I., et al. (2008). Estimation of HIV incidence in the United States. *Journal of the American Medical Association, 300*, 520–529.
2. The American College Health Association National College Health Assessment (ACHA-NCHA). (2009, March/April). Spring 2008 reference group report. *Journal of American College Health, 57*(5), *53*(5), 477–488. Reprinted by permission of the publisher (Taylor & Francis Group, http://www.informaworld.com).
3. Centers for Disease Control and Prevention. (2004, April). *Geographic distribution of malaria*. Retrieved from http://

www.cdc.gov/malaria/distribution_epi/distribution.htm
4. Centers for Disease Control and Prevention. (2010, February). *Malaria*. Retrieved from http://www.cdc.gov/malaria/
5. Cohen, S., et al. (2009). Sleep habits and susceptibility to the common cold. *Archives of Internal Medicine, 169*, 62–67.
6. Centers for Disease Control and Prevention. (Last modified 2010, December 14). *Recommendations and guidelines: 2010 Child and adolescent immunization schedules*. Retrieved from http://www.cdc.gov/vaccines/spec-grps/infants/downloads/parent-ver-sch-0-6yrs.pdf. Approved by the Centers for Disease Control and Prevention, the American Academy of Pediatrics, and the American Academy of Family Physicians.
7. Centers for Disease Control and Prevention, (2011, May). *Asthma in the US: Growing every year*. Retrieved from http://www.cdc.gov/VitalSigns/Asthma/index.html#LatestFindings
8. National Institute of Allergy and Infectious Diseases. Office of Communications and Public Liaison. (2004, December). *The common cold*. Retrieved from http://www.niaid.nih.gov/factsheets/cold.htm
9. American Lung Association. (2010). *Pneumonia fact sheet*. Retrieved from http://www.lungusa.org/lung-disease/influenza/in-depth-resources/pneumonia-fact-sheet.html
10. *How do I know if I have a cold or the flu? What are the differences?* (2010, November 1). Retrieved from http://answers.flu.gov/questions/4404
11. Centers for Disease Control and Prevention (2010, August). *Reported cases of Lyme disease by year, United States, 1995–2009*. Retrieved from http://www.cdc.gov/ncidod/dvbid/lyme/ld_UpClimbLymeDis.htm.
12. Kuehn, B. M. (2009). Sexually Transmitted Infections. *Journal of the American Medical Association, 301*, 817.
13. Baer, H., Allen, S., & Braun, L. (2000). Knowledge of human papillomavirus infection among young adult men and women: Implications for health education and research. *Journal of Community Health: Publication for Health Promotion and Disease Prevention, 25*(1), 67–78.
14. Massad, L. S., et al. (2010). Knowledge of cervical cancer prevention and human papillomavirus among women with HIV. *Gynecologic Oncology, 117*, 70–76.
15. Centers for Disease Control and Prevention. (2010, September). *Sexually transmitted diseases: Gonorrhea—CDC fact sheet*. Retrieved from http://www.cdc.gov/std/gonorrhea/STDFact-gonorrhea.htm
16. Centers for Disease Control and Prevention. (2010, September). *Sexually transmitted diseases: Syphilis—CDC fact sheet*. Retrieved from http://www.cdc.gov/std/syphilis/STDFact-Syphilis.htm
17. Centers for Disease Control and Prevention. (2010, January). *FastStats: Sexually transmitted diseases (STD)*. Retrieved from http://www.cdc.gov/nchs/fastats/stds.htm
18. El-Sadr, W. M., Mayer, K. H., & Hodder, S. L. (2010). AIDS in America—Forgotten but not gone. *New England Journal of Medicine, 362*, 967–970; Centers for Disease Control and Prevention. Sexually transmitted diseases treatment guidelines, 2010. *Morbidity and Mortality Weekly Report, 5*(RR-12).
19. UNAIDS, World Health Organization. (2010, November 23). *At least 56 countries have either stabilized or achieved significant declines in rates of new HIV infections* [press release]. Retrieved from http://unaidstoday.org/?p=1673
20. Centers for Disease Control and Prevention. (2010, July). *Sexually transmitted diseases (STDs): Genital herpes—CDC fact sheet*. Retrieved from http://www.cdc.gov/std/Herpes/STDFact-Herpes.htm
21. Report finds high rates of herpes in U.S. (2010, March 16). *The New York Times*, D6, D7.
22. Centers for Disease Control and Prevention. (2009, November). *Genital HPV infection—CDC fact sheet*. Retrieved from http://www.cdc.gov/std/HPV/STDFact-HPV.htm#common
23. Brody, J. E. (2005, October 18). Getting to know a virus, and when it can kill. *The New York Times Online*.
24. American Cancer Society. (2010, April). *American Cancer Society recommendations for human papilloma virus (HPV) vaccine use to prevent cervical cancer and pre-cancers*. Retrieved from http://www.cancer.org/Cancer/CancerCauses/OtherCarcinogens/InfectiousAgents/HPV/acs-recommendations-for-hpv-vaccine-use

Chapter 13

1. Centers for Disease Control and Prevention. (2010). *Facts at a glance*. Retrieved from http://www.cdc.gov/violence prevention/pdf/YV-DataSheet-a.pdf
2. Federal Bureau of Investigation. (2009). *Crime in the United States*. Retrieved from http://www2.fbi.gov/ucr/cius2008/data/table_20.html
3. Centers for Disease Control and Prevention. (2009, April 17). *National vital statistics reports, 57*(14).
4. Moynihan, M. M., et al. (2010). Engaging intercollegiate athletes in preventing and intervening in sexual and intimate partner violence. *Journal of American College Health, 59*, 197–204.
5. Centers for Disease Control and Prevention, National Center for Injury Prevention and Control. (2009). Understanding intimate partner violence: Fact sheet. Retrieved from https://docs.google.com/viewer?url=http://www.cdc.gov/violenceprevention/pdf/IPV_factsheet-a.pdf
6. Foran, H. M., & O'Leary, K. D. (2008). Alcohol and intimate partner violence: A meta-analytic review. *Clinical Psychology Review, 28*, 1222–1234.
7. Evans, S. E., Davies, C., & DiLillo, D. (2008). Exposure to domestic violence: A meta-analysis of child and adolescent outcomes. *Aggression and Violent Behavior, 13*, 131–140.
8. Federal Bureau of Investigation. (2009). *Hate crime statistics*. Retrieved from http://www2.fbi.gov/ucr/hc2009/incidents.html. http://usgovinfo.about.com/od/defenseandsecurity/a/hatecrimes03.htm
9. Federal Bureau of Investigation. (2010). *Latest hate crime statistics*. Retrieved from http://www.fbi.gov/news/stories/2010/november/hate_112210/hate_112210
10. Prevent Child Abuse America. (n.d.). *How many children are abused each year?* Retrieved from http://www.preventchildabuse.org/about_us/faqs.shtml#maltreatment
11. Centers for Disease Control and Prevention. (2010); CrimeinAmerica.net. (2009). *Crime against black Americans*. Retrieved from http://crimeinamerica.net/2009/06/13/crime-against-black-americans/
12. McLaughlin, K. A., et al. (2010). Childhood adversities and adult psychiatric disorders in the National Comorbidity Survey Replication II: Associations with persistence of DSM-IV disorders. *Archives of General Psychiatry, 67*, 124–132; Scott, J., Varghese, D., & McGrath, J. (2010). As the twig is bent, the tree inclines: Adult mental health consequences of childhood adversity. *Archives of General Psychiatry, 67*, 111–112.
13. *Summary campus crime data 2006–08—Criminal offenses*. Retrieved from https://docs.google.com/viewer?url=http://www2.ed.gov/admins/lead/safety/criminal2006-08.pdf
14. CollegeCampusCrime.com. (n.d.). *College campus crime*. Retrieved from http://www.collegecampuscrime.com/#
15. Trenton State College. (1991, Spring). *Sexual Assault Victim Education and Support Unit (SAVES-U) Newsletter*.
16. Basile, K. C., et al. (2007). Prevalence and characteristics of sexual violence victimization. *Violence and Victims, 22*, 437–448.
17. Federal Bureau of Investigation. (2009). *Uniform crime reports: Crimes in the United States, 2009*. Retrieved from http://www2.fbi.gov/ucr/cius2009/index.html
18. Fisher, B. S., et al. (2003). Reporting sexual victimization to the police and others: Results from a national-level study of college women. *Criminal Justice and Behavior, 30*, 6–38.

19. Campbell, R., & Wasco, S. M. (2005). Understanding rape and sexual assault: 20 years of progress and future directions. *Journal of Interpersonal Violence, 20*, 127–131.
20. Data from Dean of Students, University of North Carolina. Retrieved from http://deanofstudents.unc.edu/index.php/educational-programming-main menu-82/47-sexual-assault/114-did-you-know.html
21. Crisis Connection. (n.d.). *College campuses and rape*. Retrieved from http://www.crisisconnectioninc.org/sexual assault/college_campuses_and_rape.htm
22. Burnett, A., et al. (2009). Communicating/muting date rape: A co-cultural theoretical analysis of communication factors related to rape culture on a college campus. *Journal of Applied Communication Research, 37*, 465–485.
23. Hinrichsen, E. (n.d.). *Dangers and guidelines for social networking in college*. Retrieved from http://www.brighthub.com/education/college/articles/86893.aspx
24. McCauley, J. L., Calhoun, K. S., & Gidycz, C. A. (2010). Binge drinking and rape: A prospective examination of college women with a history of previous sexual victimization. *Journal of Interpersonal Violence, 25*(9), 1655–1668.
25. Strebeigh, F. (2009). *Equal: Women reshape American law*. New York: Norton.
26. Gannon, T. A., et al. (2008). Rape: Psychopathology, theory and treatment. *Clinical Psychology Review, 28*, 982–1008.
27. Amstadter, A. B., et al. (2010). Prevalence and correlates of service utilization and help seeking in a national college sample of female rape victims. *Journal of Anxiety Disorders, 24*, 900–902.
28. Vickerman, K. A., & Margolina, G. (2009). Rape treatment outcome research: Empirical findings and state of the literature. *Clinical Psychology Review, 29*, 431–448.
29. Stockdale, M. S., et al. (2004). Perceptions of the sexual harassment of men. *Psychology of Men and Masculinity, 5*, 158–167.
30. Adapted from Rathus, S. A., Nevid, J. S., & Fichner-Rathus, L. (2011). *Human sexuality in a world of diversity* (8th ed.). Boston, MA: Allyn and Bacon.
31. Chaiyavej, S., & Morash, M. (2009). Reasons for policewomen's assertive and passive reactions to sexual harassment. *Police Quarterly, 12*, 63–85.
32. Menard, K. S., et al. (2003). Gender differences in sexual harassment and coercion in college students: Developmental, individual, and situational determinants. *Journal of Interpersonal Violence, 18*, 1222–1239.
33. Champion, D. R. (2006). Sexual harassment: Criminal justice and academia. *Criminal Justice Studies: A Critical Journal of Crime, Law and Society, 19*, 101–109.
34. National Safety Council. (2010a). *Summary from injury facts, 2010 edition*. Retrieved from https://docs.google.com/viewer?url=http://www.nsc.org/news_resources/injury_and_death_statistics/Documents/Summary_2010_Ed.pdf; National Safety Council. (2010b). *Injury facts 2010 edition: A complete reference*. Itasca, IL: National Safety Council.
35. National Safety Council, 2010b.
36. U.S. Environmental Protection Agency. (2011). *Putting risks in perspective*. Retrieved from http://www.epa.gov/oar/oaqps/air_risc/3_90_022.html
37. National Safety Council, 2010a.
38. National Safety Council. (2003, July). *Frequently asked questions*. Retrieved from http://www.nsc.org/lrs/statfaq.htm#Question12.
39. Centers for Disease Control and Prevention. (2005, January 4). *Deaths from 113 selected causes, alcohol-induced causes, drug-induced causes, and injury by firearms, by 10-year age groups, race and sex: United States, 1999–2002*. Retrieved from http://www.cdc.gov/nchs/data/dvs/mortfinal2002_work290f.pdf
40. National Highway Safety Administration. (2005, June). *Motor vehicle occupant protection: Facts. Facts about young adults ages 16 to 20*. Retrieved from http://www.nhtsa.gov/people/injury/airbags/occupantprotectionfacts/young_adults.htm
41. White, J. B. (2010, December 15). New puzzle: Why fewer are killed in car crashes. *The Wall Street Journal*, D1.
42. Daily, L. (2005, Spring). Anatomy of a crash. *GEICO Direct*, 20–23.
43. Top 10 lifesavers. (2005, May). *Car and Travel*, 4.
44. The Associated Press. (2010, May 24). State-by-state seat belt use rate in 2009. Retrieved from http://www.boston.com/news/nation/washington/articles/2010/05/24/state_by_state_seat_belt_use_rate_in_2009/
45. Adapted from Top 10 lifesavers, 2005. Based on data supplied by NHSTA.
46. National Highway Traffic Safety Administration. (2010). *Think fast...* Retrieved from www.nhtsa.gov/.../NHTSA/Traffic%20Injury%20Control
47. Brody, J. E. (2011, April 12) Keeping eyes on distracted driving's toll. *The New York Times,* D7.
48. Parker-Pope, T. A. (2009, January 13). Problem of the brain, not the hands: Group urges phone ban for drivers. *The New York Times*, D5.
49. Brody, 2011.
50. *Distraction.gov*. (2011). Retrieved from http://www.distraction.gov/stats-and-facts/
51. National Highway Safety Administration. (2008, August). *2006 motor vehicle occupant protection: Facts. Children, youth, young adults*. Retrieved from www.nhtsa.gov/DOT/NHTSA/Traffic%20Injury%20Control/.../810654.pdf
52. Monahan, J. (2005, Spring). Wake up! *GEICO Direct*, 31.
53. *Distraction.gov*, 2011.
54. National Highway Traffic Safety Administration. (2008). *Traffic safety facts: 2008 Data. Motorcycles*. Retrieved from https://docs.google.com/viewer?url=http://www-nrd.nhtsa.dot.gov/pubs/811159.pdf
55. National Highway Traffic Safety Administration. (n.d.). *Motorcycles*. Retrieved from http://www.nhtsa.gov/Safety/Motorcycles
56. National Safety Council. (n.d.). *Protect yourself . . . wear a helmet!* Retrieved from http://www.nsc.org/library/facts/helmets-old.htm

Chapter 14

1. Soaring cost of healthcare sets a record. (2010, February 4). *Los Angeles Times*. Retrieved from http://articles.latimes.com/2010/feb/04/nation/la-na-healthcare4-2010feb04
2. U.S. Census Bureau. (2010, September). *Income, poverty and health insurance coverage in the United States: 2009*. Retrieved from www.census.gov/prod/2009pubs/p60-236.pdf
3. *Affordable health care for America*. (2010, March 18). Prepared by the House Committees on Ways and Means, Energy And Commerce, and Education and Labor.
4. Sack, K. (2010, December 14). Core of health care law is rejected by a U.S. judge. *The New York Times,* A1, A24; Pear, R., & Abelson, R. (2010, December 14). Law will proceed, administration says. *The New York Times,* A24.
5. U.S. Department of Health & Human Services. (2010, September 23). A new day for American consumers, *HealthCare.gov*; Summary of National Health Care Reform Legislation and Reconciliation Amendment Changes. (2010, March 30). *Community Catalyst*.
6. The White House. (2010). *Health reform in action*. Retrieved from www.whitehouse.gov
7. Centers for Medicare and Medicaid Services. (2008). *The nation's health dollar, calendar year 2008*. Retrieved from https://www.cms.gov/NationalHealthExpendData/downloads/PieChartSourcesExpenditures2008.pdf
8. U.S. Census Bureau. (2009a). *Income, poverty and health insurance coverage in the United States: 2009*; U.S. Census Bureau. (2009b). *People without health insurance coverage by race and Hispanic origin using 2- and 3-year averages: 2006–2007, 2008–2009, and 2007–2009*. Retrieved from http://www.census.gov/hhes/www/hlthins/data/incpovhlth/2009/race.xls+People+Without+Health+Insurance+Coverage+by+Race+and

+Hispanic+Origin+Using+2-+and +3-Year+Averages:+2006-2007, +2008-2009,+and+2007-2009&cd =1&hl=en&ct=clnk&gl=us
9. U.S. Census Bureau, 2009a.
10. Johnson & Johnson Health Care Systems, Inc. (2009). *Discover nursing*. Retrieved from http://www.discover-nursing.com.
11. Adapted from Rosenbaum, S. (2003). Managed care and patients' rights. *Journal of the American Medical Association, 289*, 906–907.
12. Barnes, P. M., Bloom, B., & Nahin, R. (2008, December). Complementary and alternative medicine use among adults and children: United States, 2007. *National Health Statistics Reports*, 12. Retrieved from www.cdc.gov/nchs/data/nhsr/nhsr012.pdf; National Center for Complementary and Alternative Medicine. (2010, November). *What is complementary and alternative medicine (CAM)?* Retrieved from http://nccam.nih.gov/health/whatiscam/
13. U. S. Commission on Civil Rights. (2005). *Broken promises: Evaluating the Native American health care system.*
14. U.S. Commission on Civil Rights, 2005.
15. Adapted from National Center for Complementary and Alternative Medicine. (2010, November). *What is complementary and alternative medicine (CAM)?* Retrieved from http://nccam.nih.gov/health/whatiscam/, and other sources.
16. National Center for Complementary and Alternative Medicine, National Institutes of Health. (2009, January). *CAM use by race/ethnicity among adults*. Retrieved from http://nccam.nih.gov/news/camstats/2007/72_dpi_CHARTS/chart3.htm
17. National Center for Complementary and Alternative Medicine, National Institutes of Health. (2009, January). *Reasons people use CAM*. Retrieved from http://nccam.nih.gov/news/images/camreason_large.gif
18. National Center for Complementary and Alternative Medicine, 2010, November.

Chapter 15

1. National Safety Council. (2008). *Lead poisoning*. Retrieved from http://www.nsc.org/news_resources/Resources/Documents/Lead_Poisoning.pdf&pli=1
2. Environmental Protection Agency (EPA). (2010, November). *Lead in paint, dust, and soil; basic information.* Retrieved from http://epa.gov/lead/pubs/leadinfo.htm
3. Koger, S. M., Schettler, T., & Weiss, B. (2005). Environment toxicants and developmental disabilities. *American Psychologist, 60*, 243–255; Hubbs-Tait, L., et al. Neurotoxicants, micronutrients, and social environments individual and combined effects on children's development. *Psychological Science in the Public Interest,* 6, 57–121.
4. Jones, R. L, et al. (2009). Trends in blood lead levels and blood lead testing among U.S. children aged 1 to 5 years, 1988–2004. *Pediatrics, 123*, e376–e385.
5. Environmental Protection Agency. (2010, September). *A citizen's guide to radon: The guide to protecting yourself and your family from radon.* Retrieved from http://www.epa.gov/radon/pubs/citguide.html
6. Environmental Protection Agency. (2010, September). *Exposure to radon causes lung cancer in non-smokers and smokers alike.* Retrieved from http://www.epa.gov/radon/healthrisks.html
7. Henry, C. R., et al. (2006). Myocardial injury and long-term mortality following moderate to severe carbon monoxide poisoning. *Journal of the American Medical Association*, 295, 398–402.
8. National Institute of Environmental Health Science, National Institutes of Health. (2007, November). *Aflatoxin and liver cancer*. Retrieved from http://www.niehs.nih.gov/health/impacts/aflatoxin.cfm
9. National Institutes of Health. (2009, May). *Asbestos exposure and cancer risk*. Retrieved from http://www.cancer.gov/cancertopics/factsheet/Risk/asbestos
10. Health and Safety Executive. (2010, August). *Asbestos related disease statistics: Frequently asked questions and answers*. Retrieved from http://www.hse.gov.uk/statistics/causdis/asbfaq.htm#fatalcount
11. Koger, Schettler, and Weiss, 2005.
12. U.S. Environmental Protection Agency. (2010, December). *DDT: A brief history and status.* Retrieved from http://www.epa.gov/opp00001/factsheets/chemicals/ddt-brief-history-status.htm
13. Galt, R. E. (2008). Beyond the circle of poison: Significant shifts in the global pesticide complex, 1976–2008. *Global Environmental Change, 18*, 786-799.
14. Agency for Toxic Substances and Disease Registry, Division of Toxicology. (2010, September). *ToxFAQs™ for methyl parathion*. Retrieved from http://www.atsdr.cdc.gov/toxfaqs/tf.asp?id=635&tid=117
15. World Health Organization. (2005). *Electromagnetic fields (EMF)*. Retrieved from http://www.who.int/peh-emf/about/WhatisEMF/en/index1.html; Zeman, G. (2009, December). *Health risks associated with living near high-voltage power lines.* Retrieved from http://www.hps.org/hpspublications/articles/powerlines.html
16. National Cancer Institute. (2010, May). *Cell phones and cancer risk*; American Cancer Society. (2010, May). *Cellular phones*. Retrieved from http://www.cancer.org/Cancer/CancerCauses/OtherCarcinogens/AtHome/cellular-phones
17. U.S. Food and Drug Administration. (2011). *Reducing radiation from medical X-rays*. Retrieved from http://www.fda.gov/ForConsumers/ConsumerUpdates/ucm095505.htm
18. Parker-Pope, T., & Barringer, F. (2011, June 1). Panel adds to debate over the cancer risk of cellphone radiation. *The New York Times*, A13.
19. National Cancer Institute. *Cell phones and cancer risk;* American Cancer Society. (2010, May). *Cellular phones*. Retrieved from http://www.cancer.org/Cancer/CancerCauses/OtherCarcinogens/AtHome/cellular-phones
20. U.S. Census Bureau. (2010, December). *International data base*. Retrieved from http://www.census.gov/ipc/www/idb/worldpopgraph.php
21. U.S. Environmental Protection Agency. (2010, April). *Risk assessment for toxic air pollutants: A citizen's guide*. [Originally published as EPA 450/3-90-024.]
22. U.S. Environmental Protection Agency. (2008, April). *Acid rain*. Retrieved from http://www.epa.gov/acidrain
23. Krantz, D., & Kifferstein, B. (2005). *Water pollution and society*. Retrieved from http://www.umich.edu/~gs265/society/waterpollution.htm
24. U.S. Environmental Protection Agency. (2010, July). *Wastes—Non-hazardous waste*. Retrieved from http://www.epa.gov/osw/nonhaz/; Walker, R. (2010, December 5). Wasted data. *The New York Times Magazine,* 20.
25. Environmental Protection Agency. (2008, November). *Municipal solid waste in the United States*. Retrieved from http://www.epa.gov/osw/nonhaz/municipal/msw99.htm
26. Kujawal, S. G., & Liberman, M. C. (2006). Acceleration of age-related hearing loss by early noise exposure: Evidence of a misspent youth. *Journal of Neuroscience, 26*, 2115–2123.
27. Johnson, C. K. (2010, August 17). 1 in 5 U.S. teens has hearing loss, new study says. Retrieved from http://www.msnbc.msn.com/id/38742752/ns/health-kids_and_parenting
28. Noonan, D. (2006, June 6). *A little bit louder, please*. Retrieved from http://www.noiseoff.org/document/msnbc.little.bit.louder.pdf
29. U.S. Environmental Protection Agency. *(2004/2005). Superfund program implementation manual FY04/05* [OSWER Directive 9200.3-14-1G-Q, Superfund Program Implementation Manual (SPIM) Fiscal Year 2004/2005]. Retrieved from http://www.epa.gov/superfund/action/process/pdfs/chap1_2.pdf
30. National Academy of Sciences Committee on the Science of Climate Change. (2001). *Climate change science: An analysis of some key questions.* Washington, DC: National Academy Press; National Oceanic and Atmospheric Administration (NCDC). (2008, August). *Global warming: Frequently asked questions*. Retrieved from http://www.ncdc.noaa.gov/oa/climate

/globalwarming.html; Doran, P. T., & Zimmerman, M. K. (2009). *Examining the scientific consensus on climate change.* American Geophysical Union. Retrieved from http://www.agu.org/journals/ABS/2009/2009EO030002.shtml

Chapter 16

1. Andersen, M. L., & Taylor, H. H. (2012). *Sociology: The essentials* (6th ed.). Belmont, CA: Wadsworth.
2. Central Intelligence Agency. (2011). *World factbook*. Retrieved from https://www.cia.gov/library/publications/the-world-factbook/
3. Sommers, M. S. (2008). Age-related changes in spoken word recognition. In D. B. Pisoni, & R. E. Remez (Eds.), *The handbook of speech perception* (pp. 469–493). Malden, MA: Blackwell Publishing.
4. U.S. Department of Health and Human Services (USDHHS). (n.d.) *Bone health and osteoporosis: A report of the surgeon general.* Retrieved from http://www.surgeongeneral.gov/library/bonehealth/docs/full_report.pdf
5. Wickwire Jr., E. M., et al. (2008). Sleep disorders. In M. Hersen & D. Michel (Eds.), *Handbook of psychological assessment, case conceptualization, and treatment. Vol 2: Children and adolescents* (pp. 622–651). Hoboken, NJ: Wiley.
6. Bopp, K. L., & Verhaeghen, P. (2010). Working memory and aging: Separating the effects of content and context. *Psychology and Aging, 24*, 968–980; Peters, E., et al. (2007). Adult age differences in dual information processes: Implications for the role of affective and deliberative processes in older adults' decision making. *Perspectives on Psychological Science, 2*, 1–23.
7. Singer, T., et al. (2003). The fate of cognition in very old age: Six-year longitudinal findings in the Berlin Aging Study (BASE). *Psychology and Aging, 18*, 318–331.
8. Goldman, J. S., Adamson, J., Karydas, A., Miller, B. L., & Hutton, M. (2008). New genes, new dilemmas: FTLD genetics and its implications for families. *American Journal of Alzheimer's Disease and Other Dementias, 22*, 507–515.
9. Jacobsen, J. S., et al. (2006). Early-onset behavioral and synaptic deficits in a mouse model of Alzheimer's disease. *Proceedings of the National Academy of Sciences, 103*, 5161-5166.
10. Gray, S. L., et al. (2008). Antioxidant vitamin supplement use and risk of dementia or Alzheimer's disease in older adults. *Journal of the American Geriatrics Society, 56*, 291–295; Meinert, C. L., & Breitner, J. C. S. (2008). Chronic disease long-term drug prevention trials: Lessons from the Alzheimer's Disease Anti-Inflammatory Prevention Trial (ADAPT). *Alzheimer's and Dementia, 4(Suppl 1)*, S7–S14.
11. Qin, W., et al. (2006). Calorie restriction attenuates Alzheimer's disease type brain amyloidosis in squirrel monkeys (*Saimiri sciureus*). *Journal of Alzheimer's Disease, 10*, 417–422.
12. Vellas, B., Gillette-Guyonnet, S., & Andrieu, S. (2008). Memory health clinics—A first step to prevention. *Alzheimer's and Dementia, 4 (Suppl 1)*, S144–S149.
13. Laumann, E. O., et al. (2006). Sexual activity, sexual disorders and associated help-seeking behavior among mature adults in five anglophone countries from the global survey of sexual attitudes and behaviors. *Archives of Sexual Behavior, 35*, 145–161.
14. Barnett, J. E., & Dunning, C. (2003). Clinical perspectives on elderly sexuality. *Archives of Sexual Behavior, 32*, 295–296.
15. Laumann et al., 2006.
16. Ibid.
17. Perls, T. T. (2005). The oldest old. *Scientific American, 272*, 70–75.
18. Zanni, G. R., & Wick, J. Y. (2011). Telomeres: Unlocking the mystery of cell division and aging. *The Consultant Pharmacist, 26*, 78–90.
19. Roth, G. S., et al. (2004). Aging in rhesus monkeys: Relevance to human health interventions. *Science, 305*, 1423–1426.
20. Hursting, S. D., et al. (2003). Calorie restriction, aging, and cancer prevention: Mechanisms of action and applicability to humans. *Annual Review of Medicine, 54*, 131–152.
21. Chong, L., McDonald, H., & Strauss, E. (2004). Deconstructing aging. *Science, 305*, 1419.
22. Sierra, F. (2009). Biology of Aging Summit report. *Journal of Gerontology, 64A*, 155–156.
23. Kalapos, M. P., et al. (2010). Methyglyoxal, oxidative stress, and aging. *Aging and Age-Related Disorders, 1*, 149–167.
24. Johnson-Greene, D., & Inscore, A. B. (2005). Substance abuse in older adults. In S. S. Bush, & T. A. Martin (Eds.), *Geriatric neuropsychology: Practice essentials (Studies on neuropsychology, neurology and cognition)* (pp. 429–451). Philadelphia: Taylor and Francis.
25. Johnson-Grene and Inscore, 2005.
26. Kübler-Ross, E. (1969). *On death and dying*. New York: Macmillan.
27. National Hospice and Palliative Care Organization (NHPCO). (2007, November). *NHPCO facts and figures: Hospice care in America*. Retrieved from http://www.nhpco.org/files/public/Statistics_Research/NHPCO_facts-and-figures_Nov2007.pdf
28. Lattanzi-Licht, M. (2007). Religion, spirituality, and dying. In D. Balk, et al. (Eds.), *Handbook of thanatology* (pp. 11–17). New York: Routledge/Taylor and Francis Group.
29. Jacobs, S. (1993). *Pathologic grief: Maladaptation to loss*. Washington, DC: American Psychiatric Press.
30. Maciejewski, P. K., et al. (2007). An empirical examination of the stage theory of grief. *Journal of the American Medical Association, 297*, 716–723.

Index

*Figures are denoted by an italic *f* following the page number. Tables are denoted by an italic *t* following the page number. Names in notes are indicated by an italic *n*.

A

B

Learning Outcomes

1. Define health and wellness
2. Explain how to strive for wellness
3. Describe the health concerns of women and men from different racial and ethnic backgrounds
4. Describe the goals of the government project *Healthy People*
5. Explain ways of thinking critically about health-related information

Chapter Outline

Additional Health APP features available online for Chapter 1:

Health Check 1-1 The Dimensions of Health: Where Do You Stand?
Diversity 1-1 Socioeconomic Status: The Rich Get Richer and the Poor Get . . . Sicker
Diversity 1-2 Women's Health Research: A History of Exclusion
Prevention 1-1 Debunking Miracle Cures and Quick Fixes from the Self-Help Aisle
Health Skills 1-2 Practicing Self-Care

HLTH Assets available online for each chapter:

Crossword Puzzles
Flashcards
Glossary
Quizzes

Figure1-1 Six Dimensions of Health

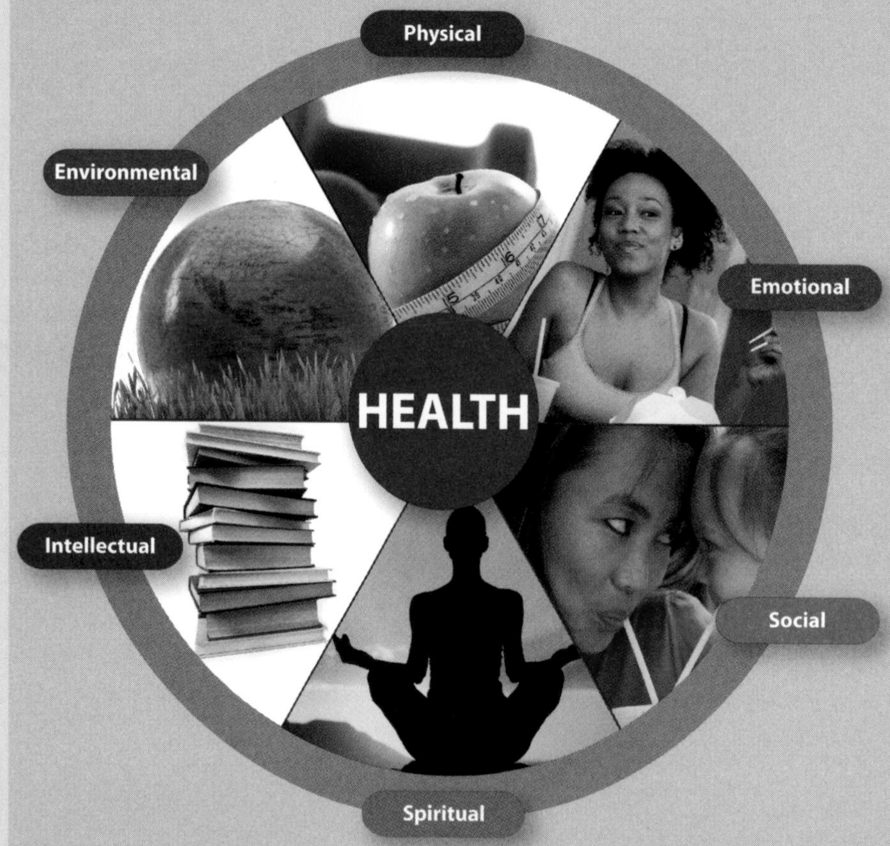

Clockwise from top: © iStockphoto.com/Ioana Davies / © iStockphoto.com/Steven Miric / © iStockphoto.com/RonTech2000 / © iStockphoto.com/Joshua Hodge Photography / © iStockphoto.com/Rick Rhay / © iStockphoto.com/Mehmet Salih Guler

Key Terms

arthritis Inflammation of a joint, typically accompanied by pain, stiffness, and swelling; results from a number of conditions affecting the structures inside and surrounding the joint. **13**

critical thinking The adoption of a questioning attitude characterized by careful weighing of evidence and thoughtful analysis and probing of the claims and arguments of others. **14**

emotional health Emotional well-being and ability to share one's feelings with others. **4**

environmental health The relationship between humans and other organisms and their physical environment that allows them to survive and flourish. **5**

ethnic group A group of people who are united by their cultural heritage, race, language, and common history. **7**

external locus of control The perception that a person's future is determined by forces beyond his or her control. **9**

health Soundness of body and mind; a state of vigor and vitality that permits a person to function physically, psychologically, and socially. **4**

hypertension High blood pressure. **12**

intellectual health The ability to use one's intellectual resources to solve problems, meet life challenges, develop personal values, and adopt healthy behaviors and lifestyles. **5**

internal locus of control The belief that one can control the outcomes that one experiences in life. **9**

osteoporosis Condition of generalized bone loss, making bones more brittle and subject to breakage. **13**

physical health Soundness of body, as represented by healthy physical functioning and the absence of disease. **4**

sickle-cell anemia An inherited blood disorder that mostly affects African Americans and is characterized by the presence of crescent- or sickle-shaped red blood cells. **12**

social health The ability to relate effectively to other people such as family members, intimate partners, friends, fellow students or workers, professors, and supervisors. **4**

socioeconomic status Relative position in terms of education and income level. **9**

spiritual health The attainment of connectedness to a higher order or purpose beyond oneself, such as commitment to a particular religion, aesthetic values, or community service. **5**

Tay-Sachs disease A fatal neurological disorder that primarily affects Jews of eastern European origin. **12**

wellness A state of optimum health, as characterized by active efforts to maximize one's physical health and well-being. **6**

Critical Thinking Questions

1. **Q: What is the difference between health and wellness?**

   A: Health is soundness of body and mind and the ability to function physically, socially and psychologically with vigor. Wellness is the state of optimum health characterized by active efforts to maximize physical health and well-being. The difference being that wellness is a process and health is the desired result of wellness behaviors.

2. **Q: To what extent does your environment either sustain or threaten your health?**

   A: We affect our environment daily by our interactions with our habitat. The environment supports us by providing air, water, and food.

   Because of our lack of consideration for the balance of nature, we are at a point of worldwide environmental crisis. The choices we as world citizens are making by, for example, destroying the rain forest and drilling for oil in the wilderness are altering the natural habitats of animals, causing some species to become extinct, and causing huge amounts of pollution in our air, water, and on land, posing monumental threats to our planet's future.

3. **Q: Describe some predisposing factors, enabling factors, and reinforcing factors that affect your health behavior. To what extent do these factors encourage/hinder healthy changes? What can you do to control these factors?**

   A: Predisposing factors either promote or hinder healthful changes in behavior. These factors include beliefs, attitudes, knowledge, expectancies, and values.

   Enabling factors promote change. These include skills or abilities, physical and mental capabilities, and the availability and accessibility of resources.

   Reinforcing factors include the praise and support you receive from others and from yourself that encourage healthy behavior.

4. **Q: Why is it important to study the relationship between ethnicity and health?**

   A: It is important to study ethnicity and its relationship to health in an effort to lessen the health disparities within different ethnicities. Health care should be effective and accessible for all Americans.

5. **Q: How would you go about determining if health claims made by a doctor, website, or magazine were accurate?**

   A: Be skeptical, examine terms, remember that correlation is not causation, examine the quality of evidence, make sure the information does not oversimplify or overgeneralize, and check citations and author credentials.

Web Exercises

1. Go to http://www.healthfinder.gov. Click on "Personal Health Tools," and explore the section titled "Online Checkups." Here you will find health quizzes and self-tests, as well as health news and links to organizations that provide more information on each topic you select. Examples include "Men's health quiz: How Well Do You Take Care of Yourself?" and "How Are Alcohol and Drugs Affecting Your Life?—A Self-Test for Teenagers." Choose three health topics that interest you and complete the quiz or self-test for each topic.
2. Go to http://www.cdc.gov, the website for the U.S. Centers for Disease Control and Prevention. Search the site for "Deaths—Leading Causes"; click on "FASTATS—Leading Causes of Death." This site lists the numbers of deaths for the 10 leading causes of death in the United States. For each cause of death listed, identify the health behaviors you can adopt to decrease your risk factors.

prepcard/ CHAPTER 2 PSYCHOLOGICAL HEALTH

Learning Outcomes

1 Describe the elements of psychological health

2 Explain what is meant by the mind–body connection

3 Discuss the contribution of spiritual health to psychological health

4 Discuss psychological disorders, focusing on anxiety and depression

5 Describe ways of treating psychological disorders

Chapter Outline

Additional Health APP features available online for Chapter 2:

Health Check 2-2 Getting in Touch with Your Self-Concept
Health Skills 2-1 Enhancing Self-Esteem
Health Skills 2-2 Assert Yourself!
Health Check 2-4 Are You an Optimist or a Pessimist?
Health Check 2-5 Are You Anxious?
Diversity 2-1 The Case of Women and Depression
Health Skills 2-3 Do You Need to Get Out of the Dumps?
Prevention 2-1 Suicide Prevention: Helping a Friend in Crisis

HLTH Assets available online for each chapter:

Crossword Puzzles
Flashcards
Glossary
Quizzes

BBC Health Video Titles available online for Chapter 2:

Cognitive Behavioral Therapy
Shyness
Sleep
Exercise and Depression

Critical Thinking Questions

1. **Q: How does leading a meaningful life help people cope with stress and disappointment?**

   A: Having a meaningful life creates an anchor when life is difficult.

2. **Q: Agree or disagree with the following statement, and support your answer: "Money can buy happiness."**

   A: [Student opinions will vary.]

3. **Q: Agree or disagree with the following statement, and support your answer: "Biology is destiny."**

   A: [Student opinions will vary.]

4. **Q: Explain how biological, psychological, and sociocultural factors are related to psychological health.**

   A: Our psychological health depends on many factors, including biological factors such as genetics and the workings of the nervous system, psychological factors such as optimism and self-confidence, and sociocultural factors such as cultural and religious heritage.

Key Terms

antidepressant Drug that combats depression by altering the availability of neurotransmitters in the brain. **34**

anxiety Emotional state characterized by body arousal, feelings of nervousness or tension, or a sense of apprehension about the future. **33**

anxiety disorders Category of psychological disorders involving excessive or inappropriate anxiety reactions. **33**

behavior therapy Type of therapy involving the systematic application of learning-based techniques to help people change problem behaviors. **40**

bipolar disorder Type of mood disorder characterized by mood swings between severe depression and mania. **37**

chromosomes Rod-shaped structures in the cell's nucleus that house the organism's genes. **30**

cognitive therapy Type of psychotherapy developed by Aaron Beck that helps clients identify and correct dysfunctional thinking patterns. **40**

delusions False, unshakable beliefs. **37**

deoxyribonucleic acid (DNA) The chemical substance in chromosomes that carries the organism's genetic code. **30**

dream analysis Technique used in psychoanalysis in which the symbolic meaning of dreams is believed to reflect upon unconscious material. **40**

ego identity The sense of who one is and what one stands for. **28**

electroconvulsive therapy (ECT) Form of therapy for severe depression involving the administration of brief pulses of electricity to the patient's brain. **41**

free association Technique used in psychoanalysis in which the patient is encouraged to verbalize any thoughts that come to mind, free of conscious efforts to censure or edit them. **39**

gamma-aminobutyric acid (GABA) A neurotransmitter that helps calm anxiety reactions by inhibiting excess firing of neurons. **33**

gene The basic unit or building block of heredity that contains the genetic code. **30**

generalized anxiety disorder Type of anxiety disorder characterized by high levels of anxiety that is not limited to particular situations and by general feelings of worry, dread, and foreboding. **34**

hallucinations Perceptual distortions that occur in the absence of external stimuli and are confused with reality, such as "hearing voices" or seeing things that are not there. **37**

Web Exercises

1. Go to http://www.cdc.gov, the website of the U.S. Centers for Disease Control and Prevention. Search the site for "suicide facts" and click on "Suicide, Facts at a Glance." Read the Suicide Fact Sheet and make a list of all the facts that were not included in your text.
2. Go to http://www.nimh.nih.gov, the website of the U.S. National Institute of Mental Health. Choose two of the psychological disorders listed under "Health Topics." Answer the following questions about each disorder: (1) What are the major symptoms? (2) What are the recommended treatments? (3) Where could I get professional help in my local area?

hormones Chemicals that are secreted by endocrine glands and are involved in the regulation of a wide range of body processes, including reproduction and growth. **30**

ideal self The mental image corresponding to what we believe we ought to be like. **24**

identity crisis A period of serious soul-searching and self-examination in an effort to achieve ego identity. **28**

manic episode Episode of extremely inflated mood and excitability. **37**

mood disorder Disturbances of mood that affect the individual's ability to function effectively, are unduly prolonged or severe, or are out of keeping with the events the person has encountered. **34**

neuron A nerve cell. **29**

neurotransmitter Chemical substance that transfers neural impulses from one neuron to another. **29**

obsessive-compulsive disorder (OCD) Type of anxiety disorder characterized by obsessions (nagging, intrusive thoughts or images) and/or compulsions (repetitive behaviors that the person feels compelled to perform). **34**

panic disorder Type of anxiety disorder characterized by episodes of sheer terror, called *panic attacks*, and by the resultant fear of such attacks occurring again. **33**

phobia An excessive or irrational fear. **33**

psychoanalysis Type of therapy developed by Sigmund Freud that helps people achieve insight into unconscious processes and conflicts believed to give rise to psychological problems. **39**

psychological disorder Abnormal behavior patterns associated with significant personal distress, impaired functioning, or disturbed thinking, perceptions, or emotions. Also called *mental disorders* or *mental illnesses*. **32**

psychological health Soundness of mind, characterized by the absence of significant psychological problems and by the ability to function effectively in meeting life demands and to derive satisfaction from work, social relationships, and leisure pursuits. **20**

psychotherapy A verbal form of therapy, or "talk therapy," based on the application of psychological principles and techniques. **39**

psychotic disorder A psychological disorder involving a break with reality. **37**

psychotropic drugs Drugs used to treat psychological or mental disorders. **40**

rational-emotive behavior therapy (REBT) Type of cognitive therapy developed by Albert Ellis that focuses on helping people dispute and correct irrational thinking. **40**

repression In Freudian theory, the process of motivated forgetting by which the unconscious mind banishes from awareness troubling ideas or impulses. **39**

schizophrenia An enduring type of psychotic disorder involving disturbances in thought processes, perception, emotion, and behavior. **37**

self-actualization Self-initiated tendency to strive to realize one's potential. **23**

serotonin A type of neurotransmitter that is involved in regulating appetite and mood states and is linked to depression. **34**

specific phobia Phobia involving specific objects or situations, such as fear of enclosed spaces (claustrophobia) or fear of small animals or insects. **33**

systematic desensitization Behavior therapy technique that attempts to help a person overcome a phobia by staging a series of imagined encounters with feared objects or stimuli while the person remains deeply relaxed. **40**

prepcard/ CHAPTER 3 STRESS AND YOUR HEALTH

Learning Outcomes

1 Describe various sources of stress

2 Describe the effects of stress on the body

3 Explain the effects of stress on the immune system

4 Explain how stress affects your health

5 Discuss the problem of insomnia and ways of getting your *Z*s.

6 Describe ways of managing stress

Chapter Outline

Additional Health APP features available online for Chapter 3:

Prevention 3-1 Ten Ways to Prevent Burnout
Health Check 3-2 Are You Type A?
Health Skills 3-1 Pain, Pain, Go Away—Don't Come Again Another Day
Diversity 3-1 "Fight or Flight" or "Tend and Befriend"? Do Men and Women Respond Differently to Stress?
Health Skills 3-2 Overcoming Insomnia

HLTH Assets available online for each chapter:

Crossword puzzles
Flashcards
Glossary
Quizzes

BBC Health Video Title available online for Chapter 3:

Sleep

Critical Thinking Questions

1. **Q: To what extent is personality style a source of stress in people's lives? What do you think they can do about it?**

   A: Type A personalities tend to be more time driven and respond to stress more dramatically, which may lead to higher levels of stress-related hormones and increased health risks. Type B personalities seem to be more relaxed and less stressed, lessening potential health issues.

   Recognizing your personality type and its associated risks can be the first step in achieving effective stress management.

2. **Q: How does the general adaptation syndrome (GAS) help us meet stressful challenges? On the other hand, how might the GAS represent a hindrance to our health or well-being?**

   A: GAS helps the body respond to danger, in essence keeping us out of harm. The alarm state may act as a motivator for action. Yet if we do not recognize or listen to the body as it moves through the stages of GAS, we may be putting our health at risk.

3. **Q: Do you find you are more likely to catch colds when you are under stress? How might you explain this relationship?**

   A: The body's ability to fight off infection is related to a healthy immune system. If the body is under attack from a variety of stressors, it is less able to fight off infection.

Key Terms

adrenal glands A pair of endocrine glands that lie just above the kidneys and produce various stress hormones. **53**

adrenocorticotropic hormone (ACTH) Hormone produced by the pituitary gland that activates the adrenal cortex (outer layer) to secrete corticosteroids (cortical steroids). **53**

alarm reaction The first stage of the general adaptation syndrome; it describes the body's initial response to stress, consisting of activation of the sympathetic nervous system and release of stress hormones. **49**

antibody Specialized protein produced by white blood cells that attaches itself to invading microbes and other foreign bodies, inactivates them, and marks them for destruction. **54**

autonomic nervous system (ANS) The part of the peripheral nervous system that functions "automatically" (without awareness or voluntary control) to control internal body processes such as heart rate, respiration, and endocrine functioning. **51**

central nervous system The central part of the nervous system, consisting of the brain and spinal cord. **51**

corticosteroids Steroidal hormones released by the adrenal cortex that increase resistance to stress by fending off allergic reactions and reducing inflammation. Also called *cortical steroids.* **53**

corticotropin-releasing hormone (CRH) Substance produced by the hypothalamus that causes the pituitary gland to release adrenocorticotropic hormone (ACTH). **52**

endocrine system A system of glands that secrete hormones directly into the bloodstream, rather than by means of ducts. **52**

endorphins Neurotransmitters that have opiate-like effects of deadening pain and producing states of pleasure by directly stimulating pleasure centers in the brain. **49**

exhaustion stage The third and final stage of the general adaptation syndrome; characterized by depletion of body resources and lowering of resistance to stress-related illness. **50**

general adaptation syndrome (GAS) The body's three-phase general response to persistent or intense stress. **49**

homeostasis The maintenance of a steady state in the body. **50**

hypothalamus The small brain structure in the lower middle part of the brain that is involved in regulating a range of body processes, including motivation, emotion, and body temperature. **52**

immune system The body's system for identifying and eliminating disease-causing agents, such as bacteria and viruses, and for ridding the body of diseased, mutated, or worn-out cells. **54**

insomnia Difficulty falling asleep, remaining asleep, or achieving restorative sleep. **56**

parasympathetic nervous system Branch of the autonomic nervous system involved in body processes, such as digestion, that preserve and replenish the body's stores of energy. **51**

peripheral nervous system The part of the nervous system comprising a system of nerves that connect the brain and spinal cord to the other body parts, including sensory organs, muscles, and glands. **51**

pituitary gland A structure in the brain dubbed the "master gland" because of its key role in many body processes, including growth and the formation of sperm and egg cells. **52**

posttraumatic stress disorder (PTSD) Type of psychological disorder involving a maladaptive reaction to a traumatic experience. The disorder may not begin until months or years following the traumatic event and may last for years after its onset. **54**

resistance stage The second stage of the general adaptation syndrome, during which the body attempts to renew and conserve its resources in order to cope with prolonged stress. Also called the *adaptation stage.* **50**

somatic nervous system The part of the peripheral nervous system that involves the voluntary control of skeletal muscles and feeds information from the sense organs to the brain. **51**

stress A pressure or force placed upon a body or an object. In human terms, it refers to a demand placed upon a person to adjust. **42**

sympathetic nervous system The branch of the autonomic nervous system that accelerates body processes and releases stores of energy needed for physical exertion. The sympathetic branch is activated as part of the alarm reaction in response to stress. **51**

Type A personality A personality type characterized by impatience, time urgency, competitiveness, and hostility **48**

Web Exercises

1. Go to http://www.stress.org, the website for the American Institute of Stress. Search for the article "Type A and Coronary Disease, Separating Fact from Fiction: An Interview with Dr. Ray Rosenman." (At time of press, the article could be found here: http://www.stress.org/interview-TypeA_CoronaryDisease.htm.) As you read the interview, answer the following questions:
   - How did two doctors who treated cardiovascular problems come to "discover" Type A personality?
   - Which characteristics of Type A behavior are most important?
   - What is the significance of hostility in Type A behavior and heart disease?
2. Go to http://www.workhealth.org, the website of the Job Stress Network. Click on the "Job Strain" link. At the top of a list of links, you'll find "Interested to know if you have job strain?" This link takes you to a brief questionnaire and scoring key that will give you an indication of how much job strain you experience at work.

prepcard/ CHAPTER 4 INTIMATE RELATIONSHIPS AND SEXUALITY

Learning Outcomes

1. Describe the formation of intimate relationships
2. Discuss contemporary lifestyles, from being single to cohabitation to marriage and parenting
3. Discuss factors in unhealthy relationships
4. Describe female and male sexual anatomy and related health issues
5. Discuss sexual orientation
6. Discuss different types of sexual behaviors
7. Discuss sexual dysfunctions and sex therapy

Chapter Outline

continued

Additional Health APP features available online for Chapter 4:

Diversity 4-1 Sex Differences in Preferences for Mates across 37 Cultures
Health Skills 4-1 Using Small Talk and Opening Lines to Jump-Start Relationships
Health Skills 4-2 Loneliness and Health: "All the Lonely People, Where Do They All Come From?"
Health Skills 4-3 Resolving Conflicts in Relationships
Diversity 4-3 Clitoridectomy—Tradition, Mutilation, or Both?
Prevention 4-1 Preventing Cystitis and Vaginitis
Prevention 4-2 The Pelvic Exam: What to Expect
Health Skills 4-4 How to Handle Menstrual Discomfort

HLTH Assets available online for each chapter:

Crossword Puzzles
Flashcards
Glossary
Quizzes

BBC Health Video Title available online for Chapter 4:

Etiquette: Art of Small Talk

Critical Thinking Questions

1. **Q: Critical thinkers pay attention to definitions of terms. Does each of Sternberg's kinds of love strike you as a recognizable form of love? Why or why not?**

   A: [Student answers will vary.]

2. **Q: How do you determine which kinds of sexual behavior are appropriate for you and which are not? What are your criteria, or standards, for making these judgments?**

   A: [Student answers will vary.]

3. **Q: Do you believe that sex differences in aggression and nurturance are inborn or the result of cultural influences? Why?**

   A: [Student answers will vary.]

4. **Q: When does a sexual problem become a sexual dysfunction?**

   A: When sexual problems become persistent and cause distress, they may be labeled as sexual dysfunctions.

5. **Q: Do you believe that sexual orientation is a matter of choice? What does the evidence suggest?**

   A: [Student answers will vary.]

Web Exercises

1. Go to http://health.discovery.com, the website of the Discovery TV channels. In the top links, click on "Sexual Health." On the Sexual Health page, click on "Quiz." Take this 10-item quiz about sexuality and intimacy and read the explanations for the correct answers.
2. Go to http://www.sexhealth.org, the website of the Sexual Health InfoCenter. Click "Enter InfoCenter." In the left column, click on the topic of "Masturbation" and read "A Brief History of Masturbation." Using examples from TV shows and friends' comments, compare our current view of masturbation with historical views.
3. Go to http://www.apa.org, the website for the American Psychological Association (APA). Type "sexual orientation" in the search box. From the list of search results, choose "Answers to Your Questions For a Better Understanding of Sexual Orientation and Homosexuality." Read the article and answer the following questions:
   - What does the APA say about the origins of sexual orientation?
   - What is the APA's position on whether therapy can change a person's sexual orientation?

Key Terms

cervix The lower end of the uterus. (Latin for "neck.") **75**

circumcision Surgical removal of the foreskin of the penis. (From the Latin *circumcidere*, meaning "to cut around.") **81**

clitoris A female sex organ consisting of a shaft and glans located above the urethral opening. It is extremely sensitive to sexual sensations. **74**

cohabitation Living together as though married but without legal sanction. **70**

corpus luteum The follicle that has released an ovum and then produces copious amounts of progesterone and estrogen during the luteal phase of a woman's cycle. (From Latin roots meaning "yellow body.") **78**

endometrium The innermost layer of the uterus. (From Latin and Greek roots meaning "within the uterus.") **75**

epididymis A tube that lies against the back wall of each testicle and serves as a storage facility for sperm. (From Greek roots meaning "upon testicles.") **80**

excitement phase The first phase of the sexual response cycle, which is characterized by erection in the male, vaginal lubrication in the female, and muscle tension and increases in heart rate in both males and females. **81**

homogamy The practice of marrying people who are similar in social background and standing. (From Greek roots meaning "same" [*homos*] and "marriage" [*gamos*].) **71**

hymen A fold of tissue across the vaginal opening that is usually present at birth and remains at least partly intact until a woman engages in coitus. (Greek for "membrane.") **74**

hysterectomy Surgical removal of the uterus. **75**

labia majora Large folds of skin that run downward from the mons along the sides of the vulva. (Latin for "large lips" or "major lips.") **74**

labia minora Hairless, light-colored membranes, located between the labia majora. (Latin for "small lips" or "minor lips.") **74**

mammary glands Milk-secreting glands. (From the Latin *mamma*, which means both "breast" and "mother.") **75**

menopause The cessation of menstruation. **79**

menstrual phase The fourth phase of the menstrual cycle, during which the endometrium is sloughed off in the menstrual flow. **78**

orgasmic phase The third phase of the sexual response cycle, characterized by the rhythmic contractions of orgasm. **82**

ovaries Almond-shaped organs that produce ova and the hormones estrogen and progesterone. **75**

ovulation The release of an ovum from an ovary. **76**

ovulatory phase The second stage of the menstrual cycle, during which a follicle ruptures and releases a mature ovum. **76**

perimenopause The beginning of menopause, as characterized by 3 to 11 months of amenorrhea or irregular periods. **79**

plateau phase The second phase of the sexual response cycle, which is characterized by increases in vasocongestion, muscle tension, heart rate, and blood pressure in preparation for orgasm. **82**

premature ejaculation A sexual dysfunction in which ejaculation occurs too rapidly or with minimal sexual stimulation. **85**

premenstrual syndrome (PMS) A combination of physical and psychological symptoms (e.g., anxiety, depression, irritability, weight gain from fluid retention, and abdominal discomfort) that regularly afflicts many women during the 4- to 6-day interval that precedes their menses each month. **78**

proliferative phase The first phase of the menstrual cycle, which begins with the end of menstruation and lasts about 9 or 10 days. During this phase, the endometrium proliferates. **76**

prostate gland The gland that lies beneath the bladder and secretes prostatic fluid, which gives semen its characteristic odor and texture. **80**

refractory period A period of time following a response (e.g., orgasm) during which an individual is no longer responsive to stimulation (e.g., sexual stimulation). **82**

resolution phase The fourth phase of the sexual response cycle, during which the body gradually returns to its prearoused state. **82**

secretory phase The third phase of the menstrual cycle, which follows ovulation. Also referred to as the *luteal phase,* after the *corpus luteum,* which begins to secrete large amounts of progesterone and estrogen following ovulation. **76**

semen The whitish fluid that constitutes the ejaculate, consisting of sperm and secretions from the seminal vesicles, prostate, and Cowper's glands. **81**

serial monogamy A pattern of involvement in one exclusive relationship after another, as opposed to engaging in multiple sexual relationships at the same time. **70**

sexual dysfunction Problems with sexual interest, arousal, or response. **85**

sexual orientation The directionality of one's sexual interests—toward members of the same gender, the opposite gender, or both genders. **82**

urethral opening The opening through which urine passes from the female's body. **74**

uterus The organ in which a fertilized ovum implants and develops until birth. Also called the *womb*. **75**

vagina The tubular female sex organ that contains the penis during sexual intercourse and through which a baby is born. (Latin for "sheath.") **75**

vas deferens A tube that conducts sperm from the testicle to the ejaculatory duct of the penis. (From Latin roots meaning "a vessel" that "carries down.") **80**

vasocongestion The swelling of the genital tissues with blood, which causes erection of the penis and engorgement of the area surrounding the vaginal opening. **81**

vulva The external sexual structures of the female. **74**

prepcard/ CHAPTER 5 REPRODUCTIVE CHOICES

Learning Outcomes

1 Describe the process of conception

2 Discuss the problem of infertility and alternate methods of having children

3 Discuss the pros and cons of various methods of contraception

4 Discuss methods of abortion

5 Discuss health issues in pregnancy and prenatal development

6 Describe health issues associated with methods of childbirth

7 Discuss health issues in the postpartum period

Chapter Outline

Additional Health APP features available online for Chapter 5:

Diversity 5-1 Where Are the Missing Chinese Girls?
Health Skills 5-1 Talking with Your Partner about Contraception
Health Skills 5-2 Selecting a Method of Contraception
Health Skills 5-3 Selecting an Obstetrician
Prevention 5-1 Safeguarding Your Baby against Low Birthweight, Stillbirth, Birth Defects, and Disease
Diversity 5-2 Advice for Expectant Fathers
Diversity 5-3 Maternal and Infant Mortality around the World

HLTH Assets available online for each chapter:

Crossword Puzzles
Flashcards
Glossary
Quizzes

BBC Health Video Title available online for Chapter 5:

Abortion Incidence and Sex Education

Critical Thinking Questions

1. **Q: Sex selection raises many moral and ethical questions. Many people wonder whether people have the "right" to select the sex of their children, either for religious reasons or because sex selection is usually sexist (that is, males are usually preferred). What is your view?**

   A: [Student answers will vary.]

2. **Q: Do any methods of overcoming infertility strike you as "unnatural"? Explain. Would your view affect your willingness to try one or more of them? Explain.**

   A: [Student answers will vary.]

3. **Q: Are the minipill and the IUD methods of contraception or abortion? Does it matter? Explain your view.**

   A: [Student answers will vary.]

4. **Q: One of the issues concerning abortion is whether it is the taking of a human life. How do *you* define *human life*? When do *you* believe human life begins? At conception? When the embryo becomes implanted in the uterus? When the fetus begins to assume a human shape or develops human facial features? When the fetus is capable of sustaining independent life? Explain.**

   A: [Student answers will vary.]

Key Terms

amniotic sac The sac containing the fetus. **106**

artificial insemination The introduction of sperm in the reproductive tract through means other than sexual intercourse. **92**

cesarean section A method of childbirth in which the fetus is delivered through a surgical incision in the abdomen. (Formerly spelled *Caeserean.*) **110**

diaphragm A shallow rubber cup or dome, fitted to the contour of a woman's vagina, that is coated with a spermicide and inserted prior to coitus to prevent conception. **96**

dilate To open or widen. **107**

dilation and curetage (D&C) An operation in which the cervix is dilated and uterine contents are scraped away. **101**

dilation and evacuation (D&E) An abortion method in which the cervix is dilated prior to vacuum aspiration. **101**

efface To become thin. **107**

embryonic stage The stage of prenatal development that lasts from implantation through the eighth week, and which is characterized by the differentiation of the major organ systems. **105**

episiotomy A surgical incision in the perineum that widens the birth canal, preventing random tearing during childbirth. **109**

gamete intrafallopian transfer (GIFT) A method of conception in which sperm and ova are inserted into a fallopian tube to encourage conception. **92**

general anesthesia The use of drugs to put people to sleep and eliminate pain, as during childbirth. **109**

germinal stage The period of prenatal development prior to implantation in the uterus. **105**

human chorionic gonadotropin (HCG) A hormone produced by women shortly after conception, which stimulates the corpus luteum to continue to produce progesterone. The presence of HCG in a woman's urine indicates that she is pregnant. **104**

infertility The inability to conceive a child. **91**

intra-amniotic infusion An abortion method in which a substance is injected into the amniotic sac to induce premature labor. Also called *instillation.* **102**

intrauterine device (IUD) A small object that is inserted into the uterus and left in place to prevent conception. **94**

in vitro fertilization (IVF) A method of conception in which mature ova are surgically removed from an ovary and placed in a laboratory dish along with sperm. **92**

Lamaze method A childbirth method in which women learn about childbirth, learn to relax and to breathe in patterns that conserve energy and lessen pain, and have a coach (usually the father) present at childbirth. Also termed *prepared childbirth.* **109**

local anesthetic Anesthetic that eliminates pain in a specific area of the body, as during childbirth. **109**

neural tube A hollow area in the blastocyst from which the nervous system will develop. **106**

oral contraceptive A contraceptive, consisting of sex hormones, which is taken by mouth. **93**

oxytocin A pituitary hormone that stimulates uterine contractions. **107**

perineum The area between the vulva and the anus. **109**

placenta An organ connected to the fetus by the umbilical cord. The placenta serves as a relay station between mother and fetus, allowing the exchange of nutrients and wastes. **106**

postpartum Following birth. **111**

postpartum depression (PPD) Persistent and severe mood changes during the postpartum period, involving feelings of despair and apathy and characterized by changes in appetite and sleep, low self-esteem, and difficulty concentrating. **111**

preterm Born prior to 37 weeks of gestation. **110**

prophylactic An agent that protects against disease. **96**

prostaglandins Uterine hormones that stimulate uterine contractions. **107**

respiratory distress syndrome A cluster of breathing problems, including weak and irregular breathing, to which preterm babies are especially prone. **111**

spontaneous abortion The involuntary expulsion of the embryo or fetus from the uterus before it is capable of independent life. Also called *miscarriage.* **90**

sterilization Surgical procedures that render people incapable of reproduction without affecting sexual activity. **98**

transition The process during which the cervix becomes nearly fully dilated and the head of the fetus begins to move into the birth canal. **109**

tubal sterilization The most common method of female sterilization, in which the fallopian tubes are surgically severed to prevent the meeting of sperm and ova. **99**

umbilical cord A tube that connects the fetus to the placenta. **106**

vacuum aspiration Removal of the uterine contents by suction. An abortion method used early in pregnancy. **101**

zygote A fertilized ovum. **90**

5. **Q: What types of research could you conduct to determine whether or not there are an excessive number of cesarean sections?**

   A: [Student answers will vary.]

6. **Q: Critical thinkers tackle controversial issues. If a new mother who is experiencing postpartum depression with psychotic features harms her child, should she be held responsible by the law?**

   A: [Student answers will vary.]

Web Exercises

1. Go to http://www.arhp.org, the website of the Association of Reproductive Health Professionals. Click on "Publications & Resources." In the left column, click on "Interactive Tools" and then on "My Method." Take this 5- to 10-minute interactive quiz, and you will get a list of birth control options that appear best suited to you, based on your medical history and lifestyle.
2. Go to http://www.marchofdimes.com, the website of the March of Dimes. Search for "Your Pre-Pregnancy IQ" (at press, retrieved from here: http://marchofdimes.com/pregnancy/getready_quiz.html). Take this short quiz to see if you have accurate knowledge about the effect on a baby of a woman's choices before and during her pregnancy.
3. Go to http://www.healthfinder.gov, a service of the National Health Information Center, U.S. Department of Health and Human Services. Click on "Personal Health Tools" and then "Online Checkups." Click on the letter "P." Click "Pregnancy." Take the quiz "Pregnancy Know-How Quiz," and find out how much you know about being pregnant.

Learning Outcomes

1. **Discuss the concept of addiction and describe various addictive behaviors**
2. **Discuss various kinds of drugs, including prescription and over-the-counter drugs**
3. **Discuss different types of psychoactive drugs and their effects**
4. **Discuss who uses psychoactive drugs**
5. **Explain how people respond to drugs in different ways**
6. **Describe pathways to drug abuse and dependence**
7. **Discuss ways of becoming and remaining drug free**

Chapter Outline

continued

Additional Health APP features available online for Chapter 6:

Health Skills 6-1	What To Do about Compulsive Spending
Prevention 6-1	Using Medications Wisely
Health Check 6-2	Are You a Codependent?
Health Check 6-3	Warning Signs of Drug Dependence
Prevention 6-2	Preventing Drug Abuse
Health Skills 6-3	Self-Help Organizations

HLTH Assets available online for each chapter:

Crossword Puzzles
Flashcards
Glossary
Quizzes

BBC Health Video Titles available online for Chapter 6:

Drug Abuse
Drug Addiction

Critical Thinking Questions

1. **Q: Why is it correct to say that the effects of a drug depend upon the person, not just the drug itself?**

   A: Social setting, the user's frame of mind, gender, and weight can alter the drug's effect on the user.

2. **Q: Agree or disagree with the following statement and support your answer: "I have control over any drugs I am using."**

   A: [Student opinions will vary.]

3. **Q: Agree or disagree with the following statement and support your answer: "The most dangerous drugs are legal and widely available."**

   A: [Student opinions will vary.]

4. **Q: Some people argue that marijuana should be legalized or at least decriminalized. Take one side or the other in this debate and support your argument with evidence supporting your position.**

   A: [Student opinions will vary.]

5. **Q: Many teenagers today have parents who themselves smoked marijuana or used other drugs when they were younger. If you were one of those parents, what would you tell your kids about drugs?**

   A: [Student opinions will vary.]

Web Exercises

1. Go to http://www.acde.org, the website of the American Council for Drug Education. Click on the picture labeled "Youth." Then, choose the "Got the smarts?" knowledge quiz. Take this 20-item quiz about drugs used today and their effects. Answers are provided for each question.
2. Go to http://www.collegedrinkingprevention.gov, a website of the U.S. National Institute on Alcohol Abuse and Alcoholism. Click on the "College Students" section. Choose the "Interactive Body" to trace the flow of alcohol through your body and see how it affects your organs and systems. Or, click on "Alcohol Myths" and find out the facts behind several widely held myths about alcohol.

Key Terms

abstinence syndrome A cluster of withdrawal symptoms that is characteristic of abrupt cessation of use of a particular drug. **116**

amphetamine psychosis An acute psychotic reaction induced by the ingestion of amphetamines that mimics acute episodes of paranoid schizophrenia. **124**

amphetamines A class of synthetic stimulants. **124**

anabolic steroid Synthetic version of the male sex hormone testosterone. **129**

antagonist A drug that blocks or neutralizes the effects of another. **133**

antihistamine A drug that blocks the actions of histamine, a substance released in the body during an allergic reaction. **130**

caffeine A mild stimulant found in coffee beans, tea, cola beverages, and chocolate. **126**

club drugs (designer drugs) Synthetic drugs manufactured in illicit labs that are chemical analogues (drugs having similar properties and effects) of illegal drugs. **128**

cocaine psychosis An acute psychotic reaction induced by the use of cocaine, often involving paranoid delusions. **125**

codependent A person involved in a close relationship with a drug-dependent person who plays a part in enabling or maintaining the other person's chemical dependency. **136**

deliriant A substance that induces delirium, or a state of gross mental confusion, excitability, and disorientation. **127**

depressants Drugs such as barbiturates, tranquilizers, opiates, and alcohol that lower the rate of nervous system activity. **123**

detoxification The process of eliminating drugs from a person's body, usually taking place under supervised conditions where withdrawal symptoms can be monitored and controlled. **137**

dose-response relationship The relationship between the dosage level of a drug and its effects on the individual, usually expressed in the form of a graph showing the drug's effects at specific dosage levels. **132**

drug Chemical agent that affects biological functions. **119**

drug abuse Persistent use of a drug despite the fact that use of the drug is harmful to the user's health, impairs the user's ability to function, or exposes the user or others to dangerous situations. **133**

drug misuse The use of a drug for a purpose for which it was not intended, or in ways that deviate from the correct use of the drug. **119**

endorphins Naturally occurring chemicals in the body that are similar in their effects to opiates. **135**

gateway drug A drug serving as a "stepping-stone" or gateway to use of other, usually "harder," drugs. **136**

hallucinogenic A drug that produces hallucinations. **127**

inhalants Chemical fumes that are inhaled for their psychoactive effects. **128**

marijuana Derived from the *cannabis sativa* plant, a drug with relaxant and mild hallucinogenic effects. **128**

methadone A synthetic opiate that is used as a substitute for heroin in the treatment of heroin addiction. **137**

narcotics Drugs, primarily opiates, that have sleep-inducing and pain-relieving effects with a high potential for addiction. **123**

over-the-counter (OTC) drug A drug available for sale without a prescription. **119**

pharmacology The study of drugs and their role in medicine. **119**

pharmacy The discipline relating to the preparation and dispensing of drugs. **119**

physiological addiction A state of physical need for a drug, characterized by the development of a withdrawal syndrome following abrupt cessation of the use of the substance. **116**

potentiate Relating to drugs, to enhance a drug's effects or potency. **133**

psychoactive drugs Drugs that act on the brain to affect mental processes. **120**

psychological addiction A pattern of compulsive behavior or habitual use of a drug indicating impaired control but without physiological signs of dependence. **115**

sedative A central nervous system depressant that has calming and relaxing effects. **123**

stimulant Psychoactive drug that increases the level of activity of the central nervous system. **124**

synergistic effect As applied to drug interactions, the action of two or more drugs operating together to enhance the overall effect to a level greater than the sum of the effects of each drug operating by itself. **133**

tolerance A feature of drug dependence in which the user comes to need larger amounts or doses of the drug to achieve the same effect. **116**

toxicity The quality or degree of being poisonous. **133**

Learning Outcomes

1 Explain what alcohol is

2 Explain which segments of the population are most likely to drink

3 Describe the effects of alcohol

4 Define *alcohol abuse* and *dependence*

5 Discuss the causes of alcoholism

6 Describe various methods of treating alcoholism

7 Explain which segments of the population are most likely to smoke

8 Explain why people smoke

9 Describe the effects of smoking on health

10 Discuss the health benefits of quitting smoking

Chapter Outline

continued

Additional Health APP features available online for Chapter 7:

Health Check 7-1	Why Do *You* Drink?
Prevention 7-2	Preventing Youthful Drinking and Driving
Diversity 7-2	Ethnicity and Alcoholism
Health Skills 7-1	Getting a Handle on the ABCs of Your Drinking
Prevention 7-3	Preventing Smoking
Diversity 7-4	Smoking and Ethnic Minorities
Health Check 7-3	Are You Addicted to Nicotine?
Health Skills 7-2	Becoming an Ex-Smoker

HLTH Assets available online for each chapter:

Crossword Puzzles
Flashcards
Glossary
Quizzes

Critical Thinking Questions

1. **Q: Jamie does something while drinking that Jamie would not otherwise do. Is Jamie responsible for his or her behavior while drinking? Explain your view.**

   A: [Student opinions will vary.]

2. **Q: What is the lure of drinking to underage students? What do you think can be done to change the attitudes of young people toward drinking?**

   A: [Student opinions will vary.]

3. **Q: Do you believe that people who were addicted to alcohol can never touch another drop without becoming addicted again? Why or why not?**

   A: Student opinions will vary, although the medical model supports this premise.

4. **Q: Recognizing that smoking is the most preventable cause of premature death, what should society do, if anything, to protect the health of its citizens?**

   A: [Student opinions will vary.]

5. **Q: Have you heard smokers claim that they could give up their habits anytime they want to? Do you believe them? Why or why not?**

   A: Student opinions will vary, although tolerance, physical dependence, and withdrawal all occur, making it difficult to quit.

6. **Q: What should society do, if anything, about protecting children from secondhand smoking in the home? Do we need additional laws to protect children from tobacco smoke? Or should we focus on public health campaigns targeting parents to draw attention to the problem? What do you think? Support your answer.**

   A: [Student opinions will vary.]

Key Terms

alcohol abuse A pattern of misuse of alcohol in which heavy or continued drinking becomes associated with health problems and/or impaired social functioning. **149**

alcohol dependence A physical dependence on, or addiction to, alcohol that is characterized by a loss of control over the use of the substance. Also called *alcoholism*. **149**

alcoholic hepatitis An inflammation of the liver caused by viruses, chronic alcoholism, or exposure to toxic materials. **148**

aversive conditioning A technique of behavior therapy involving the pairing of noxious stimuli, such as nausea or electric shock, with undesirable behavior, for the purpose of acquiring a conditioned aversion to the stimuli associated with the undesirable behavior. **153**

blackout Episode involving a loss of consciousness. **150**

carbon monoxide An odorless, poisonous flammable gas produced from the burning of carbon with insufficient air. **154**

carcinogenic Cancer-causing. **160**

chewing tobacco Tobacco leaves that have been prepared for chewing or sucking when lodged between the cheek and gum. **154**

chronic obstructive pulmonary disease (COPD) A disease process that results in diminished capacity of the lungs to perform respiration. Chronic bronchitis and emphysema are among the leading causes. **159**

cirrhosis of the liver A disease of the liver in which scar tissue comes to replace healthy liver tissue. **148**

delirium tremens A withdrawal syndrome in chronic alcoholics occurring following a sudden reduction or cessation of drinking; denoted by extreme restlessness, sweating, disorientation, and hallucinations. **150**

distillation As applied to the making of distilled spirits, a process of boiling out the alcohol from the fermentation process and then condensing the vapors back into a liquid form. **141**

dopamine A type of neurotransmitter that is believed to be involved in brain mechanisms regulating states of pleasure as well as other functions. **153**

ethanol Another term for ethyl alcohol. **140**

fatty liver A condition involving an accumulation of fat in the liver, causing enlargement of the organ. **148**

fermentation As applied to the making of alcoholic beverages, a process by which yeast plants are used to convert sugar in grains into ethyl alcohol and carbon dioxide. **140**

intoxication A state of drunkenness brought on by the use of alcohol or other intoxicating drugs. **144**

nicotine A stimulant drug found naturally in tobacco. **153**

proof The alcoholic strength of a beverage, expressed by a number that is twice the percentage of alcohol in the beverage. **141**

seizure A sudden attack involving a disruption of brain electrical rhythms, as in the type of convulsive seizures occurring during epileptic attacks. **150**

sidestream smoking Ingestion of tobacco smoke from other people's lit cigarettes. **156**

smoker's face A characteristic wrinkling of the face due to smoke, denoted by the appearance of many fine wrinkles emanating in spoke-like projections from the lips and eyes. **160**

snuff A powdered form of tobacco that can be inhaled through the nose or sucked when placed inside the cheek. **154**

tar The sticky residue in tobacco smoke, containing many carcinogens and other toxins. **154**

tobacco A member of a family of plants containing nicotine whose leaves are prepared for smoking, chewing, or use as snuff. **153**

Wernicke-Korsakoff's syndrome A form of memory impairment related to chronic alcoholism and deficiencies of the vitamin thiamine. **148**

Web Exercises

1. Go to http://www.mayoclinic.com, sponsored by the Mayo Clinic. From the bar at the top, choose "Diseases and Conditions" and then choose "Alcoholism." From the top tab choose "In Depth" and then select "Alcohol-use: Do you have a drinking problem?" Take this eight-item self-assessment to rate your drinking habits and explore solutions.
2. Drinking too much? Go to this site to test your use or abuse of alcohol: http://counsellingresource.com/lib/quizzes/drug-testing/alcohol-mast. This 22-question quiz is based on the current revised version of the Michigan Alcohol Screening Test (MAST), one of the most widely used measures for assessing alcohol abuse, designed to provide a rapid and effective screening for lifetime alcohol-related problems.
3. Go to http://www.healthfinder.gov, a service of the National Health Information Center, U.S. Department of Health and Human Services. Click on the letter "S." Click "Secondhand Smoke." Choose the "Secondhand Smoke Quiz." Take this 10-item quiz and find out how much you know about secondhand smoke and respiratory disease.

prepcard/ CHAPTER 8 FITNESS FOR LIFE

Learning Outcomes

1. Describe the physical and psychological health benefits of exercise
2. Explain how to begin to get fit
3. Describe the uses of aerobic exercise
4. Describe the uses of anaerobic exercise
5. Discuss the benefits of stretching
6. Describe exercise injuries—how to prevent them, how to treat them

Chapter Outline

Key Terms

aerobic exercise Strenuous physical activity that requires a sustained increase in the use of oxygen by the body. **167**

afterburner effect The increased rate of metabolism of fat following exercise. **171**

anaerobic exercise Exercise involving short bursts of intense muscle activity. **173**

cardiac output The amount of blood the heart pumps per minute. **171**

Additional Health APP features available online for Chapter 8:

Health Skills 8-1	How Much Exercise Do You Need?
Health Skills 8-2	Which Kinds of Exercise Are Right for You?
Health Skills 8-3	Guidelines for Muscle-Strengthening Exercises
Health Skills 8-4	Take a Hike! Walking for Fitness
Health Skills 8-5	Making Exercise Part of Your Lifestyle
Prevention 8-1	Overtraining: Are You Doing Too Much of a Good Thing?
Prevention 8-2	Preventing Exercise-Related Injuries

HLTH Assets available online for each chapter:

Crossword Puzzles
Flashcards
Glossary
Quizzes

BBC Health Video Titles available online for Chapter 8:

Workout Mistakes
Exercise and Depression
Sports Nutrition

Exercise Demonstration Videos (see entire list on CourseMate for HLTH)

Strength-Training Exercises with Weights
Strength-Training Exercises without Weights
Stability Ball Exercises
Exercise Test Videos

Critical Thinking Questions

1. **Q: What are the benefits of exercise on physical and psychological health?**

A: Physically inactive people have double the risk of developing heart disease than their active peers. Exercise helps to maintain a healthy weight and improve body composition. It boosts the functioning of the immune system. Exercise may reduce the risk of some forms of cancer and increases energy levels.

Regular exercise can enhance mood, lessening feelings of tension and depression. Completing a work-out can act as a stress reliever and increase self confidence.

cardiorespiratory fitness The ability of the heart, lungs, and blood vessels to provide muscles with sufficient amounts of oxygen to sustain vigorous activity for an extended period of time. Also called *aerobic fitness* or *aerobic endurance.* **168**

cardiovascular system The system composed of the heart, lungs, and blood vessels that carries oxygen-rich blood through the body and delivers oxygen to all body tissues, including muscles. **166**

cartilage Tough, flexible type of connective tissue that covers the surface of a joint, serving as padding or a "shock absorber" for the joint. **178**

exercise A structured sequence of movements performed consistently over a period of time sufficient to build the components of fitness. **166**

fitness The ability to perform moderate to vigorous levels of physical activity without undue fatigue. **166**

flexibility The ability of the joints to move through their entire range of motion without undue stress. Flexibility is measured by the length and amount of stretch in the tissues surrounding the joints. **175**

fracture A broken bone. **178**

immune system The body's system of defense for identifying and eradicating invading bacteria and viruses as well as diseased, mutated, and worn-out cells. **167**

insulin A hormone produced by the pancreas that plays an essential role in the metabolism of blood sugar (glucose) and the maintenance of a proper level of blood sugar. **168**

isokinetic exercise Exercise in which muscles contract against resistance that varies with the user's level of exertion throughout the range of motion; requires use of exercise machines. **175**

isometric exercise Working a muscle by contracting it in a stationary position, such as by pushing against a wall or other immovable object. **174**

isotonic exercise Exercise in which muscles repeatedly contract under constant resistance throughout the range of motion; most weight-training exercises are of this type. **174**

ligament Tough, fibrous tissue that connects two bones together at a joint. **177**

muscle atrophy Deterioration or loss of muscle tone. **174**

muscle endurance The ability to contract muscles repeatedly over time. **169**

muscle strength The amount of force, or power, a person can apply with one or more muscles in a single contraction. **169**

natural killer (NK) cell A type of white blood cell that kills viruses. **167**

2. Q: Why can you experience gain from exercise without incurring pain?

A: When exercising, it is important to allow your body to adjust to increased demands slowly. Employ the general principles of training: specificity, overload, warm-up, cool-down, and regularity.

3. Q: How can you tell if an exercise injury requires medical attention?

A: Seek medical assistance for any injury that produces sharp pain, persistent swelling, fracture, ruptured tendon, weather-related injuries, or any other injury that you feel should be evaluated by a health-care professional. Remember, "when in doubt, check it out".

Web Exercises

1. Go to http://www.caloriecontrol.org, the website of the Calorie Control Council. Click on the section titled "Get Moving! Calculator." Choose your favorite activity or exercise from a list of dozens, type in the number of minutes you plan to do this activity, and your weight. Click "compute," and the site will provide an estimate of the number of calories you will burn based on moderate, not vigorous, activity. This site also provides a "Calorie Counter" that tells you the number of calories and fat grams in a serving of various foods.
2. Go to http://www.americaonthemove.org. America on the Move is a national initiative to help people improve their health and quality of life. The goal is to get individuals and various types of groups (community, work, and faith groups, for example) to register and follow their program by making two basic daily changes: Take 2,000 more steps (about one mile) and eat 100 fewer calories (about a pat of butter). Individuals or groups who register will get an e-program for setting health goals, motivation tools, links to health information, a health e-newsletter, a place to record progress, and daily health tips. Begin becoming more active today!

osteoarthritis A chronic, degenerative disease of the joints that produces pain and restricted movement. More commonly called *arthritis.* **168**

osteoporosis A degenerative condition of the bones characterized by the loss of bone density, which makes bones more brittle and prone to break. **168**

overloading The process of gradually increasing the stressful burden placed on the body to achieve a training effect. **169**

range of motion The arc of motion of a joint, or the extent to which a joint can be moved through its normal spectrum. **169**

resistance training Muscle training involving repeated movement or lifting against an opposing force or weight. **168**

resting heart rate The number of times per minute the heart beats while the person is resting. **171**

R.I.C.E. principle A program of rest, ice, compression, and elevation used in the treatment of exercise-related injuries. **179**

shin splints Injuries similar to stress fractures but involving tears in muscle fibers rather than tiny breaks in bone. **179**

sprain An injury caused by a sudden joint twist that stretches or tears a ligament. **177**

static stretching Slowly stretching a muscle to an extended stretch and holding it for 10 to 30 seconds. **175**

strain A stretch (or muscle pull) or actual tear in muscle fibers or surrounding tissue. **177**

stress fracture A microscopic break in a bone (such as in the foot, shin, or thigh) caused by repeated and excessive pressure or pounding. **178**

stress test A medical test for determining cardiorespiratory fitness by measuring oxygen consumption and heart functioning during strenuous exercise; commonly involves the use of a treadmill or stationary bicycle. **177**

target heart rate (THR) The recommended range of heartbeats per minute during vigorous exercise intended to improve cardiorespiratory fitness. **171**

tendon Fibrous connective tissue that attaches muscle to bone in the body. **178**

tendonitis Inflammation of a tendon. **178**

tibia The larger of the two bones of the lower leg, extending from the knee to the ankle. **179**

training The gradual adjustment of the body to increasingly higher demands through a structured sequence of repetitive and progressive movements. Also called *conditioning.* **169**

training effect The benefits to the heart, lungs, muscles, and bones produced by overloading. **169**

triglycerides A type of lipid or fatty substance found in the blood. **167**

prepcard/ CHAPTER 9 NUTRITION FOR LIFE

Learning Outcomes

1 Describe tips for eating right based on the *Dietary Guidelines for Americans*

2 Describe the functions and sources of proteins

3 Describe the functions, types, and sources of carbohydrates

4 Describe the functions of fats and health implications of excess fat intake

5 Describe the functions of vitamins and how to obtain them

6 Describe the functions of minerals and how to obtain them

7 Describe the nutritional roles of water and electrolytes and the risks of excess sodium intake

Chapter Outline

continued

Additional Health APP features available online for Chapter 9:

Health Skills 9-2	How to Cut Fat from Your Diet
Diversity 9-1	Ethnic Food—Eating Out, Eating Smart
Prevention 9-2	Preventing Vitamin Deficiency Syndromes
Prevention 9-3	Should You Take Vitamin Supplements?
Prevention 9-4	Minerals
Health Skills 9-4	Cutting Back on Sodium
Prevention 9-5	Ensuring Food Safety

HLTH Assets available online for each chapter:

Crossword Puzzles
Flashcards
Glossary
Quizzes

BBC Health Video Titles available online for Chapter 9:

Eating for Exercise
America and Diets
Eating Disorders and the Media
Eating Disorders and Talking Therapy
Food Poisoning

Critical Thinking Questions

1. **Q. Do you believe that government should have a role in helping people adopt healthier diets? Why or why not?**

   A: [Student opinions will vary.]

2. **Q: Agree or disagree with the following statement, and support your answer: "People generally don't consume enough protein in their diet."**

   A: [Student opinions will vary.]

3. **Q: What are the two major types of carbohydrates? How do carbohydrates contribute to our health?**

   A: The two major types of carbohydrates are complex starches and simple sugars; they contribute to your health by providing energy.

4. **Q: What might you say to someone who claims that carbohydrates are unhealthy for you?**

   A: Student opinions will vary, but note that nutritionists recommend that complex carbohydrates should comprise about half of our diet.

5. **Q: Agree or disagree with the following statement, and support your answer: "Megadosing on vitamins is too much of a good thing."**

   A: [Student opinions will vary.]

6. **Q: How do the different kinds of minerals contribute to our health?**

   A: Ingesting adequate levels of vitamins prevents vitamin deficiency syndromes, reduces the risk of osteoporosis, reduces the risk of aggressive prostate cancer, relieves PMS symptoms, and relieves asthma in some cases.

7. **Q: How do water and electrolytes contribute to your health?**

   A: Water transports nutrients, removes waists, and regulates body temperature. Electrolytes conduct electrical currents in the body through the nervous system.

Web Exercises

1. Go to http://www.nal.usda.gov/fnic, a site sponsored by the Food and Nutrition Center (FNIC) at the National Agricultural Library (NAL). Select the Search function and type, "Do you know your vitamin ABCs?" Click on this title at the top of the result list. Take this 30-item quiz to check your knowledge of the role of vitamins and minerals in body health.
2. Go to http://www.eatsmart.org, a site sponsored by the Washington State Dairy Council. From the left-hand topic bar, choose "Nutrition Cafe." Play each of the three nutrition games: Nutrition Sleuth (clues lead you the nutrient the character is missing), Grab a Grape (provides the answer to a nutrition question, and you click on the question), and Have-a-Bite Café (choose the components of a meal, and find out if you chose wisely).
3. Go to http://www.healthfinder.gov, a site sponsored by the National Health Information Center, U.S. Department of Health and Human Services. Under "Personal Health Tools" click "Online Checkups." Under N, choose Nutrition, and then click on the quiz titled "Test Your Food Label Knowledge!" Test how well you can read food labels for nutrition facts.

Key Terms

amino acids Organic compounds that are the building blocks from which proteins are made. **185**

anemia A condition involving a lack of hemoglobin in the blood, causing such symptoms as weakness, paleness, heart palpitations, shortness of breath, and lack of vigor. **200**

antioxidants Agents that prevent or inhibit oxidation; they are believed to have healthful benefits by reducing the build-up of free radicals in the body. **197**

calcium A mineral essential to the growth and maintenance of bones. **198**

calorie A measure of food energy, which is equivalent to the amount of energy required to raise the temperature of one gram of water by one degree Celsius. **185**

carbohydrates Organic compounds forming the structural parts of plants that are important sources of nutrition for animals and humans. **185**

cholesterol A natural, fat-like substance found in humans and animals. **189**

complex carbohydrates A class of carbohydrates that includes starches and fibers. **185**

dietary fiber Complex carbohydrates that form the structural parts of plants, such as cellulose and pectin, that cannot be broken down by human digestive enzymes. **185**

electrolyte A substance that conducts electricity. **200**

essential amino acids Amino acids essential to survival that must be obtained from the food we eat since the body is unable to manufacture them on its own. **185**

fat Organic compound that forms the basis of fatty tissue of animals, including humans ("body fat"), and is also found in some plant materials. **188**

flavonoids A group of antioxidant compounds found in plants that may have healthful benefits. **198**

folic acid A B vitamin, also known as *folate*, which helps prevent neural-tube defects and may play a role in preventing heart disease. **198**

free radical Metabolic waste product produced during normal oxidation, which may damage cell membranes and genetic material. **197**

hemoglobin A protein in red blood cells, which gives blood its reddish color and transports oxygen to body cells. **198**

high-density lipoprotein (HDL) The so-called good cholesterol because it sweeps away cholesterol deposits from artery walls for elimination from the body, thereby lowering the risk of cardiovascular disease. **192**

insoluble fiber Type of dietary fiber that is not dissolvable in water. **186**

iron An essential mineral, it is a metallic element that forms part of the makeup of hemoglobin. **199**

lipoprotein A compound or complex of fat and protein by which fats are transported through the bloodstream. **191**

low-density lipoprotein (LDL) The so-called bad cholesterol because it can stick to artery walls, forming fatty deposits that restrict the flow of blood to vital body organs, setting the stage for heart attacks and strokes. **191**

metabolism The organic process by which food is changed into energy and assimilated into bodily tissue to sustain life and promote growth. **195**

minerals Inorganic elements obtained from the food we eat that are essential to survival. **198**

phytochemical Naturally occurring plant chemical. **198**

protein Organic molecule that forms the basic building blocks of body tissues. **185**

simple carbohydrates A class of carbohydrates consisting of small molecules, including various sugars. **200**

sodium A metallic element that functions as an electrolyte in the body. **186**

soluble fiber A type of dietary fiber that is dissolvable in water. **186**

starch A complex carbohydrate that forms an important part of the structure of plants such as corn, rice, wheat, potatoes, and beans. **185**

sugar A sweet-tasting simple carbohydrate, present in different forms in many of the foods we eat. **187**

trans-fatty acid A type of fatty acid produced in the hardening process of margarine that can raise blood cholesterol levels. **191**

vitamins Organic substances required in minute amounts to serve a variety of vital roles in metabolism, growth, and maintenance of bodily processes. **195**

prepcard/ CHAPTER 10 MANAGING YOUR WEIGHT

Learning Outcomes

1. Describe the relationship between calories and weight
2. Explain theories and evidence as to why people become overweight
3. Discuss the eating disorders, their origins, and their treatment

Chapter Outline

Additional Health APP features available online for Chapter 10:

Health Skills 10-1 Skills of Effective Weight Management

HLTH Assets available online for each chapter:

Crossword Puzzles
Flashcards
Glossary
Quizzes

BBC Health Video Titles available online for Chapter 10:

Diet
Diet Crazes
America and Diets
Eating Disorders and the Media
Eating Disorders and Talking Therapy

Critical Thinking Questions

1. **Q: What is the connection between calories and weight?**

   A: Calories in food > calories used = weight gain
   Calories in food < calories used = weight loss
   Calories in food = calories used = weight control

2. **Q: Why does the text emphasize achieving a healthy weight rather than a slender build?**

   A: BMI is used as an indicator of weight ranges. Each of us should seek to be healthy within our body's parameters.

3. **Q: Agree or disagree with the following statement, and support your answer: "Obese people simply lack willpower."**

   A: Obesity is a complex problem consisting of an interrelationship between heredity, body metabolism, and activity level.

4. **Q: What happens to metabolism when people restrict their calorie intake?**

   A: The body conforms to the metabolic needs and regulates itself at a lesser level.

5. **Q: Why do you think women are more likely than men to develop anorexia and bulimia?**

   A: In our society, social cultural pressures to conform to the media's ideal slender body, desire to remain a young girl to avoid adult responsibilities, perfectionism, and control intertwine to cause the complexity of eating disorders.

Key Terms

adipose tissue The body tissue in which fat is stored. **209**

amenorrhea Absence of menstruation. **217**

anorexia nervosa An eating disorder characterized by the maintenance of an unusually low and unhealthy body weight and accompanied by an intense fear of gaining weight, a distorted body image, and, in females, an absence of menstruation (*amenorrhea*). **216**

basal metabolic rate (BMR) The minimum amount of energy needed to maintain bodily functions, apart from digestion. **204**

behavior modification A set of psychological interventions that apply the principles of learning to help people change their behavior. **220**

binge-eating disorder A type of eating disorder characterized by recurrent binges that are not accompanied by purging. **220**

bioelectrical impedance analysis A method of measuring body fat composition by analyzing the changes in electrical conductance (impedance) as a mild electric current is passed through the body. **207**

body mass index (BMI) A measure of obesity that takes into account both weight and height. It is calculated by dividing body weight (in kilograms) by the square of the person's height (in meters). **205**

bulimia nervosa An eating disorder characterized by repeated episodes of binge eating followed by purging, and accompanied by persistent fears of gaining weight. **217**

eating disorder Disturbance of eating behavior, including anorexia nervosa and bulimia nervosa. **211**

fat cell Body cell that stores fat. **209**

hydrostatic weighing A method of measuring body weight by weighing a person both underwater and on dry land and comparing the results. **207**

hypothalamus A structure in the midbrain that is involved in regulating body temperature, emotional states, and motivational states such as hunger and thirst. **209**

obesity A condition of excess body fat. **206**

overweight A body weight exceeding desirable weight for an individual of a given age, height, and body frame, usually based on a criteria of a weight exceeding 20% above the desirable weight. **206**

resting metabolic rate (RMR) The minimum energy that the body requires to maintain bodily functions including digestion. **204**

skinfold thickness The thickness of the folds of skin, usually of the underarms, waist, or back, which is used to estimate the percentage of body fat. **209**

set point theory The theory that the brain regulates body weight around a genetically predetermined level or "set point." **207**

Web Exercises

1. Go to http://familydoctor.org, a website from the American Academy of Family Physicians. Click "Health Tools" and click on "BMI Calculator." Type in your height, weight, and gender, and click on "Body Mass Index Calculator." The site provides your BMI as well as your possible risk of health problems.
2. Go to http://www.eatright.org, the website of the American Dietetic Association. Search for the feature "Rate Your Plate" and take the interactive quiz to determine if you're on the right track with your eating habits (at time of press, the quiz was found at this URL: http://www.eatright.org/nnm/games/quiz/index.html).
3. Go to http://www.ftc.gov, the website of the U.S. Federal Trade Commission. Search for and read the article "Weighing the Evidence in Diet Ads" (at time of press, the URL was http://ftc.gov/bcp/edu/pubs/consumer/health/hea03.shtm). Find at least three online, newspaper, magazine, or TV ads that rely on the false claims listed in the article.

Figure 10-1 Heavier than Ever

Americans have eaten themselves into a situation in which two-thirds of all adults are overweight, and more than half of the overweight are obese.

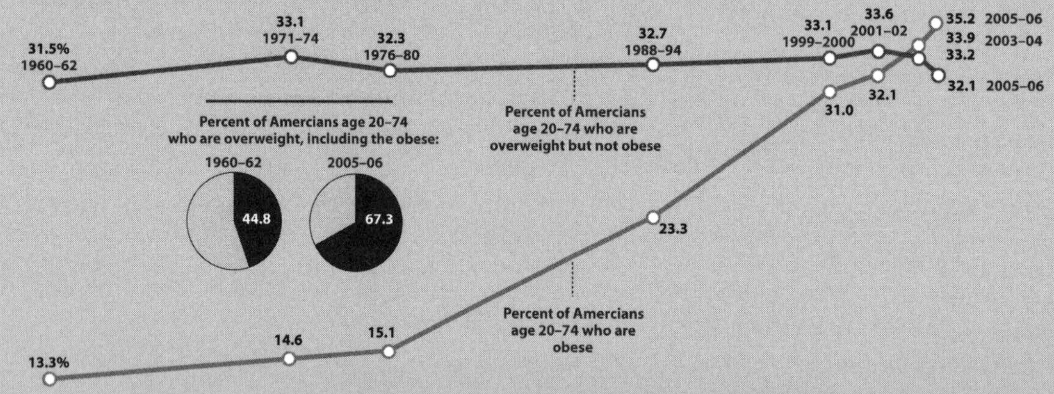

1960s 1961: The Kennedy administration revamps the President's Council on Youth Fitness.

1970s 1974: Richard Simmons opens the Slimmons exercise studio.

1980s 1982: Jane Fonda releases her first exercise video.

1990s 1996: Madonna takes up yoga to get back in shape following the birth of her daughter.

2000s 2006: Nintendo introduces the Wii, ushering in "lounge fitness."

2010s 2010: Michelle Obama introduces Let's Move, a campaign to fight childhood obesity.

Source: Adapted from graphic in *The New York Times*, accessed online at http://www.nytimes.com/interactive/2011/01/30/weekinreview/30marsh.html?ref=weekinreview

prepcard/ CHAPTER 11 COMBATING CARDIOVASCULAR DISEASE, CANCER, AND OTHER MAJOR DISEASES

Learning Outcomes

1. Describe the cardiovascular system
2. Discuss the major forms of cardiovascular disease
3. Describe methods of diagnosing and treating cardiovascular disease
4. List and discuss the risk factors for cardiovascular disease
5. Discuss the nature of cancer and how it develops.
6. List and discuss the causes of cancer
7. Discuss the similarities and differences among various types of cancer
8. Discuss the nature, incidence, and control of diabetes
9. Discuss the major forms of chronic obstructive pulmonary disease

Chapter Outline

continued

Additional Health APP features available online for Chapter 11:

Health Check 11-1 Heart Quiz
Diversity 11-1 High Blood Pressure and Ethnicity
Prevention 11-1 Aspirin: Not Just for Headaches Anymore
Health Check 11-2 Estimating Your Risk of a Heart Attack
Health Skills 11-1 Dieting to Cut Your Cholesterol Level
Diversity 11-3 Racial/Ethnic Differences in Cancer Risk
Health Skills 11-2 New Methods of Combating Cancer
Health Skills 11-3 Living with Cancer
Health Skills 11-4 Protecting Yourself from Cancer and Other Chronic Diseases

Key Terms

angina Heart pain arising from insufficient blood flow to the heart. **227**

arrhythmia An irregular heart rhythm. **230**

arteries Blood vessels that carry blood from the heart and connect to capillaries that deliver oxygen-rich blood to body tissues. **225**

arteriosclerosis A condition in which the walls of arteries become thicker and harder and lose elasticity. Commonly called *hardening of the arteries*. **226**

atrium The upper chamber in each half of the heart. **224**

basal cell carcinoma (BCC) A form of nonmelanoma skin cancer; it is easily curable if detected and treated early. It appears as translucent, pearly raised tumors, usually found on the skin of the face, neck, hands, and trunk. **253**

cancer Any of more than 100 diseases characterized by the development of malignant tumors, which may invade surrounding tissues and spread to other sites in the body through they lymphatic system and bloodstream. **238**

capillaries Tiny blood vessels that carry blood from the smallest arteries directly to the cells and connect to the tiniest veins for transport of deoxygenated blood and cellular waste products. **225**

carcinogen A cancer-causing substance. **240**

carcinoma Cancer that originates in the epithelial tissues of the body. **244**

cardiomyopathy A disease of the heart muscle or myocardium. **234**

cardiopulmonary resuscitation (CPR) An emergency medical treatment used to restore coronary and pulmonary functioning following cardiac arrest. **230**

cardiovascular disease A disease of the heart or blood vessels. **223**

circulatory system The system or network of blood vessels that carries blood throughout the body. **224**

congenital heart defect A heart defect that is present at birth. **229**

congestive heart failure A condition in which the heart is unable to pump out as much blood as it receives, leading to a backing-up or pooling of blood in the veins, lungs, and extremities. **229**

coronary heart disease (CHD) A disease usually caused by damage to coronary arteries in which the blood supply to the heart is reduced to a level that is insufficient to meet the heart's needs. **225**

diabetes mellitus A metabolic disease involving insufficient production of insulin or a failure of cells to utilize the insulin that is produced, which leads to high glucose levels building up in the blood while cells remain starved for the glucose they need. **255**

diastolic blood pressure (DBP) The minimum pressure that remains in the arteries when the heart relaxes between beats. **228**

emphysema A lung disease involving destruction of the walls of the air sacs (alveoli) in the lungs. The most common symptom of emphysema is breathlessness upon exertion. **257**

erythrocytes Red blood cells; they carry oxygen to cells. **225**

gestational diabetes Diabetes developed during pregnancy. **257**

Hodgkin's disease A rare type of lymphoma characterized by enlargement of the lymph nodes, named after Thomas Hodgkin (1798–1866), a London physician who described its symptoms. **255**

hypertension High blood pressure, generally determined by a blood pressure reading of 140 (systolic)/90 (diastolic) or higher. **228**

insulin A hormone produced by the pancreas that allows cells to take up glucose from the bloodstream. **256**

ionizing radiation Powerful, high-energy radiation capable of causing atoms to become electrically charged or ionized. **243**

leukemia Cancer that forms in the blood and blood-forming tissues of the body. **244**

leukocytes White blood cells; they combat infection. **225**

lymphoma Cancer that forms in the cells of the lymphatic system. **244**

melanoma A potentially deadly form of cancer involving the formation of cancerous growths in melanin-forming cells, most commonly in the skin but sometimes in other parts of the body containing such cells, such as the eye. **244**

metastases Secondary tumors that arise from the primary growth in a new location in the body. Cancers that metastasize are those that spread from one body part to another. **239**

myocardial infarction (MI) A condition involving damage or death of heart tissue due to insufficient blood flow to the heart, usually as the result of a blockage in one or more coronary arteries. **226**

non-Hodgkin's lymphomas All forms of lymphoma (cancers of the lymphatic system) other than Hodgkin's disease. **255**

oncogenes Genes involved in regulating cell growth that in mutated form can promote the development of cancerous growths. **240**

pancreas A gland located near the stomach that secretes a digestive fluid into the intestines and manufactures the hormone insulin. **256**

Pap test The scraping of a "smear" of cells from the vagina and cervix for microscopic examination to reveal the presence of cancer. Also called a *Pap smear*; named after its developer, George Papanicolaou (1883–1962). **248**

platelets Round or oval disks in the blood that help blood clot when there is a wound or injury. **225**

polyps Bulging masses of tissue in the colon, which may become cancerous. **250**

sarcoma Cancer that originates in connective tissues of the body. **244**

squamous cell carcinoma (SCC) A form of nonmelanoma skin cancer, which like basal cell carcinoma, is easily curable if detected and treated early. It appears as a reddish or pinkish raised nodule, usually on the face, hands, or ears. **253**

stroke The sudden loss of consciousness and resulting paralysis, loss of sensation, and other disability or death resulting from blockage of blood to a part of the brain or bleeding in the brain. Also called a *cerebrovascular accident* or *CVA*. **226**

suppressor genes Genes that curb cell division and suppress development of tumors. **240**

systolic blood pressure (SBP) The maximum pressure in the arteries that occurs when the heart contacts with each heartbeat. **228**

triglycerides The main type of fat carried through the bloodstream and stored in the body's fatty tissue. **237**

tumor A mass of excess body tissue or growth that may or may not be cancerous **239**

Type 1 diabetes A form of diabetes that usually develops in childhood or young adulthood in which the person requires daily doses of insulin to make up for the deficient production by the pancreas. Previously called *juvenile diabetes* or *insulin-dependent diabetes mellitus (IDDM)*. **256**

Type 2 diabetes A type of diabetes that usually develops in middle or later life involving a breakdown in the body's use of insulin. Previously called *adult-onset diabetes* or *noninsulin-dependent diabetes mellitus (NIDM)*. **256**

ultraviolet A (UVA) A form of ultraviolet radiation from sunlight that can damage the skin and eyes. **253**

ultraviolet B (UVB) A more dangerous form of ultraviolet radiation from sunlight that is principally responsible for sunburns. **253**

veins Blood vessels that carry blood back to the heart. **225**

vena cava The largest veins, which carry blood directly into the heart. **225**

ventricle The lower chamber in each half of the heart. **224**

prepcard/ CHAPTER 12 INFECTION AND IMMUNITY

Learning Outcomes

1. Discuss the nature of infection, types of pathogens, and the course of infections
2. Describe the body's defenses against infection
3. Discuss immunity and immunization
4. Describe common infectious diseases
5. Discuss the causes, transmission, symptoms, diagnosis, and treatment of sexually transmitted infections

Chapter Outline

Additional Health APP features available online for Chapter 12:

Prevention 12-1 Wash Those Hands!
Diversity 12-1 Children and Immunizations—Many Aren't Protected
Prevention 12-3 Protecting Yourself from Lyme Disease
Health Skills 12-2 Toward Safer Sex

HLTH Assets available online for each chapter:

Crossword Puzzles
Flashcards
Glossary
Quizzes

BBC Health Video Titles available online for Chapter 12:

HIV Virus and Children
HPV Virus Vaccine
Tuberculosis Vaccine

Critical Thinking Questions

1. **Q: Agree or disagree and support your answer: "People provide their personal best defense against most infectious illnesses."**

   A: [Student opinions will vary.]

2. **Q: Why do you think it is important to understand what the incubation period of an infectious disease is?**

   A: [Student opinions will vary.]

3. **Q: Why do you think it is important to consult a health care provider if you suspect that you may not be fully recovered from an infection?**

   A: [Student opinions will vary (e.g. if one has not recovered, additional illness may be the issue or the original treatment was not effective).]

4. **Q: How can you make a distinction between a cold and the flu? Why is it important to make the distinction?**

   A: About 200 different viruses cause the common cold. Symptoms include nasal congestion, sore throat, fatigue, headache, and perhaps a low-grade fever. Colds typically last one to two weeks.

   Influenza, or "the flu," is a highly contagious viral disease that affects the lungs and other parts of the body. People with the flu experience an abrupt onset of a fever between 102° and 104° Fahrenheit, chills, headache, general aches and pains, fatigue, weakness, and possibly a sore throat, dry cough, nausea, and burning eyes. Flu symptoms may last two to three weeks.

Key Terms

allergens Commonly occurring antigens such as dust, food, pollen, and dander that trigger an allergic reaction in persons with allergies. **272**

allergic rhinitis One of the most common kinds of allergies, caused when airborne allergen particles (pollen, dust, mold, animal dander, and so forth) enter the nose and throat of an allergic person. Also called *hay fever.* **272**

anaphylaxis A severe allergic reaction ranging from hives and wheezing to convulsions; treated with injections of adrenaline. **272**

antibodies Protein molecules that mark antigens for destruction by other cells. Also called *immunoglobulins*. **265**

antigen Any substance that the immune system recognizes as foreign to the body and which induces it to produce antibodies. **268**

antihistamines Medications designed to counter the effects of histamine, the chemical produced in an allergic reaction. **274**

autoimmune disorder Disease in which the immune system mistakenly identifies the body's own cells as foreign and attacks them. **274**

bacteria Microscopic, single-celled organisms that live in air, soil, food, plants, animals, and humans (singular: bacterium). **263**

endogenous microorganisms Organisms normally living within the body that constitute its natural flora; if growth patterns are disturbed, it can cause infection. **263**

epidemic The occurrence of disease above usual levels in a given group or community. **260**

exogenous microorganism An organism that does not normally inhabit the host. **263**

fungi Primitive vegetable organisms such as yeasts and molds. **265**

gamma globulin Antibody-rich serum (blood fluid) from the blood of another person or animal used to induce passive immunity. **270**

helminths Multicellular parasites, or worms (flat or round) ranging in size from tiny microscopic flukes to 20-foot-long tapeworms that flourish in the intestines. **266**

histamine A powerful inflammatory chemical that causes symptoms of allergies and asthma. **272**

immune system The body system that recognizes and destroys invasive disease-causing agents and rids the body of diseased or worn-out cells. **263**

impetigo A contagious skin disease, primarily affecting the skin around the mouth and nose, caused by different types of bacteria including streptococci. **264**

infectious mononucleosis A viral disease caused by the Epstein-Barr virus and characterized in the acute stage by enlarged lymph nodes and spleen, fever, and sore throat. **277**

influenza An acute lower-respiratory-tract infection caused by several viruses. Abbreviated form: *flu.* **275**

Lyme disease An infectious disease spread to people and animals by ticks; caused by the bacterium *Borrelia burgdorferi*. **276**

lymph The fluid, usually clear or colorless, found in lymphatic vessels. **269**

lymph nodes Lymphatic glands located throughout the body, primarily under the arms and in the groin, neck, and elbow, that produce and store lymphocytes and serve an immune system function by filtering out infectious agents. **269**

lymphatic system The system of vessels, nodes, ducts, organs, and cells that manufactures and stores lymphocytes and helps destroy infectious agents. **269**

lymphocytes White blood cells of the immune system that attack antigens; may be T-lymphocytes ("T cells") or B-lymphocytes ("B cells"). **268**

memory cell A type of B cell that recognizes and disposes of antigens that are reintroduced in the body, sometimes years after initial infection. **270**

meningitis An inflammation of the membranes (meninges) of the spinal cord or brain. **262**

natural killer (NK) cell A type of white blood cell that destroys many kinds of antigens, especially viruses and tumor cells. **268**

pandemic An epidemic affecting a whole country, continent, or the entire world. **275**

pathogen Disease-causing organism, including bacteria, viruses, fungi, and parasites. **261**

phagocytes A major class of white blood cells that seek out and destroy antigens in the bloodstream. Also called *cell eaters*. **268**

pneumonia An acute infectious disease of the respiratory tract that results from pathogens causing fluids to build up in tiny air sacs called *alveoli*, making breathing difficult. **275**

rabies A viral disease that primarily affects the central nervous system and can lead to paralysis and death if not treated immediately with the rabies vaccination. **265**

rickettsiae Bacterial-like organisms that grow inside insects and other parasites; transmitted to humans via bites by lice, fleas, ticks, and mites. **264**

ringworm A fungal skin infection characterized by red patches, itching, and scaling, such as athlete's foot. **265**

strep throat A bacterial infection caused by streptococcal bacteria; characterized by a painful and reddish sore throat, fever, ear pain, and enlarged lymph nodes. **264**

suppressor T cells Immune cells that regulate the activities of T and B cells; suppressor T cells prevent lymphocytes from damaging healthy cells near the site of infection. **270**

toxic shock syndrome (TSS) A rare and sometimes fatal bacterial infection linked to tampon use. **264**

tuberculosis (TB) A bacterial infection that usually affects the lungs and sometimes other parts of the body, including the brain, kidneys, or spine. **276**

vaccination A means of introducing a weakened or partial form of an infectious agent into the body so as to produce immunity without incurring the full-blown illness caused by the infectious agent. **264**

viruses Submicroscopic particles consisting of a core of nucleic acid containing DNA or RNA and a surrounding coat of protein; incapable of replicating outside of cells of living plants or animals. **264**

white blood cells Specialized blood cells that comprise part of the body's immune system by combating invading pathogens. Also called *leukocytes*. **268**

Web Exercises

1. Go to http://www.betterhealth.vic.gov.au, an Australian government website that provides consumer health information. Search the site for "immune system quiz" and complete the quiz. As you click your answer for each of the eight questions, a pop-up window will provide the correct answer and an explanation of immune system function.
2. Go to http://www.cdc.gov/vaccines, the website of the U.S. Centers for Disease Control and Prevention National Immunization Program. From the section labeled "Immunization Schedules," "Teens & College Students," scroll down and select "Vaccines Quiz." Complete the "Adolescent and Adult Vaccine Quiz" to get a list of vaccines you may need. Print out the results and discuss them with your health care professional.
3. Go to http://www.smartersex.org, a website on safe and smart sex, developed in conjunction with the Planned Parenthood Federation of America. Locate "X & Y of STIs" in the menu bar near the top of the page. From its drop-down menu, choose "Test Your STI Smarts." Answer this 13-item quiz, and then submit your answers. The scoring key provides the correct answer and further information on each topic.

Learning Outcomes

1. Discuss crimes of violence in America and ways to avoid becoming a victim
2. Discuss crime on campus and its prevention
3. Explain what is meant by sexual coercion and discuss the problems of rape and sexual harassment
4. Discuss various kinds of unintentional injuries—injuries from accidents—and how to prevent them

Chapter Outline

Additional Health APP features available online for Chapter 13:

Health Skills 13-1 Anger Management
Prevention 13-1 Rape Prevention
Health Skills 13-4 Combating Sexual Harassment
Health Skills 13-5 Making Your Home a Safer Place
Prevention 13-2 Eating while Driving? Really?
Health Skills 13-6 How NOT to Sleep when Driving

HLTH Assets available online for each chapter:

Crossword Puzzles
Flashcards
Glossary
Quizzes

Critical Thinking Questions

1. **Q: Should government restrict the ability of people to use handheld cell phones while driving? What about hands-free phones? What do you think? Support your answer.**

   A: [Student opinions will vary.]

2. **Q: Why do you think the United States has such a high homicide rate?**

   A: [Student opinions will vary.]

3. **Q: Agree or disagree with the following statement and support your answer: "Schools should require students to take parent training classes to help prepare them for parenting roles."**

   A: [Student opinions will vary.]

4. **Q: What can we as a society and as individuals do to reduce the incidence of rape? To combat sexual harassment?**

   A: [Student opinions will vary (for example, Insist on greater societal respect for women, offer rape and harassment prevention workshops, create and enforce laws that do not tolerate rape or harassment).]

Web Exercises

1. Go to http://www.aaafoundation.org, the website for the AAA Foundation for Traffic Safety, a foundation dedicated to research and education aimed at reducing injuries on the roads. From the banner along the top, choose "Quizzes." Take the 10-question quiz "Drowsy Driving." Submit your answers, and then click on an item to get a full explanation of the answer. Then take the 40-item "Aggressive Driving" quiz, and get your Driver Stress Profile.

Key Terms

batterer A person who inflicts violent physical abuse upon his or her intimate partner. **290**

forcible rape Sexual intercourse with a nonconsenting person achieved by force or threat of force. **294**

identity theft Impersonating another person for criminal purposes by means of using the person's social security number, bank account information, or other personally identifying information. **293**

sexual harassment Unwelcome comments, gestures, demands, overtures, or physical contact of a sexual nature. **294**

statutory rape Sexual intercourse with a person who is below the age of consent, even if the person cooperates. **298**

2. Go to http://www.fvpcgc.org, the website for the Family Violence Prevention Center of Greene County, Ohio. Select "Get Informed" from the top links, and drop down to "Take Our Quiz." The "Domestic Violence Quiz" asks respondents to identify each of the 12 statements as either fact or myth. Scroll down for the answers and to get the facts and the sources for the information.
3. Go to http://www.aboutdaterape.nsw.gov.au/index.html, a site set up by the NSW (New South Wales) Attorney-General's Department Crime Prevention Division to provide information to women and girls about date rape. Select "Test Your Knowledge" from the links on the left-hand side of the page. Take one of the three quizzes that test what you know about date rate (this site is not interactive; students will print out the quiz and check answers at the bottom of the quiz). (There is a section for men and boys, too. Click "Finding Help" on the left, and then select the link "Guys as Victims.")

Figure 13-4 Top 10 Lifesavers on the Road

This list identifies the 10 innovations in automotive safety that have saved the most lives over the last four decades.

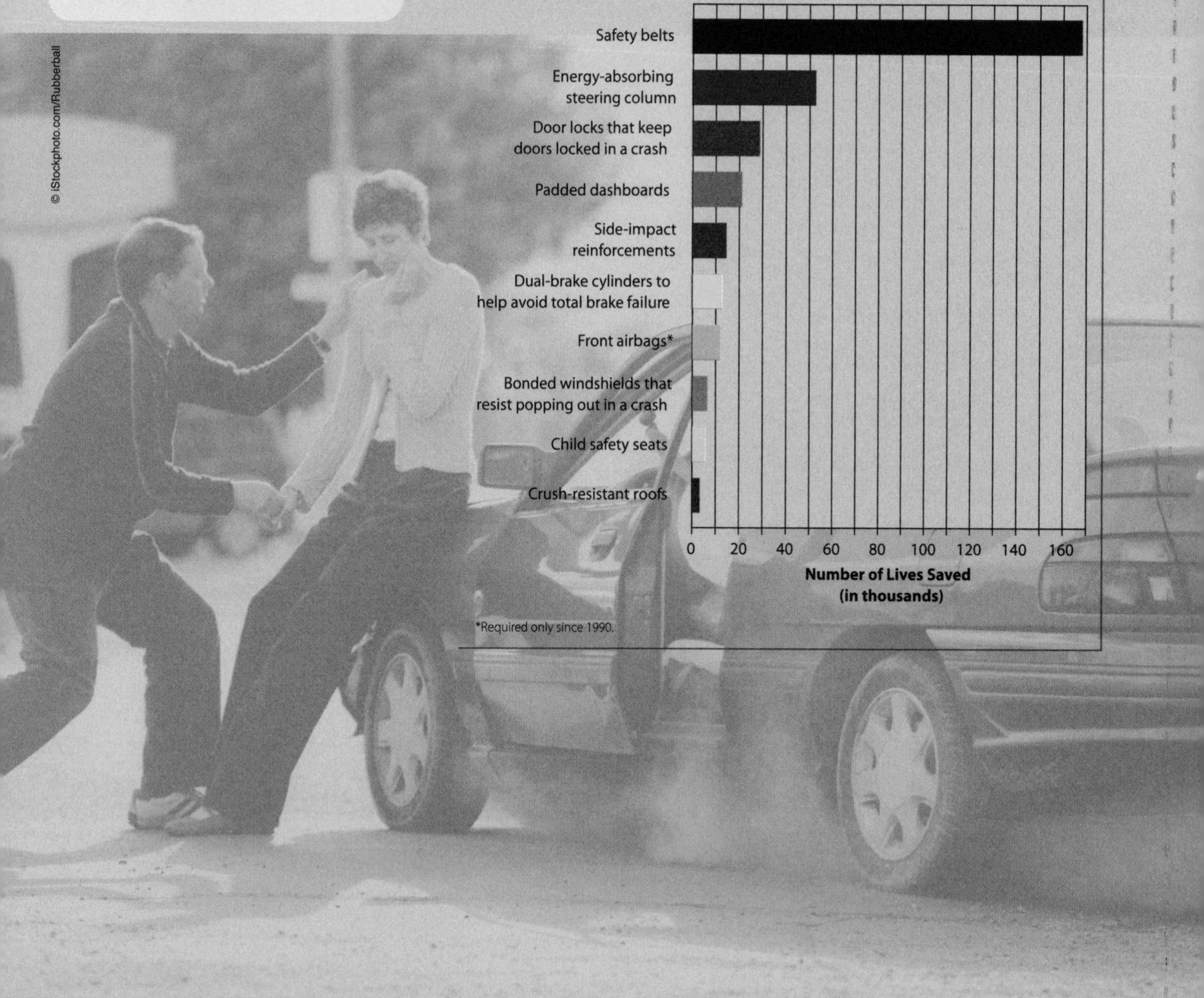

*Required only since 1990.

prepcard/ CHAPTER 14 MANAGING YOUR HEALTH CARE

Learning Outcomes

1 Discuss ways of managing your own health care

2 Describe the health care system in the United States

3 Discuss the benefits of health care insurance along with its drawbacks and inequities

4 Discuss complementary and alternative medicine (CAM)

Chapter Outline

Additional Health APP features available online for Chapter 14:

Prevention 14-1 Your Health Checkup—What Happens and Why
Health Skills 14-1 Choosing a Health Care Plan
Prevention 14-2 Treatment Yes, Prevention Definitely

HLTH Assets available online for each chapter:

Crossword Puzzles
Flashcards
Glossary
Quizzes

Critical Thinking Questions

1. **Q: How can you determine whether a medical exam, test, or procedure is necessary?**
   A: You could get a second opinion about the need for the procedure and conduct personal research.
2. **Q: Agree or disagree with the following statement and support your answer: Managed care places HCPs in a conflict of interest.**
   A: [Student opinions will vary.]
3. **Q: What factors should you consider in choosing a health care plan?**
   A: The best way to select an insurance plan is to acquire information and carefully weigh the advantages and disadvantages of a variety of plans. Issues to consider include outcomes and performances, costs, treatment when away, and long-term care. Research your insurance needs and match them with the most appropriate program for you.
4. **Q: Are there any barriers in your efforts to obtain adequate health care? What are they? What can you do about them?**
   A: [Student opinions will vary.]
5. **Q: Do you know people who "swear by" a method of CAM? What is their evidence? Do you find their evidence to be satisfactory? Why or why not?**
   A: [Student opinions will vary.]
6. **Q: Are you comfortable that you would be able to evaluate the safety and effectiveness of a method of CAM? If not, what can you do to become comfortable?**
   [A: Student opinions will vary.]

Web Exercises

1. Go to http://www.insurance.state.pa.us/naic/quiz_health.html, the website of The Pennsylvania Insurance Department. Take the quiz "Are You Smart about Health Insurance," to test your knowledge about health insurance choices.

Key Terms

alternative medicine Health care practices and products that are used instead of conventional medicine. **322**

capitated In the context of managed care, a fixed dollar amount that the individual or the employer must pay for membership in the plan, regardless of how much medical services the individual uses. **318**

coinsurance The percentage of costs for medical services that the insured person must pay after deductibles are met. **317**

complementary medicine Health care practices and products that are used along with conventional medicine. **322**

copayment A predetermined set amount the individual must pay for medical services. **318**

deductible The annual amount that the individual must pay for medical expenses before the health insurance plan starts contributing its share. **317**

health maintenance organization (HMO) A prepaid type of managed care plan in which the costs are usually capitated according to a fixed amount of money per enrollee. **319**

hospice Interdisciplinary health care program that provides services to terminally ill patients, either in the home or in a hospice facility, that address the medical, spiritual, emotional, and economic needs of patients and their families. **316**

indemnity A traditional type of insurance plan in which the insurance carrier or employer (for self-insured employers) pays for a predetermined percentage of all medical bills after deductibles and barring any limitations or exclusions. Also called *fee-for-service (FSS)* plan. **317**

malpractice Failure of a professional to render proper treatment, especially when injury or harm occurs as a result. **312**

managed care A system of controlling health care costs by eliminating waste and unnecessary medical procedures. **304**

Medicaid A federal program that provides health care benefits to the poor. **322**

Medicare A federally sponsored program that provides health care coverage for older Americans and people with disabilities. **321**

Medigap policy An insurance policy with a private carrier that fills gaps in Medicare coverage. **321**

point-of-service (POS) A type of HMO that offers its members the choice of using doctors within its network of providers or choosing their own doctors at higher cost. **319**

2. Go to http://www.nccam.nih.gov, the government website for the National Center for Complementary and Alternative Medicine (NCCAM). Click on "Health Info" in the top links. On this page, examine the "FDA Alerts and Consumer Advisories" section; it provides information on drug interactions with CAMs, harmful side effects of CAMs, and public health advisories. If anyone you know is using one of the CAMs that has an alert or an advisory, read the information and forward it to him or her. Additional information and research on CAMs can be found at http://www.aafp.org, the website of the American Academy of Family Physicians. Type "Complementary and Alternative Medicine: A Primer" into the search engine and choose that title from the list. This article describes CAMs, presents research on the effectiveness of CAMs, and emphasizes that patients should tell their physicians about any CAM they are using.

Figure 14-1 Our Health Dollars

About 40% of our health care health dollars come from private sources. The single largest expense is for hospital care, followed by physician and clinical services and prescription drugs.

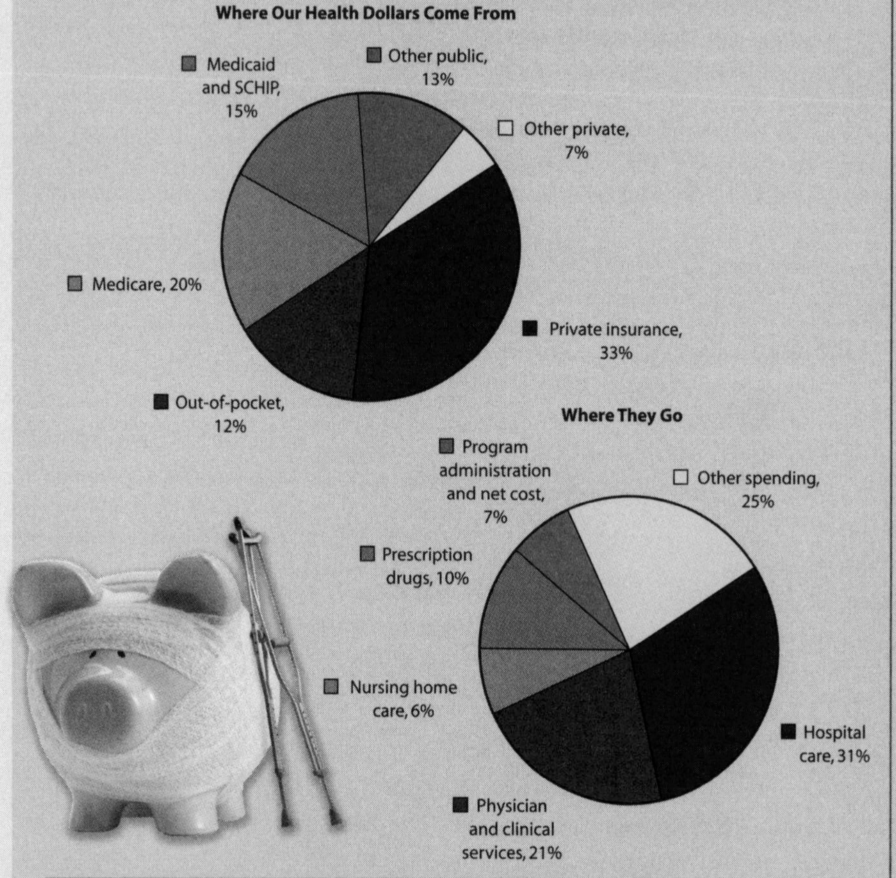

preferred provider organization (PPO) A group of health care providers who agree to provide health care services to members of a managed care plan for a discounted rate. **318**

rehabilitation center Health care facility that provides comprehensive medical, physical therapy, occupational therapy, and mental health services to help people with disabilities achieve a maximum level of functioning. **316**

sliding scale A system for adjusting fees according to the patient's income level. **322**

staff model HMO A type of HMO that offers comprehensive health care services within a free-standing clinic or health center that employs its own doctors, nurses, and allied health professionals. **319**

Learning Outcomes

1. **Discuss health hazards in the home environment**
2. **Discuss health hazards in the community environment**
3. **Discuss the hazards of various kinds of radiation**
4. **Discuss the relationship between population growth and health**
5. **Discuss the health hazards of various kinds of pollution and what can be done about them**
6. **Discuss the relationship between climate change and health**

Chapter Outline

continued

Additional Health APP features available online for Chapter 15:

Prevention 15-1 Protecting Our Families from Lead Poisoning
Health Check 15-1 Rating Environmental Hazards—What's the Risk?
Prevention 15-3 Protecting Our Drinking Water
Health Skills 15-2 Doing Your Part to Make the Environment Safer and Healthier
Health Skills 15-3 Renewable Sources of Energy in the United States

HLTH Assets available online for each chapter:

Crossword Puzzles
Flashcards
Glossary
Quizzes

BBC Health Video Title available online for Chapter 15:

Mobile Phones and Health

Critical Thinking Questions

1. **Q: How can we raise people's awareness about the possible hidden dangers in their homes? What is the role of schools in this process? Government? Media? Health professionals?**

   A: [Student opinions will vary.]

2. **Q: How has technology improved the quality of life? How has it threatened the environment and health?**

   A: Technology has improved our lives by increasing our ability to communicate through a variety of mediums and lessening the time needed to complete many tasks, but there are issues of concern: microwaves and cell phones may leak radiation, toxic waste may leach into our water supplies, and global pollution may contribute to climate change.

3. **Q: Agree or disagree with the following statement and support your answer: "A good way to protect yourself from air pollution is to stay indoors."**

   A: [Student opinions will vary.]

4. **Q: What are the potential effects of global warming on our health? Why?**

   A: Due to global warming, we can expect a rising sea level, changes in rainfall patterns, and more extreme weather patterns, leading to more droughts and flooding and reduced crop yields, which will increase the threat of starvation. Temperature changes increase the potential for tropical diseases such as malaria, yellow fever, and dengue to spread to previously more temperate areas. We can also expect more heat-related deaths from killer heat waves. With further global warming, the numbers of heat-related illnesses and deaths will likely increase.

Key Terms

acid rain Polluted precipitation that results when pollutants such as sulfur dioxide and nitrogen oxide combine with water molecules in the atmosphere. **341**

aquifer Geological formation that holds water. **343**

carbon monoxide An odorless, colorless gas that is a major source of air pollution and is produced from the burning of carbon with insufficient air. **332**

chlorofluorocarbons (CFCs) Organochlorine chemicals used as coolants, aerosol propellants, and solvents; the primary culprit in the depletion of the ozone layer. **343**

electromagnetic fields (EMFs) Energy fields resulting from the movement of electrical charges and that represent a source of nonionizing radiation. **338**

extremely low frequency (ELF) electromagnetic radiation A source of nonionizing radiation emitted by computer monitors, TVs, radios, and other appliances that is characterized by extremely low frequency electromagnetic waves. **339**

fossil fuels Carbon-based sources of energy derived from deposits in the Earth, including oil, natural gas, and coal. These are considered nonrenewable sources of energy because they cannot be replenished. **341**

global warming The gradual increase in global temperatures. **348**

greenhouse effect The rise in atmospheric temperature resulting from the release of heat-trapping gasses produced by the burning of fossil fuels. **348**

groundwater Water below the land surface from snow and rain that collects in porous rock formations. **343**

hazmats Industrial wastes that are considered hazardous (ignitable, corrosive, reactive, or toxic) and pose risks to health and environment. **344**

ion Atom or molecule having a positive or negative electrical charge. **337**

ionizing radiation Powerful, high-energy radiation that is capable of causing atoms to become ionized or electrically charged. **337**

microwave A form of nonionizing radiation consisting of very high frequency electromagnetic waves that cause molecules to vibrate rapidly, thereby producing heat that can rapidly cook food or boil water. **339**

mutagen Substance that induces genetic mutations. Ionizing radiation and ultraviolet light are known mutagens. **334**

neurotoxin Poisonous substance that affects the brain and central nervous system (CNS). **334**

nonbiodegradable Substances that do not decay naturally in the environment. **336**

nonionizing radiation Radiation that lacks sufficient energy to cause atoms to become ions. **338**

nuclear medicine The branch of medicine that uses forms of radiation in the diagnosis and treatment of illness. **338**

organochlorines A class of petrochemicals, including some pesticides and other toxic substances, that is used widely in industrial settings. **336**

organophosphates A class of potentially dangerous chemical compounds used as pesticides and sometimes as chemical weapons. **336**

ozone An extremely reactive form of oxygen that is harmful to humans when inhaled and forms a major constituent of smog. **342**

petrochemical Chemical substance derived from petroleum or natural gas. **336**

rad Short for *radiation-absorbed dose*, a measure of exposure to radiation. **337**

radioisotope Radioactive material used in medical diagnosis and treatment. **338**

secondary air pollution Pollution produced by chemical interactions involving primary pollutants, such as sulfur dioxide, hydrocarbons, and nitrogen oxide. **342**

surface water Water found in aboveground bodies such as ponds, lakes, rivers, streams, and reservoirs. **343**

X-ray Ionizing radiation that can penetrate most solid objects and is used to project images of the body on photographic film. **338**

5. Q: Why do you think toxic waste sites are more likely to be located near communities inhabited by ethnic minority groups and poor people?

A: [Student opinions will vary.]

Web Exercises

1. Go to http://www.keepkidshealthy.com, a pediatrician's guide to your children's health and safety. Under "Online Resources" in the left column, click on "Lead Screening." Complete the 14-item "Lead Poisoning Screening Quiz" to evaluate the risk of lead exposure to your family members.

2. Go to http://www.webmd.com/health-ehome-9/default.htm, WebMD's site in collaboration with the Healthy Child Healthy World, a national nonprofit organization dedicated to educating the public about environmental toxins. Click "Get Started" to complete the "Health eHome Check". When you complete this six-page quiz, you'll receive a personalized assessment of your family's risk factors due to unhealthy chemicals and substances inside your home.

3. Go to the website of the British Broadcasting Corporation at http://news.bbc.co.uk/2/hi/science/nature/4086947.stm, and take the quiz "Do You Know Your Pollution?" This eight-item quiz will help you see how much you know about the effects of everyday substances in your environment. Then, check out the quiz at this url: http://news.bbc.co.uk/2/hi/science/nature/3579492.stm "Are You Clued Up on Climate?" Take this quiz to test your knowledge of global climate change. Both quizzes provide correct answers and explanations when you submit your answers.